DYSPHAGIA

DYSPHAGIA
Foundation, Theory and Practice

Edited by
JULIE A Y CICHERO
BRUCE E MURDOCH

John Wiley & Sons, Ltd
Chichester · New York · Weinheim · Brisbane · Toronto · Singapore

Other Wiley Editorial Offices

John Wiley & Sons Inc., 111 River Street, Hoboken, NJ 07030, USA

Jossey-Bass, 989 Market Street, San Francisco, CA 94103-1741, USA

Wiley-VCH Verlag GmbH, Boschstr. 12, D-69469 Weinheim, Germany

John Wiley & Sons Australia Ltd, 42 McDougall Street, Milton, Queensland 4064, Australia

John Wiley & Sons (Asia) Pte Ltd, 2 Clementi Loop #02-01, Jin Xing Distripark, Singapore 129809

John Wiley & Sons Canada Ltd, 6045 Freemont Blvd, Mississauga, ONT, L5R 4J3

Wiley also publishes its books in a variety of electronic formats. Some content that appears in print
may not be available in electronic books.

Library of Congress Cataloging-in-Publication Data

Dysphagia: foundation, theory, and practice / [edited by] Julie Cichero and Bruce Murdoch.
     p. ; cm.
   Includes bibliographical references and index.
   ISBN-13: 978-1-86156-505-1 (pbk.: alk. paper)
   ISBN-10: 1-86156-505-4 (pbk.: alk. paper)
   1. Deglutition disorders.   I. Cichero, Julie. II. Murdoch, B. E., 1950-.
   [DNLM: 1. Deglutition Disorders.   2. Deglutition–physiology.   WI 250 D9985 2006]
   RC815.2.D97 2006
   616.3'23–dc22

                                                                              2006001186

British Library Cataloging in Publication Data

A catalogue record for this book is available from the British Library

ISBN:13 978-1-86156-505-1 (PB)

Typeset in 10/12pt Times by Thomson Digital.
Printed and bound in Great Britain by TJ International Ltd, Padstow, Cornwall.
This book is printed on acid-free paper responsibly manufactured from sustainable forestry in which
at least two trees are planted for each one used for paper production.

Contents

Contributors

Rodd Brockett, MBBS, FRACP, FJFICM.
Consultant general physician.
Brisbane, Australia.

Jonathan Cichero, BDSc.
Dental surgeon.
Brisbane, Australia.

Julie Cichero, BA, BSpThy, PhD.
School of Health and Rehabilitation
  Sciences.
The University of Queensland, Australia.

Neila Donovan, PhD, CCC-SLP.
Department of Communicative Disorders.
University of Florida, Gainesville,
  United States of America.

Peter Halley, BE(Chem), PhD, F I
  Chem E.
School of Engineering/Australian
  Institute for Bioengineering and
  Nanotechnology.
The University of Queensland,
  Australia.

Hilary Johnson, DipSpThy, MA(Ed).
School of Human Communication
  Sciences, La Trobe University.
Melbourne, Australia.

Susan Langmore, MA, PhD, CCC-SLP,
  BRS-S.
Department of Otolaryngology,
  University of California.
San Francisco, United States of
  America.

Angela Morgan, BSpPath, PhD.
Institute of Child Health,
  University College London.
London, United Kingdom.

Sheena Reilly, BAppSc(SpPath), PhD.
Professor–Director Paediatric Speech
  Pathology
School of Human Communication
  Sciences, La Trobe University &
Royal Children's Hospital Healthy
  Development Theme, Murdoch
  Children's Research Institute.
Melbourne, Australia.

Bruce E Murdoch, PhD.
Professor and Head of Department of
  Speech Pathology and Audiology.
The University of Queensland, Australia

Nathalie Rommel, MA(Sp-LPath), PhD.
Centre for Paediatric and Adolescent
  Gastroenterology, Women's and
  Children's Hospital.
Adelaide, Australia.

John Rosenbek, PhD, CCC-SLP.
Department of Communicative
  Disorders, University of Florida.
Gainesville, United States of America.

Amanda Scott, BAppSc(SpPath), PhD.
Speech Pathology Department, The
  Alfred Hospital.
Melbourne, Australia.

Justine Joan Sheppard, PhD, CCC-SLP,
  BRS-S.
Department of Biobehavioural Studies,
  Teachers College, Columbia University.
New York, United States of America.

Sarah Starr, BAppSc(SpPath),
  MHlthSc(Ed).
Speech Pathology Services.
Burwood, New South Wales, Australia.

Part I Foundations of Swallowing

1 Applied Anatomy and Physiology of the Normal Swallow

JONATHAN CICHERO

The ability to swallow safely is paramount in the care and management of the dysphagic patient. To help the patient achieve this the clinician must first understand how a normal swallow occurs. This chapter looks at the important features involved in controlling the passage of a bolus, and their intricate integration.

THE ANATOMY OF DEGLUTITION

To develop a clear mental picture of the internal representation of the oropharynx and how it works we are going to adopt a 'first person' perspective of a bolus (for example a biscuit or cookie) on its journey towards the oesophagus. Once a firm mental picture is achieved we can take a closer look at how the structures we pass are innervated and coordinated.

Looking posteriorly upon entering the oral cavity, the bolus is thrust sideways into the teeth by the movement of the tongue (Figure 1.1; arrow 3) and cheeks. It is being prepared to a consistency that the brain, using feedback loops based on previous experience, is happy to swallow. During this stage there is no access for us (as the bolus) to the pharynx because the soft palate (Figure 1.1; arrow 2) has been drawn down towards an elevated posterior portion of the tongue. Once we have been prepared to an appropriate viscosity, the tongue starts to raise us up towards the hard palate (Figure 1.1; arrow 1) and then compresses us backwards towards the pharynx. This is the primary force required to deliver the bolus on its path. We can also feel forces pulling us towards the pharynx, as lower pressure levels have developed there due to changes in respiration prior to the swallow and the opening of the upper oesophageal sphincter.

Tipping over the edge of the posterior third of the tongue, we find ourselves sliding down towards the valleculae (Figure 1.1; arrow 7), that area bounded by the base of the tongue (at the level of the hyoid – Figure 1.1; arrow 5) and the epiglottis (Figure 1.1; arrow 6). However, we do not see too much of the valleculae as the entire larynx by this time has been elevated superiorly and anteriorly (Figure 1.1; arrow 4 – mylohyoid) towards the base of the tongue, out of the path of the bolus. Laryngeal elevation and tongue pressure cause the epiglottis to tip over and assist in protecting the entrance to the larynx. We, the bolus, are split into two, with each half going lateral to the epiglottis, and being

Dysphagia: Foundation, Theory and Practice. Edited by J. Cichero and B. Murdoch
© 2006 John Wiley & Sons, Ltd.

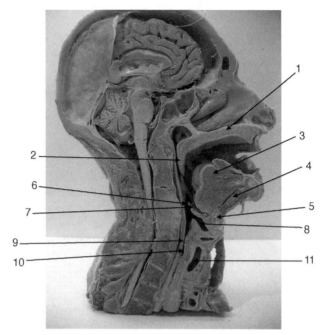

Figure 1.1   Sagittal head and neck section

directed into the steep chutes that are the pyriform recesses (Figure 1.1; arrow 8). The aryepiglottic folds have been stretched up into a 'curtain' by the movement of the arytenoid cartilages, with each aryepiglottic fold forming one medial wall of each pyriform sinus. We are being pushed from the sides all of this time as the pharyngeal constrictors squeeze laterally towards the midline, pushing us ever downwards.

Our final destination is approaching, as the cricopharyngeus (Figure 1.1; arrow 9), the opening to the oesophagus, has relaxed completely. It has been stretched wide open by the upward and anterior movement of the larynx and relaxation of the muscles and allows us to enter the oesophagus successfully. Prior to the relaxation of the cricopharyngeus, this muscle remains in a tonic state of contraction, a state necessary to keep gastric contents enclosed within the oesophagus (Figure 1.1; arrow 10). Inhibiting any possible reflux of contents into the pharynx is crucial in reducing the risk of aspiration, which is the penetration of material into the airway (Figure 1.1; arrow 11 – trachea). Upon entering the oesophagus, we can turn around and see the upper oesophageal sphincter (the cricopharyngeus) contract and close off our escape route as the entire system returns to rest.

Having taken a 'first person' approach to the passage of a bolus, we have noticed some important scenery along the way. In reality, however, once the swallow is initiated, the time taken to travel from the mouth to the oesophagus is approximately one second, so the scenery passes by very quickly. The coordination of this event in such a short time frame has been the subject of volumes of work over the years and an understanding of how it is achieved is essential for the clinician. This chapter will now explore more deeply into each of the components responsible for a successful swallow, starting with the neural control. A firm grasp of the brain and neural network controlling the swallow will aid the clinician in the diagnosis and treatment of the dysphagic patient.

CORTICAL MAPPING

The above is a simplistic description of an extremely complex process requiring the precise coordination of a myriad of muscles and a nebula of nerves. In recent years researchers have made great inroads into understanding the brain and its role in many human functions. Through various mapping techniques such as positron emission studies and functional magnetic resonance imaging, the human cortex has begun to give up its secrets. It is imperative that the clinician gain a sound understanding of loci within the cortex in order to predict safely what the patient might experience given a specific injury, and hence to develop an appropriate treatment philosophy.

To visualize the three-dimensional nature of the cortex and the various loci in relation to each other, a basic list of terminology is used, which can be found in the glossary at the end of this chapter.

In addition to understanding the terminology used when discussing the human brain, it is important that a clear picture of its gross anatomy is present in the clinician's mind. Referring to the figures in this chapter will enable readers to visualize and understand the areas of the brain in this discussion. Figure 1.2 shows the external topography of the brain laterally, and Figure 1.3 shows the topography in a midline sagittal plane. Figure 1.4 shows a lateral dissection, exposing the insula, or '5th lobe', and Figure 1.5 is a coronal section at the level of the diencephalon. Figure 1.6 is a horizontal section through the ventricles.

Armed with a layout of the human brain, we can now start to focus on specific areas involved in specified tasks, and then how they may interact with each other.

THE NEED FOR SUSTENANCE

Swallowing is a major step in the process of refuelling our bodies. Our desire to eat, along with what we wish to eat, are the first two activities the brain focuses on. In the treatment and management of a dysphagic patient, it is important to look at the entire process of sustenance or nutrition, rather than focus purely on the process of passing the bolus safely. Important connections exist between the body's need for food and what we choose to eat, knowledge of which will help the clinician understand the dysphagic patient better, while possibly providing treatment modalities.

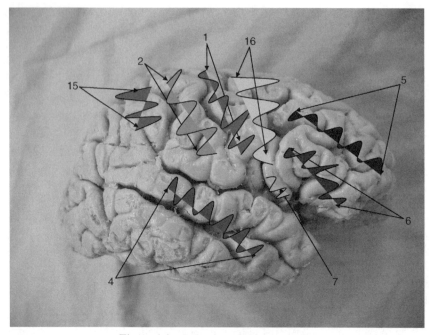

Figure 1.2   Lateral cerebral topography

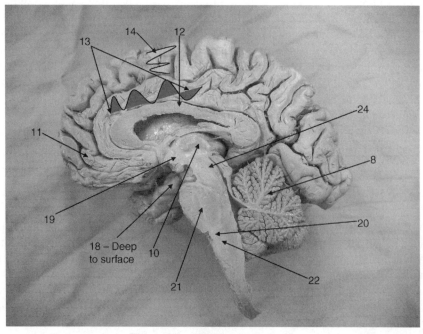

Figure 1.3   Mid-line sagittal split

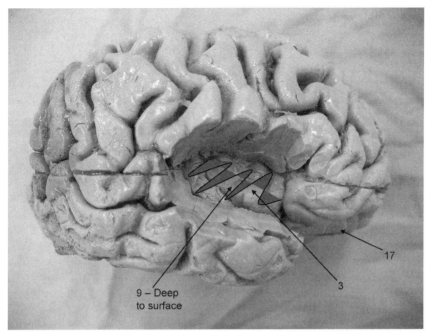

Figure 1.4 Lateral dissection of insula

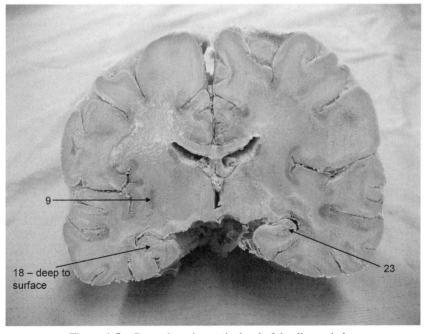

Figure 1.5 Coronal section at the level of the diencephalon

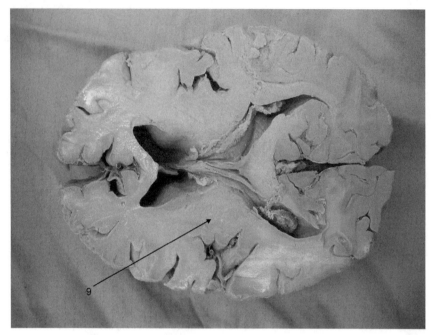

Figure 1.6   Horizontal section through the ventricles

1. Lateral precentral gyrus and primary motor cortex
2. Lateral postcentral gyrus and primary sensory cortex
3. Insula
4. Superior temporal gyrus
5. Middle frontal gyrus
6. Inferior frontal gyrus
7. Frontal operculum
8. Cerebellum
9. Putamen
10. Thalamus
11. Anterior cingulate cortex
12. Corpus callosum
13. Cingulate gyrus
14. Supplementary motor cortex
15. Secondary sensory cortex or posterior parietal cortex
16. Premotor cortex
17. Orbitofrontal cortex
18. Amygdala
19. Hypothalamus
20. Reticular formation
21. Pons
22. Medulla
23. Hippocampus
24. Mesencephalon or Mid brain

HUNGER AND THIRST

Sewards and Sewards (2003) provide a strong understanding of the cortical representation of hunger and thirst. The food drive comes from the *lateral nuclei of the hypothalamus*, also known as the 'hunger centre'. This area of the brain controls the quantity of intake and excites lower centres in the brain stem to perform the mechanical motions of food consumption. In addition to this, the *ventromedial nuclei of the hypothalamus* causes the feeling of 'fullness', and acts on the lateral nuclei of the hypothalamus to inhibit the drive for food. However, satiation is associated with neuronal activity in the prefrontal cortex. The sensation of 'thirst' is also located in the lateral nuclei of the hypothalamus and is triggered when electrolytes in the centre become too concentrated, causing a strong need to drink until the electrolyte concentration returns to normal.

The lateral nuclei of the hypothalamus are in turn affected by strong connections from the *amygdala*. Zald and Pardo (2000) show that the dorsomedial portion of the amygdala receives fibres from the olfactory bulb and is part of the lateral olfactory area. Herein lie important connections that allow us to smell food and immediately experience hunger for it.

The hypothalamus is also excited directly by ascending pathways from the spinal cord and brain stem, conveying information from the viscera and the gastrointestinal tract. The empty stomach can also indicate a need for food through these connections. Once excited, the hypothalamus casts many shadows across the autonomic nervous system. Impulses reach the autonomic nuclei of the brain stem and spinal cord, both directly and via relays in the reticular formation.

TASTE, SMELL AND FLAVOUR

De Araujo et al. (2003) have shown that taste and smell information converges onto singular neurones in the *caudal orbitofrontal cortex* and immediately adjacent *agranular insula*. It would appear that this may be the site where 'flavour' is processed. However, regions that become activated by both taste and smell in addition to the areas mentioned above include the *amygdala*, *insular cortex*, and *anterior cingulate cortex*. The *anteromedial aspect of the temporal lobe* (taste quality) and the *opercular aspect of the superior temporal lobe* (taste perception) show additional activation during the oral presence of stimuli.

The *frontal operculum/insula* is responsive to taste stimuli alone, and the combination of taste and smell result in activation of a *lateral anterior part of the orbitofrontal cortex*. Interestingly each of these stimuli in isolation causes no activation of this area.

It is important to appreciate the connections between hunger, thirst, taste, smell and flavour because each of these areas plays a role in preparing the body for the complex task of coordinating a swallow. These strong connections also provide an insight into effective treatment modalities for the dysphagic patient, using stimuli such as smell and taste to excite cortical areas involved in the preparation of a coordinated swallow (see Chapters 3 and 12).

From the preceding information, the overriding clinical message that must be understood is that there are many areas of the brain that become active during the preparatory phase of eating. These areas are interdependent, but physically independent, located throughout the central nervous system. Some of the areas have an integral effect on taste, smell and flavour, whereas others offer only assistance. For the clinician attempting to rehabilitate the dysphagic patient, the task will be significantly easier if there is an understanding that hunger, thirst, taste, smell or flavour could have been affected by the original event, and therefore may also need management for the overall treatment to succeed.

CORTICAL CONTROL OF SWALLOWING

The human swallow is initiated and controlled by areas within the brain stem. Terms such as a 'central pattern generator' were used in the past to describe the area of the brain stem where the afferent (sensory) inputs from central and peripheral sources were relayed to the efferent (motor) system to coordinate the appropriate musculature, after being influenced by an interneuronal network designed to 'programme' the process. This thinking suggests that swallowing is primarily a 'reflex arc' involving limited regions of the central nervous system. Parts of this thinking remain relevant but researchers have now shown that the control of the swallow goes far beyond a brain stem reflex arc.

Mosier and Bereznaya (2001) provided some ground-breaking research into understanding the cortical control of swallowing. They report that there are five distinct clusters involved in the cortical control of the swallow, with each cluster consisting of independent regions of the brain. Each region is anatomically separate from the other and regions within each cluster work in excitatory and inhibitory parallel loops to provide the overall desired effect.

The five clusters are:

- *A* – primary motor cortex; primary sensory cortex; supplementary motor cortex and cingulate gyrus;
- *B* – inferior frontal gyrus; secondary sensory cortex; corpus callosum; basal ganglia and thalamus;
- *C* – premotor cortex; posterior parietal cortex;
- *D* – cerebellum;
- *E* – insula.

Cluster A is the common point between the two loops. The cortical regions of the brain included in this cluster are usually involved in voluntary motor behaviour, planning and execution of sequential movements based on internally stored information or 'remembered' sequences. As such, it is believed this cluster might act as the sensorimotor output.

Cluster B is positively affected by cluster A, and may serve to integrate sensory information about the bolus (e.g. viscosity, inertial properties) with the internal representation of swallowing movements. Activation of this cluster will have an inhibitory effect on cluster D.

Cluster C provides an excitatory effect on cluster A, and as such could involve cortical strategies for movement planning and implementation.

Cluster D (the cerebellum) negatively and preferentially influences clusters A and B, possibly to modulate the internal representation for swallowing and coordination among the multiple effector states. It organizes the timing through sensory input and motor output. The cerebellum also acts to change the tongue and pharynx musculature toning, to counteract variable intraluminal pressures.

Cluster E (the insula) negatively and preferentially influences clusters A and C, possibly to synchronize the kinematics of movement.

As detailed above, clusters A, B and C are groupings of independent areas of the cortex, working together to achieve a common goal. Some of the areas within each group have been investigated further, to identify a more specific role that they might play in the control of swallowing. Martin et al. (2001) identified roles for these areas in the control of both voluntary and automatic swallowing.

The *lateral postcentral gyrus* (primary sensory cortex, found in cluster A) is involved in the *processing* of oropharyngeal sensory inputs. This role is subsequent to the brain stem receiving the afferent signals. The processing here requires sensory inputs that monitor saliva accumulation or bolus delivery and transport, which is converted into the appropriate stimulation of the jaw, tongue, palate and pharyngeal musculature required for swallowing.

The *frontal operculum* has classically been regarded as subserving motor speech production as part of Broca's area. However, studies have now shown that it also has a role in the control of non-speech orofacial sensorimotor behaviours.

The *anterior cingulate cortex* (cluster A) is a multifunctional region processing sensory, motor and cognitive information. Differing parts of the cortex are activated in reference to a swallow that is autonomic or volitional. An autonomic swallow is a swallow that occurs without any conscious effort on the patient's behalf. The best example of this is a saliva swallow during sleep. A volitional swallow is a swallow initiated by a conscious decision from the patient. In the autonomic swallow, the rostral region of the anterior cingulate cortex is activated, while in the volitional swallow it is the caudal and intermediate regions. These latter two regions possibly reflect premotor and/or attentional processing.

In looking through the list of cortical regions involved in the swallowing process, we can see that many of these regions overlap or are intimately related to those areas involved in taste, thirst, hunger, smell and flavour. If we find that the area of injury in a dysphagic patient is isolated in these regions, rehabilitation may be possible using taste, smell or flavour to reignite these damaged areas, and rehabilitate the swallow (see Chapter 12).

Those areas critical to this concept are as follows.

• *The insula* exists as cluster E, influencing clusters A and C, and is also involved in taste and smell in isolation, or together as flavour.

• *The cingulate cortex* is a member of cluster A, the motor behaviour group, and is involved in taste and smell in isolation, or together as flavour.

UPPER AND LOWER MOTOR NEURONES

Following our discussion of the cortical control of swallowing, it is an appropriate time to discuss the concept of upper and lower motor neurones. Kiernan (1998) helps to explain these two terms, which are primarily related to clinical discussions. They are often used as 'all-encompassing' terms for neurones that, by neuroanatomy standards, should be more clearly defined. For simplicity, however, our discussions will be framed in these clinical terms.

Upper motor neurones are those neurones of the descending pathways of the brain involved in voluntary control of the musculature. This term encompasses all higher level connections (such as the cortex, cerebellum and thalamus) where the neural message ultimately affects the relevant nucleus of the lower motor neurone. These neurones are often bundled together into tracts, such as the corticospinal tract, and carry the impulse from the cortex to the motor nucleus in the brain stem.

Lower motor neurones are those neurones that extend from the motor nuclei of the brain stem to the effector musculature. Examples of this are the lower motor neurones from the facial motor nucleus, which convey the impulses to the muscles of facial expression.

The clinician will need to understand the implications of upper versus lower motor neurones when it comes to diagnosing the patient's condition. An upper motor-neurone lesion will result in weakened or absent voluntary movements of the affected muscle, with subsequent increase in muscle tone tending towards spasticity. Reflex movement can become jerky and exaggerated. Lower motor-neurone damage will result in complete paralysis of the affected muscle, with ultimate atrophy of the muscles due to an absence of use.

During the discussion of the cortical control of swallowing we saw that many different regions of the brain have a role to play. All of this control is directed, via upper motor neurones, towards what was once considered the region where a swallow was initiated and controlled. The brain stem does hold an extremely important place in the swallowing process, but as we have seen, the role is more of a relay station rather than the generator.

THE BRAIN STEM AND CRANIAL NERVES

The brain stem houses the motor and sensory nuclei of the cranial nerves whose distributions blanket the oral and pharyngeal passageways. Afferent fibres return to this region carrying information from mechanoreceptors and free nerve endings, and efferent fibres impart the necessary stimulation to coordinate the musculature. The clinician and student of dysphagia must have an intimate understanding of the cranial nerves involved, i.e. trigeminal (V), facial (VII), glossopharyngeal (IX), vagus (X) and hypoglossal (XII), their pathways, and associated brain stem nuclei.

Perlman (1991) and Donner et al. (1985) have helped to summarize this complex area. Following their lead, we shall consider six types of nerve fibres existing within these five nerves:

- *General somatic efferent (GSE).* These send motor fibres to the skeletal muscles of the eye and tongue – muscles that have developed from myotomes of the embryonic somites, and are voluntary muscles.
- *Special visceral efferent (SVE).* These are the motor fibres for the striated muscles controlling chewing, facial expression, the larynx and pharynx. These are muscles derived from the branchial arches of the embryo, and are also under voluntary control.
- *General visceral efferent (GVE).* These fibres are motor to the smooth muscles, the blood vessels and the glands of the head and neck. They are autonomic or involuntary fibres.
- *General somatic afferent (GSA).* These fibres relay impulses from general sensory endings, primarily concerned with pain, temperature, touch and proprioception.
- *Special visceral afferent (SVA).* These neurones carry taste after innervation of the taste buds.
- *General visceral afferent (GVA).* These fibres convey sensations of fullness in hollow organs, and for our purposes, also carry sensations from visceral organs such as the larynx and pharynx.

Not every type of fibre is represented in each cranial nerve, which helps to dictate the specific role that each of these cranial nerves play. We will now analyse the five cranial nerves of interest to us in greater detail.

TRIGEMINAL (V)   *sensory*

This is primarily the general sensory nerve for the head, with a motor component for the muscles of mastication and several smaller muscles. There are three sensory branches, the ophthalmic, maxillary and mandibular. The maxillary and mandibular branches are of interest to us as they supply all sensory information from the mouth, lips, chin, teeth, tongue and palate. The motor component runs along the mandibular branch, and innervates the muscles of mastication – temporalis, masseter, lateral pterygoid and medial pterygoid. The several smaller muscles innervated by the trigeminal are the tensor tympani, tensor veli palatini, mylohyoid and anterior belly of digastric.

There are four nuclei associated with the trigeminal, one motor and three sensory. The three sensory nuclei run continuously from lateral to the cerebral aqueduct (the mesencephalic), through the pontine tegmentum (the chief sensory nuclei) and down to the inferior part of the pons through the medulla (the spinal nucleus). The motor nucleus is medial to the chief sensory nuclei, in the dorsolateral area of the pontine tegmentum.

FACIAL (VII)

The facial nerve comprises two distinct parts, a mixed-motor part and special sensory part. The motor nerve supplies the muscles of facial expression, the buccinator, the posterior belly of digastric, platysma, stylohyoid and stapedius. There is also a parasympathetic motor component (secretomotor) to the sub-mandibular, sublingual and lacrimal glands as well as the glands of the nasal and palatine mucosa. The sensory component conveys taste from the anterior two thirds of the tongue and soft palate via the chorda tympani and greater petrosal nerves respectively.

The facial motor nucleus is located caudally to the motor nucleus of the trigeminal nerve, in the ventrolateral part of the tegmental area of the pons. The secretomotor component of the facial nerve is directed from the superior salivatory and lacrimal nuclei, which are located medial to the facial motor nucleus.

The special sensory fibres run from their origins in the mouth, and terminate in the solitary nucleus, adjacent to the solitary tract.

Glossopharyngeal (IX)

This nerve is a mixture of special sensory (taste), general sensory, secretomotor and motor. The general motor component supplies one muscle, the stylopharyngeus, and the secretomotor supplies the parotid gland. The general sensory component cov-ers the mucous membranes of the oropharynx, palatine tonsils, faucial pillars and posterior third of the tongue.

The motor fibres to the stylopharyngeus arise from the rostral portion of the nucleus ambiguous, and the secretomotor fibres begin from the inferior salivatory nucleus, located caudally to the superior salivatory nucleus.

The sensory afferents of taste terminate in the nucleus of the solitary tract, and the general sensory component terminates in the spinal nucleus of the trigeminal spinal tract.

Vagus (X)

Like the glossopharyngeal, the vagus is a mix of special sensory, general sensory, visceromotor, and parasympathetic motor fibres to the abdomen and thorax.

The general visceral motor component supplies all the muscles of the soft palate (except *tensor veli palatini – V*), all the muscles of the pharynx (except *stylopharyngeus – IX*) and all the muscles of the larynx.

Sensory components for the vagus relate primarily to the mucosa of the pharynx, epiglottis, joints of the larynx, mucosa of the larynx and mucosa of the oesophagus. The taste fibres from the epiglottis are initially carried by the vagus but ultimately travel with the special sensory fibres of the glossopharyngeal.

The nuclei of the vagus are dominated by the largest parasympathetic nucleus of the brain stem, the *dorsal nucleus of the vagus nerve*. In addition to this nucleus, the nucleus ambiguus provides the motor component for the special visceral efferent fibres to the pharynx and larynx, the spinal trigeminal tract for the general visceral afferents, and the solitary nucleus for taste. These last three nuclei are the same as those involved for the glossopharyngeal nerve.

Hypoglossal (XII)

This nerve is motor to the intrinsic and extrinsic muscles of the tongue, and there is some belief that a form of sensory feedback via muscle spindle proprioception is conveyed as well. The fibres originate from the hypoglossal nucleus in the medulla, an elongated nucleus lying between the dorsal nucleus of the vagus nerve and the midline of the medulla.

A tabular summary of the cranial nerves involved in deglutition is included below, which may help some to recall and compare the various roles of the nerves.

MUSCLE ACTIONS

Having discussed which muscles are innervated by each of the five cranial nerves, it is important to understand what action each muscle, once activated, is trying to achieve. An understanding of this process will help the clinician and student appreciate at what level the patient may be experiencing problems, and subsequently arrive at appropriate compensatory manoeuvres to aid the patient. While reviewing these muscles, bear in mind that many of the muscles of the oropharynx are supplied by the *pharyngeal plexus*, which is itself made up of various branches from cranial nerves IX, X and XI.

Muscles supplied by trigeminal (V)

- The *masseter, temporalis, medial pterygoid* and *lateral pterygoid* work together to masticate a bolus, moving the mandible from side to side, elevating and protruding the jaw.
- The *tensor tympani* is innervated by the trigeminal nerve, however this muscle plays no role in swallowing. Rather, it helps to protect the tympanic membrane of the ear from damage by loud noises.
- The *tensor veli palitini* tenses the soft palate prior to its elevation.
- The *mylohyoid* elevates the hyoid bone, floor of mouth and tongue.
- The *anterior belly of digastric* depresses the mandible, raises the hyoid bone and stabilizes the hyoid bone.

Muscles supplied by facial (VII)

- The *muscles of facial expression*. Those muscles surrounding the mouth are of most importance, responsible for an adequate lip seal.
- The *buccinator* aids mastication by pressing the bolus laterally into the molar teeth.
- The *posterior belly of digastric* raises the hyoid bone and stabilizes the hyoid bone.
- The *platysma* depresses the mandible.
- The *stylohyoid* elevates the hyoid and retracts the hyoid distally.
- The *stapedius* plays no role in swallowing. Rather, it controls the movement of the stapes bone in the inner ear.

Table 1.1 Cranial nerves involved in deglutition

Nerve	Nuclei	GSE	SVE	GVE	GSA	SVA	GVA
V trigeminal	Three sensory nuclei: mesencephalic, chief sensory and spinal. They run continuously from lateral to the cerebral aqueduct, through the pontine tegmentum, down through the medulla to the inferior region of the pons. There is one motor, which lies medial to the chief sensory nucleus, in the dorsolateral area of the pontine tegmentum.		Motor to four muscles of mastication, and four additional muscles: 1. temporalis; 2. masseter; 3. medial pterygoid; 4. lateral pterygoid; 5. tensor tympani; 6. tensor veli palitini; 7. mylohyoid; 8. anterior belly of digastric.		Three branches: 1. opthalmic; 2. maxillary; 3. mandibular between the 2nd and 3rd branches, this nerve innervates the mucous membranes of the nasopharynx, hard and soft palates, anterior 2/3rds of tongue, cheeks, floor of mouth, teeth, gums, the skin of the lips and jaw.		
VII facial	The motor nucleus for the SVE fibres lies caudal to the motor nucleus of V, in the ventrolateral part of the pontine tegmentum. The salivatory nucleus and lacrimal nucleus are the nuclei for the GVE, and are located medial to the facial		Motor to: 1. muscles of facial expression (five branches); 2. buccinator; 3. posterior belly of digastric; 4. platysma; 5. stylohyoid; 6. stapedius.	Secretomotor to: 1. sublingual gland 2. submandibular gland 3. lacrimal gland 4. nasal mucosa 5. palatal mucosa		Taste from anterior 2/3rd of the tongue via the chorda tympani, and from the soft palate from the greater petrosal.	

Table 1.1 (Continued)

Nerve	Nuclei	GSE	SVE	GVE	GSA	SVA	GVA
	motor. The SVA fibres return to the solitary nucleus, which lies adjacent to the solitary tract.						
IX glosso-pharyngeal	The SVE motor fibres emanate from the rostral part of the nucleus ambiguus, located deep in the superior part of the medulla, caudal to the inferior salivatory nucleus. The GVE fibres originate from the inferior salivatory nucleus (lying caudal to the superior salivatory nucleus). GSA neurones terminate in the spinal trigeminal nucleus, and the SVA fibres relay taste back to the caudal section of the solitary nucleus adjacent to the solitary tract, toward the midline of the medulla.		Motor to stylopharyngeus	Secretomotor to parotid gland		Taste from the posterior 2/3rd of tongue. Fibres from the carotid body and carotid sinus are also carried. Although they play no role in deglutition they are included for completion.	Sensory from: 1. mucous membrane of oropharynx; 2. palatine tonsils; 3. faucial pillars; 4. posterior 2/3rd tongue.

Table 1.1 (*Continued*)

Nerve	Nuclei	GSE	SVE	GVE	GSA	SVA	GVA
X vagus	SVE fibres originate from the nucleus ambiguus, and the coronal root of the accessory nerve. GVE motor neurons are derived from the dorsal nucleus of the vagus nerve, the largest parasympathetic nucleus in the brain stem, located medial to the solitary nucleus. The taste SVA fibres travel along with IX to the solitary nucleus		Motor to: 1. all muscles of the soft palate, *except* tensor veli palatini, via the pharyngeal branch; 2. all muscles of the pharynx, *except* stylopharyngeus, via pharyngeal branch; 3. all intrinsic muscles of the larynx via the recurrent laryngeal; 4. the cricothyroid via the external branch of superior laryngeal; 5. the cricopharyngeus also via the external branch of the superior laryngeal.	Parasympathetic. Motor to the abdomen and thorax.		Taste from buds on the epiglottis, which travel with fibres from IX. Fibres from the aortic body and viscera of thorax and abdomen are also relayed, included here for completion.	Sensory relay from four main branches: 1. pharyngeal – to mucosa of levator tor veli palatini, superior and medial constrictors; 2. internal branch of superior laryngeal – mucosa of laryngopharynx, epiglottic and aryepiglottic folds, laryngeal mucosa *above* the vocal folds, and joint receptors in the larynx; 3. recurrent laryngeal – mucosa *below* the vocal folds, mucosa of inferior constrictors and oesophagus;

Table 1.1 (*Continued*)

Nerve	Nuclei	GSE	SVE	GVE	GSA	SVA	GVA
							4. oesophageal branch – mucosa and striated muscles of the oesophagus.
XII hypoglossal	The hypoglossal nucleus (motor) lies between the dorsal nucleus of the vagus, and the midline of the medulla.	Motor to the intrinsic muscles of the tongue, and the three extrinsic muscles: 1. genioglossus; 2. styloglossus; 3. hyoglossus. Combination with fibres from C1 to C3 to create the Ansa Cervicalis which innervates: 1. geniohyoid; 2. thyrohyoid; 3. sternohyoid; 4. sternothyroid; 5. omohyoid.					

Muscles supplied by the glossopharyngeal (IX)

• The *stylopharyngeus* elevates the pharynx and larynx.

Muscles supplied by the vagus (X)

• The *levator veli palatini* elevates the soft palate.
• The *palatoglossus* elevates the posterior part of the tongue and draws the soft palate onto the tongue.
• The *palatopharyngeus* tenses the soft palate and draws the pharynx superiorly, anteriorly and medially.
• The *musculus uvulae* shortens the uvula, pulling it superiorly.
• The *superior, middle and inferior constrictors* constrict the walls of the pharynx.
• The *salpingopharyngeus* elevates the pharynx and larynx.
• The *intrinsic muscles of the larynx* oppose the vocal cords to protect the airway during swallowing.
• The *cricothyroid* tips the thyroid cartilage anteriorly, helping to protect the airway during swallowing.
• The *cricopharyngeus* inhibits the reflux of gastric contents.

Muscles supplied by the hypoglossal (XII)

• The *intrinsic muscles of the tongue* change the shape of the tongue to allow bolus movement.
• The *genioglossus* depresses the tongue and also allows protrusion.
• The *hyoglossus* depresses and retracts the tongue.
• The *styloglossus* retracts the tongue and also draws up the lateral borders to generate a chute.
• The *geniohyoid* pulls the hyoid anteriorly and superiorly, widening the pharynx and pulling the larynx out of the bolus path.
• The *sternohyoid, omohyoid, sternothyroid and thyrohyoid* – the infrahyoids – depress the hyoid bone after swallowing or depending on other muscle movements, stabilize the hyoid, and elevate the larynx.

Now that we have a firm grasp of the sensory and motor neurone pathways and the muscles that are innervated with their actions, we can discuss the various reflexes and patterned responses that we find in the oral cavity, oropharynx and pharynx.

REFLEXES, ARCS AND PATTERNED RESPONSES

Prior to any discussion of reflexes of the oral and pharyngeal regions it is important to discuss exactly what defines a reflex. A true reflex is a neural arc that, once initiated, cannot be stopped. Previous definitions have merely stated that a reflex is indicated when specific sensory inputs subconsciously induce a motor response. This is not entirely correct, as seen in the case of the patellar tendon reflex. A firm tap of the patellar tendon of the knee will result in an immediate and uncontrollable extension of the leg. We are fully conscious of the reflex and can feel our quadriceps contract, but we are unable to stop this contraction. Accordingly, a 'subconscious motor response' is not a clear guide as to what constitutes a reflex.

A more appropriate term to use in relation to our current field of study is the *patterned response*. A patterned response is a motor activity, exhibiting elements of subconscious programming and repetition but in which the programming can be overridden voluntarily (cortical control). It is important to understand the difference between the two concepts, in order to aid diagnosis dependant on the presence or absence of each.

Traditionally the swallow has been regarded as a reflex, whereas conventional research leans more towards the concept of a programmed or patterned response. A look at the neurological control of swallowing as outlined earlier clearly shows that the human swallow is a little bit of both. This is most easily explained in the case of an automatic swallow in a decerebrate laboratory animal. Such animals were historically used to justify the entire swallow as a reflex. In the absence of a cerebrum, the test animal could still elicit a swallow following stimulation of the internal branch of the superior laryngeal nerve. At this point in the pharynx, the *continuation* of the swallow is involuntary and not under cortical control. Prior to this point, however, the motor pattern of swallowing can be overridden. This situation can be shown using biofeedback mechanisms while undergoing a fibreoptic endoscopic examination of swallowing (FEES) (see Chapter 8). A patient watching the fibreoptic picture of a bolus in the pharynx can suppress the urge to commence the swallow. Once the bolus reaches a critical point (e.g. areas innervated by the internal branch of the superior laryngeal nerve) cortical control cannot be maintained and the reflex occurs.

There are some true reflexes in the oral and pharyngeal areas. Jaw reflexes promote opening of the mouth in cases where the periodontal ligaments supporting the teeth are stimulated by biting on something too hard. The 'gag reflex' is *not* a reflex, but rather a response that exists in some people and not in others and can be limited voluntarily. The *cough reflex* is a true reflex, instigated by the presence of a stimulus at or below the vestibule of the larynx. These last two physiological events are discussed in greater details in later chapters (see Chapters 4 and 7).

THE SWALLOW IN DETAIL

Armed with the information outlined above we can now look at integrating the entire swallowing process. Tying the feedback loops, cortical control, and neural networks with the anatomy and physiology will help the student and clinician calculate exactly which part of the deglutition process has failed in the dysphagic patient, and allow a starting point for the exploration of treatment modalities.

Once again we will adopt the 'first person' viewpoint of bolus preparation and swallowing, clarifying our original discussion of surface anatomy by including the musculature and neural involvement.

Stage 1: hunger

The smell of food, an empty stomach or an electrolytic imbalance informs sections of the brain (lateral walls of the hypothalamus) of the need to eat. Connections to the brain stem activate the nuclei of CN VII and IX, to promote secretion of salivary juices in preparation of a bolus.

Stage 2: chewing

As food is placed in the oral cavity, CN VII ensures a good lip seal (orbicularis oris) while CN V relays the sensory information back to the brain stem, constantly modifying the fine motor control of bolus preparation. Cortical processing provides motor activity to CN V, VII, IX, X and XII, creating an enclosed environment within the mouth to prepare the bolus. The cheeks provide tone (buccinator, CN VII), the soft palate is tensioned and drawn down towards the tongue (tensor veli palatini, CN V; palatopharyngeus, CN IX) and the tongue is drawn up towards the soft palate (palatopharyngeus, CN X; styloglossus, CN XII). At the same time, the hyoid bone is stabilized (infrahyoid muscles, CN XII and C1–C3) to allow free movement of the mandible. The bolus is prepared by closing (temporalis, masseter, medial pterygoid, lateral pterygoid; CN V) and opening (mylohyoid and anterior belly of digastric, CN V; geniohyoid, CN XII and C1–C3) of the mandible. The bolus is also pushed around the mouth by the actions of the tongue in order to create a consistent and homogenous texture (hyoglossus, genioglossus, styloglossus and the four groups of intrinsic muscles of the tongue; CN XII). While this is happening, taste sensations (CN VII and IX) are providing additional information to the cortex, contributing to the stimulation of those areas of the brain required to coordinate the swallow (insula and cingulate cortex).

Stage 3: voluntary initiation

The patient can voluntarily initiate the swallow once the bolus has been adequately prepared. The soft palate elevates slightly (levator veli palatini and palatopharyngeus, CN X), along with slight elevation of the hyoid bone (suprahyoid muscles contracting on a rigid mandible, combined with slight relaxation of the infrahyoid muscles). At this point the entire pharyngeal tube is elevated (stylopharyngeus, CN IX; palatopharyngeus and salpingopharyngeus, CN X). Now the tongue gets to work to deliver the bolus. The movements involved force the bolus distally towards the posterior wall of the pharynx in a 'piston-like' manner, using the hard palate for resistance. It was believed that once the bolus reaches the oropharynx that the swallow cycle could not be stopped and became a reflex. We can appreciate now that this is not entirely the case.

At this stage, sensations from the passage of the bolus are conveyed mainly by CN IX, but also by CN X. Many authors discuss the concept of the 'pharyngeal plexus' to describe the areas supplied by CN IX and X throughout the mucosa of the pharynx, and such a description is appropriate here. Both nerves also convey taste from this area continuing the higher level information feedback loops.

Stage 4: laryngeal elevation

The first motion of the tongue in preparation for propelling the bolus into the oropharynx is in an elevated anterior direction toward the roof of the mouth (mylohyoid and anterior belly of digastric, CN V; stylohyoid and posterior belly of digastric, CN VII; palatoglossus, CN X; genioglossus, hyoglossus and styloglossus, CN XII; geniohyoid, CN XII and C1–C3). It is clear to see that this motion has a follow-on effect of elevating the hyoid bone in an anterior direction, and subsequently the larynx as well. By this time the soft palate has sealed off the nasopharynx, and the superior constrictors have begun their medialization of the lateral walls. The larynx is elevated and moved anteriorly in relation to the hyoid bone by the thyrohyoid (CN X).

Stage 5: laryngeal closure

While the larynx is being elevated, the vestibule closes and rises relative to the thyroid cartilage (cricothyroid and intrinsic laryngeal muscles, CN X). The apposition and elevation of the arytenoid cartilages provide the medial 'curtains' of the pyriform recesses. These 'curtains' are the aryepiglottic folds. At the same time the pressure exerted on the base of the epiglottis, in combination with laryngeal elevation from below, causes the epiglottis to tip over the apposed cords and cover the vestibule.

The medial constrictors (CN X) have continued the 'stripping' of the pharynx by medialization, following on from the superior constrictors. The palate has started to descend (palatopharyngeus, CN X) as the constrictors begin the 'stripping' process, and the tongue moves posteriorly (styloglossus, CN XII) to participate in the closure of the oropharynx. Once the bolus has reached the pharyngeal areas innervated by the internal branch of the superior laryngeal nerve, the swallow becomes reflexive and cannot be halted.

The elevation and anterior movement of the larynx have allowed stretching of cricopharyngeus (upper oesophageal sphincter) to open the entrance into the oesophagus. The inferior constrictor has finished its process of medialization after the bolus has passed through, and the bolus is delivered safely into the oesophagus.

Stage 6: resting state

Cricopharyngeus resumes its tonic state of closure once the bolus has passed. The absence of any stimulus in or around the vestibule will allow reopening of the glottis, and the larynx to lower. All of these actions are covered by a reflex arc involving only CN X. Presence of a stimulus in the region should result in a reflex cough. The tongue and hyoid return to their resting position, as does the palate.

When studying the physiological sequence of a swallow it must be remembered that all of this occurs with split-second timing. Our outline above suggests that one event follows neatly after the next and then the next. In reality the timing of the oral phase for a liquid bolus is a second, and the timing of the pharyngeal phase for *all* boluses is also a second.

SUMMARY

The aim of this chapter has been to provide an understanding of the integration of many muscles and nerves to perform the complex task of swallowing. New research has opened our eyes to the crucial role the cortex and other parts of the brain all play in execution of this task, while offering an insight into many clinical manifestations of dysphagia that until recently have been incorrectly explained. In addition, an appreciation of exactly where a swallow becomes automatic has been gained, increasing the need for a clinician to understand, for example, that residual pooling of material in the valleculae may in fact be normal (see Chapter 3).

As you progress through this text, let your grounding in what is normal be your guide in order that your diagnosis and treatment of dysphagia be achieved from first principles.

ACKNOWLEDGEMENTS

The author wishes to acknowledge and thank the assistance of the Anatomy Department at the University of Queensland, Australia, for the plasticized dissections used in the figures of this chapter.

GLOSSARY

Axial: a slice laterally, from one side to the opposite side, perpendicular to a sagittal section.
Caudal: towards the inferior or tail end of the body.
Coronal: a horizontal slice.
Dorsal: towards the back or top-most of the body.
Lateral: towards the side or outside of the body.
Medial: towards the middle of the body.
Rostral: towards the anterior of the body.
Sagittal: a slice from the front or anterior, through to the back or posterior.
Ventral: towards the belly or underside of the body.

REFERENCES

De Araujo IET, Rolls ET, Kringelbach ML, et al. (2003) Taste-olfactory convergence, and the representation of the pleasantness of flavour, in the human brain. European Journal of Neuroscience 18: 2059–68.

Donner M, Bosma JF, Robertson DL (1985) Anatomy and physiology of the pharynx. Gastrointestinal Radiology 10: 196–212.

Kiernan JA (1998) Barr's The Human Nervous System: An Anatomical Viewpoint (7th edn). Philadelphia: Lippincott-Raven.

Martin RE, Goodyear BG, Gati JS, et al. (2001) Cerebral cortical representation of automatic and volitional swallowing in humans. Journal of Neurophysiology 85: 938–50.

Moore KL, Dalley AF II (1999) Clinically Oriented Anatomy (4th edn). Philadelphia PA: Lippincott Williams & Wilkins.

Mosier K, Bereznaya I (2001) Parallel cortical networks for volitional control of swallowing in humans. Experimental Brain Research 140: 280–9.

Perlman AL (1991) The neurology of swallowing. Seminars in Speech and Language 12(3): 171–83.

Sewards TV, Sewards MA (2003) Representations of motivational drives in mesial cortex, medial thalamus, hypothalamus and midbrain. Brain Research Bulletin 61: 25–49.

Zald DH, Pardo JV (2000) Functional neuroimaging of the olfactory system in humans. International Journal of Psychophysiology 36: 165–81.

FURTHER READING

Broussard DL, Altschuler SM (2000) Brainstem viscerotopic organization of afferents and efferents involved in the control of swallowing. The American Journal of Medicine 108(4a): 79s–86s.

Broussard DL, Altschuler SM (2000) Central integration of swallowing and airway-protective reflexes. The American Journal of Medicine 108(4a): 62s–67s.

Crossman AR (2000) Neuroanatomy: An Illustrated Colour Text (2nd edn). Edinburgh, New York: Churchill Livingstone.

Del Parigi A, Gautier J, Chen K, Salbe AD, Ravussin E, Reiman E, et al. (2002) Neuroimaging and obesity: Mapping the brain responses to hunger and satiation in humans using positron emission tomography. Annals of the New York Academy of Sciences 967: 389–97.

Hamdy S, Rothwell JC, Aziz Q, Thompson DG (2000) Organization and reorganization of human swallowing motor cortex: implications for recovery after stroke. Clinical Science 98: 151–7.

Jafari S, Prince RA, Kim DY, Paydarfar D (2003) Sensory regulation of swallowing and airway protection: a role for the internal superior laryngeal nerve in humans. Journal of Physiology 550(1): 287–304.

Jean A (2001) Brain stem control of swallowing: Neuronal network and cellular mechanisms. Physiology Reviews 81(2): 929–69.

Miller AJ (2002) Oral and pharyngeal reflexes in the mammalian nervous system: Their diverse range in complexity and the pivotal role of the tongue. Critical Reviews in Oral Biology and Medicine 13(5): 409–25.

Moore KL, Dalley AF II (1999) Clinically Oriented Anatomy (4th edn). Philadelphia PA: Lippincott Williams & Wilkins.

Sawczuk A, Mosier KM (2001) Neural control of tongue movement with respect to respiration and swallowing. Critical Reviews in Oral Biology and Medicine 12(1): 18–37.

Yamamoto F, Nishino T (2002) Phasic vagal influence on the rate and timing of reflex swallowing. American Journal of Respiratory and Critical Care Medicine 165: 1400–3.

Yutaka W et al. (2004) Cortical regulation during the early stage of initiation of voluntary swallowing in humans. Dysphagia 19: 100–8.

Zald DH, Pardo JV (2000) Functional neuroimaging of the olfactory system in humans. International Journal of Psychophysiology 36: 165–81.

2 Swallowing from Infancy to Old Age

JULIE CICHERO

So far we have discussed the anatomical features and physiology of the normal swallow in general terms (see Chapter 1). There are, however, some important differences between the adult and infant swallow and even between adult and infant oropharyngeal structures. The paediatric swallow is fascinating not least because it is evident in the foetus from 12 weeks' gestational age. The infant must learn to adapt to different foods, fluids and textures – a process the child manages very well by about 3 years of age. This chapter will cover the process of suckle, suck and swallow in the infant and will also discuss transitional feeding. Humans, do not, however, reach a stable state once normal chewing and swallowing patterns have been achieved. The ageing process takes a toll on swallowing. Some physiological parameters of the swallow alter as we age. Many of these are discussed in other chapters of this text; however, the broad changes that occur with ageing will be highlighted here.

THE EMBRYO, THE INFANT AND THE CHILD

Breathing and swallowing are two of the most important functions necessary to sustain life. As noted above, the human foetus is able to swallow from 12 weeks' gestational age. The very early development of this function alerts us to its importance. Infants begin life by sucking and swallowing liquids. This involves a high degree of coordination in order to feed effectively and, at the same time, to protect the airway. Infants begin by suckling, and then move onto the more mature pattern of sucking. Similarly, the actions of chewing develop from a less mature munching pattern. As infants grow they also develop skills that allow them to move from thin liquids to the wide variety of textures that adults enjoy. Excellent texts have been devoted to the paediatric feeding and swallowing mechanism, pattern of development, and pathology (Wolf and Glass, 1994; Arvedson and Brodsky, 2002). This section serves to alert the reader to some important considerations when examining the infant swallow and its maturation.

THE BRANCHIAL ARCHES AND THEIR SIGNIFICANCE

Many paediatric dysphagia texts begin with a discussion of the branchial arches. Certainly it seems like overkill to start as far back as embryologic development;

Dysphagia: Foundation, Theory and Practice. Edited by J. Cichero and B. Murdoch
© 2006 John Wiley & Sons, Ltd.

however, there is at least one very important reason for revisiting the branchial arches: it helps us to understand congenital swallowing disorders and craniofacial abnormalities (e.g. Treacher Collins syndrome and also cleft palate). These are elaborated in Chapter 13. More importantly, the branchial arches also help us to understand why certain functions are so closely linked – like swallowing and respiration, for example. The following brief discussion highlights aspects of the development of the branchial arches that may be of interest to the dysphagia clinician.

BRANCHIAL ARCH DEVELOPMENT

Three weeks after conception there are three germ layers present. These are the ectoderm, mesoderm and endoderm and they are otherwise known as the neural crest cells. These layers provide the basis for the development of the skin and nervous system (ectoderm), smooth muscle, connective tissue and blood vessels (mesoderm), and digestive and respiratory systems (endoderm). The three germ layers give rise to all tissues and organs of the embryo (Moore, 1973). Early in the fourth week after conception, the branchial arches develop from these neural crest cells. All vertebrae, and specifically the head and neck, develop from the branchial arches and their constituents. More specifically the face, neck, nasal cavities, mouth, larynx and pharynx along with muscular attachments for the head and neck are all derived from the branchial arches (Arvedson and Brodsky, 2002). There are six pairs of branchial arches with each being separated from each other by obvious branchial grooves (also known as clefts). A simple figure illustrating the branchial arches is shown in Figure 2.1.

Each branchial arch develops into specific skeletal structures and muscles and their nerve supply. The development of the branchial arches explains how, for

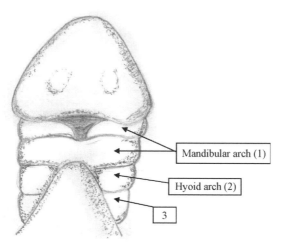

Figure 2.1(a)   Antero-posterior view of the brachial apparatus 28 ± 1 day (adapted from Moore, 1973)

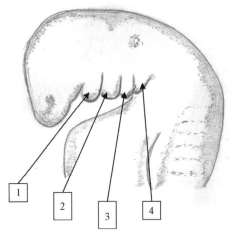

Figure 2.1(b)   Lateral view of the brachial apparatus 28 ± 1 day (adapted from Moore, 1973)

example, a single structure like the tongue receives innervation from a number of different nerves (i.e. CN. V, VII, IX and XII). In short, this is because the tongue is formed by a number of the branchial arches. The motor supply to the muscles of the tongue is provided by the hypoglossal nerve (CN. XII), which emanates from myoblasts from the occipital myotomes (Moore, 1973). As noted in Chapter 1, sensory nerve supply is provided to the mucosa of the anterior two-thirds of the tongue by the lingual branch of the mandibular division of the trigeminal nerve (CN V – first branchial arch). Taste for the anterior two-thirds of the tongue is supplied by the facial nerve (second branchial arch), whereas taste for the posterior third of the tongue is supplied by the glossopharyngeal nerve (third branchial arch). In addition, a small area of the tongue anterior to the epiglottis is supplied by the superior laryngeal nerve of the vagus nerve (fourth branchial arch) (Moore, 1973). Although it is confusing it helps to explain the many dimensions of this single structure.

The first branchial arch gives rise to the upper and lower jaw, the malleus and incus of the inner ear and the trigeminal nerve. The second branch provides portions of the hyoid bone and stapes of the inner ear, among other structures, and the facial nerve. The first and second arches provide the mouth, tongue and muscles of mastication, and the facial nerve (Moore, 1973; Tuchman, 1994). The third brancial arch contributes portions of the hyoid bone, the posterior third of the tongue and a portion of the epiglottis and pyriform sinuses, while the fourth and sixth arches give rise to the tongue, laryngeal cartilages, epiglottis and inferior pharyngeal constrictors (fourth arch). The third branchial arch provides the glossopharyngeal nerve and the hypoglossal nerve. The fourth and sixth branchial arches give rise to the vagus nerve and specifically the recurrent laryngeal nerve and the superior laryngeal nerve (Arvedson and Brodsky, 2002). Pairs of pharyngeal pouches also develop between the branchial arches. There are five pharyngeal pouches. Briefly, these pouches develop into the Eustachian tube, the tonisllar fossa region, the parathyroid glands and the thymus (Moore, 1973).

The respiratory system and the digestive system develop from the same embryonic structure – that of the endoderm. The fact that these systems develop from the one embryonic structure shows that these systems are by nature linked together. Both systems develop from the laryngotracheal groove in the primitive pharynx. The underbelly of the laryngotracheal tube eventually becomes the larynx, trachea, bronchi and lungs. The back of the laryngotracheal groove develops into the oesophagus. This early development (fourth week) shows that the respiratory and deglutitory systems are tightly woven together from the very early stages of gestation. It is hardly surprising to find the two systems working in the harmony that is required to sustain life, both by breathing and swallowing. It also provides excellent reason to look at the syncrhonization of the respiratory and swallowing systems (see Chapter 4). Koempel and Holinger (1998) also note that the limbs develop at the same time as the orofacial structures (approximately 6 weeks' gestation). They indicate that this would account for the concurrent limb abnormalities found in children with orofaciodigital syndromes.

Some interesting markers of embryonic development as they relate to swallowing

The very importance of the act of swallowing is evident in that the reflex is present by 12 weeks' gestational age. The epiglottis and larynx are clearly identifiable by day 41 of life (approximately 6 weeks) (Koempel and Holinger, 1998). By the end of the first trimester (i.e. 12 weeks) the foetus can swallow (Arvedson and Brodsky, 2002), absorb and discharge fluids. Within the next week the vocal folds form. By 10 weeks all organs are present and the heart is almost completely developed. Taste buds are forming on the tongue by 7 weeks' gestation and taste receptors are noted by 12 weeks (Arvedson and Brodsky, 2002). By 20 weeks the taste buds can distinguish sweet from bitter (Stoppard, 1993). The gag reflex is present at 26 to 27 weeks' gestational age and the rooting reflex is noted by 32 weeks gestation (Arvedson and Brodsky, 2002). The coordination between swallowing and breathing is not fully organized until after 34 weeks' gestational age.

ANATOMICAL DIFFERENCES

Infants and older children have a number of anatomical differences. These mostly concern the relative size of the various structures relating to swallowing. These are the oral cavity, the pharynx, larynx and oesophagus. Table 2.1 provides a ready reference to these differences. Beginning with the oral cavity, note that the distance between the velopharyngeal region and tongue base increases from around 20 mm at 3 months to 27 mm at 4 years. The distance between the tongue base and the

Table 2.1 Orofacial and functional swallowing differences between (a) infants and (b) the older child and adults

Anatomic location or physiological variable	Infant	Older child/adult
Mouth	Tongue fills the mouth. Cheeks have sucking pads. Small mandible proportionate to the cranium.	The mouth is large and the tongue rests on the floor of the mouth. No sucking pads. More proportionate mandible.
Pharynx	Gentle curve from the nasopharynx to the hypopharynx, hence no definite or distinct oropharynx. Pharynx found at the level of the third cervical vertebrae.	During maturation the gentle curve becomes a 90° angle between the nasopharynx and oropharynx, distinguishing the two regions from each other. Pharynx found at the level of the sixth cervical vertebrae.
Larynx	Located at the third and fourth cervical vertebrae. Arytenoids are nearly mature in size in comparison with remainder of laryngeal structures which are a third of the adult size. Vocal cord length: 6 mm to 8 mm. Glottis width at rest: 3 mm. Maximum glottis: 6 mm. Narrow vertical epiglottis.	Descends to the sixth cervical vertebrae during childhood and comes to rest at the seventh cervical vertebrae during puberty. Vocal cord length: Males: 17 mm to 23 mm. Females: 12.5 mm to 17 mm. Glottis width at rest: males 8 mm; females 6 mm. Maximum glottis: males 19 mm; females 13 mm. Flat, wide epiglottis.
Trachea	Diameter of a pencil (~0.8 cm).	Diameter of 2.5 cm.
Oesophagus	5 mm diameter, 11 cm long	2 cm diameter, extends from sixth cervical vertebrae to eleventh thoracic vertebrae (23 cm to 25 cm long)
Volume per swallow	0.2 ml (± 0.11 ml)	20 ml to 25 ml per mouthful.
Swallows per day	600 to 1000	600+

Source: Lear et al. (1965); Aronson (1985).

entrance to the larynx increases from around 5 mm at 3 months to 9 mm at 4 years (Rommel, 2002).

In infants, the tongue is very large compared to the oral cavity. The hyoid bone sits very high in the infant, right up under the mandible. The hyoid is similarly set high and the thryroid cartilage is 'continguous' with the hyoid bone. This arrangement explains why there is less vertical distance travelled in the motion of laryngeal elevation in the infant. In the adult there is an obvious space between the mandible and the hyoid bone, and the distance travelled makes the vertical movement more obvious. A prominent pharyngeal pressure wave is also noted in infants whereas this is not normally seen in adults (Tuchman, 1994).

The pharynx consists of three 'geographical' regions – the nasopharynx (behind the nose), the oropharynx (behind the mouth) and the hypopharynx (closest to the larynx). In infants, the pharynx shows a gentle curve from the nasopharynx to the hypopharynx. As infants grow, however, the gentle curve gradually changes to become closer to a 90° angle between the nasopharynx and oropharynx as seen in adults. In infants, the small oral cavity in combination with the close proximity of the tongue, soft palate and pharynx with the larynx appear to facilitate nasal breathing (Rommel, 2002).

The base of tongue and larynx descend during the first year of life. In the newborn, the larynx and pharynx are initially located at the level of the third and fourth cervical vertebrae, and descends to the level of the sixth cervical vertebrae during childhood, reaching the seventh cervical vertebrae by 15 to 20 years (Aronson, 1985). The larynx grows steadily until about 3 years of age, and then remains relatively stable until 12 years of age. At the onset of puberty the laryngeal cavity grows larger, the vocal folds lengthen and thicken. In addition, the laryngeal prominence becomes more noticeable in males as the thyroid alae narrows to 90°, as opposed to females, where it remains the same (Aronson, 1985; Moore and Dalley, 1999). The larynx continues to descend throughout life. The trachea similarly grows from the diameter of a pencil in infancy to the adult size of 2.5 cm (Moore and Dalley, 1999).

In the infant, the arytenoids are nearly mature in size, when compared with the small size of the remainder of the laryngeal structures. Our understanding of glottic closure patterns in normal adult swallowing shows that closure and anterior movement of the arytenoids is critical to protection of the airway (see also Chapter 4). The relatively large size of the arytenoids in comparison to the laryngeal region may well explain why relatively little epiglottic tilt is required until the child reaches 5 years 9 months of age. Closure of the arytenoids would provide primary protection from aspiration (Rommel, 2002).

The oesophagus in the infant is 5 mm in diameter and approximately 11 cm long. By adulthood it is 2 cm in diameter. It extends from the upper oesophageal sphincter (UES) at the level of the sixth cervical vertebrae to the level of the lower oeopheageal sphincter (LES) where it meets the stomach at the level of the 11th thoracic vertebrae. The UES is fully functional in the newborn infant and varies in length between 5 mm and 10 mm in the newborn while the adult dimensions are in the order of 20 mm to 44 mm in length (Rommel, 2002).

PHYSIOLOGICAL DIFFERENCES

While there are many anatomical differences between infant and adult oropharyngeal structures, there are also some physiological differences relating to swallowing. Newborn infants have a poorly developed cough reflex (Bamford et al., 1992). The infant response to a laryngeal irritant such as water is to have a period of apnoea, then a swallow, and then possibly a cough (see Table 2.2). The average volume of milk taken by an infant in each suck is 0.2 ml (±0.11 ml), requiring 300 sucking and

Table 2.2 Maturation of infant reflexes

Skill	From 0 to 5 months	Five months to 1 year	Two years	Adult
Biting[1] stimulated by pressure on upper and lower gums.	Reflexive action – vertical bite, release pattern.	Integration of biting and chewing. Rotary chewing begins at 1 year.	Mature biting and chewing development evident. Rotary chewing motion evident and ability to use tongue to keep oral contents between the tooth surfaces.	Adult efficiency of chewing realized at 16 years.
Gag[1,2] stimulated by touching the posterior three-quarters of the tongue or pharyngeal walls.	Causes tongue protrusion, head and jaw protrusion and pharyngeal constriction and elevation. Usually very strong.	By 6 to 9 months the stimulus-sensitive area moves to the posterior half of the tongue and the pharyngeal walls.	Persists.	Sensitivity shifts to back quarter of the tongue and the pharyngeal wall by adulthood.
Tongue[1] protrusion stimulated by touching the tongue or lips.	Causes the tongue to protrude.	This reflex disappears between 4 and 6 months.		
Rooting reflex[1,2] stimulated by touching the cheeks or corner of the mouth.	Causes the infant to turn its head towards touch.	This reflex disappears between 3 and 6 months.		
Cough reflex[3] can be stimulated by both mechanoreceptors (touch/pressure) and chemoreceptors (water, milk, saline, secretions, gastric acid).	Brief apnoea and swallowing, followed by a cough. By one month of age 80% of infants are reported to cough instead of using the apnoic response.	Persists.	Persists.	Persists.

[1]Tuchman and Walter (1994).
[2]Arvedson and Brodsky (2002).

swallowing motions to consume 60 ml (Selley et al., 1990). The amount of fluid an infant draws in has also been measured to be as small as 0.04 ml, which is the size of a drop commonly seen if one watches the drop rate in intravenous infusions (Selley et al., 1990). Wolf and Glass (1992) reported that in breast-fed infants, the milk volume early in the feed is closer to 0.14 ml/suck, whereas at the end of the feed it dips as low as 0.01 ml/suck. Healthy infants swallow six times per minute while awake and six times per hour while asleep (Arvedson and Brodsky, 2002). Adults swallow on average 600 times per day but preserve the ratio of highest swallow rates during food intake (mean rate of 296 swallows/hour) and lowest swallow rates during sleep (mean rate of 7.5 swallows/hour) (Lear et al., 1965).

SUCKLE, SWALLOW AND RESPIRATION – A PATTERNED SEQUENCE

In healthy infants the actions of suckle, swallow and respiration are discrete yet finely timed and sequenced. Suckle movements occur to propel fluid into the oral cavity before the swallow. Swallow-respiratory coordination is then instrumental in impeding respiration. The pattern of bolus collection in the oral cavity, swallow, and apnoea during the swallow is described fully in Chapter 4. The usual swallow-respiratory pattern is one of inspiration-swallow-expiration (Bamford et al., 1992), although Selley et al. (1990) have also reported that inspiration-expiration-swallow-expiration is another common pattern. The primary form of nourishment in infants comes from milk (breast or bottle), which is a thin liquid. It is fascinating that infants begin their gustatory journey with thin fluids, rheologically the most difficult of bolus types to control (see Chapter 3). It is imperative, then, that the suckle-swallow-breathe pattern be finely executed (see Chapter 4). Note that with the breastfed infant, milk is *ejected* from the alveoli to the nipple. This is different from bottlefeeding where the milk *passively* flows from the teat. The breastfed infant requires significant coordination during the early phase of feeding as there is a high flow rate of milk once the letdown reflex (milk ejection reflex) has been activated. Swallowing must occur immediately to clear the oral cavity in preparation for the next bolus being ejected into the oral cavity.

THE NORMAL FEEDING PATTERN

The normal feeding pattern is characterized as follows. The infant will normally commence with a rooting reflex to find a nipple or teat and then latch onto the nipple or teat (see Table 2.2). Once the infant has latched on, nutritive suckling commences. During nutritive suckling, fluid is obtained from the nipple or teat as a result of the combination of (a) intraoral suction and (b) external pressure on the nipple or teat by the closing mandible, which facilitates the flow of liquid into the oral cavity. That is, something pushes the milk out of the nipple or teat (the jaw) and something pulls the milk into the mouth (loosely, the tongue and oral cavity) (Wolf and Glass,

1992). Jaw movement is a combination of forward and backward movements on top of opening and closing actions (Selley et al., 1990). Peak milk flow and maximum reduction in intraoral pressure occur as the jaw opens widely. Jaw closure occurs at the time of swallowing. This coincides with both the apnoeic period and normalization of intraoral pressure. Generation of intraoral pressure, which assists in bringing the bolus into the oral cavity, occurs because the oral system is 'closed'. It is closed anteriorly with the lips sealing around the teat, and posteriorly by the tongue rising up posteriorly and meeting with the soft palate. The reduction in intraoral pressure is then mediated by the sucking action which will bring the bolus into the oral cavity. The intraoral pressure is quite strong. In breastfeeding it is necessary to break the seal (e.g. by placing the little finger into the corner of the infant's mouth) to release the pressure and detach the infant from the nipple.

The bolus collects between the tongue and hard and soft palates. It collects onto a depression in the tongue. When the posterior part of the tongue is depressed, the buccal mucosa moves inwards and then outwards during the compression phase. The buccal mucosa is supported by the buccinator muscles and fat pads (Arvedson and Brodsky, 2002). The 'fat pads' or 'sucking pads' provide the rounded profile of the infant's cheeks and offer stability to the otherwise unstable mandible (Wolf and Glass, 1992). The soft palate, in conjunction with the most posterior part of the tongue, forms a seal to contain the bolus within the oral cavity until such time as the infant is ready to swallow. Logan and Bosma (1967) reported that the bolus may be contained between the posterior part of the tongue and the soft palate, but also collected as far down as the epiglottis in young infants. There is a rolling front-to-backwards direction of the tongue against the palate. The bolus then enters the pharynx. It is prevented from entering the nasal cavity by upward and backward displacement of the soft palate and the superior pharyngeal constrictor muscles moving towards each other in a squeezing motion. The tongue continues its backward motion making contact with the soft palate and then the posterior pharyngeal wall. The pharyngeal muscles (middle and inferior constrictors) also sequentially move towards each other behind the bolus and encourage the bolus's advancing movement towards the cricopharyngeus. As with the adult swallow, the cricopharyngeus is assisted in opening by anterior and superior movement of the hyoid and larynx complex. With the initiation of the swallow, respiration ceases (Logan and Bosma, 1967). Protection of the airway is afforded by elevation of the larynx under the base of the tongue, and anterior movement of the arytenoids towards the base of the epiglottis. Previous researchers have reported that the epiglottis closes over the laryngeal opening to afford additional protection, as is the case for the adult swallow (Logan and Bosma, 1967; Wolf and Glass, 1992). However, Rommel (2002) reported, that infants and children do not show a consistent pattern of epiglottic tilting until 5 years, 9 months of age. This is an interesting finding. Rommel (2002) also found that infants have significantly less epiglottic titling than children over one year of age. It may be that the anterior movement of the arytenoids in this very small laryngeal space is generally sufficient to protect the airway. It may also be that titling of the epiglottis is in fact a maturational factor that progresses with growth of the pharyngeal structures and vertical growth of the laryngopharyngeal region (Rommel, 2002).

The suck-swallow-breathe pattern in healthy infants should be well coordinated. Generally the suck and swallow pattern should occur in a 1:1 ratio. Infants will suck and swallow in that 1:1 sequence anywhere between 10 and 30 times before they take a breath and then continue feeding (Arvedson and Brodsky, 2002). Bamford et al. (1992) report, however, that breath-to-breath intervals range from 1.3 s to 2.0 s in infants (14 hours to 48 hours after birth). This shows that the usual suck:swallow: breath ratios are closer to 1:1:1. Breathing rate during feeding is slower than it is before feeding commences, at least initially (i.e. in the initial 30 s of feeding) (Bamford et al., 1992). The reduction in breathing rate in those initial seconds of the feed is also accompanied by a faster, regular swallowing rhythm. Mild desaturation has been noted to occur (85% to 90%), however full saturation was restored within a few seconds in healthy infants (Bamford et al., 1992). Oxygen saturation is discussed in detail in Chapter 7. Bamford et al. (1992) suggest that there is evidence for correlations between unstable breathing patterns and inefficient feeding. It is essential that the infant has the capacity to breathe nasally. After the bolus leaves the pharynx, air flows in through the nose and the next suck-swallow-breathe cycle commences.

There are also some subtle differences in the sucking and swallowing of breastfed infants. As noted above, the 'letdown' reflex causes milk to be ejected from the nipple. Sucking stimulates the 'letdown' reflex (see Chapter 15). Consequently there is a high sucking rate until the 'letdown' reflex is activated. The sucking rate then slows as the ejected milk is being swallowed. The sucking rate increases again as the milk flow diminishes towards the end of the feed. The same pattern in repeated when the infant takes the second breast (Wolf and Glass, 1992). Bottle-fed infants do not experience this pattern as the milk flows passively or by gravity from the bottle.

NUTRITIVE AND NON-NUTRITIVE SUCKING

Nutritive sucking (i.e. sucking giving nutrition) involves the liquid bolus being delivered to the oral cavity. Non-nutritive sucking involves rhythmic movements on a nipple or teat where there is no feeding possible (i.e. a dummy or pacifier). Nonnutritive suckling is characterized by rapid sucks at irregular intervals of varying length. The respiratory pattern also changes depending on whether nutritive or non-nutritive sucking is employed. During non-nutritive sucking, the breathing pattern switches to alternating inspiration and exhalation. There is no apnoeic period and the breathing and sucking systems appear to function independently (Selley et al., 1990). During nutritive sucking there is an apnoeic period during the swallow. The swallow-respiratory pattern is either inspiration-swallow-exhalation or inspiration-exhalation-swallow-exhalation.

Even jaw movements and intraoral pressure change depending on whether the infant is engaging in nutritive or non-nutritive sucking. During nutritive sucking, when the jaw moves there is a drop in intra-oral pressure. This pattern is not found during non-nutritive sucking.

Suck versus suckle

Sucking and suckling are in fact two different things, with the latter being the precursor to sucking. Suckling is an early pattern of development and is characterized by an extension-retraction pattern of the tongue, with only loose approximation of the lips (Walter, 1994). When watching the infant suckle, we may notice the tongue moves rhythmically in and out of the mouth just fractionally over the lips, which are parted only enough to gently sandwich the tongue between them. The backward and forward action of the tongue is combined with a pronounced opening and closing of the jaw. The backwards phase of tongue motion is more pronounced than the forward phase (Arvedson and Brodsky, 2002). This suckling pattern allows the infant to draw liquid into the mouth. The true 'suck pattern' involves a stronger pressure of the lips. In addition, the lips, tongue, jaw and hyoid move in synchrony, alternating in the direction of movement to more effectively draw the liquid into the mouth. The intrinsic muscles of the tongue allow it to be raised and lowered. Note the difference between this up-down tongue movement and the previous backward-forward movement used in suckling. The greater vertical movements of the tongue allow smaller vertical movement of the jaw. A mixture of suckling and sucking are used until the infant is roughly 6 months of age. At this stage the suck pattern is the more dominant pattern. This is most likely because the tongue has a greater ability to use the up-down motion effectively because of the elongation and forward growth of the face and oral cavity. Arvedson and Brodsky (2002) note that the transition from suckling to sucking is an important developmental step to allow the infant to manipulate thick fluids and soft foods that are spoonfed. In these cases, good lip closure is important as is more finely mastered tongue movement.

FEEDING AND COMMUNICATION

Selley et al. (1990) provided a compelling argument for looking at successful feeding as something of a predictor for normal communication. The authors stated that normal feeding and speech both depend on several common factors:

- rhythm;
- breath control;
- lip tone;
- finely coordinated tongue movements;
- speed of muscle movements; and
- well developed sensory feedback systems.

In swallowing, the muscles of the lips, tongues and cheeks should become coordinated. If they fail to become coordinated it is conceivable that difficulties in speech might follow as the muscles employed during the oral phase of the swallow are also employed for speech. Arvedson and Brodsky (2002) concur that the ability to manipulate the various textures of food during transitional feeding are common with parallel gains in speech development, and trunk, head and neck stability.

Transitional feeding

'Transitional feeding is the term used to describe the intermediary steps from sucking to chewing, and encompasses the process of taking purees from a spoon' (Walter, 1994: 32). Healthy normal infants can begin taking solids (i.e. foodstuffs other than breast milk or formulae) between 4 and 6 months of age. At this stage smooth, pureed fruits, vegetables and rice cereals are usually introduced. In these early stages of transitional feeding, the infant may cough, splutter and spit food out. Remember that the texture has changed significantly and infants cannot suck and swallow as they have done previously, although they will certainly try this to begin with! They have to learn how to use the lingual and buccal muscles to cope with this new food. Between 6 and 9 months 'chunky' purees are introduced, allowing the infants to begin to explore texture. This is important for desensitizing the gag reflex. Meat, chicken, fish and finger foods are usually added to the diet at around this stage. This is also the time when the deciduous or baby teeth are beginning to erupt.

Interestingly, the eruption of teeth appears to have more of a role in providing sensory information to the brain than the motor pattern that adults use to break food down. It is possible for example, for infants who have late eruption of their deciduous teeth to 'chew' quite effectively using the gums in the molar region (Arvedson and Brodsky, 2002). Chewing at this stage is usually referred to as 'munching' to differentiate it from the adult pattern of rotary movements of the jaw in combination with a grinding action of the teeth. The sucking pads that were important to effective suckling and sucking are also gradually absorbed during this transitional feeding time. At 9 to 12 months of age chopped food and finger food are introduced. At this stage cheese, yoghurt and cow's milk are also added to supplement the infant's breast milk or formulae intake. After the child's first birthday, the child is usually ready to enjoy soft foods and food that requires chewing. The child also progresses to independent cup drinking and utensil use. This is further discussed in terms of therapeutic intervention in the child with dysphagia in Chapters 13 and 15. Details regarding spoonfeeding and cup drinking can also be found in Chapter 13.

With the introduction of pureed food, the infant uses the tongue to mash the food against the palate. As the infant's oral cavity grows there is more space in the oral cavity (due to descent of the jaw and recession of the buccal fat pads). This allows the food to be moved by the tongue towards the gums where the up-down munching pattern allows the infant to mash the food. Somewhere between 3 and 6 years of age infants develop the adult coordination of vertical and lateral movements of the jaw to allow effective mastication of food. Table 2.3 provides a feeding progression table for summary purposes.

The swallowing mechanism remains reasonably stable (barring assault or injury) for many years after this stage. At approximately 45 years of age nature changes the anatomical system that we work with and the physiology of the swallow responds accordingly. We see an increase in total swallowing time, and in fact changes to all phases of the swallow that occur as a direct result of ageing. The section that follows expands upon the anatomical and physiological changes that occur as individuals age.

Table 2.3 Feeding progression table

Age	Food	Oral preparation and 'oral events'	Feeding utensil
Birth to 6 months	Milk, liquids	Suckling and then sucking.	Breast or bottle.
4 to 6 months	Cereals, purees	Initially sucking, then tongue to palate movement, may eject food from spoon involuntarily, gags on new textures.	Spoon.
6 to 9 months	Chunky puree, mashed food, soft finger foods	Emerging munching pattern, desensitization of gag reflex. Lateralization of food to gums. Deciduous teeth erupting. Coordinated lip, tongue, jaw movements.	Spoon, drinking from cup ~ 9 months.
9 to 12 months	Chopped food and finger food	Licking food off lips, biting of objects. Controlled sustained bite on hard food (e.g. biscuit/cracker).	Spoon, cup. Self finger feeding. Weaning from breast/bottle as cup drinking increases.
15 to 24 months	Full diet with some exclusionary items (e.g. nuts)	Licks food from lips, increased maturity of adult rotary chew pattern, jaw stability in cup drinking. Independence in self-feeding. Straw drinking.	Spoon, cup, fork. Self-feeding predominates.

Source: adapted from Walter (1994), Arvedson and Brodsky (2002).

THE AGEING SWALLOW

The pattern of adult chewing and swallowing is discussed in Chapter 1 and Chapter 3. As we age, the muscles and cartilages that we rely on for efficient swallowing also age. The ageing process causes some changes to the physiology of the swallow. This section will highlight the major changes one might expect of the ageing swallow. It is imperative to have a good appreciation of the ageing swallow and to be aware of its differences from the swallows of younger or middle-aged individuals so that ageing is not mistaken for pathological function. It is important that we can differentiate normal from abnormal function, particularly when there are certain diseases that cause swallowing problems as these are also typically associated with older age (e.g. stroke) (see also Chapter 9).

ANATOMICAL CHANGES THAT OCCUR WITH AGEING

The larynx grows until approximately 3 years of age, after which little growth occurs until roughly 12 years of age, or the onset of puberty. The hyoid bone is the earliest to ossify and this begins at 2 years of age. At the time of puberty the laryngeal cavity becomes bigger, the vocal folds lengthen and thicken and the growth of the laminae of the thyroid cartilages become quite noticeable in males as the 'Adam's apple'. By about 25 years of age the cartilages of the larynx (thyroid and cricoid cartilages) begin to ossify, with the arytenoids beginning to ossify in the late 30s (Aronson, 1985). By 65 years of age these laryngeal cartilages, with the exception of the cuneiform and corniculate cartilages, are often visible on radiographs due to their ossification (Aronson, 1985; Moore and Dalley, 1999). In addition, there is atrophy of the intrinsic laryngeal muscles, dehydration of the laryngeal mucosa, loss of elasticity of laryngeal ligaments, and flaccidity and bowing of the vocal folds (Aronson, 1985).

Most obviously there are changes with tooth loss and the fitting of dentures that are associated with ageing. These will affect the individual's ability to prepare adequately the bolus and will affect the types of boluses older individuals choose to eat. There are also sensory changes that occur in the pharyngeal region with increasing age. Aviv et al. (1994) found there to be a progressive reduction in sensory capacity in the laryngopharyngeal region associated with increasing age. A statistically significant reduction in sensory capacity was found between the 41 to 60 year age group and the 61 to 90 year age group. This is further supported by histology and morphology findings that as individuals age, there is a reduction in the number of small myelinated fibres of the superior laryngeal nerve. These fibres are thought to be sensory in nature and may account for a reduction in the ability to perceive sensation in the area the superior laryngeal nerve supplies. These findings have implications for the ability to detect and clear residue post-swallow in older individuals. The reduction in hypopharyngeal sensation associated with ageing may contribute to aspiration in older individuals. Indeed, Donner and Jones (1991) report that the surface epithelium of the larynx appears to be less sensitive to aspirated material as individual's age. It was reported that the threshold for coughing on an aspirated chemical irritant was six times higher in individuals in their eighties and nineties, when compared to individuals in their twenties (Donner and Jones, 1991).

Some of the age-related changes to swallowing may be accounted for by tissue and muscle laxity (Donner and Jones, 1991). Ageing of the suspensory muscles of the larynx causes a lack of maximum vertical excursion of the hyolaryngeal complex. Reduced hyolaryngeal elevation causes the larynx to be insufficiently protected during swallowing, and may allow penetration of the bolus into the larynx. Older people require more time to move the hyoid to its maximal anterior position (Sonies et al., 1988). Tissue laxity also causes the tongue and hyoid to be anatomically positioned lower. The lower position provides the opportunity for liquids to leak into the pharynx prior to swallow reflex initiation. In the majority of cases, the swallow reflex triggers in time to avoid penetration (Donner and Jones, 1991; Robbins et al., 1992; Logemann et al., 2000). Even the epiglottis becomes less pliable with advancing age, likely due to a breakdown of elastic fibres (Donner and Jones, 1991).

Changes in the oesophagus are also reported to be associated with ageing. Gastroesophageal reflux, compression of the oesophagus by 'a tortuous thoracic aorta', and mechanical obstruction of the oesophagus due to skeletal changes (hyperostosis) of the cervical vertebrae (e.g. cervical osteophytes) may all contribute to dysphagia in the elderly (Donner and Jones, 1991). A reduction in oesophageal tone may result in air filling the aged oesophagus, resulting in oesophageal dilation (Donner and Jones, 1991).

Physiological changes that occur with ageing

Several investigators have studied what effect ageing has on the timing of events in the normal oropharyngeal swallow. Studies that have investigated the effect of age on the physiology of swallowing have been reasonably consistent in separating individuals into 'young', 'middle aged', and 'old' groups. For argument's sake, the consensus appears to be as follows: individuals aged 18–40 years are classified as *young*; 40–60 years are classified as *middle aged*, and persons over the age of 60 years are classified as *old*. This generic classification is the 'best fit' for the current literature, and consistency of terminology.

The current literature is in agreement that individuals over the age of 65, swallow more slowly than people under the age of 45 (Sonies et al., 1988; Tracy et al., 1989; Robbins et al., 1992; Logemann et al., 2000). Tracy et al. (1989) explain that when young people swallow, the oral and pharyngeal phases of the swallow are closely linked, to the point of overlap. With advancing age, the coupling of these two phases is weakened. Robbins et al. (1992) reported that swallowing begins to slow gradually some time after 45 years of age. By 70 years, swallowing was significantly slower than it was at age 45. In addition to the anatomical changes outlined above, an alternative reason for uncoupling of the oral and pharyngeal phases may relate to slowing of neural processing time with ageing (Rademaker et al., 1998). The way in which ageing affects each phase of the swallow is elaborated below.

Anticipatory phase

There is a reduction in the sense of smell and taste with age. This is because there is a loss of olfactory neurosensory cells in the olfactory epithelium that occurs with ageing (Moore and Dalley, 1999). In order to taste food, however, we rely on a sense of smell. Some older people will complain that food is tasteless. This is because the *flavour* of food depends on a normal olfactory (smell) system. Interestingly it is possible to have unilateral and bilateral loss of the sense of smell. Injury to the nasal mucosa, olfactory nerve fibres, olfactory bulb and olfactory tract may also impair the sense of smell (Moore and Dalley, 1999). In individuals who complain of a loss or alteration of taste, clinical studies often reveal that the perception of taste is not altered but the problem is with the olfactory system (Moore and Dalley, 1999). A reduction in the amount of saliva output has also been associated with ageing (Donner and Jones, 1991). A reduction in the pleasure of eating and drinking will probably have a detrimental effect on nutritional input.

Oral phase

Chewing itself does not change with age. Poor dentition or poorly fitting dentures may mean that an increased number of chewing strokes is needed to masticate the bolus safely. Moreover, there is an increase in connective tissue in the tongue and a decrease in masticatory strength (Jaredah, 1994). Consequently, there is a longer oral phase duration in older individuals. Sonies et al. (1988) found that the oral phase of swallowing increases with advancing age. In addition to an increased number of chewing strokes, the longer oral phase may also be accounted for by Caruso and Max's (1997) finding that older persons use multiple lingual movements to form a bolus. In addition, non-swallowing lingual pressure is reported to be significantly greater in younger individuals than older individuals in all directions of movement (i.e. elevation, depression, side-to-side and protrusion (Shaker and Lang, 1994). If the tongue pressure is reduced in the elderly for non-swallowing acts, the assumption is made that it is similarly reduced during the act of swallowing.

There is also a small increase in the amount and extent of post-swallow oral residue in individuals over the age of 60 years (Tracy et al., 1989; Robbins et al., 1992). Rademaker et al. (1998) found that oral residue increased from values of approximately 10% in younger women to values of approximately 30% in very old women (80+ years of age). When the tongue driving force is reduced, as it is in some elderly, this has the effect of increasing the likelihood of retention of the bolus in the valleculae (Dejaeger et al., 1997). Effortful swallowing (see Chapter 11) or squeezing the bolus forcefully with the tongue reduces valleculae residue. Lower peak suction pressure during straw drinking has also been implicated as an effect of ageing (Rademaker et al., 1998).

Pharyngeal phase

There is a mild delay in triggering the swallow reflex, which is considered to be normal for the ageing swallow (Tracy et al., 1989).

Tracy et al. (1989) also found that two other pharyngeal variables that were affected by age. These were:

- shorter pharyngeal swallow response time (time from onset of laryngeal excursion until the bolus tail passes through the UES); and
- shorter cricopharyngeal opening durations.

Interestingly, Rademaker et al. (1998) found that UES opening time and velopharyngeal closure time increased with age. Pharyngeal transit time is longer in older women than in younger women (Rademaker et al., 1998). Tongue base movement also diminishes with age in older women (Logemann et al., 2002). Pharyngeal contraction is variously reported to be, unaffected by age (Shaker and Lang, 1994) slowed with age (Jaradeh, 1994) or reduced with age (Dejaeger et al., 1997). Interestingly, Perlman et al. (1993) found that the duration of the pharyngeal pressure wave was longer in elderly persons. This is further supported by Shaker et al. (2003) who suggested that higher pharyngeal amplitudes compensate for the reduction in UES opening in the elderly. This may be a compensatory technique that the ageing body employs to assist efficient transport of the bolus into the oesophagus to overcome the reduction in UES opening that accompanies old age.

Donner and Jones (1991) noted an increase in pharyngeal residue in older subjects. Rademaker et al. (1998) also noted that the percentage of pharyngeal residue post swallow increased as a function of age from 18% in young women to 38% in women over the age of 40 years. An increase in the amount and extent of pharyngeal residue post swallow has also been reported to occur with ageing (Robbins et al., 1992; Tracy et al., 1989). It should not be surprising, then, to find then that there is also an increased rate of second (bolus free) swallows in older individuals. That is, it is normal for older individuals to employ a second 'clearing swallow' to cleanse the oral and pharyngeal cavities of residue, after their primary swallow of a spoonful of food or a mouthful of fluid. Note, however, that the limited retention of material in the valleculae or pyriform sinuses is not accompanied by aspiration. Retention of material in the pyriform sinuses or diffuse retention in the pharynx (valleculae + pyriform sinuses) is associated with inadequate pharyngeal shortening during the swallow (Dejaeger et al., 1997). Pharyngeal shortening is largely attributed to stylopharyngeal muscle contraction and is implicated in effectively opening the UES.

The duration of laryngeal closure and the duration of laryngeal elevation hits a peak between 60–79 years of age in healthy women, then tends to decrease in the 80+ years group (Rademaker et al., 1998). That these functions remain quite stable until the eighties is testament to their importance and resilience in protecting the airway. Note also, that a larger volume of water is required to trigger glottic closure and trigger a reflexive pharyngeal swallow in the elderly as compared with younger individuals. The threshold for triggering both glottic closure and reflexive pharyngeal swallow was 0.34 ml (±0.06 ml) in the elderly and 0.16 ml (±0.02 ml) in young individuals. These are suggestive of sensory changes in the larynx and pharynx that occur with age (Shaker et al., 2003).

As age increases, there is an increase in penetration of material into the vestibule but not an increase in aspiration (Robbins et al., 1992; Tracy et al., 1989). That is, the material may enter the laryngeal vestibule to the area above the vocal cords more often in an older swallow but does not pass below the level of the cords. Robbins et al. (1992) found that laryngeal penetration occurred more frequently in the 65- and over 70-year groups, than the 25- and 45-year groups. Sonies et al. (1988) reported that 80% of older persons exhibit multiple hyoid gestures during swallowing. In contrast, only 64% of middle-aged persons showed multiple hyoid gestures, and few, if any young subjects exhibit double or triple motions. Nilsson et al. (1996) noted that 74% of the elderly needed more than one swallow to clear a bolus.

Older men are noted to elevate the larynx just enough to open the UES and no more. Younger men, on the other hand, continue laryngeal elevation beyond when the UES has opened (Logemann et al., 2000). Logemann et al. (2000) contest that older men do not exhibit any 'reserve' hyolaryngeal function. They are able to use their muscles to achieve precisely what had to be achieved and no more. This phenomenon is peculiar to men only (Logemann et al., 2002). Individuals without reserve will come unstuck if something, for example illness, upsets their ability to use the system effectively. The lethargy that often accompanies illness in the older person may be sufficient to reduce their ability to move the hyolaryngeal system sufficiently out of the way of the incoming bolus. Hence for the period of illness the older person may potentially be at risk of transient penetration/aspiration. Note that any illness may be sufficient to cause this effect, not just those that affect the head and neck region.

Oesophageal phase

Oesophageal transit and clearance are slower and less efficient in the ageing individual. Older individuals have lower amounts of subatmospheric pressure preceding UES opening. This shows a reduced compliance or reduced resting pressure of the UES in the elderly (Dejaeger et al., 1997). Non-propulsive, repetitive contractions are commonly seen in the elderly (tertiary contractions). The following abnormal findings are also often reported for older individuals: delays in oesophageal emptying and dilatation of the oesophagus (Shaker and Lang, 1994). Although the duration and velocity of the oesophageal peristaltic wave are similar between young and older individuals, the amplitude of the pressure wave is reportedly reduced in older men (over 80 years) (Shaker and Lang, 1994).

Other changes

There is a deficit in the perception of thirst *and* in the regulation of fluid intake in healthy elderly men. After a period of 24 hours without fluids, elderly men showed a lack of thirst and discomfort. In addition, in a study where water was freely available after a 24-hour fluid deprivation trial older men did not drink enough fluid to dilute their plasma to pre-deprivation levels (Phillips et al., 1984). These are important factors in the development of dehydration in the elderly. Fluid intake is the only way to replace lost body water and if the body does not 'feel thirsty' it will not replenish the body with water efficiently. There is some suggestion that a reduction in thirst may be due to cerebral cortical dysfunction or 'reduced physiologic sensitivity to osmotic or volume stimuli' (Phillips et al., 1984: 758). This study highlights a potential predisposition to dehydration in elderly men.

The changes that occur with ageing can, therefore, be seen to affect the total swallowing continuum from the drive for thirst, through the oral, pharyngeal and oesophageal phases of swallowing. The major changes are provided in Table 2.4 for easy reference. While there are anatomical and physical changes that occur with normal ageing, the clinician should also be aware of two things. Firstly, plastic abilities of the elderly nervous system do not appear to be reduced with age. Thus, even though there is general cerebral atrophy, loss of neurones and a reduction in the ability to synthesize neurotransmitters, the aged brain still has the capacity to form and strengthen synapses among neurones (Caruso and Max, 1997). This fact has

Table 2.4 Effects of ageing on swallowing function: normal variables

Phase of swallow	Normative change with ageing
Anticipatory	↓ sense of smell
	↓ sense of taste
	↓ perception of thirst (men)
	↓ regulation of fluid intake (men)
Oral	↑ number of chewing strokes
	↑ time to complete oral phase
	↑ retention post swallow
	↓ tongue driving force (necessary to propel the bolus into the oropharynx)
	↓ suction pressure during straw drinking
Pharyngeal	Delay in triggering the swallowing reflex
	↑ pharyngeal transit time (women); possibly higher pharyngeal contraction amplitudes
	↑ pharyngeal residue post-swallow
	↑ penetration no increase in aspiration
	more than one swallow needed to clear the bolus
	↓ laryngeal excursion reserve (men)
	↓ laryngeal and pharyngeal sensation
Oesophageal	↓ oesophageal transit speed
	↓ oesophgeal clearance efficiency
	↓ amplitude of the oesophageal pressure wave, but no change to duration (time) and velocity (speed) of the pressure wave.

implications for rehabilitation of swallowing function (see Chapter 12). Secondly, research shows that there are some microscopic changes associated with 'pathological ageing' that are also seen in normal ageing (for example, senile plaques and neurfibrillary tangles). Some of the differences between normal and pathological ageing appear to be in the number and degree of changes rather than the actual kind of change per se.

It is also impossible to look at ageing in isolation. There are many medical problems common in the elderly and these may be more profound on the background of an ageing swallowing system. Kendall et al. (2004) found that elderly individuals who presented with medical problems were more likely to be associated with delays in pharyngeal transit of the bolus. In particular, individuals with hypertension had statistically significant pharyngeal stage delays associated with swallowing a 1 ml bolus. Note, the same effect was not found for a 20 ml bolus, however. A 20 ml bolus most closely equates with a 'mouthful' of a liquid bolus, whereas a 1 ml bolus more closely approximates a small saliva bolus. The difference between the two bolus sizes is important and its clinical implications are discussed more fully in Chapter 4. Kendall et al. (2004) also suggest that the medications used to treat medical conditions found in the aged population (e.g. treatments for Parkinson's disease, hypertension and diabetes) may also contribute to a change in swallowing function due to medication side effects. The effect of medication on swallowing is discussed further in Chapter 9.

SUMMARY

This chapter emphasized that swallowing is not a static function. It changes quite rapidly in the infant and child, and then again as individuals age. The clinician needs to be aware of the various changes that occur with maturation and ageing to ensure that normal swallowing anatomy and physiology are differentiated accurately from pathology. Normal variations are exactly that, normal. Clinicians must be able to discriminate normal from pathological function. Where pathology truly exists, treatment should be aimed at the cause rather than the symptoms.

REFERENCES

Aronson AE (1985) Clinical Voice Disorders: An Interdisciplinary Approach (2nd edn). New York: Thieme.

Arvedson JC, Brodsky L (2002) Pediatric Swallowing and Feeding: Assessment and Management (2nd edn). Albany NY: Singular Publishing.

Aviv JE, Martin JH, Jones ME, et al. (1994) Age-related changes in pharyngeal and supraglottic sensation. Annals of Otology Rhinology and Laryngology 103: 749–52.

Bamford O, Taciak V, Gewolb IH (1992) The relationship between rhythmic swallowing and breathing during suckle feeding in term neonates. Pediatric Research 31(6): 619–24.

Caruso AJ, Max L (1997) Effects of aging on neuromotor processes of swallowing. Seminars in Speech and Language 18(2): 181–92.

Dejaeger E, Pelemans W, Ponette E, et al. (1997) Mechanisms involved in postdeglutition retention in the elderly. Dysphagia 12: 63–7.

Donner M, Jones B (1991) Ageing and neurological disease. In Jones B, Donner MW (eds) Normal and Abnormal Swallowing: Imaging in Diagnosis and Therapy. New York: Springer-Verlag.

Jaredah S (1994) Neurophysiology of swallowing in the aged. Dysphagia 9: 218–20.

Kendall KA, Leonard RJ, McKenzie S (2004) Common medical conditions in the elderly: Impact on pharyngeal bolus transit. Dysphagia 19: 71–7.

Koempel JA, Holinger LD (1998) Congential absence of epiglottis. International Journal of Pediatric Otorhinolaryngology 45(3): 237–41.

Lear CSC, Flanagan JBJ, Morres CFA (1965) The frequency of deglutition in man. Archives of Oral Biology 10: 83–100.

Logan WJ, Bosma JF (1967) Oral and pharyngeal dysphagia in infancy. Pediatric Clinics of North America 14(1): 47–61.

Logemann J, Pauloski BR, Rademaker AW, et al. (2000) Temporal and biomechanical characteristics of oropharyngeal swallow in younger and older men. Journal of Speech Language and Hearing Research 43(5): 1264–74.

Logemann JA, Pauloski BR, Rademaker AW, et al. (2002) Orophayngeal swallow in younger and older women: Videofluoroscopic analysis. Journal of Speech Language and Hearing Research 45(3): 434–45.

Moore KL (1973) The Developing Human. Clinically Oriented Embryology. Philadelphia: WB Saunders Co.

Moore KL, Dalley AF (1999) Clinically Oriented Anatomy (4th edn). Philadelphia: Lippincott Williams & Wilkins.

Nilsson H, Ekberg O, Olsson R, et al. (1996) Quantitative aspects of swallowing in an elderly nondysphagic population. Dysphagia 11: 180–4.

Perlman AL, Guthmiller Schultz J, Van Daele DJ (1993) Effects of age, gender, bolus volume, and bolus viscosity on oropharyngeal pressure during swallowing. Journal of Applied Physiology 75: 33–7.

Phillips PA, Rolls BJ, Ledingham JG, et al. (1984) Reduced thirst after water deprivation in healthy elderly men. New England Journal of Medicine 311: 753–9.

Rademaker AW, Pauloski BR, Colangelo LA, et al. (1998) Age and volume effects on liquid swallowing function in normal women. Journal of Speech Language and Hearing Research 41: 275–84.

Robbins J, Hamilton JW, Lof GL, et al. (1992) Oropharyngeal swallowing in normal adults of different ages. Gastroenterology 103: 823–9.

Rommel N (2002) Diagnosis of oropharyngeal disorders in young children: new insights and assessment with manofluoroscopy. Doctoral thesis. Katholieke Universiteit Leuven.

Selley WG, Ellis RE, Flack FC, et al. (1990) Coordination of sucking, swallowing and breathing in the newborn: its relationship to infant feeding and normal development. British Journal of Disorders of Communication 25: 311–27.

Shaker R, Lang IM (1994) Effect of ageing on the deglutitive oral, pharyngeal, and esophageal motor function. Dysphagia 9: 221–8.

Shaker R, Ren J, Bardan E, et al. (2003) Pharyngoglottal closure reflex: characterization in healthy young, elderly and dysphagia patients with predeglutitive aspiration. Gerontology 49: 12–20.

Sonies BC, Parent LJ, Morrish K, et al. (1988) Durational aspects of the oral-pharyngeal phase of swallow in normal adults. Dysphagia 3: 1–10.

Stoppard M (1993) Conception, Pregnancy and Birth. Camberwell, Australia: Penguin Books.

Tracy J, Logemann J, Kahrilas P, et al. (1989) Prelininary observations on the effects of age on oropharyngeal deglutition. Dysphagia 4: 90–4.

Tuchman DN (1994) Physiology of the swallowing apparatus. In Tuchman DN, Walter RS (eds) Disorders of Feeding and Swallowing in Infants and Children. San Diego: Singular.

Walter RS (1994) Issues surrounding the development of feeding and swallowing. In Tuchman DN, Walter RS (eds) Disorders of Feeding and Swallowing in Infants and Children. San Diego: Singular Publishing Group.

Wolf LS, Glass RP (1994) Feeding and Swallowing Disorders in Infancy: Assessment and Management. Tucson AZ: Therapy Skills Builders.

3 Variations of the Normal Swallow

JULIE CICHERO and PETER HALLEY

It is very easy to take the act of swallowing for granted. It is just as easy to take the assessment of swallowing for granted and to keep doing what has always been done. We are rapidly discovering that we need to look critically at what we do. It is common sense in the typical dysphagia examination that we investigate how the individual handles food and liquids. We are, after all, trying to establish which types of foods and liquids can be managed safely by oral means. However, it is not necessarily as straightforward as that. The physiology of the normal swallow adjusts itself and its parameters depending on what we are swallowing (e.g. texture, size, taste, and temperature). Even for liquids, recent research has shown that a single swallow from a cup produces a patterned physiological response different from that of continuous cup drinking, and this is different again from drinking continuously through a straw. In assuming that it is all the same we run the risk of mistaking normal variation for pathological function. This chapter will provide a description of how the normal swallowing physiology changes as a direct result of what is being swallowed and the method of administration.

Thickened fluids have been an increasing area of interest in the literature. They are provided to dysphagic individuals for therapeutic reasons because they are cohesive and they move more slowly than regular thin fluids. These properties help to protect a swallowing system that may be delayed in its response to an incoming bolus or impaired in its ability to manage the bolus. 'Thickness' or 'thinness' of fluids, which collectively fall under the heading of *viscosity*, is not a straightforward property.

The latter portion of this chapter is devoted to an explanation of viscosity and its parent areas of *rheology* and *material characterization*. These factors affect bedside assessment, radiological assessment of swallowing and ongoing treatment of the person with dysphagia. Finally, the chapter concludes with information supplied by the chemosenses – that of taste and olfaction and even our use of pain receptors to enhance swallowing sensation. These variables are also important in changing the normal parameters of swallowing.

BOLUS VOLUME

Bolus volume critically affects the timing of the physiological events of the normal swallow (Dantas et al., 1990; Kahrilas and Logemann, 1993; Lazarus et al., 1993; Bisch et al., 1994). The oral and pharyngeal cavities change their configuration in

Dysphagia: Foundation, Theory and Practice. Edited by J. Cichero and B. Murdoch
© 2006 John Wiley & Sons, Ltd.

order to accommodate boluses of different volumes. For example, with a large bolus the position of the hyoid bone before the swallow starts tends to be lower. Wintzen et al. (1994) suggested that this is probably to create more space in the oral cavity by lowering the floor of the mouth. Not surprisingly, there are a variety of tongue movement patterns that are associated with changes to bolus volume (Kahrilas and Logemann, 1993). Moreover, the relationship between swallowing and breathing is altered when an individual swallows a large sized bolus. The critical relationship between swallowing and respiration is detailed fully in Chapter 4. Table 3.1 provides a summary of the physiological features associated with an increase in bolus volume.

Table 3.1 Changes to the timing of events when swallowing boluses of differing volumes

Physiological changes evident as bolus volume *increases*	Factors that remain the same regardless of changes in bolus volume
Oral phase • Longer period of velopharyngeal closure (Kahrilas et al., 1993). • Greater magnitude of anterior tongue movement (Dantas et al., 1990). • Increased depression of central groove of tongue (Kahrilas et al., 1996). • Obvious posterior movement of dorsal region of tongue (Tasko et al., 2002). • Increased maximum speed of tongue movement (Tasko et al., 2002). • Increased vigour of bolus expulsion and propulsion time (Kahrilas and Logemann, 1993; Perlman, 1993). • Lower position of hyoid prior to swallow initiation (Wintzen et al., 1994). • Greater anterior movement of the hyolaryngeal complex (Dodds et al., 1988; Dantas et al., 1990).	**Oral phase** • Timing and duration of muscular activity in submental region not affected by increased bolus volume (Dantas and Dodds, 1990) but others find submental muscles are affected by increased bolus volume (Jacob et al., 1988; Ertekin et al., 1997). • No increase in tongue force with a larger volume bolus (Kahrilas et al., 1996). **Pharyngeal phase** • Pharyngeal clearance times remain roughly the same regardless of volume (Tracy et al., 1989).
Pharyngeal phase • Increased bolus velocity (i.e. 5 ml bolus travels at 15 cm/s, a 20 ml bolus travels at 50 cm/s) (Logemann, 1998). • Increased arytenoid elevation with pharyngeal shortening (Kahrilas et al., 1996).	
Oesophageal phase • UES remains open for longer period of time (Dantas et al., 1990; Logemann et al., 2000).	
Swallow-respiratory coordination • Increase in laryngeal closure time (Preiksaitis et al., 1992). • Increased apneoic period with larger bolus volumes (Hiss et al., 2001).	

UES = upper oesophageal sphincter.

The features listed in Table 3.1 show that the oral and pharyngeal parts of the swallowing system change to accommodate boluses of different volumes. The changes made by the body are entirely logical. Ergun et al. (1993) found that the changes made to positioning of the structures of the oropharynx enlarge the pharyngeal chamber to be approximately, but not quite double its pre-swallow volume (pre-swallow volume 15 ml versus 24 ml during tongue loading). To place something large in the pharynx (the biological time-share space for swallowing and breathing), it is important that the respiratory system is protected early. If the respiratory system is not closed sufficiently prior to arrival of the bolus, the individual is at greater risk of liquid penetrating the larynx or even being aspirated. Hence the early closure of the larynx and increased period of laryngeal closure. The larynx also lifts higher and moves more anteriorly, under the base of the tongue, when a large bolus is swallowed. The larynx is physically moved further out of the way of a large bolus in a mechanical attempt to protect it (Logemann, 1988; Lang and Shaker, 1994). To drain the material quickly it is important it has somewhere to go. For this reason the upper oesophageal sphincter (UES) remains open longer and the soft palate closes the velopharyngeal port for longer than usual, guarding against possible nasal regurgitation.

Notice the changes to the tongue that occur. Greater tongue loading, increased depression of the central groove of the tongue, increased anterior movement and increased propulsion time are all associated with swallowing a large bolus volume. This setup is designed to give the large bolus a big push, giving it momentum, which will increase its speed through the pharynx. Consider a swimming analogy. If an individual were to swim across a river, the use of flippers would assist in getting to the other side faster and with less effort. The current in the river remains the same but we can swim faster using another means (i.e. the flippers). Similarly, the pharyngeal clearance times remain the same (i.e. the current) but the tongue changes the driving pressure to instigate movement (i.e. flippers). It is not surprising then that a large bolus moves faster than a small bolus (Ekberg et al., 1988; Jacob et al., 1989). In numerical terms, a large bolus moves at 50 cm/s through the pharynx, where a small bolus moves at 15 cm/s (Kahrilas and Logemann, 1993). Robbins et al. (1992) proposed that sensory (afferent) information about bolus volume is collected in the oral phase of the swallow before the swallow reflex is initiated. This information is then relayed to the nucleus of the tractus solitarius and then onto the nucleus ambiguous which designs or constructs a suitable 'swallowing programme' for the volume being swallowed.

Kahrilas (1993) provides an excellent illustration of how changing the bolus volume affects the timing of swallowing events. Imagine a large bolus of say 20 ml (about a metric tablespoon). When this volume is swallowed, tongue loading, velopharyngeal closure and UES opening start earlier and last for longer. The larynx also closes sooner and stays closed longer for a large volume bolus than a small volume bolus. When only 1 ml is swallowed, pharyngeal clearance commences *before* the laryngeal vestibule is closed. Volume is critical. The threat to the pulmonary system posed by 1 ml as opposed to 20 ml is negligible. Similarly if the pharynx is viewed abstractly like a drain, the UES presents as the 'plug hole'. It is obviously better if the plughole is open for a long time if there is a large volume coming through. Close it too soon and the residue is trapped. Physiologically the same is true. The UES is open for approximately one-third of the time it takes to swallow a 1 ml bolus, whereas it is open for approximately 75% of the time it takes to swallow a 20 ml bolus (Logemann, 1988).

AVERAGE VOLUME OF A MOUTHFUL

The average volume of a single mouthful is 21 ml for adults (Adnerhill et al., 1989). There are some gender differences with males taking a larger average mouthful (25 ml) than females (20 ml) (Adnerhill et al., 1989). Lawless et al. (2003) reported that gender differences may in fact be due to differences in body size. That is, if men and women were approximately the same height and weight, would they take similar mouthful volumes? Their results indicated that mean sip size was significantly correlated with height. Further research is required to better understand the gender versus body size differences associated with sip or mouthful size. Note also that the higher the temperature of the fluid, the smaller the volume that is consumed, reducing to 5 ml to 15 ml (Longman and Pearson, 1987). Minimal research has been carried out regarding quantification of mouthful volumes for children. Selley et al. (1990) reported that the average volume an infant consumes while feeding is 0.2 ml (±0.11 ml). Jones et al. (1961), while trying to determine average mouthfuls to treat accidental poisonings more effectively, found that young children (1;3 to 3;6) swallow an average 4.5 ml (±1.9 ml) per mouthful. Note that the subject numbers were very small, however. Further research is required to accurately quantify average mouthful volumes in infants and children.

CLINICAL INFERENCES

We know that the swallowing system adjusts depending on the volume being swallowed. In all cases of swallowing, the successful switching of the oropharynx from respiratory and speech mode to swallowing mode is critical. A change in bolus volume requires the system to stay in the 'safe' position for differing amounts of time. If the normal healthy system can cope with ease with this manipulation, what can we learn clinically from manipulating bolus volume? Kahrilas and Logemann (1993) suggested that a large bolus (20 ml) stresses the lingual musculature and its ability to control a bolus. It also provides the clinician with information about how the person copes with a 'normal mouthful' of fluid. There is little benefit to examining only 3 ml to 5 ml of liquid swallows during a radiographic study if, after the procedure, the individual continues to take *mouthfuls* (i.e. 20 ml volumes) of fluid. Small boluses on the other hand, test the competence of pharyngeal clearance and whether the larynx closes well enough, at the right time and for the right length of time (Kahrilas and Logemann, 1993). Bear in mind also that a small bolus is not as heavy on the tongue as a larger bolus, robbing the sensory receptors of its presence where sensory function has been disturbed. In this scenario are we testing a system that would never cope with a small volume because it cannot detect its presence and programme a response? The outcome? The patient continually aspirates small volumes and is never tested on larger volumes for fear of massive aspiration. For these reasons it is important to study both large-volume and small-volume boluses in individuals with dysphagia. It is also imperative to be as informed as possible of the patient's presenting symptoms (e.g. reduced oral sensation) and what you are hoping to discover from your assessment.

Palmer et al. (1999) also provide a very valid argument for using each person as his or her own control. As noted above, Adnerhill et al. (1989) indicated that an average mouthful is about 20 ml. They also noted a large degree of variability ranging from 15 ml to 30 ml per mouthful. This variability shows us that what one individual may consider a large mouthful may be an average or even smallish mouthful for another individual. Palmer et al. (1999) use this theory to explain why the studies looking at degree of submental muscle movement magically change in some studies of bolus volume, but not others. For clinical purposes they suggest that the people's own averages be used as their individual benchmark, with larger and smaller boluses adjusted from the benchmark, rather than supplying standard amounts (e.g. 5, 10, 15, 20, 30 ml). Alternatively, the work of Lawless et al. (2003) showed that height is well correlated with bolus volume and that studies that can determine average mouthfuls based on height may be more useful to the clinician than the rigid use of standard incremental amounts.

It was noted previously that, as bolus volume increases, healthy non-dysphagic people will lower the hyoid in order to lower the floor of the mouth and create space in the oral cavity for the larger bolus. This process does not, however, occur in individuals with Parkinson's disease (Wintzen et al., 1994). If we look at a different population, further details emerge about the way we deal with changes to bolus volume in health and pathology. Lazarus et al. (1993) looked at stroke and non-stroke subjects and their ability to accommodate changes in bolus volume. There were some interesting similarities between the two groups. Both groups kept the laryngeal region closed for longer as bolus volume increased. Both groups kept the cricopharyngeal sphincter open for longer as the volume increased. Both groups also reduced the length of time the tongue base contacted with the pharyngeal walls as volume increased. However, pharyngeal delay time reduced in the stroke group but not the healthy group with increased bolus volume. This is but one example of why clinicians cannot assume that what happens in healthy individuals also happens in dysphagic individuals.

In a paediatric example, children with cerebral palsy require more time to complete drinking tasks than healthy children (Casas et al., 1994). Eating and drinking places a considerable load on the ventilatory system of children with cerebral palsy. As a result, they take longer to recover their ventilation after the swallow. Casas et al. (1994) investigated ability to manage 5 ml sips and continuous drinking of 75 ml volumes in healthy children and children with cerebral palsy. They concluded that the 75 ml amount was sufficient to challenge ventilatory capacity of both the normal and cerebral palsy children. Both groups inhaled immediately after completing the task, indicative of a depletion of ventilatory reserve with this task. In addition, they concluded that the continuous cup-drinking activity placed too much stress on the respiratory system of the cerebral palsy children and that sips from a 5 ml volume were handled more safely.

SINGLE BOLUS SWALLOWS

The normal pattern for individual bolus swallows has been discussed in detail in Chapter 1. Indeed, most research investigates the single bolus swallow. The following is included as a brief summary and reminder.

In general the bolus is propelled to the posterior of the oral cavity by the tongue and the swallow reflex is initiated at roughly the anatomical landmark region extending from the faucial arches to the ramus of the mandible (if viewed radiologically). Velopharyngeal closure ensues and hyolaryngeal excursion occurs. Breathing momentarily ceases and there is a multilayered physical barrier utilizing the arytenoids and the true vocal folds, the epiglottis and aryepiglottic folds to protect the laryngeal vestibule. The tongue, which during the oral phase has been preventing posterior spillage by arching well back in the mouth (ski-slope style) to produce a physical barrier to a wayward bolus, drops and forcefully pushes the bolus into the pharynx, making contact with the medializing pharyngeal walls as it does so. The pharynx initially shortens and then contracts to move the bolus expediently through the pharynx. Movement from hyolaryngeal traction and excursion is instrumental in opening the UES to allow the bolus to pass out of the pharynx and into the oesophageal system. After a discrete swallow, the system returns to its resting position and the airway re-opens, allowing the resumption of respiration.

For discrete liquid swallows there has been much interest in the anatomical place where the swallow reflex is seen to be activated (i.e. onset of maximal hyoid and laryngeal excursion). Daniels and Foundas (2001) reported that the location of the bolus at the time of swallow reflex initiation provides us with the best clues to likelihood of aspiration. This is detailed in the Table 3.2.

Is this pattern *always* the case though? Are there some instances where it is quite acceptable for the bolus to present itself well into the pharynx before a swallow reflex is initiated? In the elderly, it is accepted that the bolus passes the ramus of

Table 3.2 Location of the bolus at the time of swallow reflex initiation as a prediction of risk of aspiration

Risk level for aspiration	Location of bolus at time of swallow reflex initiation
Low	Head of the bolus is superior to the ramus of the mandible at the onset of the pharyngeal swallow response.
Moderate	Head of the bolus is between the ramus of the mandible and the valleculae at the onset of the pharyngeal swallow response.
High	The head of the bolus is inferior to the valleculae at the onset of the pharyngeal swallow response.

the mandible rather than the more historical faucial pillars. This is a normal variation. Clinicians need to be aware of normal variations to avoid misdiagnosing normal function as pathological. Generally speaking, however, we do not swallow one
mouthful at a time. It is important, then, to be aware of the effects of continuous
drinking and even drinking through a straw as these modes of ingestion have their
own idiosyncratic patterns.

Note also that cup size will have an effect on the mouthful amount taken by the
individual. Sip volumes increase by about 15% with incremental increases in cup
size (e.g. 150, 300, 600 ml cup capacity). Individuals' sip size was 23.7 ml when taking a mouthful from a 150 ml cup and 27.2 ml when taking a mouthful from a 600 ml
cup (Lawless et al., 2003).

SALIVA SWALLOWS

Saliva swallows represent possibly the smallest volume that we swallow. Saliva
swallows are approximately 1 ml to 2 ml. The properties of saliva are discussed
in Chapter 6. Dua et al. (1997) examined the effects of chewing coloured gum on
saliva swallowing. Chewing promotes saliva flow in preparation to 'break down'
the bolus and assist digestion. Dua et al. (1997) found that chewing gum for 10
minutes produced approximately 117 saliva swallows. The saliva frequently entered the pharynx and accumulated in the pyriform sinuses prior to a swallow
reflex being generated. The entry of saliva into the pharynx caused brief partial
adduction of the vocal cords. The adductions lasted approximately 0.85 s, and the
cords averaged just less than half their closure distance from the fully open state.
After the partial adduction, the cords then returned to the resting open state and
saliva continued to accumulate in the pharynx. A swallow reflex was eventually
generated, although the authors do not provide details of the time lapse for the
saliva swallows.

Shaker et al. (1994) found that approximately 1.12 ml (±0.25) was the threshold
volume for triggering a swallow when water was directly perfused into the pharynx in young individuals. The threshold volume in elderly individuals was noted to
be significantly greater at 1.85ml (±0.36). Variation in temperature did not affect
threshold volumes that initiated a swallow.

Clinical inferences

In regard to saliva swallows, the information above shows us that the body can tolerate accumulation of saliva within the pharyngeal region, without necessarily adduct-
ing the cords to protect the airway. With intact pharyngeal sensation, the body can
obviously tolerate a certain amount of saliva accumulation in the pharynx before a
swallow reflex is generated. It is likely that there is a 'filling point' at which the accumulated swallow triggers a message to the brain to initiate a swallow reflex and drain
the material as noted in the Shaker et al. (1994) study. Note also Shaker et al. (1994)
suggested that elderly individuals lack the ability to discriminate between rapid and

slow fluid injection. This, in combination with a high threshold volume for initiating a pharyngeal swallow, places them at higher risk for penetration and aspiration. In individuals with dysphagia, the inability to cope with their secretions may be indicative of impaired pharyngeal sensation. Consequently, they lose the ability to use a dangerously full pyriform sinus to trigger the reflexive swallow.

Note also that saliva is important in reducing the unpleasant dry-mouth sensation associated with thirst. Saliva production has been found to increase during drinking, and this reduces the need to continue drinking to relieve mouth dryness (Brunstrom et al., 2000). This physiological effect has important implications for individuals who are wholly or predominantly tube fed. Less oral intake significantly reduces saliva production that would ordinarily occur during swallowing at meals times and may well contribute to the constant sensation of thirst in these individuals.

CONTINUOUS OR SEQUENTIAL CUP DRINKING

It is standard practice to examine people's ability to swallow by asking them to take 'a mouthful' or 'a sip' of fluid from a cup, or to provide them with a designated amount to swallow (e.g. 5 ml, 10 ml). Being mindful not to inadvertently drown the dysphagic person, we are less inclined to give them the cup and instruct them to drink the entire contents in one go. Yet in everyday situations people are more inclined to take a number of sequential swallows than drink the contents of a cup on a sip-by-sip basis. To explore the 'normalities' of continuous cup drinking, therefore, seems extremely logical.

The physiological timings of taking a discrete mouthful as opposed to continuously drinking from a cup are different. Sequential swallows have repeated cycles of the following events:

- lingual propulsion of the bolus;
- velopharyngeal closure;
- hyolaryngeal elevation and closure;
- pharyngeal clearance of the bolus; and
- UES opening (Chi-Fishman and Sonies, 2000).

It has been reported that during continuous drinking the hyoid and larynx achieve maximal elevation during the pharyngeal response, but are partially lowered after each sequential swallow. This pattern continues until the completion of the last swallow, at which time the hyoid and larynx finally return to their resting baseline positions. Chi-Fishman and Sonies (2000) describe this process as 'activation and partial de-activation', which is unique to sequential, but not discrete swallows.

The pattern of 'activation and partial de-activation' is noted for floor of mouth, velopharyngeal and laryngeal movement during sequential swallowing. Floor of mouth muscle activity as measured using electromyography (EMG) is understandably found to remain elevated at the end of each sequential swallow. It is logical that the submental muscles retain a heightened degree of tone in preparation to accommodate the next bolus. This differs from discrete swallows, where the submental muscle group returns to baseline activity, i.e. deactivates, at the end of the swallow.

In continuous swallows the higher amplitudes reflect repeating patterns of hyoid and laryngeal excursion and partial lowering (Chi-Fishman and Sonies, 2000). With regards to velopharyngeal movement, there are varying degrees of velopharyngeal elongation in combination with posterior oropharyngeal bulging that protect the nasal cavity from possible regurgitation; however, the pattern noted is not as pronounced as in single discrete swallows.

In discrete swallows the laryngeal vestibule consistently opens upon laryngeal descent. However, for sequential swallows, there is partial descent and re-elevation of the larynx with the laryngeal vestibule either (a) remaining closed throughout, or (b) evidence of a small, narrow opening of the laryngeal vestibule. Chi-Fishman and Sonies (2000) noted that when there was evidence of slit-like opening of the laryngeal vestibule during the sequential swallowing process there was evidence of trace penetration. Interestingly, the penetrated material was expelled from the larynx on the next cycle of laryngeal elevation (i.e. the next sequential swallow). For the velopharyngeal system and the hyoid-laryngeal systems, the rapid and coordinated pattern of activation and partial deactivation is a cost-effective muscular adjustment during a repeating, sequential task.

Another normal variation of sequential swallowing is the merging of two successive boluses in the hypopharynx before the pharyngeal response is initiated. The first bolus is usually accumulated deep in the pharynx, most likely the pyriform sinuses, with the incoming bolus propelled into the pharynx to merge with the accumulated bolus. The pharyngeal response is then triggered and the bolus cleared from the pharynx. Chi-Fishman and Sonies (2000) reported that when the bolus merging occurs the laryngeal vestibule is closed, but usually the hyoid and larynx are partially descended.

The UES is open for a shorter amount of time for sequential swallows than discrete swallows (Chi-Fishman and Sonies, 2000). The UES mechanical function, however, does not appear to be affected by discrete versus sequential swallowing tasks. During sequential swallows the UES shows repetitive opening and closing gestures from swallow to swallow. This effectively drains each bolus and closes the UES prior the next bolus being presented.

Sequential swallows show *faster* oral transit duration, pharyngeal response duration, UES opening duration and total swallow duration than discrete swallows. Sequential swallows show *slower* oral to pharyngeal stage transition and pharyngeal transit durations, however. This is one of the key differences between sequential and discrete swallows. In sequential swallows the bolus enters hypopharynx and may even pause/dwell there momentarily before a pharyngeal swallow response is generated – a phenomenon not observed in a discrete swallow. Other characteristics unique to sequential swallowing pattern are: 'movement momentum, prolonged sensory stimulation and a heightened motor response' (Chi-Fishman and Sonies, 2000: 1490).

Clinical inferences

Clinically there are a couple of important points to pull out from the differences between discrete and continuous swallows. As mentioned earlier, we do not usually drink in restrained single-bolus swallows; rather, we take a number of swallows at a time. In assessment there is the tendency to avoid continuous swallows for fear of massive aspiration. Certainly, if the individual has extremely poor swallow-respiratory coordination there are certain dangers to testing continuous cup drinking. However, it should not be ruled out. Continuous drinking is more the norm, and as part of a progression towards more normal swallowing, it should also be assessed where the risk of frank aspiration is not extreme. Note also that in assessment of this variation radiologically the speech pathologist should accept triggering of the swallowing reflex from deeper in the pharynx as normal, and the possibility of normal penetration, which is promptly cleared with the next swallow.

STRAW DRINKING

Straw drinking is also another normal swallow ingestion variation. Fans of the milkshake will know there is nothing better than drinking this particular beverage through a straw. Indeed many of the elderly tell us that they find it easier to drink with a straw. Is it, however, a physiologically simple or complex task? Daniels and Foundas (2001) investigated the physiology of sequential straw drinking in healthy young men. To what extent their findings can be carried over to the elderly population remains to be seen, nevertheless, they provide some important information worthy of consideration.

In its simplest form, the straw allows us to deliver the bolus to the posterior part of the oral cavity. So for individuals with poor tongue strength, there is an advantage in moving the bolus to the best point for swallow reflex initiation more expediently. Using the straw to promote posterior placement of the bolus in the oral cavity requires the buccal muscles, tongue and palatal muscles to work together to form suction, drawing the bolus into the mouth in a controlled manner. This is quite distinct from using respiratory force to 'vacuum' the bolus up through the straw and into the oral cavity. Note that if individuals inhale as they draw the liquid up the straw, they stand a very great chance of inhaling and thus aspirating the liquid.

The mean volume drawn up via a straw (11.5 ml, range 5.6 ml to 17.4 ml) is considerably smaller than that of the standard mouthful (21 ml SD ±5 ml, range 8–59) (Adnerhill et al., 1989). For healthy individuals there is approximately one swallow every second when drinking sequentially using a straw. For trivia buffs, the mean total volume swallowed in 10 s is 115 ml with a range of 62 ml to 168 ml. There are three different patterns of hyolaryngeal excursion associated with sequential straw drinking. Type I is the most consistent pattern, with roughly equal evidence of the other two patterns. Type III is a mixture of Types I and II. The three patterns are described in Table 3.3.

As noted in our discussions of the discrete bolus above, our expectation is for the swallow reflex to be initiated at least at the ramus of the mandible. In sequential straw drinking, the majority of swallows are initiated with the head of the bolus *below* the level of the valleculae. Only a small percentage of swallows are initiated

Table 3.3 Three patterns of laryngeal closure and hyolaryngeal excursion associated with straw drinking

Type I (53%)	Type II (27%)	Type III (20%)
• Epiglottis returns to upright after each swallow.	• Continued epiglottic inversion after each swallow.	• Interchangable mixture of patterns I and II.
• Opening of the laryngeal vestibule after each swallow.	• Closure of the laryngeal vestibule after each swallow.	
• Anatomical landmark for generation of swallow reflex: ○ 22% superior to valleculae; ○ 31% at level of valleculae; ○ 47% inferior to valleculae.	• Anatomical landmark for generation of swallow reflex: ○ 0.008% superior to valleculae; ○ 0.05% at level of valleculae; ○ 93% inferior to valleculae.	

as one would for a discrete swallow (i.e. above the level of the valleculae). This is an important normal variation that should not be confused with pathology.

In sequential straw drinking it is also normal to accumulate a bolus in the pharynx while the oral cavity takes up the next bolus, after which time the pharyngeal swallow reflex is usually triggered (Daniels and Foundas, 2001). This pattern of bolus accumulation was significantly associated with Type I hyolaryngeal excursion movements where the epiglottis returns to upright and the laryngeal vestibule opens after each swallow. Note, however, that aspiration is *not* a normal consequence of this pattern.

SOLIDS

Not surprisingly, the patterns generated for the preparation of solids differ from that of fluids. Of more interest, however, is that there are also significant normal differences in site of swallow reflex initiation and handling of the bolus. Differences predominantly occur in the oral/oral preparatory phase. Beginning with the oral preparatory phase, Hiiemae and Palmer (1999) found that hard solid foods are deposited on the depressed anterior surface of the tongue, whereas it was normal practice for soft foods to be scraped from a spoon by the upper incisors and collected on the anterior surface of the tongue as the spoon was withdrawn from the oral cavity. In both instances, the posterior portion of the tongue rides high in the mouth so that the overall configuration resembles something of a ski slope with the peak at the posterior portion of the mouth and the low point at the anterior end of the mouth. This type of configuration encourages the bolus to remain within the oral cavity and provides a physical barrier to premature escape into the pharynx. The tongue is instrumental in rapidly pulling the bolus back into the mouth so that it reaches the molar region.

Ingestion of a solid bolus requires mastication and rotary lateral movement of the mandible to bring the teeth edges together to break the food down. Food is pushed towards the molars by the tongue rising anteriorly and squeezing the bolus against the hard palate. It is this action that pushes it towards the molars. Food is also intermittently pulled back by the tongue for repositioning and further mastication (Hiiemae and Palmer, 1999). The food may then be segmented into portions that have been adequately masticated and portions that still require additional mastication. Portions that have been adequately masticated are 'stored' on the posterior surface of the moving tongue, with further morsels joining the accumulating bolus. Note that food can continue to be processed while 'swallow-safe' food accumulates to form a bolus. The 'swallow-safe' bolus that accumulates on the tongue appears to maintain its position on the still moving tongue *without* any particular anatomical constraints (e.g. the soft palate). In fact the tongue to soft palate contact is both intermittent and irregular (Hiiemae and Palmer, 1999).

The addition of food to the oral cavity and the actions of mastication also activate the salivary glands. Saliva mixes with the bolus to moisten it, which acts as a binding agent, allowing the food to be formed into a cohesive bolus, and enzymes within the saliva assist in chemically breaking the bolus down, thereby initiating the 'digestive process'. Note also that mechanical stimulation of saliva (i.e. by chewing) results in a higher salivary flow rate than stimulation by liquids (Guinard et al., 1998). (See also Chapter 6.)

For liquid swallows we appreciate that a normal 'oral phase' should be approximately one second. Note that for a solid bolus, the act of mastication and bolus preparation significantly increases this time frame. Dua et al. (1997) found that the average duration of mastication for a bite of cheeseburger was 10.6 s (+/−0.4 s). Moreover, each bite averaged approximately 8.9 strokes to prepare the bolus adequately. There will obviously be differences depending on what is being masticated. Hiiemae and Palmer (1999) reported average total swallowing sequences (i.e. oral plus pharyngeal stages combined) of approximately 22 s for hard solids (e.g. peanuts and hard cookies/biscuits) and approximately 9 s for soft solids (e.g. banana and chicken spread). Guinard et al. (1998) reported that males took from 5.8 to 38 s to chew and process crackers before initiating a swallow, whereas females took between 9.7 and 26.8 s to achieve the same goal. The gender difference was significant. Another variation between liquids and solids is that we can consume liquids at higher temperatures than solids (Longman and Pearson, 1987). For solids, chewing sequences may involve multiple swallows to clear the bolus from the oral cavity (Hiiemae and Palmer, 1999).

As noted above in the discussion of single bolus swallows, it is accepted that the swallow reflex should be initiated at the faucial arches or when the bolus crosses the anterior margin of the manidibular ramus as seen radiographically (Bisch et al., 1994). In the swallowing of solid materials the pattern changes. Material frequently enters the pharynx and resides for a time in the valleculae while the masticatory process continues (~40% of cases). However, it rarely reaches the pyriform sinuses before a swallow response is initiated (Dua et al., 1997). Dua et al. (1997) report that the vocal folds perform a partial adduction for a short period of time (0.7 s) when food is held in the valleculae prior to completion of the masticatory process. It would also appear that the swallowing system is more tolerant of foodstuffs squirrelled in the valleculae or even the pyriform sinuses than that of the epiglottal edges. The bolus would, on average, dwell for between 2.1 and 3.2 s at the valleculae (solids and liquids respectively) and 1.4 and 1.5 s at the pyriform sinuses (liquids and solids respectively) before a swallow reflex was generated. However, the bolus was limited to a dwell time of 0.3 s to 0.4 s (liquids and solids respectively) if resting on the epiglottal edges or upper epiglottal surfaces. These actions are sound physiologically. The epiglottis is one of the physical 'gatekeepers' to ensure safety of the respiratory system. One other interesting difference is that the solid bolus passes over the midline of the laryngeal structures and into the UES, whereas a liquid bolus is usually divided around the larynx before rejoining to form a singular stream entering the UES (Dua et al., 1997).

Clinical inferences

The normal physiological differences detailed above must be borne in mind when performing both the clinical bedside and radiographic assessments of swallowing. It is *normal* for food to enter the upper portion of the pharynx prior to a swallow reflex being initiated. This should not be mistaken for 'premature spillage' (Dua et al., 1997). It is *normal* to take 10 s or more to masticate a mouthful or bite of a solid food and for multiple swallows to be used to clear the oral cavity of food. Normal variations must not be confused with pathology. Poor understanding of the normal physiology can place individuals on unnecessary modified diets.

BOLUS VISCOSITY

It is essential that we ingest fluids in order to remain hydrated. Regular thin fluids require excellent muscle control (oral and pharyngeal) and accurate timing between the swallowing system and the respiratory system to ensure that they are safely ingested. When an individual presents with dysphagia, they often lack the necessary muscular control and/or the sensory input integral to generating a timely and efficient muscular response. The problems with thin fluids are that

- they are not particularly cohesive and consequently tend to fracture or 'fall apart' en route if not swallowed efficiently; and
- because of their fracturability they are highly volatile and move very quickly.

Either may result in thin fluids being aspirated. If it is not possible to 'fix' the swallowing problem, then one looks at ways of compensating for it (see Chapter 11). One way to compensate is to improve the cohesiveness of the fluid and to slow it down. Thickening the fluid achieves both of these goals. Speech pathologists have been using thickened fluids therapeutically for years in an attempt to maintain oral hydration. Thickened fluids are rarely a diet of choice but they are a diet of necessity if the person is to maintain the intake of fluids orally when the swallowing system is compromised.

As noted above, the various permutations of thin fluids can significantly alter the physiological programming of the swallowing sequence. Thickened fluids provide a new set of parameters to bear in mind. Two of the important properties of thickened fluids are that they have cohesiveness, which allows them to 'hang together' and be less likely to fracture, and also that they move more slowly than regular fluids. Rheologically, all fluids are described in terms of:

- viscosity;
- density (weight per unit area); and
- yield stress (critical force required to initiate flow of the fluid).

This combination of variables distinguishes one fluid type from another. Oral afferent receptors may transmit bolus viscosity information to the central nervous system (CNS) in the same way that bolus volume information is conveyed to the CNS. For swallow programming, oral afferent receptors are most likely to evaluate variables such as bolus volume, consistency, size, shape, pH, temperature, texture, odour and familiarity to the CNS (Coster and Schwartz, 1987). The nervous system and oral afferents relay this information in a continuous feedback cycle until the bolus is swallow safe and ready for transport to the oesophagus (see also Chapter 1). The swallow needs to be customized depending on all of these variables. Initiation of the swallow is a result of the *cohesiveness* of the bolus rather than just the size of the particles of food/fluid. This viscous cohesion is the result of particles being broken down by chewing in the oral phase and mixing with saliva as a binding agent to produce a bolus that is both lubricated and cohesive. In healthy non-dysphagic individuals it is our ability to receive sensory information and to respond to it that ensures we can drink anything along the scale from ice slushies to the mixed textures of minestrone soup or a hot cup of tea with ease. The unique parameters of each bolus necessitate that a particular swallowing pattern is generated that will allow the bolus to be prepared so that it is 'swallow safe'.

THICKENED FLUIDS

As noted above, changes to the oral and pharyngeal phase of the swallow are mediated by the amount and type of bolus being swallowed. Considerably more tongue movement is required to manipulate a thickened fluid bolus and transport it to the posterior of the oral cavity in preparation for the pharyngeal part of the swallow than for thin fluids. There is more variability in lingual movement amplitude with thickened fluids than with thin fluids (Steele and Van Lieshout, 2004). Increased viscosity requires increased *tongue force* and increased *pharyngeal contraction* (Shaker et al., 1988; Shaker et al., 1994; Miller and Watkin, 1996). While the duration of the *lingual pressure wave* is not influenced by viscosity (Shaker et al., 1988; Perlman et al., 1993), duration of the *pharyngeal pressure wave* is influenced by viscosity (i.e. longer pharyngeal transit duration) (Robbins et al., 1992; Shaker et al., 1994). Increased submental and infrahyoid muscle activity is also recorded with increased bolus viscosity (Reimers-Neils et al., 1994). Note that the most significant results have been found for differences between liquids and thick pastes (cheese spread or peanut butter) but not for liquids and thin pastes (sauce or pudding) as measured via EMG. The time for transition from the oral phase to the pharyngeal phase increases with an increase in bolus viscosity (Robbins et al., 1992).

There is some controversy about whether the UES is open for a longer or shorter period of time when a thickened bolus is swallowed as opposed to a thin liquid bolus. Dantas et al. (1990) reported that when thickened fluids are swallowed the timing and relaxation of the UES is affected such that it has a larger dimension of opening and a longer duration of opening. However, Robbins et al., (1992) found that duration of UES opening was shorter for a viscous bolus than a thin liquid bolus. This may be because a liquid bolus has less stability and elastic cohesion allowing it to disintegrate easily during its passage through the pharynx, necessitating the UES to be open for sufficient time to capture all of the thin fluid. With a paste or semi-solid bolus, its ability to maintain cohesion and the slowing effect of a higher viscosity mean that there would be less risk of it disintegrating en route and as a result having a more efficient entry into the UES. This would result in a shorter UES opening time and shorter duration of hyolaryngeal excursion. Laryngeal closure does not appear to be affected by bolus viscosity. Duration of laryngeal closure for a liquid bolus as compared with a pudding bolus was comparable at 0.42 s and 0.45 s respectively (Bisch et al., 1994). Due to increases in oral preparation time and increased duration in the pharynx, it is not surprising to find that the total swallow duration for thick fluids is longer than for thin fluids (Robbins et al., 1992; Reimers-Neils et al., 1994).

The physiological changes that occur when swallowing thickened fluids have been detailed above. Thickened fluids are not, however, straightforward. Although health professionals working in the area of dysphagia describe fluids as either 'thick' or 'thin' in nature, the field of rheology has a more detailed way of describing a fluid's properties. The following section aims to provide the speech pathologist with an introduction to rheology and material characterization as it influences the types of fluids we swallow.

AN INTRODUCTION TO RHEOLOGY AND MATERIAL CHARACTERIZATION

As noted above, there are more technical ways of describing fluids rather than the very simple dichotomy of 'thick' or 'thin'. When we consider thick fluids more carefully there is quite a range of 'thick'. It can be as runny as nectar or thick enough so that it can no longer be poured, but requires a spoon for ingestion purposes or anywhere in between! Some of the problems with thickened fluids are:

- there is limited consistency in terminology (Cichero et al., 2000a);
- variability in the way 'thickness' is measured (Cichero et al., 2000a and b);
- the properties of the thick fluids change depending on the base substance (water, juice or dairy) and when barium is added to it for radiographic use (Cichero et al., 1997; Christoffersen et al., 2002).

In order to understand more about the nature of thick fluids the following areas will be described:

- Definitions – what are viscosity, density and yield stress and what are their measurement units?
- Newtonian and non-Newtonian fluids – what are they and why is it important?
- What are shear rates and how are they mediated in the swallowing system (i.e. tongue and pharynx)? How do shear rates affect viscosity?
- How does the addition of barium affect the fluid and what are the implications of this?

For now let us just assume that fluids are 'thin' (like water, tea, coffee) or 'thick' (consistency of nectar, pouring yoghurt, thickshake, runny pudding). Thickened fluids and modified diets are also discussed in Chapter 11 in regard to compensation for swallowing difficulty.

DEFINITIONS OF MATERIAL PROPERTIES AFFECTING SWALLOWING – VISCOSITY, DENSITY AND YIELD STRESS

Three measures have been used to characterize swallowing fluids objectively:

- viscosity;
- density; and
- yield stress (Cichero et al., 2000b).

Viscosity is defined as 'the internal friction of a fluid, or its tendency to resist flow' (Coster and Schwartz, 1987: 115). More strictly the viscosity of a fluid is defined by the ratio of the shear stress (the stress transmitted by a fluid during flow) divided by the shearing rate (or the rate by which the material is being sheared) (Macosko, 1995). Thus you can see that viscosity is essentially a measure of 'thickness' or 'thinness' of a fluid. Typically a viscometer or rheometer is used to test the viscosity of the fluids. An example of a rheometer and the cone and plate attachment for the rheometer is shown in Figure 3.1.

Here the bottom plate rotates at a constant speed (or shear rate) and a torque generated by the test fluid from the motion of the bottom plate, is transmitted through the test fluid to the top truncated cone. A shear stress, and hence viscosity, may be determined from this torque signal. The unique geometry of the cone and plate configuration allows it to generate a constant shear rate across the diameter of the sample and accurately measure the viscosity of all types of fluids (e.g. Newtonian

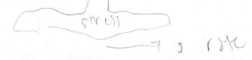

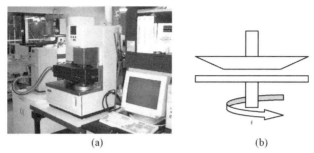

(a)   (b)

Figure 3.1   (a) Typical rheometer (Rheometrics ARES rheometer) and (b) close-up sketch of cone and plate fixture used in rheometer

and non-Newtonian fluids). The mechanics of the cone and plate system have been described in detail previously (Cichero et al., 1997).

Apart from viscosity, a fluid should also be examined for *density*. Density of a fluid is the mass per unit volume inherent in that material and most closely relates to the *weight* of the fluid. Clearly, if two fluids are of different density, there will be differences in the amount of force required to generate fluid movement. Density of the fluids is typically determined by accurately weighing a graduated cylinder of known volume.

In order to complete the rheological and material property characterization of a given fluid for swallowing studies, one should also examine the *yield stress* of the fluid. A fluid that has a yield stress is typically a particle-filled fluid or a gel. A fluid that has a yield stress has an inherent structure that must be broken down to allow the fluid to flow. The yield stress is defined as the stress that must be transmitted to a fluid above which flow occurs but below which no flow occurs. As an analogy, consider pouring a tub of yoghurt and a tub of water onto a bench. The yoghurt probably will need significantly more effort to allow it to spread, when compared with the water. This is due to the inherent structure, or yield stress, in the yoghurt. Yield stress is typically determined by measurements from a plot of viscosity versus shear stress (where shear stress is the force per unit area applied to the fluid surface) which can be obtained from the rheometer (Figure 3.1). If on the plot of viscosity versus shear stress, viscosity was seen to approach infinity as the shear stress approaches zero, then a yield stress is present (Figure 3.2).

The values of the yield stress can be read off the shear stress axis at the point where viscosity approached infinity. Other methods of direct yield stress measurements of fluids using rheometers are discussed in the literature (Gupta, 2000).

Viscosity, density and yield stress are obviously linked to the swallowing of fluids, as discussed in the following scenarios. A thick, heavy fluid (high viscosity, high density) will require more effort to initiate and maintain flow, than a thin, relatively light fluid (low viscosity, low density). A highly structured, thick material (high viscosity, high yield stress) will require higher initial force to move than a less

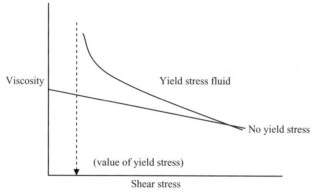

Figure 3.2   Yield stress determination of fluids from viscosity-shear stress data

structured, thin material (low viscosity, low yield stress). Thus it is important that all three variables (viscosity + density + yield stress) are measured in order to describe accurately the rheological and material property characteristics of a given fluid.

NEWTONIAN AND NON-NEWTONIAN FLUIDS

Clinicians generally differentiate fluids as either 'thin' or 'thick' but the field of rheology (or viscometry) has a far more detailed way of describing a fluid's flow properties. Fluids may be classified as either *Newtonian* or *non-Newtonian* in nature. Newtonian fluids are characterized by the fact that the force required to make the fluid flow is *directly proportional* to the resultant amount of flow (Coster and Schwartz, 1987). Fluids such as water, milk and honey are examples of Newtonian fluids. However, not all fluids are Newtonian in nature. For example, the addition of a suspension (e.g. barium) to water (a Newtonian fluid) results in a *non-Newtonian* fluid. Food-thickening agents added to thin fluids also tend to result in non-Newtonian fluids. Non-Newtonian fluids behave differently from Newtonian fluids. With a non-Newtonian fluid the 'shear stress' (i.e. the force per unit area applied to the fluid surface) is not proportional to the amount of flow or 'rate of strain' (i.e. the velocity as a result of stress applied to the fluid surface).

Another way of thinking about Newtonian and non-Newtonian fluids is to look at their viscosities. For Newtonian fluids, viscosities are independent of strain rate (mixing rate or flow rate) and it is sufficient to provide a single value for viscosity, as it will characterize the resistance to flow for all conditions of flow for that material. This is because the force required to make the fluid flow is directly proportional to the amount of flow. For non-Newtonian fluids, however, where the relationship between shear stress and rate of strain is not proportional, or where the viscosity (shear stress divided by strain rate) is not a constant value, it is not possible to provide a single value for viscosity. In fact typically for non-Newtonian fluids, the fluid is more viscous when stirred slowly and less viscous when stirred rapidly. Hence, it is not correct to provide a single viscosity value for a non-Newtonian fluid as it will not characterize the resistance to flow for all conditions of flow for that material. For non-Newtonian fluids it is more accurate to provide a *viscosity range or a viscosity profile over a range of shear rates.* This gives the viscosity of the fluid over a range of shear rates from low to high. For Newtonian fluids, no such differences exist, consequently there is only one viscosity (or score) to report. Schematically the difference between non-Newtonian and Newtonian viscosities is shown in Figure 3.3.

As can be seen from Figure 3.3 a Newtonian fluid has a constant viscosity that is independent of shearing rate, whereas non-Newtonian fluids have a viscosity that is affected by how fast the material is being sheared. Specifically in this case the non-Newtonian fluids sketched can further be described as (3a) shear thickening or (3b) shear thinning with respect to shearing rate.

Clinical inferences

The use of a viscosity range acknowledges that the viscosity of the fluid may be altered by tongue propulsion or oropharyngeal shearing during swallowing. For example, a thick fluid might have quite a viscous consistency at rest or very low shear rates within the oral cavity. However, as the fluid gains velocity due to the shearing action of the lingual and oropharyngeal systems, the viscosity of the fluid will decrease, and provide a less viscous reading. This behaviour is common to non-Newtonian fluids. In general, thickened fluids exhibit non-Newtonian behaviour (Cichero et al., 1997; Coster and Schwartz, 1987). Investigators have used shear rates from 1 s to 100 s^{-1} (inverse seconds) to accommodate the differences between low shear rates, such as those during little movement within the oral cavity, and high shear rates, such as those during maximum velocity during passage of the bolus through the oropharynx. Previous research has shown that typical shear rates during swallowing range from 5 s to 50 s^{-1} (Borwankar, 1992).

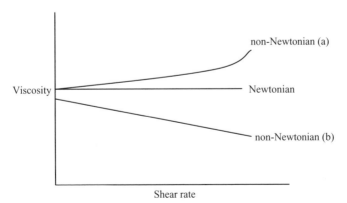

Figure 3.3   Viscosity profiles of Newtonian and non-Newtonian fluids (a) shear thickening, (b) shear thinning

CASE STUDIES IN MATERIAL CHARACTERIZATION OF SWALLOWING FLUIDS

To demonstrate the importance of fluid properties in swallowing fluids it is instructive to highlight some of our previous work.

CASE STUDY 1 – MEALTIME FLUIDS AND VIDEOFLUOROSCOPY FLUIDS: VARIABILITY BETWEEN HOSPITALS

The aim of the first case study was to examine various mealtime fluid and videofluoroscopic fluid properties from ten hospitals located in a single Australian city (Cichero et al., 2000a,b). It was hypothesized that there were quantifiable differences between the thickened fluids offered at the various hospitals. It was also hypothesized that the mealtime fluids would have different rheological properties from fluids used during videofluoroscopy. Videofluoroscopy fluids are barium-enriched fluids that are given to dysphagic patients during radiological assessments of swallowing function. Mealtime fluids are those fluids that are given to dysphagic patients as part of their normal oral diet. There were three levels of mealtime fluids. These were:

- *full thick*, subjectively described as 'slow pourable' (i.e. they should not pour rapidly or drop in lumps from the spoon);
- *half thick*, subjectively described as 'smooth yoghurt-like consistency'; and
- *quarter thick*, subjectively described as 'fruit nectar consistency' (e.g. apricot nectar).

Each hospital had its own recipes for each level of fluid thickness. Fluids were prepared according to the hospital recipe by kitchen staff. Internal classifications were also given (Table 3.4). Note that the internal classifications varied from being descriptive (e.g. 'thick syrup') to nondescript (Category I–III). Each of the 10 participating hospitals provided samples of the thickened fluids used at (a) mealtimes (n = 56) and (b) during videofluoroscopy (n = 34).

The methods used to analyse the fluid samples have been described elsewhere (Cichero et al., 1997, 2000a and b). Our rheological studies showed that for the mealtime fluids, the viscosity range for full thick was 475 cP at high shear rates and 21,000 cP at low shear rates. For half-thick fluids, we recorded a viscosity range of 283 cP at high shear rates and 11,000 cP at low shear rates. Nectar thick fluids recorded a viscosity range of 114 cP at high shear rates and 4,200 cP at low shear rates. Recall that thickened fluids are non-Newtonian and hence behave differently at high and low shear rates. They tend to be thicker when stirred or moved slowly, and become thinner when stirred or moved quickly.

Videofluoroscopy fluids were those fluids, containing barium, given to dysphagic patients during videofluorscopy procedures. Videofluoroscopy fluids were prepared by a hospital speech pathologist. The clinician added sufficient barium solution to a prepared mealtime fluid, to ensure that the new fluid would be radiopaque. In most cases, clinicians added barium 'by eye'. That is, they did not have set and

Table 3.4 Generic classification of thickened fluids used by investigators and hospital specific names of thickened fluids

Gener. name	H1	H2	H3	H4	H5	H6	H7	H8	H9	H10
Full thick	Stage I	Thick	Full thick	Cat. I	Thick	Thick	Paste	Thick	Thick	Stage I
Half thick	Stage II	Half thick	Half thick	Cat. II	Half thick	Half thick	Thick syrup	*n/a*	*n/a*	Stage II
Quart. thick	*n/a*	Quart. thick on request only	Quart. thick	Cat. III	*n/a*	*n/a*	Nectar	Nectar	Nectar	Stage III

Gener. = generic; Quart. = quarter; Cat. = category; n/a = not applicable – hospital does not provide this consistency of fluid; H = hospital.

measured amounts of barium solution that were added to measured amounts of mealtime fluids. Videofluoroscopy fluids were also subcategorized as (a) full thick, (b) half thick, and (c) quarter thick, in accordance with the descriptions provided above. Videofluoroscopy fluids were found to be more viscous than their mealtime counterpart at both high and low shear rates.

Clinical and research implications

One of the most routine parts of dysphagia assessment and treatment is the provision of thickened fluids. However, little thought has been given to the comparability of thickened fluids across institutions. If the fluids provided by the hospitals are vastly different, then the patient is at risk of being placed on an incorrect fluid consistency on interhospital transfer. The results of the Cichero et al. (2000a,b) investigation confirms suspicions that there are indeed quantifiable differences between the thickened fluids provided by different hospitals. 'Many individuals who work in flawed systems expend considerable energy to overcome these flaws in order to render a quality service' (Frattali, 1998: 175). Rather than have the clinicians continue to compensate for the flawed system, it makes more sense to improve the process itself. To ascertain whether the system is in fact flawed one must first assess the current system. The Cichero et al. (2000a and b) studies provided a means of measuring the 'current system'.

Classification and discussion of rheological differences

In the past, many investigators have addressed fluid viscosity in isolation of density and yield stress (Ku et al., 1990; Li, et al., 1992; Stanek et al., 1992; Robertson and Patillo, 1993; Zenner et al., 1995; Hamlet et al., 1996; Miller and Watkins, 1996). However, in order to characterize a fluid accurately the combined effects of viscosity, density and yield stress must be taken into account.

For the mealtime fluids reported in this study, density measurements between hospitals were comparable over all three fluid thicknesses (full thick, half thick and quarter thick) (see Table 3.5). Yield stress measures were reasonably comparable, with some variable scores being recorded (see Table 3.6). Viscosity was recorded for both low shear rates and high shear rates. Viscosity readings at low shear rates were reasonably comparable. Low shear rates represent very low levels of fluid movement within the oral cavity. At rest these fluids appeared to be fairly similar in terms of viscosity. At high shear rates, however, considerable variability was noted between hospitals for all three levels of fluid thickness. That is, at maximum velocity within the oropharyngeal system, the fluids from the different hospitals behaved in an idiosyncratic fashion rather than in a uniform fashion. For some hospitals, this means that the fluid remained thicker at high shear rates than that of their compatriot hospitals. When examined as a rheological and material property package there is noticeable variation between the hospitals for full thick, half-thick and quarter-thick mealtime fluids.

Table 3.5 Density measurements for all mealtime
fluids (g/cm^3) (Cichero et al., 2000a)

Hospital	Full thick	Half thick	Quarter thick
Mean	0.935	0.936	0.99
SD	0.04	0.06	0.04
H1	0.91	0.92	n/a
H2	0.93	0.95	n/a
H3	0.89	0.94	0.97
H4	0.9	1.0	1.05
H5	0.96	0.92	n/a
H6	1.03	1.02	1.04
H7	0.96	n/a	0.94
H8	0.96	n/a	0.94
H9	0.9	0.82	1.0
H10	0.91	0.92	n/a

n/a = not applicable – hospital does not provide this consistency of
fluid. H = Hospital.

More substantial inter-hospital variation was noted for the videofluoroscopy fluids. The yield stress measures were reasonably stable between hospitals but more significant differences were noted for viscosity (low and high shear rates) and density
measures (see Tables 3.7 and 3.8). In terms of viscosity, low shear rate measures
were more favourably consistent than high shear-rate measures. The density measures that were well matched for mealtime fluids were not comparable on an inter-
hospital basis for the videofluoroscopy fluids. Given that the videofluoroscopy fluids
were prepared by taking a quantity of mealtime fluid and adding 'sufficient' barium

Table 3.6 Yield stress measurements for all
mealtime fluids (Pa) (Cichero et al., 2000a)

Hospital	Full thick	Half thick	Quarter thick
Mean	18.6	10.6	3.5
SD	5.0	3.5	2.6
H1	18	9	n/a
H2	16.5	16	n/a
H3	8	4.3	2
H4	16.5	10.5	2
H5	21	12.5	n/a
H6	14	9	1.5
H7	22.5	n/a	7
H8	22.5	n/a	7
H9	25	14	2
H10	22	10	n/a

n/a = not applicable – hospital does not provide this consistency of
fluid. H = Hospital.

Table 3.7 Density measurements for all videofluoroscopy fluids (g/cm^3) (Cichero et al., 2000a)

Hospital	Full thick	Half thick	Quarter thick
Mean	1.22	1.26	1.39
SD	0.12	0.24	0.35
H1	1.21	1.29	n/a
H2	1.1	1.1	1.1
H4	1.3	1.34	1.35
H5	1.3	1.15	n/a
H6	1.2	1.7	1.96
H7	1.12	n/a	1.09
H8	1.45	n/a	1.49
H9	1.09	1.03	n/a

n/a = not applicable – hospital does not provide this consistency of fluid. H = Hospital.

solution to the fluid to make it radiopaque, the rheological and material property differences found may be a function of the barium solution used. Of the hospitals that provide videofluoroscopy services (n = 8), five different brands of barium, each with differing weight/weight percentage and weight/volume percentage measures, were used to prepare the videofluoroscopy fluids. Note too that where standard recipes are followed for the manufacture of the mealtime fluids, no such uniformity exists within the hospitals for the preparation of the videofluoroscopy fluids, with barium often added 'by eye'.

The rheological and material property differences noted for all fluids may also be accounted for by the method in which clinicians determine fluid thickness. Subjective measures are most common. Clinicians often stir a fluid to check its texture and resistance to the spoon and then note its flow rate as it drops from the spoon.

Table 3.8 Yield stress measurements for all videofluoroscopy fluids (Pa) (Cichero et al., 2000a)

Hospital	Full thick	Half thick	Quarter thick
Mean	26.22	10.5	6.9
SD	19.6	5.3	4.3
H1	10	2.5	n/a
H2	20	12	14
H4	18.5	9	2.5
H5	73	14	n/a
H6	29	18	7
H7	16	n/a	6
H8	24	n/a	5
H9	19.3	8	n/a

n/a = not applicable – hospital does not provide this consistency of fluid. H = Hospital.

Such techniques are hardly scientific. Borwankar (1992) showed that the rate of fluid deformation was substantially different depending on whether the fluid was (a) poured from a bottle, (b) used during basting, (c) observed for adhesion or cling, and (d) tested for mouthfeel. Visualizing and pouring showed the narrowest shear rate range, while basting and tasting exhibited the largest shear rate range. Based on this data, it is not possible to say that just because two fluids look alike or stir in a similar fashion they will create the same physiological response during swallowing. Stirring the fluids appears to give some information about viscosity at low shear rates. It does not give the valuable information required for what happens at high shear rates, such as that which occurs when the bolus moves through the oropharynx. Glassburn and Deem (1998) have also confirmed that speech pathologists showed extreme variability in their ability to mix solutions to their perceptions of nectar and honey consistencies. Both intersubject and intrasubject variability was reported. If individuals cannot repeat their own mixing consistencies, between subject variability will only make matters worse (Glassburn and Deem, 1998).

Appropriate objective assessments, such as those used in the current investigation are required to characterize fluid thickness accurately. Hospitals should be encouraged to perform regular objective measurements of their thickened fluid range. Both mealtime fluids and videofluoroscopy fluids should be assessed. Hospitals are advised to use suitably qualified personnel, and rheological equipment that is appropriate to the type of fluids being tested.

The Brookfield rheometer, the line spread test and the consistometer

Previous investigators have used a Brookfield rheometer to measure the viscosity of thickened fluids (Li et al., 1992; Robertson and Patillo, 1993; Zenner et al., 1995; Hamlet et al., 1996). The Brookfield rheometer is calibrated for use with Newtonian fluids. As noted earlier, Newtonian fluids are those where the force required to make the fluid flow is directly proportional to the resulting amount of flow (Coster and Schwartz, 1987). Most thickened fluids, however, are non-Newtonian in nature. That is, the force applied to the fluid (shear stress) is not proportional to the resulting velocity of the fluid, as a result of the stress applied to the fluid surface (shear rate) (Coster and Schwartz, 1987). Saliva, custard, yoghurt and baby food are all examples of non-Newtonian fluids. As some Brookfield rheometers are calibrated only for Newtonian fluids, it cannot be used accurately to measure the viscosity of non-Newtonian fluids.

The line spread test has also been touted as an inexpensive yet accurate measure of viscosity (Mann and Wong, 1996). The line spread test is a measure of product flow over a flat template of concentric rings measuring 0 cm to 25 cm. A 50 ml portion of fluid is placed into a hollow tube (3.5 cm high, 5 cm internal diameter). The tube is lifted and the fluid is permitted to flow for 1 minute. The distances travelled are measured at each 90 degree interval and averaged to produce a line spread reading. Thicker fluids tend to travel quite slowly, and so a smaller number is associated with a thick fluid (6.4 cm), whereas a larger number is associated with a thinner fluid

(14.3 cm). Mann and Wong (1996) found that line spread values of fluid thickness as judged by a sensory panel were well correlated with values of thickness measured using the line spread test. Note, however, that Mann and Wong (1996) used potato flakes, vegetable cereal and modified corn starch as the thickening agents. Yet the results of their assessments have been applied by clinicians to guar and xanthan based thickeners. There is no evidence to support the view that the gum-based thickeners behave in the same manner as the starch-based thickeners. A fluid that flows uniformly for a minute may well have the same eventual reading as the fluid that flows fast initially and then slows to the same reading at the end of a minute. The properties of these fluids are obviously different (probably due to differences in density or yield stress or both) yet they will provide the same 'magic number' on the line spread test. Are these fluids really equivalent?

A consistometer has also been used to provide a relatively inexpensive and somewhat objective measure of viscosity (Germain et al., 2005). Its principles are the same as for the line spread test although the method is different. The consistometer consists of a rectangular stainless steel bath. A portion at one end can be sealed from the rest of the bath by way of a guillotine. The fluid sample is placed in the separated portion. The guillotine is released and the fluid allowed to flow for a set amount of time (e.g. 30 s). A graduated measure in centimetres is taken at the end of the desired period.

The consistometer has also been touted as a reliable objective measure of fluid viscosity, however, the same arguments regarding fluid characterization levelled at the line spread test also apply to this testing procedure. Thickness is affected by the amount of thickener added (even small amounts can make a large difference in fluid thickness) and the temperature of the fluid. Fluids are more viscous at low temperatures than at high temperatures. One need only think of the toothpaste tube for confirmation – in summer it is very easy to squeeze the toothpaste out of the tube. In winter, when it is cold, toothpaste appears thicker and more force is required to squeeze it out of the tube. The toothpaste remains the same; the temperature alters the viscosity. Mann and Wong (1996) rightly state that separate formulations are need for each different type of food and beverage to ensure standard viscosity for individuals with dysphagia.

The potential effect of inter-hospital differences in thickened fluids for dysphagic patients

The rheological differences found in this study suggest that the care of dysphagic patients transferred between these facilities could be affected. At the most basic level, there were notable differences in the names the hospitals gave each of the three levels of fluid thickness (see Table 3.4). The diet recommendation of a patient transferred between H1 and H8 could pose considerable confusion for nursing and kitchen staff. Stage II (H1) fluids have no equivalent at H8. In fact, names such as 'stage I' or 'category II' do not give any indication as to the thickness or presumed thickness of the fluid being mentioned. The arbitrary names used by the hospitals do not aid in smooth transfer of diet recommendations. A common classification system for thickened fluids would be a good start to the process of rheological refinement.

Extreme variation in fluid thickness between hospitals also poses considerable medical risks. In this study, the patients assessed and treated at hospitals H5 and H6 are in considerable trouble if transferred to H3. The fluids at H3 are considerably less viscous at both low and high shear rates than at all of the other hospitals. Less extreme variation between other individual hospitals can also be seen. The variability of the fluids between hospitals is unacceptable if safe and high quality services are to be achieved.

These problems also affect videofluoroscopy services. There were two hospitals (H3 and H10) that did not have their own videofluoroscopy services and relied on the videofluoroscopy services of another hospital (H2). In this scenario it is important to compare the mealtime fluid values for H3 and H10 with the videofluorscopy fluid values of H2. The results of the study showed that H10 could reliably use the videofluoroscopy fluids at H2 to predict, in general terms, the mealtime fluid that will be most beneficial for their patients. For H3, however, there are stark differences between the viscosity, density and yield stress measures of their mealtime fluids, and that of H2's videofluoroscopy fluids. This data suggests that H3 cannot use H2's videofluoroscopy fluids to accurately ascertain the correct level of fluid thickness for their patients due to the extreme differences between the test fluid and the treatment fluid.

Remedying the problem

Quality improvement projects and further research could be applied to address the issues raised by this research. This investigation has identified a problem in inter-hospital variability of thickened fluid rheology. The cause of the problem may be related to a lack of objective assessment of fluid thickness, and inconsistencies in the preparation of videofluoroscopy fluids (Cichero et al., 2000a and b). Speech pathology and dietetic associations might also wish to take an active role in the quality improvement of dysphagic services. National associations could implement the studies outlined above to provide state-by-state or national recommendations of generic thickened fluid names and their associated rheological characteristics. Such guidelines could be incorporated into accreditation manuals to ensure quality service. Note that the fluid thickness differences outlined in this study are unlikely to be confined to the 10 hospitals surveyed but are indicative of a much larger problem.

Future directions for viscosity research

The current investigations indicate that there is a veritable 'Pandora's box' of viscosity related research waiting to be done. It is apparent that benchmarks for viscosity (low and high shear rates), density and yield stress need to be set up. The wide variation recorded between the hospitals indicates that further research for accurate benchmarking needs to take place. Chemical engineers should be involved in developing these benchmark values for viscosity, density and yield stress for fluids of different thicknesses.

It is also important to note that physical (i.e. measurable) viscosity and orally perceived viscosity do not have a one-to-one correlation. Smith et al. (1997) noted that oral sensation of viscosity grows at approximately one-third of the rate of actual viscosity. Hence it is not possible to directly compare instrumental and sensory values of viscosity because, although the values are related, they are not equivalent (Christensen, 1984). Therefore, substantially more research needs to be carried out using a combination of sensory values and instrumental values to arrive at appropriate benchmark values for full-thick, half-thick and quarter-thick fluids.

The following factors need to be considered when designing thickened fluids:

1. Type of thickening agents.
2. Whether the fluid's properties change with differences in temperature.
3. Reaction of the fluid with saliva.

Factors 1. and 2. will be easier to measure, factor 3. might prove to be more difficult. Saliva is more than 99% water and so differing amounts of saliva mixed with thickened fluids will cause changes to the viscosity and material property characteristics of the fluid. To make things more complicated, there are large individual differences in salivary flow rate. It can vary more than eightfold in healthy individuals (Christensen, 1984). The influence of viscosity and the material property characteristics of thickened fluids on both normal and dysphagic oropharyngeal swallowing also require further research.

CASE STUDY 2 – DIFFERENCES IN PREPARING SAME FORMULATIONS AT ONE HOSPITAL AT DIFFERENT TIMES

In this study the properties of dietary fluids prepared at different times at the one hospital were examined (Christoffersen et al., 2002). Dietary fluids were described as sample A or B, representing two dietary fluids from the same batch of dietary fluids. Samples A and B were collected for each of:

- thickshake;
- apple juice; and
- lemon cordial.

A matched videofluoroscopy fluid was also collected during each sampling. As in the previous study, videofluoroscopy fluids were prepared by a clinician and sufficient barium was added to the dietary sample to ensure that the new fluid would be radiopaque (i.e. it was 'added by eye'). Recipes used in this study are shown in Table 3.9.

Clinical and research implications

The current investigation aimed to establish whether there was batch-to-batch variation in the preparation of dietary and videofluoroscopy fluids as measured over

Table 3.9 Recipes for the preparation of dietary fluids used in this study (Christoffersen et al., 2002)

Thickshake (Stage I)	Apple juice (Stage I)	Lemon Cordial (Stage II)
120 ml full cream milk 100 ml ice cream 16 g skim milk powder 2 g guar gum (thickener)	200 ml apple juice 2.5 g guar gum (thickener)	200 ml diet lemon cordial 2 g guar gum (thickener)

a 4-week period. This study was the result of a single centre-experiment and one should be cautious about overinterpretation of the results. In order to classify accurately the rheological and material property characteristics of a fluid, objective measures of viscosity, density and yield stress needed to be carried out. This study found that even when recipes are used to prepare dietary fluids, viscosity and to a lesser degree density variables are shown to vary on a week-to-week basis. Note, however, that the variations recorded depended on the fluid base. That is, the lemon cordial samples were very well matched each week for the 4-week period. This result was consistent for both the dietary fluids and the videofluoroscopy fluids. The apple juice samples showed small variations from week to week for the dietary fluids, with large fluctuation between the videofluoroscopy samples on a week-to-week basis. The widest variance was recorded for the thickshake fluids. This fluid type was quite viscous at both low and high shear rates (see Figures 3.4–3.6). There was noticeable variability between the dietary samples from week to week and the match between videofluoroscopy fluids and dietary fluids was no better than chance (50%). Smaller variations were noted for the density measures (see Tables 3.10 and 3.11).

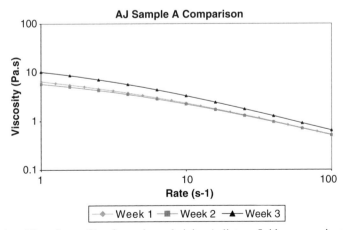

Figure 3.4a   Viscosity profile of sample apple juice A dietary fluid – comparison over weeks 1 to 3. Graph shows viscosity (Pa.s) versus rate (s^{-1})

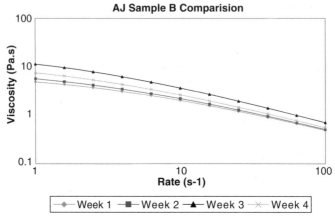

Figure 3.4b   Viscosity profile of apple juice sample B dietary fluid over weeks 1 to 4. Graph shows viscosity (Pa.s) versus rate (s^{-1})

Based on the small data set, the results suggest that lemon cordial provided an excellent substance for reproducibility both for mealtimes and during videofluoroscopy procedures. Apple juice appeared to be more volatile in this regard and the thickshake consistency was the most variable of all. The thickshake fluid appeared unsuitable for use during videofluoroscopy as it provided such a poor match to its dietary counterpart. The value of a radiological assessment of swallow using the barium-enriched thickshake fluid would be questionable as it is unclear how accurately it represented the swallowing function during mealtimes.

The relatively small variations in the viscosity, density and yield stress data for the apple juice and lemon cordial fluids perhaps have few clinical implications for

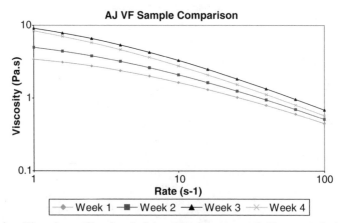

Figure 3.4c   Viscosity profile of apple juice videofluoroscopy fluid over weeks 1 to 4. Graph shows viscosity (Pa.s) versus rate (s^{-1})

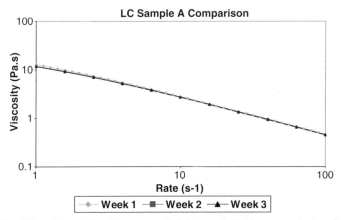

Figure 3.5a   Viscosity profile of lemon cordial dietary A fluid over weeks 1 to 3. Graph shows viscosity (Pa.s) versus rate (s^{-1})

dysphagic patients. The larger variations in the thickshake samples suggest there is potential for dysphagic patients to notice a difference in this fluid on a week-to-week basis. Larger scale studies, including those that examine patient swallowing ability, would need to be carried out to determine the degree of variability needed in the rheological and material property make-up of the fluid before swallowing function is compromised. Studies specifically linking variation in fluid viscosity, density and yield stress with patient swallowing ability have yet to be carried out.

    The comparison between the dietary fluids and the videofluoroscopy fluids provides further evidence that standard recipes of amount of barium solution added to dietary fluids should be established. In this hospital, the dietary fluid is the base

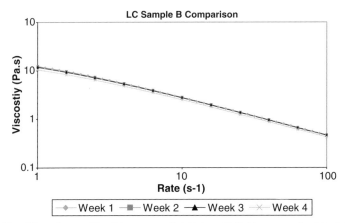

Figure 3.5b   Viscosity profile of lemon cordial dietary B fluid over weeks 1 to 4. Graph shows viscosity (Pa.s) versus rate (s^{-1})

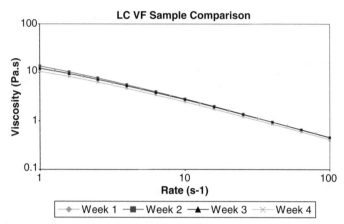

Figure 3.5c   Viscosity profile of lemon cordial videofluoroscopy fluid over weeks 1 to 4. Graph shows viscosity (Pa.s) versus rate (s^{-1})

substance with sufficient barium solution added 'by eye' to ensure that the result-ing videofluoroscopy fluid is radiopaque. Given that there was little variance in the densities of the dietary fluids (samples A and B) on a week-to-week basis but larger scale fluctuations in the density of the videofluoroscopy fluids on a week-to week basis, the effect of 'adding by eye' is well demonstrated. The results from the current investigation concur with the results of our earlier study (Cichero et al., 2000b).

Of most concern was the incidental finding of the differences between the fluid profiles of the apple juice and thickshake samples. Both fluids had been categorized by the hospital as 'Stage I' consistency. A patient receiving either thickshake or apple juice should be assured of the same level of thickness in both products. The

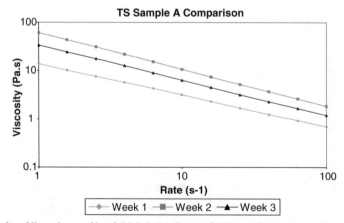

Figure 3.6a   Viscosity profile of thickshake dietary fluid sample A over weeks 1 to 3. Graph shows viscosity (Pa.s) versus rate (s^{-1})

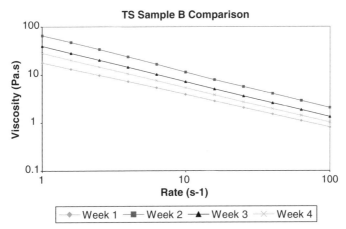

Figure 3.6b   Viscosity profile of thickshake dietary fluid sample B over weeks 1 to 4. Graph shows viscosity (Pa.s) versus rate (s^{-1})

results of the objective assessment revealed, however, that the two substances are very different rheologically. The thickshake exhibits a yield stress whereas the apple juice does not. The apple juice is more dense than the thickshake; however, the thickshake is more viscous at both low and high shear rates than the apple juice. One can hardly say, then, that these two fluid types are equivalent and interchangeable on a dysphagia diet sheet. If this degree of variation exists between these two fluid bases there is also the potential that it exists with other fluid bases – e.g. water based versus dairy based and juice based. The results from the current investigation suggest that fluids deemed to be of the same 'degree of thickness' should be objectively measured to see whether this is in fact the case. Further research is required to determine the

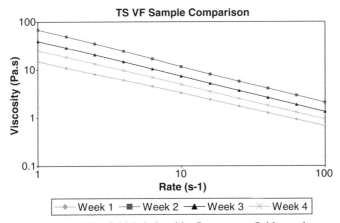

Figure 3.6c   Viscosity profile of thickshake videofluoroscopy fluid sample over weeks 1 to 4. Graph shows viscosity (Pa.s) versus rate (s^{-1})

Table 3.10 Density measurements for apple juice, lemon
cordial and thickshake samples for weeks one to four (g/ml)

	Week 1	Week 2	Week 3	Week 4
Apple juice				
Sample A	1.04	1.05	1.07	1.10
Sample B	1.05	1.05	1.05	1.10
VF fluid	1.13	1.16	1.10	1.20
Lemon cordial				
Sample A	1.06	1.09	1.06	1.09
Sample B	1.04	1.06	1.06	1.04
VF fluid	1.11	1.18	1.13	1.15
Thickshake				
Sample A	0.85	0.87	0.79	0.75
Sample B	0.82	0.87	0.80	0.76
VF fluid	0.85	0.86	0.80	0.77

amount of variation in viscosity, density and yield stress that dysphagic individuals
can tolerate before swallowing safety is compromised.

Table 3.11 Yield stress values (Pa) over four weeks for apple
juice, lemon cordial and thickshake samples

	Week 1	Week 2	Week 3	Week 4
Apple juice				
Sample A	0	0	0	—
Sample B	0	0	0	0
VF fluid	0	0	0	0
Lemon cordial				
Sample A	0	0	0	—
Sample B	0	0	0	0
VF fluid	0	0	0	0
Thickshake				
Sample A	11	58	32	—
Sample B	15	62	36	25
VF fluid	11	64	36	25

TASTE AND SMELL: RELATIONSHIP TO SWALLOWING

Taste and smell are physiologically and anatomically complex. Both senses allow
humans to determine desirable foods from bland foods and also those foods that are

noxious. As noted in Chapter 1, the smell of food, an empty stomach or an electrolyte imbalance will trigger a desire to eat. Taste has been shown in the literature to affect the rate of swallowing, as has temperature and other variables such as fluid carbonation. The sense of taste is intimately linked with olfaction (the sense of smell) and together these senses allow individuals to perceive *flavour*. Individuals will be aware that when they have a cold or influenza food tends to taste bland. In fact, it is the reduction in the ability to smell the food that causes the perception of flavour to be affected. Deficits in the chemosenses (smell and taste) may 'contribute to the failure to recognize and consume nutritious food, avoid hazardous environments, or derive pleasure from a variety of personal experiences' (Hoffman et al., 1998: 716–17). In an American population it was found that chronic smell problems increased significantly with age as did chronic taste problems (Hoffman et al., 1998). Chronic smell problems appear to be more prevalent than chronic taste problems; however, chronic taste *and* smell problems together are greater than just chronic smell problems alone. The physiology and anatomy of taste and smell and their clinical implications as they relate to swallowing will be briefly described below.

TASTE

There are four primary sensations of taste. These are:

• sour;
• salty;
• sweet; and
• bitter.

Sour taste is caused directly by acids and salty taste is elicited by ionized salts. Sweet and bitter tastes, however, are not caused by a *single class* of chemicals (Guyton, 1991). A fifth unique taste has also been identified and it is the taste associated with glutamic acid. It is referred to as 'umami taste' and is found in various foods and vegetables. Note also that human breast milk also has relatively high concentrations of glutamate. It appears that in specific flavour combinations or foods, umami substances enhance our flavour perceptions. In and of their own, however, they do not create a pleasant taste (Kurihara and Kashiwayanagi, 1998). Taste is perceived through taste buds on the tongue. *Taste buds* are modified epithelial cells. *Taste cells* are continuously being replaced, with a life span of approximately 10 days in lower mammals but unknown for humans (Guyton, 1991).

Taste buds are found on different regional areas of the tongue (vallate, foliate and most of the fungiform papillae). Taste buds are also found in the epithelium covering the soft palate, posterior wall of the oropharynx and epiglottis (Moore and Dalley, 1999). Sweet and salty tastes are located primarily on the tip of the tongue. Sour tastes tend to be located on the two lateral sides of the tongue and bitter tastes along the posterior of the tongue and soft palate. Even though taste buds are only found in certain locations on the tongue, taste sensations come from the entire inner surface of the mouth – that is, taste is a unitary event. This explains why we are not aware of the location of the specific taste receptors (Todrank and Bartoshuk, 1991). Adults have approximately 10,000 taste buds and children have more. After the age of 45 taste buds rapidly degenerate (Guyton, 1991). There is wide variability in normal thresholds for taste, with greater taste sensitivity in women than men (Delibasi et al., 2003). Application of a taste substance to the tongue causes a change in the polarization of the taste cells and consequently causes discharges of nerve fibres registering the taste. The nerve fibres react extremely quickly at first and then adapt within a couple of seconds to the stimuli. Saliva is instrumental in washing away taste chemicals. As noted in Chapter 1, taste from the anterior two-thirds of the tongue passes through the fifth cranial nerve, the chorda tympani, and into the facial nerve and then the nucleus of the tractus solitarius. Taste from the posterior third of the tongue comes via the glossopharyngeal nerve to the nucleus of the tractus solitarius. Areas supplied by the vagus nerve (e.g. epiglottis) project to the same tract. From here, the second-order neurones connect to the thalamus and also the post-central gyrus in the parietal cortex. The nucleus of the tractus solitarius also has connections with the superior and inferior salivatory nuclei. Gustatory sensations are transmitted to the thalamus and cortex bilaterally (Barr and Kiernan, 1988).

Taste and texture affect salivary flow rates. For example, as the pH of the stimulus decreases, signalling an increase in acidity, average saliva flow rate increases proportionately (Guinard et al., 1998). This effect has also been demonstrated for citric acid and bitter concentrations. Sweetness, however, also increases salivary flow rate and this has been demonstrated for both aspartame and sucrose (Guinard et al., 1998). Wine increases salivary flow rates by a combination of chemical sensations (mainly sour) and also trigeminal sensations (irritation and tactile) – which of these provides the greater stimulus to increased salivary flow has yet to be determined (Guinard et al., 1998). Note also that taste attributes are likely to be perceived for longer if the stimulus remains in the oral cavity longer, rather than being swallowed after intake, leaving only a faint residue in the oral cavity. For example, the perception of the taste of chewing gum will remain longer than a mouthful of food or fluid that is masticated and swallowed (Guinard et al., 1998).

Clinical implications

Even though the taste buds are anatomically located in certain positions on the tongue surface, the sensation of taste is a whole experience and does not vary in intensity as the substance is moved around the mouth. The advantage of this framework is that if there is localized damage to the taste system, for the most part, individuals do not notice large changes in taste experience. Interestingly, postmenopausal women have a decline in sensitivity to sucrose (sweet) perception. Delilbasi et al. (2003) warn that a reduction in the ability to perceive sweet foods may cause individuals with this problem to sweeten foods with serious consequences for those with diabetes, cardiac disease or obesity.

Multiple sensory receptors are excited to trigger a swallow response and these then send signals to the nucleus of the tractus solitarius. Given that taste sensations are part of this set of multiple sensations, it has been hypothesized that taste may facilitate swallowing by providing additional sensory input to the nucleus of the tractius solitarius. In healthy individuals, application of glucose, isotonic saline and distilled water does not affect latency of swallowing response (Kaatzke-Mc-Donald et al., 1996). Neither did the investigators find any differences between warm and cold chemical solutions (Kaatzke-McDonald et al., 1996). In neurologically impaired dysphagic individuals, however, application of a sour bolus causes oral tongue initiation of the swallow to occur faster, and the pharyngeal response to occur sooner (Logemann et al., 1995). Lazarus (1996) suggests that an acidic chemical may heighten sensory awareness and act as a stimulant for the brain stem and cortical swallowing areas. The one disadvantage of a sour bolus is that it may be unpalatable, making its use in a therapeutic sense limited. In fact soft drinks have sugar added to tone down the bitter taste of caffeine (Day, 2003). Pelletier and Lawless (2003) investigated a modification of the sour bolus by using mixture suppression to enhance flavour. The investigators used a citric acid and sucrose mix to improve palatability. Unfortunately, the improved flavour did not generate the same improvement in airway protection (i.e. decreased aspiration/penetration) found with the citric solution alone in an elderly neurologically dysphagia population. Both taste stimuli did, however, trigger significant increases in the number of spontaneous swallows after initial swallowing of the flavoured substances when compared with water (Pellteier and Lawless, 2003). Therapeutically this may be of benefit in giving dysphagic individuals increased practice of swallowing saliva boluses. Pelletier and Lawless (2003) also raise the point that personal 'taste likes and dislikes', or 'hedonics' may influence swallowing physiology, however this area has yet to be investigated. Using taste to improve swallowing function will be discussed further in Chapter 12. Note also that if taste perception varies as a function of duration of the stimulus within the oral cavity, as noted above, the clinician may choose to use gauze wrapped and tethered chewing gum to improve oral stimulation via taste in the dysphagic individual. Sweet tastes are also shown to increase salivary flow rates, and so lollipops may be useful therapeutically in:

• providing a tastant, using sensory feedback as a stimulus;
• encouraging lip closure around the stimulus; and
• enhancing salivary flow thereby encouraging individuals to swallow their secretions.

Clinicians should be mindful to encourage strict oral hygiene after such exercises, however, to minimize the formation of dental disease. Poor oral hygiene has been identified as a possible predictor of aspiration (Langmore et al., 1998).

Note also that pharmaceutical drugs have been reported to affect the sense of taste (Schiffman et al., 1998). Drugs are secreted into saliva and appear to affect taste perception either by producing a taste of their own or by modifying the mechanisms needed to perceive taste. Schiffman et al. (1998) found that concentrations as small as 0.1 mM or less of six psychotropic drugs could be detected by both young and elderly individuals (all non-smokers, taking no medications themselves).

The psychotropic drugs were found to have their own taste and also altered perception of other tastes. These results help to explain why elderly individuals who take medications have a greater loss of taste perception than those not taking medications. The dysphagia clinician needs to be cognizant of the effect of medications not only on oromotor abilities but also on sensory abilities. In combination, these may have a profound affect on swallowing ability and the amount and type of food ingested (see also Chapter 9).

The ability to taste depends heavily upon the ability to smell. It is the combination of these two senses that allows humans to perceive flavour. Without the ability to appreciate flavour individuals may be more prone to inadequate food intake and consequently malnutrition and weight loss (Schiffman et al., 1998).

SMELL

The olfactory system consists of the olfactory epithelium, olfactory bulbs and tracts and the cerebral olfactory areas (Barr and Kiernan, 1988). Olfactory cells are located in the olfactory epithelium. The olfactory epithelium covers an area of $2.5\,cm^2$ in the roof of each nasal cavity (lateral walls and nasal septum). Olfactory glands beneath the epithelium provide the epithelium with a surface layer of mucous fluid. For an odour to be perceived the substance needs to enter the nasal cavity as a gas or aerosol. It must also be water soluble so that it can be taken up by the mucous layer of the epithelium (Barr and Kiernan, 1988). Small cilia at the end of olfactory neurosensory cells project through the epithelium. These are special bipolar neurones that can serve as sensory receptors and also conduct neural impulses. Each olfactory neurosensory cell lasts for about 2 months before being replaced. Thus 'there are always new axons growing along the olfactory nerves into the olfactory bulb' (Barr and Kiernan, 1988: 260). The unmyelinated bundles of axons of the olfactory cells collectively constitute the olfactory nerves. These nerves pass through the foramina of the cribriform plate to enter the olfactory bulb. Axons from cells in the olfactory bulb project into the olfactory tract and from here into the central nervous system (CNS). There are two main areas associated with olfaction in the CNS, these being the medial and lateral olfactory areas. The medial olfactory area eventually feeds into the hypothalamus and the limbic system. The lateral olfactory area is composed of the pyriform cortex (temporal lobe) and a cortical portion of the amygdala. These areas then feed again into the limbic system but especially the hypocampus (Guyton, 1991). In addition, there are nerve fibres that pass back from the olfactory portions of the brain to the periphery – these are used to inhibit the sense of smell.

The olfactory system reacts quickly to continuous stimuli. Notice that if you walk into a bakery the initial smell of baking bread will be strong but your perception of it quickly dissipates due to the inhibitory process described above. Olfactory stimuli induce visceral responses – for example, we increase our saliva flow rates with the aroma of food. When testing the sense of smell, individuals should have both right and left nares investigated. Each should be occluded while the other is tested (Moore and Dalley, 1999). The best ability to detect odour occurs between the ages of 20 and

40 years (Kovacs, 2004). The general prevalence of olfactory impairment is 24% but in the elderly it may be as high as 70% (Kovacs, 2004). Older individuals have a reduced acuity of smell, possibly due to a reduction, with ageing, in the population of neurosensory cells in the olfactory epithelium and a general reduction in the olfactory epithelial surface (Barr and Kiernan, 1988; Kovacs, 2004). The number of mitral cells in the olfactory bulb reduces from 60,000 in individuals aged 25 years, to 14,500 in individuals aged 95 years. A drying out of the mucous layer and calfication of the ethmoid bone that houses the cribriform plate have also been implicated in the decline in the ability to perceive odour with increasing age (Vroon et al., 1997). Because the decline is gradual, older individuals may not be particularly aware of a change in their ability to smell.

Clinical inferences

In severe head injuries, mechanical damage to the olfactory bulbs or cribriform plate through trauma may produce a complete loss of smell on the affected side (Moore and Dalley, 1999). It has recently been noted that in the early stages of Alzheimer's disease odour identification is mildly altered whereas impaired odour detection is a feature of a late stage of the disease. The loss of olfactory identification has been significantly related to the Mini mental scores in individuals with Alzheimer's disease (Kovacs, 2004). Odour identification is the ability to identify specific smells whereas odour discrimination is the ability to differentiate between odorants. Moreover, damage to the olfactory bulb has been shown in individuals with Alzheimer's disease. Odour detection and identification are also damaged in individuals with Parkinson's disease, with damage to the amygdala and olfactory bulb implicated (Kovacs, 2004). The unique anatomy of the olfactory system may be critical in the investigation of neurological disorders where impairment of smell has been found. Recall that the olfactory cells are constantly regenerating and that these fibres connect with the central nervous system. The vulnerability of the olfactory structures may well be implicated as a method of entry and access to the CNS (Kovacs, 2004). Smokers have also been implicated as having worse olfactory capacity than non-smokers (Vroon et al., 1997). This may be due to adaptation to the smoke (if tested shortly after smoking) or due to direct damage to the olfactory system. Paint thinners, glues and other solvents, when inhaled, cause damage to the olfactory system (painters and cleaners are at risk).

The interplay between taste and smell is critical to the perception of flavour and hence our enjoyment or displeasure with food. Taste chemicals are released when a piece of chocolate is placed into the mouth and chewed. Escaping molecules from the mouth also waft into the nose. Without the sense of smell chocolate actually tastes quite bitter. It is the combination of taste and smell that provides individuals with flavour. Notice also that in eating generally individuals do not mix everything up together but take successive mouthfuls of various foods. This process allows stimulation of both taste and smell and fluctuating adaptation and inhibition of both senses (Vroon et al., 1997). Note also that the concentration of the smell will affect its perception. Subtle changes to the chemosenses that can occur with injury or ageing can affect the individual's ability to enjoy food and fluids. Modified diets and thickened fluids have been described as bland and unappetizing. These qualities have an effect on patient compliance and thus on nutrition and general wellbeing. Reduced compliance with thickened fluids places individuals at risk of dehydration. Whelan (2001) reported that for individuals with a diagnosis of acute stroke the mean daily intake of thickened fluids was 455 ml/day, representing an average of only 22% of daily fluid requirements. As a result, individuals required supplementary feeding to improve hydration. An understanding of the chemosenses provides the clinician with a more holistic outlook on individuals with dysphagia.

The discussion above has highlighted the chemosenses in relation to swallowing. Touch and pressure receptors are also implicated in modulating swallowing physiology. This has been noted above in the discussions of bolus volume and viscosity. Interestingly, pain receptors and nociceptors (i.e. pain or injury receptors) are also regularly stimulated by various foods or food compounds. Carbonation of fluids triggers nociceptors within the oral cavity and presumably pharynx (Dessirier et al., 2000). Pepper also stimulates pain receptors in the oral cavity (Akal et al., 2004). It may be possible to use these naturally occurring methods of sensory perception to improve the swallowing function.

EFFECTS OF CARBONATION ON SWALLOWING

As noted above, taste can affect swallowing physiology due to the provision of sensory information to the nucleus of the tractus solitarius. The nucleus ambiguous receives afferents from sensory nuclei of the brain stem and importantly from:

- the nucleus of the spinal tract of the trigeminal and
- the nucleus of the tractus solitarius (Barr and Kiernan, 1988).

Neurones from the nucleus ambiguous connect with motor neurones involved in swallowing. In individuals with dysphagia, increasing sensory awareness of the bolus may improve swallowing outcome. Carbonated water has been found to activate lingual nociceptors by converting CO_2 to carbonic acid. The nociceptors in turn excite trigeminal neurones involved in signalling oral irritation (Dessirier et al., 2000). It is interesting that a sensation that so many people enjoy is actually caused by the excitation of nociceptors! Importantly for the purposes of the dysphagia clinician, the fact that carbonated beverages excite the trigeminal neurones, with their connections to the nucleus ambiguous, provides potential therapeutic applications.

Due to issues such as patient compliance and fatigue and a desire to maintain hydration levels in individuals with dysphagia, Bulow et al. (2003) investigated the effects of carbonated thin fluids on the physiology of swallowing in individuals who aspirated. The authors found that carbonated thin liquids significantly reduced penetration when compared to both thickened liquids and thin liquids. Carbonated fluids were also found to have a reduced pharyngeal transit time when compared with both thin and thickened fluids. Bulow et al. (2003) noted that hyolaryngeal excursion commenced as soon as the carbonated fluids were taken into the oral cavity. In addition, it was noted that there was significantly less pooling in the pharynx post swallow with carbonated liquids. As noted in Chapter 4, the amount of time a material dwells within the pharynx will significantly influence the likelihood of it being drawn into the respiratory system. A reduction in post-swallow pharyngeal pooling with carbonated fluids makes these fluids attractive for individuals prone to valleculae or pyriform sinus pooling. Note, however, that the build up of gases from carbonated fluids may be ill advised for individuals with reflux due to pressure on the UES and distension of the stomach.

A paediatric study into the use of carbonated fluids in infants who aspirated also found the effects of carbonation to be beneficial (Newman et al. 2001). The authors found that the use of carbonated barium reduced the incidence of material in the pharynx prior to the swallow. Laryngeal penetration was also significantly reduced, although no significant effect was found for aspiration. The authors noted, however, that children who did aspirate were more inclined to cough on carbonated barium than they were on non-carbonated barium. The numbers used in this study were relatively small, however, and further research is advised. Finally, Njn and McDaniel (1991) have reported that healthy individuals perceive carbonation intensity to be higher when the fluid is colder, although it was also dependant upon the level of carbonation of the fluid. Clinically, this might suggest that a *cold* carbonated beverage may be even more therapeutically beneficial than a carbonated beverage in terms of oropharyngeal sensory excitation.

SUMMARY

This chapter serves to highlight the considerable variation there is in the normal swallow. Changes in physiology occur as a function of the bolus (volume, viscosity, solid or fluid), and vessel and method of ingestion (cup, straw etc.). Changes related to swallowing also occur due to chemosensory input (taste, smell, sensory receptors). All of this information needs to be considered by the dysphagia clinician when considering what is normal from what is pathological. Normal variation should never be confused with pathology.

REFERENCES

Adnerhill I, Ekberg O, Groher ME (1989) Determining normal bolus size for thin fluids. Dysphagia 4: 1–3.

Akal UK, Kucukyavuz R, Nalcaci T, et al. (2004) Evaluation of gustatory function after third molar removal. International Journal of Oral and Maxillofacial Surgery 33: 564–8.

Barr ML, Kiernan JA (1988) The Human Nervous System: An Anatomical Viewpoint 5th edn. Philadelphia: JB Lippincott Co.

Bisch EM, Logemann JA, Rademaker AW, et al. (1994) Pharyngeal effects of bolus volume, viscosity, and temperature in patients with dysphagia resulting from neurologic impairment and in normal subjects. Journal of Speech and Hearing Research 37: 1041–9.

Borwankar RP (1992) Food texture: a tutorial review. Journal of Food Engineering 16: 1–16.

Brunstrom JM, Tribbeck PM, MacRae AW (2000) The role of mouth state in the termination of drinking behaviour in humans. Physiology and Behaviour 68(4): 579–83.

Bulow M, Olsson R, Ekberg O (2003) Videoradiographic analysis of how carbonated thin liquids and thickened liquids affect the physiology of swallowing in subjects with aspiration on thin liquids. Acta Radiologica 44: 366–72.

Casas MJ, Kenny DJ, McPherson KA (1994) Swallowing/ventilation interactions during oral swallow in normal children and children with cerebral palsy. Dysphagia 9: 40–6.

Chi-Fishman G, Sonies BC (2000) Motor strategy in rapid sequential swallowing: new insights. Journal of Speech, Language and Hearing Research 43(6): 1481–92.

Christensen CM (1984) Food texture perception. Advances in Food Research 29: 159–99.

Christoffersen C, Sargent A-L, Cichero JAY, et al. (2002) What we don't know could hurt us: a single centre study of batch-to-batch variability of dietary fluids and 'matched' videofluoroscopy fluids. Journal of Medical Speech-Language Pathology 10(3): 159–71.

Cichero JAY, Hay G, Murdoch BE, et al. (1997) Videofluoroscopic fluids versus mealtime fluids: differences in viscosity and density made clear. Journal of Medical Speech-Language Pathology 5(3): 203–15.

Cichero JAY, Jackson O, Halley PJ, et al. (2000a) Which one of these is not like the others? An inter-hospital study of the viscosity of thickened fluids. Journal of Speech and Hearing Research 43: 537–47.

Cichero JAY, Jackson O, Halley PJ, et al. (2000b) How thick is thick? A multi-centre study of the rheological and material property characteristics of mealtime and videofluoroscopy fluids. Dysphagia 15(4): 188–200.

Coster ST, Schwartz WH (1987) Rheology and the swallow-safe bolus. Dysphagia 1: 113–18.

Daniels SK, Foundas AL (2001) Swallowing physiology of sequential straw drinking. Dysphagia 16: 176–82.

Dantas RO, Kern MK, Massey BT, et al. (1990) Effect of swallowed bolus variables on oral and pharyngeal phases of swallowing. American Journal of Physiology 258: G675–G681.

Day S (2003) Researchers seek to trick bitter taste buds. New York Times, 26 August.

Delilbasi C, Cehiz T, Akal UK, et al. (2003) Evaluation of gustatory function in postmenopausal women. British Dental Journal 194: 447–9.

Desirier JM, Simons CT, Cartsens MI, et al. (2000) Psychophysical and neurobiological evidence that oral sensation elicited by carbonated water is of chemogenic origin. Chemical Senses 25(3): 277–84.

Dodds WJ, Man KM, Cook IJ, et al. (1988) Influence of bolus volume on swallow-induced hyoid movement in normal subjects. American Journal of Roentgenology 150: 1307–9.

Dua KS, Ren J, Bardan E, et al. (1997) Coordination of deglutitive glottal function and pharyngeal bolus transit during normal eating. Gastroenterology 112: 73–83.

Ekberg O, Olsson R, Sundgren-Borgstrom P (1988) Relation of bolus size and pharyngeal swallow. Dysphagia 3: 69–72.

Ergun GA, Kahrilas PJ, Lin S, et al. (1993) Shape, volume, and content of the deglutitive pharyngeal chamber imaged by ultrafast computerized tomography. Gastroenterology 105(5): 1396–1403.

Ertekin C, Aydoggdu I, Yuceyar N, et al. (1997) Effects of bolus volume on oropharyngeal swallowing: an electrophysiologic study in man. American Journal of Gastroenterology 92: 2049–53.

Frattali CM (1998) Quality improvement. In Frattali CM (ed.) Measuring Outcomes in Speech-Language Pathology. New York: Thieme, pp. 172–85.

Germain I, Dufresne T, Ramaswamy HS (in press) Rheological characterization of thickened beverages used in the treatment of dysphagia. Journal of Food Engineering.

Glassburn D, Deem JF (1998) Thickener viscosity in dysphagia management: Variability among speech-language pathologists. Dysphagia 13: 218–22.

Guinard J-X, Zoumas-Morse C, Walchak C (1998) Relation between parotid saliva flow and composition and perception of gustatory and trigeminal stimuli in food. Physiology and Behaviour 63(1): 109–18.

Gupta RK (2000) Polymer and Composite Rheology. New York: Marcel Dekker.

Guyton AC (1991) Textbook of Medical Physiology (8th edn). Philadelphia: W.B. Saunders.

Hamlet S, Choi J, Zormeier M, et al. (1996) Normal adult swallowing of liquid and viscous material: scintigraphic data on bolus transit and oropharyngeal residues. Dysphagia 11: 41–7.

Hiiemae KM, Palmer JB (1999) Food transport and bolus formation during complete feeding sequences on foods of different initial consistency. Dysphagia 14: 31–42.

Hiss SG, Treole K, Stuart A (2001) Effects of age, gender, bolus volume, and trial on swallowing apnoea duration and swallow/respiratory phase relationships of normal adults. Dysphagia 16: 128–35.

Hoffman HJ, Ishi EK, Macturk RH (1998) Age-related changes in the prevalence of smell/taste problems among the United States Population. In Murphy C (ed.) Olfaction and Taste XII: An International Symposium. Annals of the New York Academy of Sciences, volume 855. New York: New York Academy of Sciences, pp. 716–22.

Jacob P, Kahrilas PJ, Logemann JA, et al. (1989) Upper esophageal sphincter opening and modulation during swallowing. Gastroenterology 97: 1496–78.

Jones DV, Work CE, Cincinnati MD (1961) Volume of a swallow. American Journal of Dieases of Children 102(173): 427.

Kaatzke-McDonald MN, Post E, David PJ (1996) The effects of cold, touch, and chemical stimulation of the anterior faucial pillar on human swallowing. Dysphagia 11: 198–206.

Kahrilas PJ (1993) Pharyngeal structure and function. Dypshagia 8: 303–7.

Kahrilas PJ, Lin S, Chen J, et al. (1996) Oropharyngeal accommodation to swallow volume. Gastroenterology 111: 297–306.

Kahrilas PJ, Logemann JA (1993) Volume accommodation during swallowing. Dysphagia 8: 259–65.

Kovacs T (2004) Review: mechanisms of olfactory dysfunction in aging and neurodegenerative disorders. Ageing Research Reviews 3: 215–32.

Ku DP, Ma P-P, McConnel FM.S, et al. (1990) A kinematic study of the oropharyngeal swallowing of a liquid. Annals of Biomedical Engineering 18: 655–69.

Kurihara K, Kashiwayanagi M (1998) Introductory remarks on umami taste. In Murphy C (ed.) Olfaction and Taste XII: An International Symposium. Annals of the New York Academy of Sciences (Vol 855). New York: New York Academy of Sciences, pp. 393–7.

Lang I, Shaker R (1994) An update on the physiology of the components of the upper esophageal sphincter. Dysphagia 9: 229–32.

Langmore SE, Terpenning,MS, Schork A, et al. (1998) Predictors of aspiration pneumonia: How important is dysphagia? Dysphagia 13: 69–81.

Lawless HT, Bender S, Oman C, et al. (2003) Gender, age, vessel size, cup vs. straw sipping, and sequence effects on sip volume. Dysphagia 18: 196–202.

Lazarus CL (1996) Comments on the effects of cold, touch, and chemical stimulation of the anterior faucial pillar on human swallowing. Dysphagia 11: 207–8.

Lazarus CL, Logemann JA, Rademaker AW, et al. (1993) Effects of bolus volume, viscosity, and repeated swallows in nonstroke subjects and stroke patients. Archives of Physical Medicine and Rehabilitation 74: 1066–70.

Lear CSC, Flanagan JBJ, Morres CFA (1965) The frequency of deglutition in man. Archives of Oral Biology 10: 83–100.

Li M., Brasseur JG, Kern MK, et al. (1992) Viscosity measurements of barium sulfate mixtures for use in motility studies of the pharynx and esophagus. Dysphagia 7: 17–30.

Logemann JA (1988) Swallowing physiology and pathophysiology. Otolaryngologic Clinics of North America 21(4): 613–23.

Logemann JA (1998) Efficacy, outcomes, and cost effectiveness in dysphagia. In CM Frattali (ed.) Measuring outcomes in speech-language pathology (pp. 321–33). New York: Thieme.

Logemann JA, Pauloski BR, Colangelo L, et al. (1995) Effects of a sour bolus on oropharyngeal swallowing measures in patients with neurogenic dysphagia. Journal of Speech and Hearing Research 38: 556–63.

Logemann JA, Pauloski BR, Rademaker AW, et al. (2000) Temporal and biomechanical characteristics of oropharyngeal swallow in younger and older men. Journal of Speech and Hearing Research 43: 1264–74.

Longman CM, Pearson GJ (1987) Variations in tooth surface temperature in the oral cavity during fluid intake. Biomaterials 8: 411–14.

Macsoko CW (1995) Rheology. New York: VCH Publishers.

Mann LL, Wong K (1996) Development of an objective method for assessing viscosity of formulated foods and beverages for the dysphagic diet. Journal of the American Dietetic Association 96: 585–8.

Miller JL, Watkin KL (1996) The influence of bolus volume and viscosity on anterior lingual force during the oral stage of swallowing. Dysphagia 11: 117–24.

Moore KL, Dalley AF (1999) Clinically Oriented Anatomy. 4th edn. Philadelphia: Lippincott Williams & Wilkins.

Newman L, Armstrong R, Rogers T, et al. (2001) The effect of carbonation on sensory dysphagia in the pediatric population. Dysphagia 16: 146–50.

Njn Y, McDaniel MR (1991) The effect of temperature on carbonation perception. Chemical Senses 16(4): 337–48.

Palmer PM, Luschei ES, Jaffe D, et al. (1999) Contributions of individual muscles to the submental surface electromyogram during swallowing. Journal of Speech, Language and Hearing Research 42(6): 1378–91.

Pelletier CA, Lawless HT (2003) Effect of citric acid and citric acid-sucrose mixtures on swallowing in neurogenic oropharyngeal dysphagia. Dysphagia 18: 231–41.

Perlman AL, Guthmiller Schultz J, Van Daele DJ (1993) Effects of age, gender, bolus volume and bolus viscosity on oropharyngeal pressure during swallowing. Journal of Applied Physiology 75: 33–7.

Preiksaitis HG, Mayrand S, Robbins K, et al. (1992) Coordination of respiration and swallowing: Effect of bolus volume in normal adults. American Journal of Physiology 263: R624–R630.

Reimers-Neils L, Logemann J, Larson C (1994) Viscosity effects in EMG activity in normal swallowing. Dysphagia 9: 101–6.

Robbins J, Hamilton JW, Lof GL, et al. (1992) Orophayngeal swallowing in normal adults of different ages. Gastroenterology 103: 823–9.

Robertson HM, Patillo MS (1993) A strategy for providing food to the patient with neurologically based dysphagia. Journal of the Canadian Dietetics Association 54: 198–201.

Schiffman SS, Graham BG, Suggs MS, et al. (1998) Effect of psychotropic drugs on taste responses in young and elderly persons. In C Murphy (ed.) Olfaction and Taste XII: An International Symposium. Annals of the New York Academy of Sciences, volume 855. New York: New York Academy of Sciences, pp. 732–7.

Selley WG, Ellis RE, Flack FC, et al. (1990) Coordination of sucking, swallowing and breathing in the newborn: its relationship to infant feeding and normal development. British Journal of Disorders of Communication 25: 311–27.

Shaker R, Cook IJS, Dodds WJ, et al. (1988) Pressure-flow dynamics of the oral phase of swallowing. Dysphagia 3: 79–84.

Shaker R, Ren J, Zamir Z, et al. (1994) Effect of aging, position, and temperature on the threshold volume triggering pharyngeal swallows. Gastroenterology 107: 396–402.

Smith CH, Logemann JA, Burghardt WR, et al. (1997) Oral sensory discrimination of fluid viscosity. Dysphagia 12: 68–73.

Stanek K, Hensley C, Van Riper C (1992) Factors affecting use of food and commercial agents to thicken liquids for individuals with swallowing disorders. Journal of the American Dietetics Association 92(4): 488–90.

Steele CM, Van Lieshout PHHM (2004) Influence of bolus consistency on lingual behaviours in sequential swallowing. Dysphagia 19: 192–206.

Tasko SM, Kent, RD, Westbury JR (2002) Variability in tongue movement kinematics during normal liquid swallowing. Dysphagia 17(2): 126–38.

Todrank J, Bartoshuk LM (1991) A taste illusion: taste sensation localized by touch. Physiology and Behaviour 50: 1027–31.

Tracy JF, Logemann JA, Kahrilas PJ, et al. (1989) Preliminary observations on the effects of age on oropharyngeal deglutition. Dysphagia 4: 90–4.

Vroon, P, Van Amerongen A, De Vries H (1997) Smell: The Secret Seducer. Translated from the Dutch by Paul Vincent. New York: Farrar, Straus & Giroux.

Whelan K (2001) Inadequate fluid intakes in dysphagic acute stroke. Clinical Nutrition 20(5): 423–8.

Wintzen AR, Badrising UA, Roos RA, et al. (1994) Influence of bolus volume on hyoid movements in normal individuals and patients with Parkinson's disease. Canadian Journal of Neurological Sciences 21(1): 57–9.

Zenner PM, Losinski DM, Mills RH (1995) Using cervical auscultation in the clinical dysphagia examination in long-term care. Dysphagia 10: 27–31.

4 Respiration and Swallowing

JULIE CICHERO

INTRODUCTION

So far we have viewed swallowing as an isolated event. Certainly this is a good place to start but it is by no means the whole picture. Swallowing is intimately related to respiration. This chapter focuses on a significant set of information relating to the relationship between swallowing and respiration. Specifically, this chapter addresses:

- the swallow-respiratory cycle;
- neural regulation of respiration for swallowing;
- details of glottic closure during swallowing;
- deglutition apnoea;
- respiratory factors that contribute to or prevent aspiration; and
- the clinical relevance of the interplay between swallowing and respiration.

THE SWALLOW-RESPIRATORY CYCLE

Selley et al. (1989a) aptly describe swallowing and respiration as possessing a type of 'biological time share'. Time share is a term that was very popular in the 1980s and used to describe the concept of a group of individuals purchasing a holiday unit, for example. One family might stay in the unit for a couple of weeks, another family for another few weeks and so on. They key to the concept was that although everyone owned the unit, only one group was in residence at any one time. The same concept can be applied to the laryngopharyngeal region. The pharynx in particular is the common pathway (the unit if you like), which is at times used for swallowing, but for the most part used for respiration. It is also true to the time-share concept in that when we swallow, we do not breathe and when we breathe, we do not swallow. When swallowing and respiration co-occur, aspiration is the usual outcome.

THE SWALLOW-RESPIRATORY CYCLE OF HEALTHY INDIVIDUALS

Selley et al. (1989a) found that there is a swallow-respiratory pattern that is activated during drinking. This pattern has been observed in babies and is also evident throughout the age continuum to individuals in their nineties. Selley et al. (1989a) describes

Dysphagia: Foundation, Theory and Practice. Edited by J. Cichero and B. Murdoch
© 2006 John Wiley & Sons, Ltd.

the cycle as follows. As a spoon approaches an individual's lips there is a small inhalation. There is then a small exhalation and then apnoea (cessation of breathing) ensues while the swallow occurs. After the swallow there is an immediate exhalation. This pattern of a swallow immediately followed by an exhalation occurs in 95% of all swallows (Selley et al., 1989a). There is a small difference that occurs with cup drinking – when taking a liquid bolus from a cup there is a period of apnoea while the bolus is transferred into the oral cavity. Nishino et al. (1985) also reported a pattern of swallows occurring during the expiratory phase of respiration. When swallows occurred during the inspiratory phase, the swallow halted the inspiration and was immediately followed by a short exhalation. This is supportive of Selley et al.'s (1989a) results. Nishino et al. (1985) also reported that there was a significant increase in tidal volume in the breaths immediately occurring after swallowing. The same result was found regardless of whether a saliva bolus or a fluid bolus was swallowed.

It is not a chance happening that we usually exhale immediately after a swallow. It also proves that we do not simply 'stop breathing' when we swallow. The relay system for the respiratory system, the nucleus of the tractus solitarius, is also critical for the regulation of swallowing. This is no accident. Physiologically it is imperative that these two systems communicate with each other. Consider the exhalation that occurs after swallowing. If there is trace residue in the pharynx, then it makes sense that that residue be expelled upwards towards the mouth via an exhalation, rather than drawn into the airway during an inhalation. The ramifications extend further, however. Selley et al. (1990b) contend that without adequate triggering of the swallow reflex, this special 'swallow-respiratory' sequence may be delayed in activation or may not be activated at all. If the respiratory system is not expecting a swallow and the bolus 'sneaks up' on it, the respiratory system is left in jeopardy. Situations like this may occur if there are deficits in sensory input (see Chapter 1 for further details on triggering the swallowing reflex). If sensory input is inadequate, it is unlikely that there will be successful communication between the swallowing centre and the respiratory centre. The vagus nerve and the glossopharyngeal nerve provide this information. Thus the usual biomechanical events may be improperly timed, or worse still not timed at all, allowing food to be ingested while the respiratory system is unprotected. Selley et al. (1990a) noted that when topical anaesthetic was applied to the soft palate, dorsum of the tongue and pillars of fauces, the overall regularity of the swallow-respiratory pattern was reduced. Increased oral transit time was noted and post-swallow respiration was not always expiratory in nature. Post-swallow coughing occurred, which indicated potential laryngeal penetration or aspiration. Although based on a small number of subjects, this experiment serves to show the importance of oral afferents in providing sensory information to the swallowing centre and the subsequent effect this has on the respiratory centre. In short, poor oral sensory perception adversely affects swallow-respiratory coordination. Interestingly, blindfolding the subjects, denying them visual perception of an incoming bolus did not affect swallow-respiratory patterns.

Hiss et al. (2001) have reported lower values of expectation for the 'exhalation-swallow-exhalation' pattern. In a study of 60 individuals they found that exhalation preceded swallowing in 75% of cases and exhalation followed swallowing in 86% of cases. They cited differences in method of bolus delivery to account for differences between their results and researchers such as Selley et al. (1989a). In another study, Hirst et al. (2002) reported that 91% of swallows were followed by an exhalation. This data is more in keeping with the Selley et al. (1989a) results.

THE SWALLOW-RESPIRATORY CYCLE OF DYSPHAGIC INDIVIDUALS

Selley et al. (1989b) have also investigated the swallow-respiratory patterns of dysphagic individuals with neurological impairment. They found that individuals with stroke, motor neurone disease and multiple sclerosis had different swallow-respiratory patterns from those of healthy individuals. Importantly, they found the swallow-respiratory patterns appeared to be aetiology specific. For example, the stroke group showed variable respiratory patterns upon spoon contact with the mouth, a variable length of time from the end of spoon contact to the swallow and variable respiration immediately after the swallow. In fact 43% of respiratory events immediately post swallow were *inspiratory* in nature, compared with only 5% in the healthy population. Similar results have also been reported by Leslie et al. (2002) who found that fewer stroke patients 'always breathed out' post swallow and some did not breathe out at all when compared with a control group. Any residue left in the pharyngeal or laryngeal region could potentially be drawn into the respiratory system, rather than expelled. In addition, where healthy individuals showed a fairly consistent pattern of swallow-respiratory behaviour from one swallow to the next, this consistency was lost in the stroke population. The multiple sclerosis group also showed an individual pattern. This latter group showed variable inhalation or exhalation at spoon contact, a prolonged and variable amount of time between spoon contact and the swallow and apnoea beginning earlier and lasting for longer than in the healthy group. The motor neurone disease group had essentially the same swallow-respiratory pattern as for healthy individuals except that they produced multiple and rapid swallows per teaspoonful of fluid. For all other groups (both normal and dysphagic), only one swallow per teaspoon of 5 ml was recorded.

By way of explanation, Selley et al. (1989b) suggested that the swallow pattern is mediated through the swallowing centre. If the swallowing centre does not receive appropriate information about an incoming bolus, it will not send appropriate messages to the respiratory centre. For both the stroke and MS subgroups, damage to nerves important to swallowing (e.g. cranial nerves V, VII, IX, X or XII) means that there is either insufficient sensory information to trigger the swallow or insufficient motor action available to complete the swallow safely (see also Chapter 9). The swallowing areas of the brain stem are unable to communicate effectively with the respiratory system, leading to abnormalities of the swallow-respiratory cycle as outlined above. For the motor neurone disease group, there may be some difficulty in clearing a bolus due to reduced tongue strength, which would afford bolus residue. The residue is picked up by the intact afferent (sensory) receptors, which alert

Table 4.1 Summary: the swallow-respiratory cycle

Timing of events	Healthy swallow-respiratory cycle	Dysphagic swallow-respiratory cycle
Immediately before the swallow	Small inhalation ↓ small exhalation	Stroke. Variable respiratory pattern
During the swallow	Apnoea(swallow)	Apnoea(swallow)
Immediately after the swallow	Immediate exhalation	Variable respiratory pattern post-swallow

the CNS that the bolus has not been adequately cleared and further swallows are triggered.

Individuals presenting with chronic obstructive pulmonary disease (COPD) present as another interesting group. During exacerbation of their disease state, these individuals interrupt the inspiratory phase and resume respiration more often in the inspiratory phase (Shaker et al., 1992). This is quite the opposite to what we know to be the normal pattern for healthy individuals. In the COPD group, the coordination between respiration and swallowing appears to be 'reset' during their disease exacerbation. It is possible that during an acute exacerbation of COPD, the body dictates that respiration is the most important function. The provision of sufficient oxygen may necessarily come at the expense of swallowing safety. The swallow-respiratory cycle patterns for healthy and dysphagic individuals are summarized in Table 4.1.

NEURAL REGULATION OF RESPIRATION FOR SWALLOWING

Giving due importance to the task of breathing, there are in fact three respiratory centres in the brain. The *inspiratory* and *expiratory* centres are located in the reticular formation of the medulla (Kiernan, 1998). These are associated with the nucleus of the tractus solitarius and the nucleus ambiguous (Sawczuk and Mosier, 2001). There is also a *pneumotaxic* area at the level of the junction between the pons and the medulla in the nucleus parabrachialis. The pneumotaxic centre regulates the rhythm of inspiration and exhalation and the switch between expiratory and inhalatory phases (Kiernan, 1998; Sawczuk and Mosier, 2001).

Inspiration is set in motion via carbon dioxide in the circulating blood. The amount of circulating carbon dioxide is relayed to the inspiratory centre, which uses reticulospinal connections to activate the diaphragm and intercostals muscles. There are also chemoreceptors, which respond to decreases in circulating *oxygen* in the blood. Alerted by carotid bodies (these are paired and near the bifurcation of the carotid arteries) and aortic bodies (near the aortic arch), impulses are transmitted to the nucleus of the tractus solitarius, which then relays this information to the

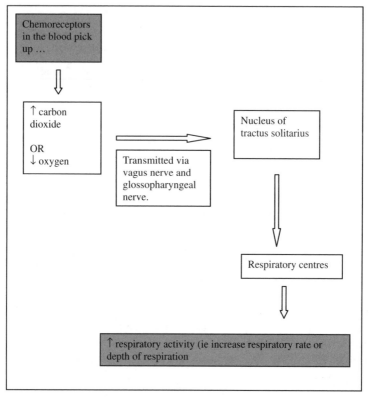

Figure 4.1   Schematic representation of the process of inhalation

respiratory centres. The chemoreceptors are sensitive to a reduction in circulating oxygen and also an increase in carbon dioxide. Excitation of the chemoreceptors causes an increase in respiratory activity – i.e. increased respiratory rate. Interestingly, the peripheral chemoreceptors respond more rapidly than for central stimulation (Guyton, 1991). Recall that the inspiratory and expiratory respiratory centres are located in the reticular formation and that the vagus and glossoppharyngeal nerves have their nuclei in the nucleus of the tractus solitarius. The nucleus of the tractus solitarius is adjacent to and synaptically linked with the reticular formation. The chemoreceptors use the vagus and glossopharyngeal nerves to relay impulses through the nucleus of the tractus solitarius to the respiratory centres. The response to a reduction in circulating oxygen is for an increase in rate and depth of breathing. This reflex operates under any circumstances that produce asphyxia. A schematic diagram of the respiratory process of inhalation is found in Figure 4.1.

Exhalation occurs when sensory endings in the bronchial tree signal that the lungs are inflated. Sensory neurones in the vagus nerve transmit this information to the expiratory centre through the nucleus of the tractus solitarius. Neurones in the expiratory centre then inhibit the actions of inspiration and the predominantly

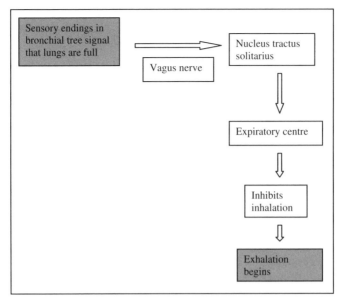

Figure 4.2   Schematic representation of the process of exhalation

passive process of exhalation begins. Figure 4.2 is a schematic diagram of the process of exhalation. The nucleus of the tractus solitarius plays a critical role as a relay system for the inspiratory centre and the expiratory centre and also, via reflex arcs, for the pneumotaxic centre. The vagus and glossophayngeal nerves provide key sensory inputs to this nucleus. These same nerves and nuclei are also critical for swallowing. For example, stimulation of the internal branch of the superior laryngeal nerve (a branch of the vagus nerve), can cause swallowing, apnoea and resetting of respiratory rhythm (Jafari et al., 2003). Note that changes to oxygen concentration have very little direct effect on the respiratory centre. What directly affects the respiratory centre and regulates breathing rate is in fact an increase in carbon dioxide levels.

The discussion above points to the fact that neurones controlling breathing and swallowing communicate at the level of the brain stem. True to the biological time-share concept, it has been suggested that the different functions required of the larynx (during breathing and swallowing) are assisted by reorganization of shared neural networks. This is significant as it suggests reorganization rather than a course of separate pathways (Sawczuk and Mosier, 2001). Recently, the hypoglossal nerve has been implicated in the link between the brain stem swallowing centre and the respiratory centres (Broussard and Altschuler, 2000; Sawczuk and Mosier, 2001). More specifically, inspiratory drive is said to influence protrusive tongue movement. When we inhale we require maximum air passage through the upper airway and into the trachea. This is achieved by opening the laryngeal and pharyngeal regions mediated by genioglossus, palatal elevator muscles, palatoglossus, palatopharyngeus and the posterior cricoarytenoid, which causes the vocal folds to open (abduct) (Sawczuk and Mosier, 2001). Tongue protrusion (via action of genioglossus) is tied to this act of maximizing air passage. Individuals who mouth-breathe may be seen to have their mouths open and tongue slightly protruding. In contrast, tongue retraction is necessary for initiating orpharyngeal swallowing and the commencement of airway protective measures such as laryngeal excursion. Given the tongue's dual role in both respiration and swallowing, Sawczuk and Mosier (2001: 18) suggest that 'subtle changes in the neural control of tongue movement may signal the transition between respiration and swallowing'.

ADVANCED CONSIDERATIONS – NEURAL INTERPLAY BETWEEN RESPIRATION AND SWALLOWING

There are a number of small but significant pieces of information that the clinician may find useful in dealing with complex neurogenic, surgical or neurosurgical cases. These relate to:

• the role of laryngeal irritant receptors;
• removal of laryngeal irritants; and
• protection of the airway during retching and vomiting.

Laryngeal irritant receptors

Laryngeal irritant receptors are unrelated to the respiratory cycle. They appear to be superficial as topical anaesthetics can block them. They are activated by mechanical and chemical stimuli (e.g. cigarette smoke). Interestingly, there appear to be different irritant receptors in the larynx to those in the tracheobronchial tree (Sant'Ambrogio et al., 1995). This has important implications for our understanding of dysphagic individuals with 'silent aspiration'. Individuals who 'silently' aspirate do not cough, clear their throat or have wet phonation so as to indicate that material has been aspirated. The irritant receptors in the larynx differ from those in the tracheobronchial tree, which may enable us to begin to unravel the conundrum of the 'silent aspirator'. This is illustrated by heart-lung transplanted individuals who have a poor or absent cough reflex to the inhalation of distilled water (Higgenbottam et al., 1989). The larynx of individuals with heart-lung transplants remains innervated but the tracheobronchial tree is no longer innervated (Higgenbottam et al., 1989). In an experiment where these individuals inhaled distilled water aerosol, the majority was reported to be deposited in the central airways (56%) with only a small amount deposited in the laryngeal/tracheal region (10%). When the vocal folds were directly stimulated by dropping distilled water directly onto their surface, all heart-lung transplant patients coughed. This suggests that the vocal folds need to be directly stimulated in order to provoke a cough reflex in individuals where the afferent receptors of the tracheobroncial tree or the neural connections from the tracheobronchial tree may be faulty.

Removal of laryngeal irritants

The cough reflex is a defensive reflex designed to remove irritant stimuli. The irritant could be either chemical or mechanical. Apnoea on the other hand is a protective reflex designed to prevent material from being aspirated in the first place. The cough reflex has both inspiratory and expiratory components. First, the individual breathes in. Then the epiglottis inverts and the vocal folds come together to trap the air within the lungs. Following this the abdominal muscles contract quite strongly, pushing against the diaphragm and against a closed glottis. Other expiratory muscles also contract to assist the process of coughing. The result of these events is a build up of pressure in the lungs. Once the pressure has built up the epiglottis and vocal folds open up suddenly and widely and the air that has been under pressure in the lungs explodes upwards into the pharynx. The compression of the lungs also causes the bronchi and the trachea to 'collapse towards each other' and produce narrow slits for the fast moving air stream to pass through. As a result of this action, any foreign material is carried on the fast-moving air stream up through the bronchi and trachea towards the pharynx (Guyton, 1991). When the sudden obstruction of the closed glottis is released, the 'linear velocity of air through the larynx is said to approach the speed of sound' (Lumb, 2000).

Protecting the airway during retching and vomiting

Gastric contents are high in acid content. If this acidic material is aspirated into the lungs it will rapidly damage the lung tissue. Aspiration of gastric contents is more life threatening than aspiration of food or fluid during swallowing. It is discussed further in Chapter 5. It is imperative that this material be kept out of the lungs. Vomiting and retching are two occasions where there is the potential to aspirate acidic gastric contents. The healthy body, is however, well designed to protect the airway from aspiration of gastric contents. During retching the airway is protected by glottic closure. This is a very tight glottic closure that is subtly different to the closure experienced during swallowing. During the effort closure that occurs during vomiting there is actual adduction of the laryngeal walls including both the true *and* false vocal folds. During normal swallowing the false vocal folds do not adduct. The thyroid cartilage is elevated during effort closure and approximates the hyoid bone as subglottic pressure increases (Aronson, 1985). Between retches the hyolaryngeal complex and pharyngeal constrictors elevate and the upper oesophageal sphincter closes, which helps to protect the airway (Lang et al., 2002). Vomiting occurs during the ascending phase of the retch. In addition, there are phases of ascending and descending hyolaryngeal and pharyngeal muscular movement. Reverse activation of the oesophagus and pharyngeal muscles occurs in order to expel gastric and/or refluxed intestinal contents towards the mouth. The laryngeal adductors are maximally activated in all phases of the vomit (Lang et al., 2002). The effort closure function of the larynx is also activated during coughing, throat clearing, urination, defecation and parturition (Aronson, 1985).

GLOTTIC CLOSURE DURING SWALLOWING

Glottic closure is critical to protecting the airway during swallowing. The first event of glottic closure is the movement of the arytenoids towards each other (adduction). After this the arytenoids come together and contact with each other. It is only *after* these events that the vocal folds come together. They do not completely come together until the larynx has begun elevating. In fact it has been observed endoscopically that the bolus can have reached the pyriform sinuses before true vocal fold closure has been realized (Ohmae et al., 1995). It has been suggested that the adduction of the arytenoids creates more space at the posterior end of the airway entrance for the divided bolus to safely enter the pyriform sinuses (Ohmae et al., 1995). The arytenoids also present as a mechanical barrier to the bolus. In addition, their movement lifts the aryepiglottic folds like a fist lifts a curtain up high. By pulling the aryepiglottic folds to height it assists in directing the bolus down into the pyriform sinuses. This is critical because, as stated above, the true vocal folds don't close until the bolus is well into the pharyngeal region.

Closure of the true vocal folds is the 'last frontier' in protection of the trachea and airway. The cords have three different closure patterns. Interestingly, only one closure pattern results in closure of the cords along their entire length. The other two patterns leave a separation between the cords, either (a) slit-like along the entire length, or (b) leaving a small gap at the posterior region (Shaker et al., 1990). This is an important point – this 'last frontier' is not the full mechanical barrier we might imagine it to be, and this is entirely normal. In healthy individuals it rarely presents a problem. In dysphagic individuals poor vocal fold mobility is a contributing factor to reduced airway protection (Sellars et al., 1999). It is also important to note that the false vocal folds generally do not come together during swallowing (Shaker et al., 1990).

Until this point, the role of the epiglottis has not been mentioned. The epiglottis is a broad flat structure with its base attached to the medial surface of the thyroid cartilage via the thyroepiglottic ligaments. It is also attached to the base of the tongue via a mucous membrane (Aronson, 1985). During swallowing the epiglottis descends to cover the laryngeal inlet. Movement of the epiglottis is predominantly a biomechanical event. It has little choice in the matter. The epiglottis covers the laryngeal inlet as a result of pressure from the tongue base above, in combination with lifting of the laryngeal system from below. The tongue base exerts pressure below it when delivering the bolus to the pharynx. The epiglottis is subject to the pressures from the tongue base, and these push the epiglottis away from the tongue base and towards the posterior pharyngeal wall. At the same time, laryngeal elevation effectively knocks the 'feet' of the epiglottis out from under it due to its connection with the thyroid cartilage. The combination of pressure from above and upward movement from below causes the epiglottis to move like a trap door and to come down over the top of the laryngeal inlet. This is not to say that it fits like a cork and forms a tight seal in this position. It is merely a mechanical barrier. Much like a rock in a stream, the epiglottis provides an obstacle to the fluid. The fluid will tend to move around the epiglottis and follow the path into the pyriform sinuses. In addition to arytenoid movement and epiglottic movement detailed above, these two structures also move towards each other to help achieve airway closure (Logemann et al., 1992).

Succinctly, then, to achieve glottic closure the following events occur in order:

- the arytenoids move towards each other and then come into contact with each other;
- the vocal folds start to come together and the larynx begins its upward and forward movement;
- the epiglottis begins its descent as a combination of pressure from above (tongue) and movement from below (laryngeal excursion);
- the arytenoids tilt or lurch forwards towards the base of the epiglottis and the epiglottis moves towards the arytenoids effecting arytenoid to base of epiglottic closure;
- the epiglottis assumes its horizontal position.

The true vocal folds may or may not be completely adducted along their full length when the bolus moves through the pharynx. Return to rest of the epiglottis depends on release of the tongue base movement and the elastic properties of the epiglottic cartilage (Logemann et al., 1992).

Airway closure is important in protecting the airway during the act of swallowing. An efficient swallow, however, is also dependent upon the respiratory system; namely adequate subglottic air pressure. The lack of subglottic pressure is most keenly demonstrated in the tracheostomized population. In this population, the airway is brought forward via a tracheostomy tube to the anterior neck region. The individual breathes directly through the tracheostomy tube and there is nothing to impede the flow of air into and out of the trache tube (i.e. no subglottic pressure). The tracheostomy population is discussed in detail in Chapters 5 and 9. Researchers have found that when subglottic pressure is restored in the tracheostomized population that aspiration is markedly reduced (Eibling and Gross, 1996; Suiter et al., 2003) and that the velocity of bolus transit through the pharynx appears to be improved (Eibling and Gross, 1996). Eibling and Gross (1996) state that subglottic pressure peaks during swallowing. During speech, air flows out from the lungs and causes pressure under the glottic 'shelf' (the vocal folds). A certain amount of pressure will force the vocal folds open but then a sudden drop in pressure below the cords causes a suction effect and with the aid of elasticity of the ligaments, the cords are drawn back together again. This is the basic principle behind the production of speech. Successive bursts of air are released into the space above the vocal folds and these puffs of air vibrate the vocal folds and cause phonation to occur. A change in subglottic pressure, then, is intimately linked to whether the vocal folds come together or not. We know that the vocal folds are drawn together during swallowing to assist in protection of the airway. Subglottic pressure is, therefore, very important to the vocal folds being able to achieve closure during swallowing. There are a number of mechanisms by which subglottic closure can be improved. In the person with a tracheostomy these include: decannulation or use of a one way speaking valve. For non-tracheostomized individuals it may include use of the 'supraglottic swallow technique' (discussed in Chapter 11) and muscle strengthening targeting this region (e.g. Valsalva manoeuvre). Surgical interventions to optimize glottic closure include medialization thyroplasty and vocal fold injection (Eibling and Gross, 1996). These techniques are also discussed in Chapter 11.

DEGLUTITION APNOEA

Two mechanisms have been proposed to explain the occurrence of deglutition apnoea. Deglutition apnoea is a result of either

• a glottic closure mechanism; or
• a centrally mediated response during swallowing.

The trigger produces an apnoeic period where respiration ceases, however, the glottis may or may not be closed during this apnoeic interval (Perlman et al., 2000). Deglutition apnoea should occur before the bolus is propelled into the pharynx and should also be maintained for as long as there is any material in the pharynx. The bolus should have left the pharynx before deglutition apnoea finishes and normal tidal respirations recommence. Variations to deglutition apnoea as a result of volume and viscosity are also provided.

TWO MECHANISMS OF DEGLUTITION APNOEA

Does deglutition apnoea occur because the laryngeal mechanism is mechanically 'shut down' during swallowing, or does it occur secondary to a neural command? Hiss et al. (2003) found a novel way of addressing the issue. Individuals who have undergone a laryngectomy have anatomically separate respiratory and swallowing systems. In brief, the larynx is removed and the opening to the trachea is rerouted to the anterior of the neck. The individual with laryngectomy breathes through a stoma in the neck. Food, however, continues to be ingested through the mouth, into the pharynx and via the oesophagus into the stomach. If deglutition apnoea is *only due to mechanical closure forces* of the larynx during swallowing (i.e. closure of the arytenoids, closure of the vocal folds, and closure of the epiglottis), then deglutition apnoea should no longer be seen in individuals who have undergone a laryngectomy. Physiologically there is no longer a need for deglutition apnoea – there is no longer a shared respiratory and swallowing pathway. So Hiss et al.'s (2003) question was simple – was deglutition apnoea maintained in the laryngectomy population? The answer was that it was. Without a larynx, and with no physiological need for deglutition apnoea, individuals with laryngectomy still exhibited deglutition apnoea. In fact, their periods of deglutition apnoea were nearly triple that of intact healthy individuals. There are two important pieces of information to take from this study. Firstly, that deglutition apnoea exists in individuals who physiologically no longer need it points to a neural command that is activated for deglutition apnoea to occur. It shows that the mechanics of closing the larynx are not (solely) responsible for initiating and maintaining deglutition apnoea.

Why then do individuals with laryngectomy produce longer periods of deglutition apnoea? Hiss et al. (2003) report that deglutition apnoea is most likely associated with the duration of the pharyngeal phase and or the opening of the upper oesophageal sphincter. If material remains in the pharynx or if the UES fails to open sufficiently, material will remain in a precarious position – to be breathed in the moment a large inspiratory breath occurs. Information about the pharyngeal phase is most likely mediated by mechanoreceptors in the pharynx and these provide an afferent feedback loop to the brain stem. Individuals with laryngectomy are reported to have pharyngeal phases twice as long as those of healthy intact individuals (0.6 s healthy; 1.2 s laryngectomy) (Hiss et al., 2003). The reasons for increased pharyngeal phase include:

- an absence of hyolaryngeal excursion to open the UES thus delaying and inhibiting entry of the bolus into the oesophagus; and
- increased pharyngeal resistance.

Both of these events will increase the amount of time that the bolus spends in the pharynx. Hiss et al. (2003) suggest that mechanoreceptors in the pharynx are alerted that a bolus remains in the pharynx and pass this information to the brain stem. The brain stem responds by continuing to inhibit respiration. This explains the significantly longer periods of deglutition apnoea in individuals with laryngectomy compared with healthy intact individuals. It is interesting to note, however, even 1 year post-laryngectomy deglutition apnoea was preserved. Hiss et al. (2003) suggest that in addition to the concept of a dedicated neural command for deglutition apnoea emanating from the brain stem, that deglutition apnoea may also be a habitual motor response. It would be interesting to see if individuals with very long-term laryngectomies still produced an apnoeic response during swallowing. The concept of neural plasticity and the potential abolishment of deglutition apnoea is fascinating. Investigation of individuals who had undergone a pharyngectomy or laryngopharyngectomy and received a jejunal graft may throw some light on the concept of deglutition apnoea being mediated by sensory receptors in the pharynx as outlined above.

FACTORS AFFECTING DEGLUTITION APNOEA

Having established that even individuals with laryngectomy continue to produce deglutition apnoea, even when it is no longer required physiologically, what other variables influence deglutition apnoea? Hiss et al. (2001) investigated the effects of age, gender and bolus volume on deglutition apnoea. All of these variables were found to affect deglutition apnoea. Hiss et al. (2001) found that swallowing apnoea duration increased with increasing age. This is complimentary to physiologic information of changes in aged swallowing – elderly swallows are slower than younger swallows (see Chapter 2). Deglutition apnoea was shown to be on average, 0.84 s for young individuals (20–39 years); 0.92 s for middle aged individuals (40–59 years) and 1.10 s for elderly individuals (60–83 years). This data is complimented by the results of Hirst et al. (2002). Hiss et al. (2001) also found that deglutition apnoea was longer in females than in males. The reason for this may be due to anatomical differences between males and females. Females are reported to have a longer UES opening time than males and so boluses of similar size may take a longer period of time to pass through the relatively smaller UES in the female as opposed to the male. Interestingly, however, the gender differences noted for bolus swallows were different to what happened with saliva swallows. In swallowing saliva males showed decreased deglutition apnoea duration as they aged, whereas women showed an increased period of deglutition apnoea as they aged. These results suggest that saliva should be considered as a physiologically independent bolus. Indeed the deglutition apnoea associated with saliva swallows was often many times longer than the swallow apnoea duration recorded for a 20 ml swallow, regardless of age. This is an interesting finding given that the average bolus size for a saliva swallow is approximately 1 ml. The reasons for the differences between saliva swallows and bolus swallows are not well understood. As hinted at above, deglutition apnoea also changes as a function of bolus volume. Specifically deglutition apnoea increases with an increase in bolus volume.

Deglutition apnoea and bolus volume

Martin et al. (1994) reported that the duration of apnoea is quite similar for 3 ml, 10 ml and 20 ml bolus volumes; i.e. it was approximately 1 s (1.09 ± 0.27 s). These results are similar to those reported by Perlman et al. (2000). This is contrary to the results of Hiss et al. (2001) who found that deglutition apnoea duration increases with increases in bolus volume. However, for a very large volume, such as 100 ml as ingested during continuous straw drinking, the apnoeic period was noted to be considerably longer (7.71 s ± 5.51 s) (Martin et al., 1994). Also of interest was the fact that these large volume swallows were more inclined to produce an inspiratory post-swallow breath, going against the norm of the expiratory post-swallow breath production. Physiologically these results should not be a surprise. After being without air for 7 s, it is likely that chemoreceptors have alerted the respiratory centres to drops in circulating oxygen and increases in carbon dioxide, hence triggering an inspiratory event. As Martin et al. (1994) note, healthy individuals do not gasp for air after swallowing or report shortness of breath. However, for dysphagic individuals, particularly those with concurrent respiratory difficulties (e.g. chronic obstructive pulmonary disease – COPD), the mere act of swallowing may jeopardize their fragile respiratory system. In this case, the likely scenario is that a swallow is interrupted in order to 'take a breath'. This act can end up doing more harm than good though if aspiration is the outcome. Any lack of coordination between respiration and swallowing, such as that which might occur after a stroke, would have similar consequences. Table 4.2 provides a summary of the healthy and dysphagic deglutition apnoea durations.

Table 4.2 Summary: healthy and dysphagic deglutition apnoea durations

Healthy individuals 3 ml, 10 ml, 20 ml boluses	Healthy individuals 100 ml boluses (continuous drinking)	Dysphagic individuals	Factors affecting deglutition apnoea
1.09 s(± 0.27 s)	7.71 s(± 5.51 s)	Stroke Some had no difference to healthy, others had apnoeic periods of between 10–20 s[1] *Laryngectomy*: Nearly triple the period of deglutition apnoea as healthy individuals	Age Gender Bolus volume

[1]Leslie et al., 2002.

Deglutition apnoea and bolus viscosity

Investigators have found that the viscosity of the bolus does not affect the duration of deglutition apnoea. Thin and thickened boluses (paste) have been found to produce similar durations of deglutition apnoea (thin 0.788 ± 0.318 s; paste 0.742 ± 0.278 s) (Perlman et al., 2000; Leslie et al., 2002). Leslie et al. (2002) compared healthy individuals with post-stroke dysphagic individuals. They found there to be no significant difference in the duration of swallowing apnoea between the two groups for water and yoghurt consistencies. Both groups maintained levels of approximately 0.75 s. These findings were consistent despite the fact that the post-stroke group showed abnormal swallow-respiratory patterns as compared with the healthy group.

RESPIRATORY FACTORS THAT CONTRIBUTE TO OR PREVENT ASPIRATION

Morton et al. (2002) investigated a group of individuals with known dysphagia in addition to poor control of respiration. They found that, for those who aspirated, the bolus or bolus residue remained in the pharynx for a significantly longer amount of time. Premature spillage or delayed swallow onset might have resulted in material entering and dwelling in the pharynx prior to the swallow. Alternatively, the material may have remained in the pharynx after the swallow due to inadequate pharyngeal clearance or poor laryngeal elevation during the swallow. For individuals who aspirated, material remained in the pharynx for approximately 6 s, whereas for non-aspirators the material only remained in the pharynx for 2.4 s. It was not merely the fact that material was left sitting in the pharynx that distinguished individuals who aspirated from those individuals who did not aspirate. Individuals were far more likely to aspirate if:

- they left material in the pharynx for a long time (i.e. 6 s);
- during the time that the material was in the pharynx the individual spent a large percentage of the respiratory cycle in the inspiratory phase (e.g. 31.1%); and
- if the individual showed severely abnormal respiratory patterns during this period characterized by high velocity or chaotic respiratory patterns.

In fact, this type of disordered breathing was likely to induce aspiration even if the time in the pharynx was quite short. Morton et al. (2002) state that in individuals with poor swallow respiratory coordination, aspiration results from an interaction between:

- the amount of time material dwells in the pharynx;
- the amount of time spent in inspiration; and
- abnormality of the respiratory rhythm.

Children with Rett syndrome often present with dysphagia. This is due to a combination of oropharyngeal abnormalities and unusual respiratory patterns characterized by hyperventilation and periods of apnoea. Individuals with Rett syndrome can present with significantly delayed oropharyngeal transit times (Morton et al., 1997). Some individuals have been reported to take up to 27 s from spoon contact with the lips to the time of the swallow. In healthy individuals this time would be 1 s. Given the significant amount of time that the bolus was held within the oropharynx, one might assume that a portion of the bolus was aspirated. However, aspiration did not occur. During oropharyngeal manipulation and transport, the individuals showed apnoea intervals interspersed with *regular and controlled* respiratory patterns before the swallow took place. Compare this with an individual who took 6 s to generate a swallow and showed intermittent apnoeas interspersed with *irregular and sharp inspirations*. The latter individual was noted to aspirate. The control and regularity of respiration appears, therefore, to be vitally important to whether the respiratory system can be protected even in situations of 'grave danger'.

During smaller volume swallows (3–20 ml) the airway is protected by the apnoeic period beginning before the swallow (0.30 s) and continuing after the onset of swallowing (1.12 s). Differences are noted, however, for the 100 ml swallow where the apnoeic period begins 0.84 s before the swallow and continues after swallow onset (0.68 s). These results indicate that respiratory activity stops just before laryngeal elevation. The apnoeic period occurs during the swallow, but then ends *before* completing the swallow. Perlman et al. (2000) concur that when apnoea begins, the bolus head is either in the oral cavity or the valleculae, and when apnoea ends, the bolus head is well into the oesophagus. Martin et al. (1994) found that the majority of subjects produced a short expiration during descent and reopening of the larynx. It is this post swallow gesture that has been termed the 'glottal release' in the discussion of cervical auscultation (see Chapter 7). Perlman et al. (2000) also reported finding a highly consistent event immediately following the period of deglutition apnoea. They reported this event to be the release of a valved seal, potentially at the level of the glottis. Lang et al. (2002) reported that during swallowing in dogs the airway is protected by laryngeal elevation and glottic closure, followed imme-diately by brief activation of the laryngeal abductors, thereby momentarily open-ing the glottis. The authors suggested that this immediate laryngeal abduction after the swallow may allow the escape of pressurized subglottal air, thereby removing material from the laryngeal vestibule. The expiratory burst post swallow may be very important in preventing trace or chronic aspiration. The action of expelling air upwards post swallow would remove residue from the immediate laryngeal region, positioning it in the pharynx. In the pharynx the material could then be swallowed, coughed up or expectorated. In any event the respiratory system is kept free from potential 'debris'.

CLINICAL RELEVANCE

If material is pooled in the pharynx, it is important that actions do not occur that will draw it into the respiratory system (i.e. the trachea and its subsystems). A longer pe-riod of apnoea or a prolonged expiration – both components of the supraglottic swal-low technique – may assist in protecting the individual from aspiration if pharyngeal pooling is a significant feature of the dysphagia. Respiratory rhythm should also be integrated into the management of dysphagic individuals. Chaotic breathing (i.e. variations in depth and rate of respiration) is only likely to increase the likelihood of aspiration. Interestingly, a careful pattern of low velocity and regular breathing can reduce the likelihood of aspiration of the pooled material, even in the presence of pharyngeal pooling. Morton et al. (2002) indicate that this pattern of integrating a safer respiratory pattern with an impaired swallowing system is common in people with Rett syndrome, and means that aspiration is often avoided.

Morton et al. (2002) stress that the respiratory system, specifically respiratory control, should be treated alongside dysphagia. They suggest that, when an indi-vidual is being fed, the caregiver should be cognizant of the timing of the respiratory phase. In addition, the caregiver should allow sufficient time for the dysphagic indi-vidual to swallow and regain respiration before the next bolus is presented. Smaller boluses may be useful in reducing the amount of material that pools in the pharynx, however, the clinician should also be aware that the bolus should be large enough to trigger a sensory response in the oral and pharyngeal phases of swallowing (see Chapter 3).

There is further evidence to suggest that it is imperative that swallowing and respiration be viewed simultaneously. Individuals who present with dysphagia post stroke should be assessed for regularity of breathing pattern, both at rest and dur-ing feeding. Leslie et al. (2002) found that more than 25% of stroke patients who presented with clinical signs of dysphagia also had disordered breathing patterns. In these individuals apnoeic periods varied between 10 s to 20 s and were then followed by eight to 12 breaths. These findings had been 'clinically silent' prior to investiga-tion of breathing patterns in the group. Recall that for healthy individuals, the period of deglutition apnoea is usually less than one second! The investigators also found that the post-stroke group had faster respiratory rates than the control group during resting respiration.

The Leslie et al. (2002) study raises some questions:

- Is the abnormal respiratory pattern a feature of stroke? If this is the case, is the chaotic breathing the catalyst for difficulty coordinating respiration and swallowing?
- Alternatively, does impaired oropharyngeal function (premature spillage or insufficient pharyngeal clearance) cause changes in respiratory patterns? In this case the dysphagia contributes to the abnormal respiratory pattern.

It may also be possible for both scenarios to occur at the same time, particularly where the nucleus of the tractus solitarius has been specifically affected.

RESTING RESPIRATORY RATE

Resting respiratory rate should also be considered. The work of Leslie et al. (2002) suggests that abnormalities in resting respiratory rate may give subclinical markers to individuals at high risk of developing chest infections. This is due to suspected lack of swallow-respiratory coordination, or impairments to the person's ability to regulate breathing, which then impact upon swallowing. Respiratory rate is measured by counting the number of breaths taken in one full minute. It is possible to count the number of breaths taken in 15 s and multiply by four; however, this method is more prone to error than measurement over one full minute. The normal resting respiratory rate for adults is 16–24 breaths/minute (Hooker et al., 1989). Women are noted to have a faster respiratory rate that men (women mean rate = 20.9; men, mean respiratory rate = 19.4). Tachypnea, or an elevated respiratory rate can be defined as a respiratory rate exceeding 24 breaths per minute (Hooker et al., 1989). Note also, that lung infections and pneumonia are associated with an increased respiratory rate (Hooker et al., 1989). Normal respiratory rates are shown in Table 4.3.

Table 4.3 Normal respiratory rates (breaths per minute)

Age	Mean	Standard deviation
0–1 years	39	11
1–2 years	30	6
2–3 years	28	4
3–4 years	25	4
4–5 years	27	5
5–6 years	23	5
6–7 years	25	5
7–8 years	24	6
Adult male	19.4	4
Adult female	20.9	3.9

Source: Hooker et al., 1989; Hooker et al., 1992.

There is also some suggestion that, in older individuals, respiratory rate may increase marginally immediately after swallowing, showing a variation from a resting respiratory rate of 15.6 breaths/minute to 17.3 breaths/minute immediately after each swallow (Hirst et al., 2002). Note that, although the difference was statistically significant, both values fall within the normal respiratory rate range for adults, according to Table 4.3.

Respiratory rate values are higher in young children. Respiratory rate is inversely related to age, that is, the younger the person, the higher the respiratory rate. In children under the age of 1 year the range was 22 to 65 breaths/minute with an average of 39. Between the ages of 1 to 2 years this falls to a mean of 30 breaths/minute. Between 2 and 3 years the rate drops again to 28 breaths/minute and for 3 to 4 years to 25 breaths/minute. From 4 to 7 years there are fluctuations between 23 to 27 breaths/minute. By 8 years of age and beyond, respiratory rate is equivalent to the adult range (Hooker et al., 1992). Respiratory rates are detailed in Table 4.3. In the paediatric populations, elevated respiratory rates have been associated with pneumonia, asthma, bronchiolitis, salicylism and sepsis (Hooker et al., 1992).

CONCLUSION

Finally it is imperative that swallowing be viewed as part of a continuum with respiration. The integrity of the swallowing system, the respiratory system and the links between the two are critical for maintaining safe swallowing.

REFERENCES

Aronson AE (1985) Clinical Voice Disorders: An Interdisciplinary Approach (2nd edn). New York: Thieme.

Broussard DI, Altschuler SM (2000) Central integration of swallow and airway-protective reflexes. American Journal of Medicine 108(4A): 62s–67s.

Eibling DE, Gross RD (1996) Subglottic air pressure: a key component of swallowing efficiency. Annals of Otology Rhinology and Laryngology 105: 253–8.

Guyton AC (1991) Textbook of Medical Physiology. Philadelphia: Harcourt Brace Jovanovich.

Higgenbottam T, Jackson M, Woolan P, et al. (1989) The cough response to ultrasonically nebulized distilled water in heart-lung transplantation patients. American Review of Respiratory Disease 140: 58–61.

Hirst LJ, Ford GA, Gibson J, et al. (2002) Swallow-induced alterations in breathing in normal older people. Dysphagia 17: 152–61.

Hiss SG, Strauss M, Treole K, et al. (2003) Swallowing apnea as a function of airway closure. Dysphagia 18: 293–300.

Hiss SG, Treole K, Stuart A (2001) Effects of age, gender, bolus volume, and trial on swallowing apnea duration and swallow/respiratory phase relationships of normal adults. Dysphagia 16: 128–35.

Hooker EA, O'Brien DJ, Danzl DF, et al. (1989) Respiratory rates in emergency department patients. Journal of Emergency Medicine 7: 129–32.

Hooker EA, Danzl DF, Brueggmeyer M, et al. (1992) Respiratory rates in pediatric emergency patients. Journal of Emergency Medicine 10: 407–10.

Jafari S, Prince RA, Kim DY, et al. (2003) Sensory regulation of swallowing and airway protection: a role for the internal superior laryngeal nerve in humans. Journal of Physiology 550(1): 287–304.

Kiernan JA (1998) Barr's The Human Nervous System: An Anatomical Viewpoint (7th edn). Philadelphia: Lippincott-Raven.

Lang IM, Dana N, Medda BK, et al. (2002) Mechanisms of airway protection during retching, vomiting and swallowing. American Journal of Physiology – Gastrointestinal and Liver Physiology 283(3): G529–G536.

Leslie P, Drinnan MJ, Ford GA, et al. (2002) Resting respiration in dysphagic patients following acute stroke. Dysphagia 17: 208–13.

Logemann JA, Kahrilas PJ, Cheng J, et al. (1992) Closure mechanisms of laryngeal vestibule during swallow. American Journal of Physiology 262: G338–G344.

Lumb AB (2000) Nunn's Applied Respiratory Physiology. Oxford: Butterworth Heinemann.

Morton RE, Bonas R, Tarrant SC, et al. (1997) Respiration patterns during feeding in Rett syndrome. Developmental Medicine and Child Neurology 39: 607–13.

Morton R, Minford J, Ellis R (2002) Aspiration with dysphagia: The interaction between oropharyngeal and respiratory impairments. Dysphagia 17: 192–6.

Martin BJ, Logemann JA, Shaker R, et al. (1994) Coordination between respiration and swallowing: respiratory phase relationships and temporal integration. Journal of Applied Physiology 76(2): 714–23.

Nishino T, Yonezawa T, Honda Y (1985) Effects of swallowing on the pattern of continuous respiration in human adults. American Review of Respiratory Disease 132(6): 1219–22.

OhmaeY, Logemann JA, Kaiser P, et al. (1995) Timing of glottic closure during swallowing. Head and Neck 17: 394–402.

Perlman AL, Ettema SL, Barkmeier J (2000) Respiratory and acoustic signals associated with bolus passage during swallowing. Dysphagia 15: 89–94.

Sant'Ambrogio G, Tsubone H, Sant'Ambrogio FB (1995) Sensory information from the upper airway: Role in the control of breathing. Respiration Physiology 102: 1–16.

Sawczuk A, Mosier KM (2001) Neural control of tongue movement with respect to respiration and swallowing. Critical Reviews in Oral Biology and Medicine 12(1): 18–37.

Sellars C, Campbell AM, Stott DJ, et al. (1999) Swallowing abnormalities after acute stroke: a case control study. Dysphagia 14: 212–18.

Selley WG, Flack FC, Ellis RE, et al. (1989a) Respiratory patterns associated with swallowing: Part 1. The normal adult pattern and changes with age. Age and Ageing 18: 168–172.

Selley WG, Flack FC, Ellis RE, et al. (1989b) Respiratory patterns associated with swallowing: Part 2. Neurologically impaired dysphagic patients. Age and Ageing 18: 173–6.

Selley WG, Flack FC, Ellis RE (1990a) The Exeter dysphagia assessment technique. Dysphagia 4: 227–35.

Selley WG, Ellis RE, Flack FC, et al. (1990b) Coordination of sucking, swallowing and breathing in the newborn: Its relationship to infant feeding and normal development. British Journal of Disorders of Communication 25: 311–27.

Shaker R, Dodds WJ, Dantas RO, et al. (1990) Coordination of deglutitive glottic closure with oropharyngeal swallowing. Gastroenterology 98: 1478–84.

Shaker R, Li Q, Ren J, et al. (1992) Coordination of deglutition and phases of respiration: effect of aging, tachypnea, bolus volume and chronic obstructive pulmonary disease. Gastroenterology 263: G750–G755.

Suiter DM, McCullough GH, Powell PW (2003) Effects of cuff deflation and one-way tracheostomy speaking valve placement on swallow physiology. Dysphagia 18: 284–92.

5 Medical Management of Patients at Risk of Aspiration

RODD BROCKETT

INTRODUCTION

Aspiration is the syndrome where either regurgitant stomach contents or oropharyngeal contents end up travelling past the larynx into the trachea and lungs. Thereafter, there may or may not be infection (tracheobronchitis or pneumonia). It has been estimated that approximately 10% of cases of community-acquired pneumonia are actually aspiration pneumonia (Moine et al., 1994). There are no data on the incidence of aspiration itself.

In this chapter we will consider the risk factors for aspiration, the outcomes of aspiration, what the signs and symptoms of aspiration are and what the alternatives to normal oral nutrition are for patients at risk of, or with, aspiration. We will also discuss tracheostomy tubes.

I have kept references to a minimum – the references cited exemplify 'consensus' viewpoints. The recommended reading article is basically a brief overview of the medical aspects of aspiration, written for general practitioners.

RISK FACTORS FOR ASPIRATION

The risk factors for aspiration include anything that impairs consciousness, gastroesophageal reflux, or any cause of dysphagia. It is more common amongst the elderly because of their increased risks of dysphagia, the events associated with impairment of consciousness and gastroesophageal reflux disease. For instance, it has been shown that the risk of aspiration pneumonia is increased threefold amongst residents of nursing homes (Marrie et al., 1986), probably because of their decreased level of consciousness and/or the presence of clinical or subclinical dysphagia.

MECHANISMS THAT PROTECT THE RESPIRATORY TRACT

The protective mechanisms for the airway during swallowing are described in detail in Chapters 1 and 4. The swallow reflex is described in greater depth in Chapters 1,

Dysphagia: Foundation, Theory and Practice. Edited by J. Cichero and B. Murdoch
© 2006 John Wiley & Sons, Ltd.

2 and 3. There are three key mechanisms to protect the respiratory tract from the aspiration of oropharyngeal or gastric secretions/contents: the cough reflex, swallowing reflexes and the oesophageal sphincters. The cough reflex is activated whenever an irritant gas or fluid or particles contact nerve receptors within the larynx. It involves the explosive contraction of expiratory muscles against the closed vocal cords that then suddenly open allowing the forced exhalation out (hopefully carrying the irritant with it). It does not matter whether the irritant is breathed in, aspirated or transported up the mucociliary escalator (see below). The oesophageal sphincters alternately relax and then contract to allow food through – this is an involuntary or reflex action that occurs once the patient has voluntarily moved the food bolus to the pharynx from the mouth. The sphincters also contract in a reflex fashion when there is distension of the stomach to keep stomach contents out of the oesophagus and ultimately the larynx/oropharynx.

GASTROESOPHAGEAL REFLUX

The importance of adequate functioning of these sphincters becomes clear in light of gastroesophageal reflux. Gastroesophageal reflux is the syndrome whereby gastric contents spontaneously move back up the oesophagus into the pharynx. This can be due to mechanical problems with swallowing (see below), due to anatomical problems such as a hiatus hernia (where part of the stomach is above the diaphragm, thereby rendering the lower oesophageal sphincter ineffective), weak lower oesophageal sphincter (especially relative weakness when opposed by gravity when bending over or opposed by obesity) and gastric stasis (also known as gastroparesis, where the stomach fails to empty and move food along in a timely fashion). Gastroparesis is particularly common in hospital patients because any severe illness will cause gastric dysmotility such that gastric emptying is slowed down.

IMPAIRED LEVEL OF CONSCIOUSNESS

There are multiple causes of impairment in level of consciousness. Head injury, therapeutic general anaesthetics or administration of sedative drugs, intentional or unintentional drug overdose, seizures, toxaemia from infection, cerebrovascular accidents or intracranial haemorrhage are just some of the many causes of deterioration in a patient's level of consciousness. A cerebrovascular accident is the interruption of blood supply to part of a patient's brain resulting in death of part of the brain and is very common. Mendelson's syndrome of aspiration pneumonitis was first described in the postoperative course of patients receiving a general anaesthetic for obstetric conditions, where the twin problems were increased abdominal pressure forcing gastric contents (in a patient who was both non-fasting and, due to labour, suffering from gastroparesis) back past the lower oesophageal sphincter and the anaesthetic abolishing the sphincter's tone and reflex contraction.

CAUSES OF DYSPHAGIA

Dysphagia, or disordered swallowing, likewise has a multitude of causes that can be further divided into mechanical (muscular) or neurological. Mechanical problems include pouches, webs, strictures and surgical changes. A muscular disorder called achalasia, which is due to a disorder of smooth muscle in the wall of the oesophagus, can cause the lower oesophageal sphincter to fail with free reflux of gastric contents back up the oesophagus with the possibility of aspiration. Neurological causes can include upper motor neurone causes such as cerebrovascular accidents, tumours, hydrocephalus and rarer disorders such as motor neurone disease, Parkinson's disease and multiple sclerosis just to name a few. Of patients who suffer a CVA, 40% to 70% will have swallowing dysfunction (Kidd et al., 1993). These are called upper motor neurone lesions because they affect the nerve cells and transmitting nerve fibres that are above the lower motor neurone system. The lower motor neurone system is the nerve cell body, transmitting nerve fibre, the junction between the nerve fibre and the muscle and the muscle itself. This is basically located in the lower part of the central nervous system known as the brain stem, which lies between the cortex and the spinal cord. Lower motor neurone diseases include myasthenia gravis, general debility, malnutrition, hypophosphataemia (refeeding a starved patient can cause this), other electrolyte abnormalities and lesions such as bleeding/trauma/stroke to the brain stem.

CONSEQUENCES OF ASPIRATION: PNEUMONIA AND PNEUMONITIS

Aspiration may or may not end up in pneumonia. Pneumonia is the active infection of lung tissue by an infectious agent – which might be bacterial, viral, fungal or other rarer organisms – with resultant inflammatory changes. Pneumonitis is the sterile inflammatory changes in the lungs without the growth of infectious agents. The two can occur simultaneously or separately but aspiration pneumonia is usually preceded by aspiration pneumonitis. Aspiration pneumonia mostly involves bacterial infection, although a small subset may have fungal agents implicated.

It is suggested that even common causes of community acquired pneumonia, such as the bacteria *Streptococcus pneumoniae, Mycoplasma pneumoniae,* and *Haemophilus pneumophila* and viruses such as adenovirus, respiratory synctial virus, influenza and parainfluenza, usually colonize the oropharynx first before being aspirated down into the lungs to cause pneumonia. The oropharynx is normally colonized by fairly benign and non-virulent organisms. Certain risk factors increase the risk of colonization of the oropharynx with more virulent organisms such as gram negative bacilli or MRSA ('golden staph'). These include prolonged hospitalization, exposure to antibiotics, significant medical diseases (chronic heart or lung disease, diabetes, renal failure, liver disease), invasive (via a tube) ventilation and smoking.

Most people do not develop complications from these subclinical aspiration syndromes because of the small amounts of fluid involved as well as the defence mechanisms that protect the tracheobronchial tree and lungs from infection. Of course, large aspirated amounts will overwhelm these defences. The defence mechanisms include coughing, active ciliary transport and immune reactions. The mucociliary escalator is the combination of the mucus lining that coats the airways and traps small particles (larger particles are usually deposited on the oropharynx or nasopharynx and are filtered out by the nostrils) in the airway, as well as bacteria, and the minute hairs that whisk the trapped small particles up the trachea to the vocal cords to be coughed out or swallowed. The immune reactions include humoral immunity, mediated by antibodies to the infectious agent, cellular immunity, mediated by cells such as T lymphocytes, and innate immunity, mediated by alveolar macrophages and secreted toxins within the alveolus (air sac). Weakening of these defences will increase the risks of acquired infection from aspiration of even these small amounts. Weakening can be done by things such as smoking, which impairs coughing and the mucociliary escalator. The mucociliary escalator can also be impaired by general anaesthetics, viral or bacterial infections, and even intubation for ventilation. Cough can be impaired by anything that affects respiratory muscle strength such as chronic obstructive lung disease, or any factor that depresses the level of consciousness, or lower motor neurone disease. Drugs such as chemotherapy to treat cancer or immunosuppressive drugs such as steroids to treat overactive immune systems can all weaken the humoral and cellular immune systems. A myriad of diseases can also damage the immune system, ranging from diabetes through heart failure to autoimmune diseases where an overactive immune system actually attacks the body. Finally, inhaled toxins (such as asbestos and those in cigarette smoke), viral infections and starvation can damage the innate immune systems.

ASPIRATION PNEUMONITIS

As mentioned earlier, pneumonitis is a sterile inflammatory change in the lungs without the growth of infectious agents. The inhalation into the lungs of sterile stomach contents causes Mendelson's syndrome. This is a chemical injury to the lung tissue caused by the acidic nature of the stomach fluids – as outlined above it was first described in pregnant patients in labour undergoing emergency operative deliveries under general anaesthetic. The acidic nature of the stomach fluids usually keeps such fluids free of organisms. However, the use of anti-ulcer therapy, particularly in ventilated patients often allows the stomach contents to become colonized with the same organisms as the oropharynx. Other factors may also increase the chances of such colonization, including use of enteral feeds (common in intensive care units), gastroparesis or small bowel obstruction. Such colonization increases the risk of pneumonia in the event of aspiration of stomach contents, although, of course, most aspiration episodes involve oropharyngeal secretions that are already colonized with such organisms.

Aspiration of sterile stomach contents leads to a chemical burn of the trachea, bronchi and lungs. It usually requires more than 30 ml to cause such a burn (James et al., 1984). Aspiration of particulate matter such as undigested or semi-digested food will increase the likelihood of pneumonia, and, in particular, lung abscesses, developing and has been suggested to increase even the severity of pneumonitis.

Aspiration pneumonitis may result in quite dramatic signs and symptoms. It may also be totally silent clinically – 63% of patients with known aspiration have been found to have no symptoms/signs (Warner et al., 1993). However, it was also suggested in the same study that those that did acquire symptoms were more likely to need more intensive support, such as ventilation and antibiotics, and were more likely to die. Symptoms that might be seen after an aspiration episode include cough, wheeze, fevers or chills, rigors, breathlessness or chest pain. Signs that might be elicited include temperatures, wheeze, crackles, bronchial breathing, reduced chest expansion, fast (often shallow) respirations, hypotension or cyanosis (a blue tinge to the skin). Bronchial breathing is where the breath sounds heard at the peripheries of the lung sound like those heard through the stethoscope over the centre of the lung. This is best noticed by observing that normally there is a small gap between the inspiratory noise and the expiratory noise at the periphery – in bronchial breathing there is no such gap. Simple testing may show a low oxygen level in the blood – low arterial or transcutaneous saturations – or radiological signs such as atelectasis (collapse) or consolidation. The natural tendency is for aspirated material to go down the right side of the tracheobronchial tree into the right lower lobe because the right main bronchus is straighter and more in alignment with the trachea. Therefore, radiological and clinical signs tend to be best seen at the right base/lower zones. These signs and symptoms are summarized in Table 5.1.

In simple terms, the principles of management of an acute episode of aspiration are as follows. The patient should be placed either head down to facilitate drainage of the fluids or in the lateral recovery position to try to minimize further aspiration. The witness should call for help, preferably trained help such as medical officers or nursing staff. Then suctioning should be done to clear the oropharynx. Antibiotics

Table 5.1 Signs and symptoms of an aspiration episode

Clinical signs	Specific respiratory signs	Radiological signs
• Cough	• Breathlessness or chest	• Lung atelectasis (collapse)
• Wheeze	pain	or consolidation
• Fevers or chills	• Wheeze	○ Specifically right base
• Rigors	• Crackles	or lower zones
• Increased temperature	• Bronchial breathing	
(38.0°C)	• Reduced chest expansion	
• Hypotension or cyanosis	• Fast (often shallow)	
	respiration	
	• Low oxygen saturation	
	levels	

may or may not be prescribed – it is my practice to withhold antibiotics unless the patient's physiological reserve is too small to tolerate the further insult of pneumonia as not all aspiration will result in infection. Chest radiographs may or may not be obtained, either as a baseline or to show the pneumonitis. If the patient produces sputum, samples should be taken and sent off to culture organisms. If impairment of gas exchange is severe enough, the patient may be moved to the intensive care unit and ventilation, either invasive via an endotracheal tube or non-invasive via a mask, may be initiated. Of course, further assessment is indicated once the patient's clinical condition stabilizes to lessen the risk of a repeat episode of aspiration (see Chapters 7, 8 and 14).

ASPIRATION PNEUMONIA

Aspiration pneumonia is an infection of the lungs caused by aspiration of oropharyngeal secretions or gastric contents down the trachea, past the glottic barrier. Aspiration can also lead to airway obstruction from laryngeal oedema (or foreign object such as a 'steak bolus'). It can also be a cause of an asthma attack (in those who are susceptible, especially asthmatics) or even a chronic cough. It can be associated with lung abscess, which can be the endpoint of a necrotizing pneumonia caused by a virulent (or more vicious) organism or due to obstruction of the airway to a part of the lung by foreign material (such as food), or even a chronic interstitial fibrosis (Irwin, 1999).

I will briefly outline the principles of medical management of aspiration pneumonia (i.e. infectious state). Antibiotic therapy is unequivocally indicated in these patients. Likewise, a chest radiograph is indicated. Surgery or thoracocentesis (drainage of the pleural/chest cavity by needle or operating telescope) may even be indicated. Otherwise, symptoms, signs, treatment and investigation are much as for aspiration pneumonitis. It can be very difficult to distinguish aspiration pneumonitis from pneumonia in the short term – with the passage of time, the difference will usually become clearer.

MANAGEMENT OF PATIENTS AT RISK OF OR WITH ASPIRATION

Unfortunately, the only dietary alternatives for the individual with aspiration or at risk of aspiration is to either (a) modify the diet mechanically to lessen the risk of aspiration or (b) to provide sustenance in an alternative form and via an alternative route. Diet modification is discussed in Chapter 11.

ALTERNATIVES TO THE ORAL DIET

Basically, the alternatives to an orally based diet come down to parenteral (into a vein) or nasogastric (this is a form of 'enteral feeding'). The diet can either be purely fluids or can be nutritional supplements. Enteral feeding is in general preferred to parenteral feeding. This is because the enteral route is definitely cheaper and easier. It is also less associated with infection – nasal tubes do cause sinusitis, but parenteral feeding lines become infected much more commonly. Enteral nutrition is felt to maintain gut integrity better than parenteral nutrition and it is therefore felt that it will probably reduce the risk of systemic infections – but the jury is still out on this issue.

Non-oral feeding

Nasogastric feeding is not the only alternative to the intravenous method – feeds can also be placed down a nasojejunal or percutaneous endoscopically placed gastrostomy (PEG) tube. A PEG tube is placed through the abdominal wall into the stomach to allow feeding. The placement of PEG or nasojejunal tubes is supposed to reduce the risk of aspiration, but unfortunately clinical practice has not borne this out. There is an increased chance of reaching nutritional targets but no decrease in the incidence of aspiration pneumonia (Park et al., 1992; Spain et al., 1995). Basically feeding tubes whether through the mouth, nose or abdominal wall only offer differences in amount of food being consumed and not in the risk of colonized oral secretions ending up down past the larynx. Oral secretions are discussed in detail in Chapter 6. Percutaneous endoscopically placed gastrostomy tubes are usually inserted for nursing convenience – particularly for nursing home care – as they are easier to maintain and less likely to dislodge. Nasojejunal tubes are usually preferred in situations where the stomach is either paralysed (gastroparesis) or has been operated on, such as in critical care units. Here, the food is instilled straight into the small bowel.

Minimum targets: nutrition and hydration

There are certain nutritional minimal targets that need to be achieved to sustain life in the first instance and ensure a healthy individual in the second instance by permitting wound healing and providing a functioning immune system. A detailed assessment of nutritional matters is beyond the scope of this chapter. In brief, one looks at body weight and recent change in weight. Muscle bulk, grip strength and skin thickness are easily assessed and a history of weight loss is a significant indicator of suboptimal nutrition.

The minimum daily water requirements are not precisely known but it is desirable to have a water intake of approximately 30 to 40 ml/kg/day for an adult (Ganong, 1995). This equates to about 2 to 3 L for the average person. The human kidney needs a minimum of 6 ml/kg/day of urine to perform the functions of excreting acids, toxins, metabolites and salts. This is maximally concentrated urine and equates to about 500 ml per day for the average person. The average person, in an air-conditioned hospital, loses about 500 ml a day in sweat. Therefore, the average person would need at least 1 L of water per day. These figures assume normal kidney function and do not include situations such as febrile patients or patients who have lost the heat and moisture exchange role of the nasopharynx by being ventilated.

It is also necessary for patients to receive electrolytes – the salts that are needed to ensure blood and extracellular volume. The major electrolytes are sodium and potassium – the human body needs approximately 2 mmoles/kg per day of sodium and 1 mmole/kg per day of potassium (Ganong, 1995) – corresponding to about 150 mmoles per day of sodium and 70 mmoles per day of potassium for the average person. This is not difficult to achieve in the average diet but has to be factored in to the equation when the only source of fluids is intravenous. A bag of 'normal saline' contains, for instance, 1 L of water and 150 mmoles of sodium. It has no potassium. So, if one were to add 60 mmoles of potassium to the bag and infuse it into a patient over a day, one would barely meet that patient's fluid requirements but one would meet all their electrolyte requirements. Other fluids can be used, such as 3% dextrose and 1/3 saline, which contains only 50 mmoles of sodium in 1 L. If one were to add 20 mmoles of potassium per bag and give 3 L per day, one would give the patient enough of both fluids and the key electrolytes. This is a simplistic view that does not take into consideration trace elements, such as selenium, copper or zinc, or even more common elements such as magnesium or calcium. Nor does it take into account vitamins.

You also need to consider calories or energy needs. The average person who has been well nourished and has no intercurrent stress (such as an infection or surgery or trauma) can survive for at least 4 weeks if fluid and electrolyte requirements are attended to (Ganong, 1995). However, this approach is likely to lead to severe protein-energy malnutrition (PEM). This has a number of consequences. There is impairment of the patient's immune defences leading to increased risk of infections (wound, lung, intravenous cannula site, and urinary tract). Patients suffer a loss of muscle bulk resulting in profound weakness leading to problems mobilizing, weakened swallowing and difficulty in weaning off ventilation. There is also impaired wound healing leading to wound dehiscences, anastomotic leaks and infections of wounds. It is frequently stated that 30% of patients are admitted to hospital with PEM, but 70% are discharged with PEM (Shronts and Cerra, 1999). The 3% dextrose and 1/3 saline fluid regimen listed above for instance would only supply about 360 calories per day. The patient lying quietly but awake at rest needs a minimum of about 25 calories per kg per day – about 1,500 to 1,800 calories per day. The postoperative or trauma patient might need up to 3,600 calories a day, even if heavily sedated and being fully ventilated. Nevertheless, it will not harm most patients to have a very reduced caloric intake for 2 to 3 days as long as fluid and electrolyte needs are attended to.

Parenteral and enteral nutrition are techniques that are used to provide the necessary calories as well as the water and electrolytes that patients need. Detailed discussion of the various formulae and their indications and complications are beyond the scope of this chapter. Roughly about 50% of the daily caloric needs are given as carbohydrates, 30% as fat and the rest as protein (the body needs approximately 1.2 to 1.5 g/kg/day of protein – 100 g per day for the average patient).

These proportions are varied according to the clinical need of the patient. Most enteral feeds are 1 calorie per ml. Parenteral feeds are usually prepacked within a sterile pharmacy and contain solutions of lipids (fats), amino acids (protein) and glucose (carbohydrate) with trace elements, electrolytes and minerals added. You may read about immunonutrition – the addition of certain amino acids (predominately glutamine and arginine) or fats (omega 3 fish oils or polyunsaturated fatty acids) – in augmenting either type of feed. These are currently not fully proven therapeutic options.

Assessment and modification of diet and other measures

Assessment of the swallowing function (including the gag reflex) in all patients who have suffered a likely aspiration syndrome (whether pneumonia or pneumonitis) is obviously essential. Assessment of swallowing function is detailed in Chapters 7, 8 and 14. When in doubt, one should carry out an assessment, as aspirations can frequently be silent.

All individuals at risk of aspiration (see above) should probably be assessed as well. Assessment should be by a qualified speech pathologist. There has been a vogue within the US critical care community to use fibreoptic endoscopic safety swallowing examination to look for food dyes in awake and non-intubated patients to diagnose silent aspiration. This was in accordance with most expert opinion until a randomized trial proved that, although patients with prolonged endotracheal intubation were at risk of aspiration after extubation, the addition of such an endoscopic examination of the larynx and trachea did not change the incidence (Barquist et al., 2001). Usual care consisting of speech pathology review and appropriate dietary modification was not inferior to the high technology of looking directly down at the vocal cords and upper trachea. Fibreoptic endoscopic evaluation of swallowing function is detailed in Chapter 8 and the clinical examination of dysphagia is discussed in detail in Chapter 7.

Further measures to reduce the risk of aspiration are basically simple, usually mechanical, things. These include regular oral hygiene care and nursing patients, especially if consciousness is reduced, either in the lateral recovery position, the 30-degree head-up position, or both. Certainly positioning ventilated patients in half-sitting posture reduces the risk of ventilator associated pneumonia (Drakulovic et al., 1999). Ventilator associated pneumonia (VAP) is only different from normal 'community-acquired' pneumonia in that the organisms involved are different and usually more virulent/toxic to the body. It is associated with a longer duration of ventilation, longer length of stay in ICU, and high mortality rate – it is therefore worth reducing the risk of its occurrence. Gastroesophageal reflux can be reduced by elevating the head of the bed and by the use of weight reduction in the long term. Drugs that lower the oesophageal sphincter's tone – such as alcohol, chocolate, peppermint, caffeine and tea – should be avoided. Anti-ulcer therapy may reduce the acidity of reflux and aspirated fluid, thus lessening the damage done by any aspirated fluids from the stomach and prokinetics such as metoclopramide and erythromycin will speed up gastric emptying thus lessening reflux. Ways of reducing gastroesophageal reflux are as follows:

• Elevation of the head of the bed.
• Positioning patients in sitting postures.
• Remain upright after meals for at least 20 minutes.
• Reduce consumption of substances that lower oesophageal sphincter tone:

  – alcohol;
  – chocolate;
  – peppermint;
  – caffeine;
  – tea.

• Anti-ulcer therapy:

  – pharmaceuticals to lessen the acidity of reflux and aspirated fluid;
  – pharmaceuticals to speed up gastric emptying, lessening the chance of reflux.

SITUATIONS REQUIRING USE OF TRACHEOSTOMY TUBES: IMPLICATIONS FOR INDIVIDUALS AT RISK OF OR WITH ASPIRATION

Tracheostomy tubes present a special situation. They are most often used to facilitate weaning from the ventilator in critical care units. Ventilation is the provision of support to a patient's lungs by the application of positive pressure (or set volumes) either through a tube, as we are discussing here, or through a mask. Endotracheal tubes, which are tubes running from outside the patient through either the nose or mouth to the trachea, have a significant amount of dead space. Resistance to gas flow to and from the patient's lungs through a tube is inversely related to the fourth power of the radius of the tube and directly related to the length of the tube. Using a tracheostomy usually eliminates about 20 cm of tube compared with an endotracheal tube. This substantially reduces the resistance offered by the tube, which becomes very important when switching from ventilator-supported spontaneous breathing to unsupported spontaneous breathing. This is the final step just before extubation or decannulation. Tracheostomies are also favoured in longer term ventilation because they allow weaning of the often heavy sedative regimens required for 'tube tolerance' in the patient with an endotracheal tube. Tracheostomies have a reduced risk of a much-feared complication of long term use of an endotracheal tube – laryngomalacia – where the larynx and/or tracheal cartilages soften to the point where they collapse during inspiration, thereby being a cause of upper airway obstruction once the tube is removed. They also allow more mobility, the possibility of discharge to the ward once off ventilatory support (thereby freeing up the bed for the next patient), and the recommencement of oral food and fluids under the guidance of the speech pathologist.

INDICATIONS FOR THE INSERTION OF TRACHEOSTOMY TUBES

The indications to insert tracheostomies are to bypass upper airway obstruction, provide easy access to the airway for aspiration of tracheobronchial secretions and for weaning from ventilatory support (Silva, 1999) (the most common reason). The causes of upper airway obstruction are most often acute – burns, foreign bodies, corrosive gas/liquid exposure, infections or trauma. Occasionally such obstructions are slower in onset, especially if neoplastic in origin. Access to the airway for aspiration of secretions is most often needed in the post-intensive care setting when patients recovering from pneumonia or infective exacerbation of chronic obstructive lung disease are still producing copious amounts of secretions. The cough is very often weakened in this situation because of the inability of intensivists to provide enough nutrition in the acute illness setting to overcome the body's tendency to break down muscles (including the diaphragm, accessory muscles and the intercostal muscles). It is debatable that even the delivery of enough calories would make a difference as the body produces certain chemical messengers (hormones and cytokines) that drive this process of muscle breakdown and prevent utilization of energy, whether delivered directly intravenously or indirectly enterally. Tracheostomy for ventilatory support has been mentioned previously.

This said, the most common reason for insertion of a tracheostomy is for the facilitation of weaning long-term ventilated patients from the ventilator. In Australia, we tend to use the cutoff of 2 weeks to define long-term ventilation – this does not mean that one necessarily waits 2 weeks, but if you think ventilation is very likely to be longer than two weeks, a tracheostomy is considered at the first clinically safe and technically feasible occasion. This is a historical practice that is currently being subjected to randomized trials of early versus late tracheostomies to try to work out the ideal time to insert one for patients with prolonged intubation. Indications for insertion of tracheostomies are as follows:

- To bypass upper airway obstruction. For example:

  - burns;
  - foreign bodies;
  - corrosive gas/liquid exposure;
  - infections;
  - trauma.

- To provide easy access to the airway for aspiration of tracheobronchial secretions. For example:

  - post intensive care when recovering from pneumonia or infection exacerbation of chronic obstructive lung disease (COAD/COPD);
  - to wean patients from ventilatory support.

It is important to note that a tracheostomy tube does not guarantee protection from aspiration. It has been reported that aspiration may occur in up to 15% of patients managed with a tracheostomy (Irwin, 1999). It is believed that tracheostomies reduce the risk of aspiration but there is very little solid scientific evidence to confirm this. Nevertheless, one must never assume that just because a tracheostomy is in place, even with the cuff balloon inflated, the patient is safe from aspiration and its consequences. A good general rule is always assume the cuff is not working and carry out all the mechanical procedures to minimize the risk of reflux and aspiration.

There are various sizes of tubes and various other technical innovations. Almost all are equipped with a cuff and are now made of a silicon based material. The cuff allows inflation and occlusion of the airway to material from above – this, as mentioned previously, does not guarantee protection from aspiration and it has been noted that even the use of suctioning ports above the cuff does not reduce that risk. Smaller tracheostomies – the so-called 'mini-trach' – are often used in those patients with a weakened cough and/or excessive secretions to facilitate 'tracheal toilet'. If the patient is not constantly on the ventilator, he or she can have a tube with holes (fenestrated) placed in or have a speaking valve put on the tracheostomy (with the cuff deflated) – these devices allow the passage of air from the lungs and up the trachea over the vocal cords. The speech pathologist's role in the assessment and management of swallowing and communication for individuals with tracheostomy tubes is detailed in Chapter 9.

Endotracheal tubes are associated with a change in the reflexes needed for swallowing due to changes in neurological sensitivity, muscular dysfunction and subacute injury even if the tube has only been in less than one day. These changes usually resolve rapidly and rarely need any formal intervention (DeLarminat et al., 1995). Should formal swallowing therapy be required, these would follow the principles outlined in Chapters 11 and 12.

COMPLICATIONS OF TRACHEOSTOMY

Complications of tracheostomy are in the order of 6% to 50% with mortality rates of 0.9% to 4.5% (Silva, 1999). The most serious complications are bleeding, misplacement of the tube and obstruction. Bleeding can occur at an early stage – this is most often likely to be local and is more of an irritation than a serious concern. If it occurs at a late stage this is often serious, with 50% being due to erosion into the innominate artery (supplying the right arm and side of the head/brain) with catastrophic consequences. Misplacement may occur after dislodgement with faulty replacement, or as an initial insertion problem, and leads to a failure to ventilate. Obstruction is most often due to dried out and viscous secretions but can also be due to bleeding. There are a multitude of other complications – stoma infections, nerve injury (particularly the recurrent laryngeal nerve), pneumothorax, lung collapse, tracheo-oesophageal fistula and laryngomalacia.

From the speech pathology point of view, the major complications of tracheostomy are dysphagia and aspiration. Dysphagia and aspiration can have potentially serious and devastating outcomes, especially if they lead to a severe aspiration pneumonitis with acute respiratory distress syndrome (ARDS), which carries a mortality rate of 40%. The cuffs are now designed to be more compliant even with high volumes of air in them resulting in less over-distension and less pressure on the airway – also most intensive care unit protocols call for either a leak test or a check of the cuff pressure to prevent excessive pressures being present in the cuff. Despite this, the cuff is often described in retrospect by patients as feeling like an orange stuck in the throat on attempting to swallow. A good general rule is to let the cuff down as soon as the patient is off the ventilator, especially when the patient is in the sitting position. Tracheostomies lead to delayed swallow triggering and pharyngeal pooling of contrast material on videofluoroscopy (DeVita and Spierer-Rundback, 1990). There is poorer anterior movement of the pharynx in swallowing and laryngeal elevation is decreased as well. This is mostly due to fixation of the trachea to the skin by the tracheostomy although compression of the oesophagus by the cuff also plays a role. As mentioned before, endotracheal tubes can desensitize the nerves of the oropharynx and, likewise, tracheostomies and prolonged fasting/nil by mouth can desensitize the nerves involved with the sensation and coordination of swallowing. This leads to a loss of protective reflexes such as the cough or gag reflex and the reflex closure of laryngeal opening, which contributes to lack of coordination of the swallowing process. This greatly increases the risks of aspiration. Techniques for the remediation of swallowing can be found in Chapter 12.

INDICATIONS FOR REMOVAL OF TRACHEOSTOMIES

Indications for removal of tracheostomies are: complications of the tracheostomy tube, successful weaning from the ventilation, strengthening cough or decreasing secretions or removal/resolution of the obstructive process in the upper airway. Basically, as soon as there is no further indication for the tracheostomy and the patient is considered safe, the tracheostomy should be removed. This decision should be arrived at after close coordination between the clinician caring for the patient and the speech pathologist reviewing the patient. It does not mean that one has to wait until the swallow is normal before removing the tracheostomy. The process of consultation and review does not stop there – depending on the underlying pathological process, the patient may never recover a normal swallowing process and most patients after decannulation will require ongoing speech pathology review.

SUMMARY

Aspiration is often clinically silent. Therefore, those at risk of aspiration should be assessed by a qualified professional (a speech pathologist) before being allowed to have oral intake. Risk factors are readily identifiable – anything that interferes with muscle coordination or strength particularly cerebrovascular accidents or anything that depresses the level of consciousness. Those that have aspirated need to be observed closely for deterioration. Aspiration can make patients very sick whether by infection (pneumonia) or by the chemical burn to the lung (pneumonitis). Patients may require intensive care support and even invasive ventilation. The care of a patient who has suffered aspiration or a patient who is coming off a tracheostomy requires close liaison between the clinician and the speech pathologist.

REFERENCES

Barquist E, Brown M, Cohn S, et al. (2001) Postextubation fiberoptic endoscopic evaluation of swallowing after prolonged endotracheal intubation: a randomized, prospective trial. Critical Care Medicine 29: 1710–13.

DeLarminat V, Montravers P, Dureuil B, et al. (1995) Alteration in swallowing reflex after extubation in intensive care unit patients. Critical Care Medicine 23: 486–90.

DeVita MA, Spierer-Rundback L (1990) Swallowing disorders in patients with prolonged orotracheal intubation or tracheostomy tubes. Critical Care Medicine 18: 1328–35.

Drakulovic MB, Torres A, Bauer TT, et al. (1999) Supine body position as a risk factor for nosocomial pneumonia in mechanically ventilated patients: a randomised trial. Lancet 354: 1851–8.

Ganong WF (1995) Review of Medical Physiology. Connecticut: Appleton & Lange.

Irwin RS (1999) Aspiration. In Irwin RS, Cerra FB, Rippe JM et al. Intensive Care Medicine. New York: Lippincott-Raven, pp. 685–91.

James CF, Modell JH, Gibbs CP, et al. (1984) Pulmonary aspiration – effects of volume and pH in the rat. Anesthesiology and Analgesia 63: 665–8.

Kidd D, Lawson J, Nesbitt R (1993) Aspiration in acute stroke: a clinical study with videofluoroscopy. Quarterly Journal of Medicine 86: 825–9.

Marrie TJ, Durnat H, Kwan C (1986) Nursing home-acquired pneumonia: a case-control study. Journal of the American Geriatric Society 34: 697–702.

Moine P, Vercken JP, Chevret S, et al. (1994) Severe community acquired pneumonia: etiology, epidemiology, and prognosis factors. Chest 105: 1487–95.

Park RH, Allison MC, Lang J, et al. (1992) Randomised comparison of percutaneous endoscopic gastrostomy and nasogastric tube feeding in patients with persisting neurological dysphagia. British Medical Journal 304: 1406–9.

Shronts EP Cerra FB (1999) Metabolism and nutrition. In Irwin RS, Cerra FB, Rippe JM, et al. (eds) Intensive Care Medicine. New York: Lippincott Raven, pp. 2239–8.

Silva WE (1999) Tracheotomy. In Irwin RS, Cerra FB, Rippe JM, et al. (eds) Intensive Care Medicine. New York: Lippincott Raven, pp. 161–73.

Spain DA, DeWeese RC, Reynolds MA, et al. (1995) Transpyloric passage of feeding tubes in patients with head injuries does not decrease complications. Journal of Trauma 39: 1100–1102.

Warner MA, Warner ME, Weber JG (1993) Clinical significance of pulmonary aspiration during the perioperative period. Anesthesiology 78: 56–62.

FURTHER READING

Paul Marik (2001) Primary care: aspiration pneumonitis and aspiration pneumonia. New England Journal of Medicine 344(9): 665–71.

6 Saliva Management

HILARY JOHNSON and AMANDA SCOTT

This chapter introduces the role of saliva in maintaining oral health and assisting the swallowing process. Drooling or saliva loss may occur where one or more of the phases of swallowing is impaired. The issues related to assessment and consequent treatment are outlined.

INTRODUCTION

Saliva is an important substance in the mouth. Many of us only discover its importance when our mouth becomes dry while presenting at an important speaking engagement. Apart from moistening our tongues and lips while speaking, saliva has several major functions, which include the lubrication of the bolus for ease of swallowing, the maintenance of oral hygiene, and the regulation of acidity in the oesophagus. Where a person has no oral motor deficits there may still be problems with saliva production, which can result in changes in saliva viscosity. This may affect swallowing, and result in increased dental caries and periodontitis. Poor saliva control can occur in people with developmental, acquired or progressive disabilities. Hypersalivation is rare and not usually a cause of drooling (Tahmassebi and Curzon, 2003). Where a person has oral motor difficulties the problems with saliva may result in saliva overflow (also called drooling or dribbling) and cause embarrassment and social isolation. Drooling is usually considered normal until a child is over 2 years of age (Morris and Dunn Klein, 2000). However some children with no obvious neurodevelopmental disabilities may drool until six or seven years (Johnson et al., 2001).

DROOLING IN CHILDREN

Drooling among children with cerebral palsy has been estimated at from 10% (Ekedahl, 1974) to 37% (Van de Heyning et al., 1980). Tahmassabi and Curzon (2003) suggested that, in children with cerebral palsy and an intellectual disability, drooling becomes less apparent after the development of permanent dentition. Thus for some children saliva overflow may decrease with age. There are no separate prevalence rates available for those with an intellectual disability or other neurological conditions.

Dysphagia: Foundation, Theory and Practice. Edited by J. Cichero and B. Murdoch
© 2006 John Wiley & Sons, Ltd.

DROOLING IN INDIVIDUALS WITH COMPLEX COMMUNICATION NEEDS OR DEVELOPMENTAL DISABILITY

An Australian study of people with complex communication needs found 29% of individuals had saliva control difficulties (Perry et al., 2002). People with acquired neurological conditions frequently encounter saliva control problems. Drooling in these conditions is related to impairment of oral control rather than an increase in saliva production. Secretion control problems are seen in adults where dysphagia occurs after multiple strokes involving both cerebral hemispheres or following a brain stem stroke. The problem is usually worse in the acute phase but may continue to be an issue depending on the site and extent of infarction (Smithhard, 1997).

People with developmental disabilities, in particular cerebral palsy, often retain immature swallowing patterns. A tongue-thrust pattern is frequently associated with drooling. In this case, instead of the tongue collecting the saliva and then elevating itself to press against the hard palate to push the saliva into the pharynx, the tongue protrudes and retracts in much the same way an infant's tongue moves. This tongue thrust pattern becomes more apparent as the person matures because the space in the oral cavity increases, resulting in protrusion of the tongue during the oral phase of swallowing and drooling.

DROOLING IN ADULTS

Progressive neurological conditions are also associated with saliva control problems. In Parkinson's disease the characteristic paucity of movement affects the usually automatic, spontaneous swallowing of saliva. Consequently saliva pools in the mouth and drooling results. The stooped posture of Parkinson's disease contributes to drooling behaviour. Drooling is most prominent when the anti-Parkinsonian medication is not effective. This is referred to as the 'off' period (Clarke et al., 1998). As Parkinson's disease progresses the individual's response to the medication diminishes and longer and more frequent 'off' periods are experienced. For this reason drooling is very common in advanced Parkinson's disease.

Impaired saliva control is also a prominent feature of motor neurone disease. This relates directly to bulbar impairment resulting in dysphagia. The tongue is particularly affected in motor neurone disease (Robbins, 1987) and consequently saliva cannot be collected and propelled into the pharynx. Because pharyngeal impairment frequently co-occurs with oral impairment, aspiration of saliva may be a problem.

Understanding the mechanism of saliva flow and production is essential if one is to understand the management of the range of difficulties with saliva.

SALIVA

Saliva is produced by three major paired sets of major salivary glands – the parotid, submandilular and sublingual glands – and by the minor salivary glands, which are

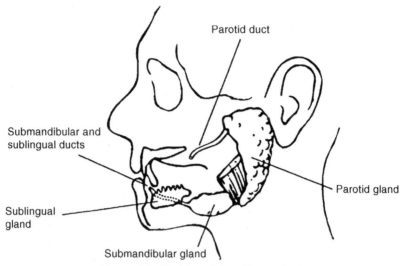

Figure 6.1 Position of the salivary glands
Source: PRO-Ed, Inc.

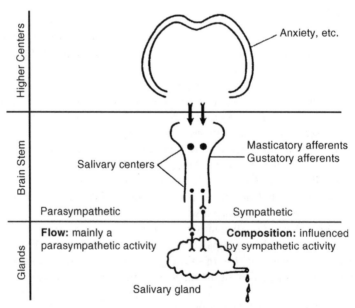

Figure 6.2 Neural control of salivary activity. Diagrammatic representation of afferent and efferent pathways that are involved in reflex salivary secretion under the coordinating control of the salivary centres. These are in turn influenced by higher centres, and in this manner anxiety, etc., may have effects on the reflex flow of saliva
Source: PRO-Ed, Inc.

scattered throughout the mucosa of the oral and pharyngeal cavities. The parotid glands are most active during chewing when the mechanical stimulation of the masseter and pterygoid muscles results in secretion of saliva via Stensen's ducts into the mouth in the region of the second molars. The submandibular glands secrete via Wharton's ducts, which are located on either side of the frenulum. Secretions from the sublingual glands flow through the ducts of Rivius, situated on the floor of the mouth (see Figure 6.1).

The structure of the salivary glands is typical of all exocrine glands, being composed of small structures called acini, into which the epithelial cells secrete saliva, and ducts that transport the saliva. The parotid glands only produce serous secretions whereas the submandibular and sublingual glands produce both serous and mucoid secretions. Salivary function is under autonomic control. Parasympathetic input increases the amount of saliva associated with eating and drinking. Sympathetic input reduces the quantity of secretion when not eating or drinking and during physical activity (see Figure 6.2).

The average person produces and swallows approximately 600 ml of saliva a day (Watanabe and Dawes, 1988). Saliva collects in the mouth and coats the surface in a thin film (0.1 mm). Saliva moves in the mouth at specific velocity (0.83–7.6 mm per min), which varies according to where it is in the mouth (Dawes et al., 1989). This movement of the saliva is important to protect the teeth from developing caries.

SWALLOWING SALIVA

Keeping the mouth moist and hygienic requires us to swallow regularly and efficiently without loosing any saliva out of the mouth onto the lips or chin. Frequent swallowing avoids the pooling of saliva in the mouth, the dribbling of saliva when we incline our head, or the spraying of saliva when we talk. It is not known whether the trigger for a saliva swallow is at the same point as for a nutritional swallow but it is possible these are different (see Chapter 3).

A mature swallow is characterized by the oral phase (a voluntary phase) and a pharyngeal phase (an involuntary phase). These phases are discussed in detail in Chapter 1. The oral phase is considered to be more influenced by cortical function whereas the pharyngeal phase is thought to be mediated within the brain stem (Bass, 1997). As with speech, the movements of the oral phase of swallowing can be defined as a learned motor sequence (Daniels, 2000). The swallowing sequence is executed so frequently that it becomes automatic; however, because it is under volitional control it is readily modifiable.

The obvious difference between swallowing saliva and swallowing food and drink is a comparative lack of anticipation when swallowing saliva. Sensory inputs of smell and vision, the proprioceptive information as the hand moves towards the mouth and pressure perception when a spoon touches the lips focuses an individual's attention onto the activity of eating of drinking and primes the swallowing mechanism for action (Selley et al., 1989a, 1989b). Once in the mouth the size, taste, temperature and texture of the bolus further stimulate the swallow sequence. Saliva is swallowed in the context of comparatively low stimulation and the amount and type of cortical input into the process may be less than for eating and drinking. These inputs lack the strong sensory input of food and fluid but effective swallowing of saliva relies on an intact sensory system that is able to detect relatively small amounts of secretions within the mouth and pharynx (see Chapter 1 for further information).

ASSESSMENT OF SALIVA SWALLOWS

The swallowing of saliva boluses has not been as rigorously studied as the swallowing of food and drink. This is partly due to the difficulty of imaging the saliva swallow. In most cases ultrasound has been used to image saliva swallows (Sonies et al., 1996). The ultasound technique was pioneered by Barbara Sonies and although it has been used elsewhere by other researchers (Kenny et al., 1989) it has not gained wide acceptance as a clinical tool. Limited use of ultrasound to study swallowing may be due to the level of skill needed to interpret the images. It is a safe non-invasive technique that can be applied to a child or adult in any position. The ultrasound transducer is placed beneath the individual's chin and a dynamic image of the swallowing process can be seen on the screen. This can be done repeatedly and audio and video recordings can be made, allowing detailed analysis. It has potential for measuring and visualizing the swallowing of saliva among individuals with various disabilities.

Cervical auscultation has shown promise for measuring swallowing frequency in different populations (Cichero, 1996; Allaire and Brown, 2004). A clicking sound can be heard when we swallow. This has been described as two or three clicks depending on whether it is a dry or wet swallow (Cichero, 1996). These sounds are best heard through a stethoscope, microphone or accelerometer. The best location for placing the stethoscope has been extensively studied (Takahashi et al., 1994). Takahashi recommended that the sensor be centrally placed just below the cricoid cartilage. This procedure is non-invasive; however, the assessor needs to be trained in listening to the sounds in order to interpret the swallow sounds. The value of this method is that it can be used on any participant who can tolerate a stethoscope on the neck for a short time, does not involve radiation exposure and is highly portable. The cervical auscultation technique is discussed in detail in Chapter 7.

Intact pharyngeal sensation is necessary for the initiation and execution of the swallow reflex. Secretions in the pharynx must be cleared regularly to ensure that they are not aspirated. Problems with secretion management are often related to dysphagia and pharyngeal impairment has potentially more serious health consequences than drooling. Consequently, information gained through videofluoroscopic assessment of swallowing function is useful when planning management strategies for secretion problems. Videofluoroscopy provides information regarding jaw closure, the ability of the tongue to propel material from the oral cavity into the pharynx. Further, it enables the effectiveness of the pharyngeal structures in clearing the material to be assessed, including determination of pharyngeal pooling of secretions (Logemann, 1998).

Pooling of secretions within the pharynx and larynx, and aspiration, can be readily observed during fibreoptic evaluation of the swallowing function. Whilst the presence of pooled secretions within the pharynx can be inferred by characteristic wet or gurgling breath and vocal sounds, it is difficult to quantify the extent and position of pooled secretions using audition alone. A fibreoptic endoscopic assessment technique is the most effective method of accurately assessing the extent of pharyngeal pooling of secretions (Murray et al., 1996; Langmore, 2001). This technique entails the insertion of a flexible endoscope through the nasal cavity and into the pharynx enabling the direct visualization of the presence of pooled secretions. Secretions within the laryngeal vestibule and trachea can also be seen, thus determining whether aspiration of secretions is occurring or at risk of occurring. Aviv et al. (1998) describe a modification of this procedure that includes the delivery of puffs of air to pharyngeal and laryngeal structures to assess sensation. Using this method the clinician can establish whether the presence of pooled secretions in the pharynx is related to poor detection of their presence. Both videofluoroscopy and fibreoptic endoscopic assessment of swallowing function are discussed further in Chapter 8.

Individuals with compromised airway protection during swallowing are at risk of developing aspiration pneumonia. A number of researchers have reported a close relationship between poor oral health, which has been found to be more prevalent in those reliant on others for oral care, and the consequent presence of harmful bacteria in saliva and the development of aspiration pneumonia (Langmore et al., 1998; Scannapieco, 1999; Terpenning et al., 2001).

FREQUENCY OF SWALLOWING

The swallowing rate varies throughout the day depending on ingestion of food and liquid (Lagerlöf and Dawes, 1984; Sheppard et al., 2003) volume of saliva flow and oral clearance (Lagerlöf and Dawes, 1984; Rudney and Larson, 1995) and the level of activity of the individual (Lear et al., 1965). Kapila et al. (1984) estimated healthy adults swallow at a rate of 1.27 +/− 0.2 swallows per minute while (Watanabe and Dawes, 1990) found the swallowing rate in five year old children was 1.6 +/− 0.6 swallows a minute. These differences relate to the amount of fluid flowing into the person's mouth.

A low rate of swallowing frequency is commonly cited as a reason for drooling. There are different opinions cited in the research into swallowing frequency in children in cerebral palsy. Sochaniwskyj et al. (1986) found that children with cerebral palsy and drooling swallowed at 45% of the normal rate and that non-drooling children with cerebral palsy swallowed at 75% of the normal rate. Lespargot et al. (1993) found that children with cerebral palsy who drooled swallowed at three times the rate as those who did not drool. They pointed out that the cerebral palsy children who drooled all had remaining liquid in their mouths after swallowing compared to the two other groups of children (typical children who did not drool and children with cerebral palsy with good saliva control) who did not have remaining wetness. Lespargot et al. (1993) suggested that the lack of an efficient oral suction phase, where there was no rapid propelling movement of the saliva such that it dripped off the posterior surface of the tongue, might have been a factor that led to remaining liquid in the mouth. Thus there was a need to swallow more frequently. Usually after a swallow some moisture (0.8 ml) will remain in the mouth and Lagerlöf and Dawes (1984) refer to this as the residual volume. This residual volume is reduced after a forced swallow.

ORAL HYGIENE AND ITS IMPORTANCE IN REDUCING THE RISK OF ASPIRATION

As mentioned previously, saliva is important for maintaining healthy gums and teeth. Extra saliva may be produced where there are irritants in mouth and this has been reported by parents in association with teething in young children (Wake et al., 1999). However, it is rare for any drooling to be associated with the eruption of permanent dentition.

The presence of dental plaque, caries and periodontitis not only leads to extra saliva but increases harmful bacteria in the saliva. If this is aspirated into the lungs it may lead to aspiration pneumonia (Langmore et al., 1988; Murray et al., 1996; Langmore et al., 1998; Langmore et al., 2002). The conditions of aspiration pneumonia and pneumotitis are described in Chapter 5. The presence of pathogenic bacteria resulting from the person experiencing gastro-oesophageal reflux can lead to the erosion of molar teeth. The regular application of good oral hygiene techniques will assist in decreasing the possibility of increased saliva due to poor dental health. Techniques such as using mouthwashes and brushing and flossing correctly can significantly reduce chronic gingivitis (Francis et al., 1987).

XEROSTOMIA

Oral dryness or xerostomia is experienced when there is damage to the salivary glands. The salivary glands are particularly susceptible to damage by ionizing radiation used to treat people with head and neck cancer. Doses required to destroy tumour cells are higher than those that destroy secretory cells within the salivary glands. Recently, the use of intensity-modulated radiotherapy has lessened the dose delivered through the region of the salivary glands by delivering radiation via a series of beams in an arch surrounding the target tumour. This enables maximum radiation doses to be summated within the tumour whilst distributing the dose throughout the non-targeted tissues (Symonds, 2001; Eisenbruch et al., 2003).

Another common cause of xerostomia is Sjögren's syndrome (see Chapter 9). This condition is a chronic autoimmune disease in which the exocrine (mucus-secreting) glands are destroyed. Sjögren's syndrome is one of the most prevalent autoimmune disorders. These disorders affect more women than men at a 9:1 ratio. Although Sjögren's syndrome occurs in all age groups, the average age of onset is late forties. People with Sjögren's syndrome experience marked xerostomia and inflammation in the salivary and lachrymal glands (Lash, 2001). Paradoxically, people with drooling problems also experience periods of excessive oral dryness. This is because the immobile tongue does not distribute the saliva around the oral cavity to lubricate the mucosa. Mouth breathing can further exacerbate this problem.

ASSESSMENT AND MANAGEMENT OF SALIVA OVERFLOW

Poor saliva control usually results from a combination of factors such as infrequent swallowing and inefficient swallowing. The first step in the process of intervention is to determine the factors involved and the importance of this impairment to the person affected, including that person's family and quality of life. This assessment process includes taking a case history and conducting a functional oral assessment. Appendices 6.1 and 6.2 present an example of two questionnaires to assist with collecting information currently used at Royal Children's Hospital saliva clinic, Melbourne, Australia. Questions on this form have been developed from studies in the literature suggesting reasons for poor saliva control (Thomas-Stonell and Greenberg, 1988). Information is sought under the headings of:

• communication and cognition;
• gross motor functioning;
• functional eating and drinking abilities;
• oral and dental health; and
• severity of the saliva management problem.

COMMUNICATION AND COGNITION

A general assessment of communication skills is important. We know that people with complex communication needs often have associated saliva control difficulties (Perry et al., 2002). The ability of the person to communicate may give important information about the person's cognitive abilities to follow instructions and also an example of purposeful oral motor skills.

GROSS MOTOR

General gross motor skills such as the ability to walk and hold the head up when either sitting, standing or walking will precede ability to perform fine motor skills. Trunk stability, for example, has implications for shoulder, head and jaw stability. Jaw stability is critical to the oral phase of swallowing. Posture and positioning are discussed further in Chapter 11.

EATING, DRINKING AND SWALLOWING

It is important to report functional eating and drinking difficulties. Although the ability to chew may not relate directly to an improvement in saliva control, recent studies indicate that the improvement of jaw stability as demonstrated in the fine motor control of eating and drinking does improve saliva control (Haberfellner and Rossiwall, 1977; Johnson et al., 2004). Straw drinking requires oral suction and lip seal, however this might not be the same suction and propelling movement described by Lespargot et al., 1993. In a study on typical children who still drool, the ability to use a straw was not a significant factor in the improvement of saliva control (Johnson et al., 2001). The ability to chew and swallow can demonstrate difficulties the person may be having at both and an automatic and volitional level. The frequency of swallowing and any difficulty swallowing is noted and a comparison made between nutritive and saliva swallows. It is important to note whether the person is aware of the saliva overflow in order to study the breakdown in the mechanism and possible interventions.

Although Sochaniwskyj et al. (1986) and Lespargot et al. (1993) disagree on the frequency of swallowing, clinical observation would suggest that infrequent swallowing results in drooling. Programmes to increase frequency of swallowing have had some long-term effects on saliva overflow (Rapp, 1980; Koheil et al., 1987; Lancioni et al., 1994).

ORAL AND DENTAL HEALTH

Oral health and structures also need to be examined. Increased or decreased saliva may be seen where there is gingivitis and /or caries. Moreover, the adequacy of the occlusion and lip seal need to be evaluated in the context of swallowing function. There is a range of more detailed oral health assessments available (Eilers et al., 1988; Foulsum, 2002).

SEVERITY OF THE SALIVA MANAGEMENT PROBLEM

Issues such as general health and attitudes to the drooling problem may assist the problem solving approach to intervention. Frequent colds and a blocked nose may contribute to mouth breathing and an open-mouth posture. Gastro-oesophageal reflux may contribute to increased saliva (Heine et al., 1996). Frequent pneumonia or severe asthma might suggest the aspiration of substances into the lungs (Vandenplas, 1997; Hilton et al., 1999; Ekberg, 2000). Some people with saliva control difficulties may have complex medical conditions which would preclude the more invasive saliva control interventions. It may also be that the saliva control problem is not considered enough of an issue to undergo certain interventions.

SALIVA OVERFLOW MANAGEMENT

The approaches to the management of saliva control are oral sensory-motor programmes; behavioural programmes; appliance therapy; assistive technology; medication, surgery and complementary medicines. This range of treatment involves professionals from different speciality backgrounds including doctor, paediatrician, gastroenterologist, plastic and ENT surgeons, dentists and dental hygienist, speech pathologist, radiologist, physiotherapist. Wherever possible the least to the most invasive hierarchy is applied when implementing programmes for saliva control.

ORAL SENSORY-MOTOR INTERVENTIONS

These include oral exercises for building strength and endurance (Jordan, 1979; Garliner, 1981; Hagg and Larsson, 2004) vibration, icing and or massage for increasing sensory awareness (Levitt, 1966; Domaracki and Sisson, 1990; Nelson and De Benabib, 1991), improving the ability to eat and drink for integrating sensory and motor functional skills (Loiselle, 1979; Gisel, 1994; Haberfellner et al., 1999) and improving oral hygiene, caries and gum disease (Walmsley, 1997; King, 2000; Griffiths, 2002). All of these programmes have limited success and the type of programme should be chosen carefully. Until recently there has been no sensorimotor therapy to increase the frequency of swallowing but recent work with E-stim shows some promise (Dilworth, 2003 personal communication) (see Chapter 12).

BEHAVIOURAL PROGRAMMES

These programmes target improving activities that are under a person's conscious control. The targeted behaviours include increasing the frequency of lip closure (Lancioi et al., 1994), swallowing (Rapp, 1980; Koheil et al., 1983), chin wiping (Drabmen et al., 1979) and the maintenance of an upright head posture. Many of these programmes work in the short term but have problems with maintenance and generalization. The person has to be well motivated for the programme to be successful.

APPLIANCE THERAPY

Several different intraoral appliances have been constructed to increase swallowing frequency and lip closure. These include vestibular screens, Innsbruck Sensori Motor Activator and Regulator (ISMAR) (Haberfellner et al., 1999; Johnson et al., 2004) and a range of plates with buttons or stimulators (Selley, 1977; Limbrock et al., 1991; Hohoff and Ehmer, 1999; Wells, 2000). The appliances aim to trigger functional oral movements to improve swallowing and are an integral part of a speech pathology programme. Assistance is needed from the speech pathologist to design, fit and alter the appliance as therapy progresses. Appliance therapy requires a close relationship between the dentist and speech pathologist and frequent clinic visits for the person wearing the appliance.

ASSISTIVE TECHNOLOGY

Recent advances in technology could provide a solution for some people. Researchers in the US (Brown and Allaire, 2000) have been developing systems that can collect saliva from inside the mouth and pump it back into the pharynx. This intraoral appliance removes the saliva through a vacuum like mechanism and stores it elsewhere for disposal. This technology is currently under trial and should be available in the next few years.

MEDICATION

Medications can be used to reduce saliva and the most commonly used medications to reduce saliva production have anticholinergic properties that block the parasympathetic innervation of the salivary glands. Several studies have demonstrated the effectiveness of these medications (Camp-Bruno et al., 1989; Reddihough et al., 1990; Blasco and Stansbury, 1996; Zeppetella, 1999). Medication has not always proved effective in reducing saliva loss and may have side effects such as change in mood and alertness, blurred vision and urinary retention.

In the last few years neurotoxin botulinum (botox) has also been used. Botulinum blocks the release of acetylcholine in the nerve terminals, at the neuromuscular junction but also in the sympathetic and parasympathetic ganglion cells and in postganglionic parasympathetic nerves. Botox is injected into specific saliva glands under the guidance of ultrasound (Porta, 2001; Suskind and Tilton, 2002; Jongerius et al., 2003).

SURGERY

Surgery for saliva loss includes denervation or excision of the salivary glands and ligation or relocation of salivary ducts (Wilkie and Brody, 1977; Frederick and Stewart, 1982; Shirley et al., 2003; Uppal et al., 2003). The most common operative technique is the relocation of the submandibular gland ducts into the pharynx and the excision of the sublingual glands (Crysdale et al., 2001). Some people may also have a ligation of one or more of the parotid ducts. Care is taken not to reduce the protective factor of saliva, which may result in increased caries (Hallet et al., 1995). People with poor oral health may not be suitable candidates for surgery and every effort to ensure good oral health practices are instituted before surgery. Surgery is usually around 75% effective in reducing the saliva loss but only a small number of people gain total control.

Alternatively the use of laser to decrease saliva production from the parotid ducts has also been used but is not a widespread technique (Chang and Wong, 2001).

MANAGEMENT OF XEROSTOMIA

The condition of a dry mouth can be alleviated by a number of interventions. These include increasing water intake and moistening mucous membranes using oral lubricants such as artificial saliva. Saliva output can be increased by chewing gum or sucking fruit lozenges, decreasing mouth breathing and reviewing medications to minimize the use of anticholinergic medications (see http://www.scopevic.org.au/therapy_crc_research_saliva_dry.html#general).

COMPLEMENTARY THERAPIES

There are many different types of complementary medicine or therapy that have been implicated in the management of saliva problems. These include Chinese herbs, acupuncture (Blom et al., 1992; Dawidson et al., 1997; Wong et al., 2001), acupressure, and kinaesiology. Many of the philosophies behind these are not based on the principles of Western medicine and there is usually only anecdotal evidence of the usefulness of these approaches. Mucolytic enzymes, such as papase, which occurs in pawpaw (papaya), are purported to reduce the viscosity of ropey secretions. These are available in tablet form from health food shops. Some people report that dietary changes have improved their saliva control and this area would benefit from further research.

SUMMARY

The area of saliva and secretion management is under-researched. People with these issues have a range of aetiologies and often complex medical histories. We are still struggling to fully understand the mechanisms that cause saliva overflow and are seeking reliable, permanent and non-invasive treatments to manage secretions. Many of the treatments are not completely successful for everyone and clothing protectors, handkerchiefs (for increased salivary flow) and chewing gum (to stimulate saliva in a dry mouth) are still used as props to alleviate this embarrassing condition.

REFERENCES

Allaire JH, Brown C (2004) Technology and saliva overflow. In Scott A, Johnson H (eds) A practical approach to the management of saliva. 2nd edn. Austin: Pro-ed.

Aviv JE, Kim T, Sacco RL, et al. (1998) FEESST: A new bedside endoscopic test of motor and sensory components of swallowing. Annals of Otology, Rinology and Laryngology 107: 378–87.

Bass NH (1997) The Neurology of swallowing. In Groher ME (ed.) Dysphagia: Diagnosis and Management. 3 edn. Newton MA: Butterworth-Heinemann, pp. 7–36.

Blasco PA, Stansbury JC (1996) Glycopyrrolate treatment of chronic drooling. Archives of Pediatrics and Adolescent Medicine 150(99): 932–5.

Blom M, Dawidson I, Angmar-Mänsson B (1992) The effect of acupuncture on salivary flow rates in patients with xerostomia. Oral Surgery, Oral Medicine and Oral Pathology 73(3): 293–8.

Brown C, Allaire JH (2000) Saliva Control and AAC: The Relationship. Paper presented at the International Society for Augmentative and Alternative Communication. Washington DC.

Camp-Bruno JA, Winsberg BG, Green-Parsons AR, et al. (1989) Efficacy of benztropine therapy for drooling. Developmental Medicine and Child Neurology 31(3): 309–19.

Chang CJ, Wong AM (2001) Intraductal laser photocoagulation of the bilateral parotid ducts for reduction of drooling in patients with cerebral palsy. Plastic and Reconstructive Surgery 107: 907–13.

Cichero J (1996) Cervical auscultation – an assessment of the sounds of swallowing. Australian Communication Quarterly (Spring): 22.

Clarke CE, Gullaksen E, Macdonald S, et al. (1998) Referral criteria for speech and language therapy assessment of dysphagia caused by idiopathic Parkinson's disease. Acta Neurologica Scandinavia 97: 27–35.

Crysdale WS, Raveh E, McCann C, et al. (2001) Management of drooling in individuals with neurodisability: a surgical experience. Developmental Medicine and Child Neurology 43(6): 379–83.

Daniels SK (2000) Swallowing apraxia: a disorder of the praxis system. Dysphagia 15(3): 159–66.

Dawes C, Watanabe S, Biglow-Lecomte P, et al. (1989) Estimation of the velocity of the salivary film at some different locations in the mouth. Journal of Dental Research 68(11): 1479–82.

Dawidson I, Blom M, Lundeberg T, et al. (1997) The influence of acupuncture on salivary flow rates in healthy subjects. Journal of Oral Rehabilitation 24(3): 204–8.

Domaracki LS, Sisson LA (1990) Decreasing drooling with oral motor stimulation in children with multiple disabilities. American Journal of Occupational Therapy 44(8): 680–4.

Drabmen R, Cordua y Cruz G, Ross J, et al. (1979) Suppression of chronic drooling in mentally retarded children and adolescents: Effectiveness of a behavioural treatment package. Behaviour Therapy 10: 46–56.

Eilers J, Berger AM, Petersen MC (1988) Development, testing, and application of the oral assessment guide. Oncology Nursing Forum 15(3): 325–30.

Eisenbruch A, Ship JA, Dawson LA, et al. (2003) Salivary gland sparing and improved target irradiation by conformal and intensity modulated irradiation of head and neck cancer. World Journal of Surgery 27: 832–7.

Ekberg O (2000) Diagnostic aspects of dysphagia. Acta Oto-Laryngologica, Supplement 543: 225–8.

Ekedahl C (1974) Surgical treatment of drooling. Acta Oto-Laryngologica 77: 215–20.

Foulsum IM (2002) Oral Health Screening Tool. Melbourne: Department of Human Services.

Francis JR, Hunter B, Addy M (1987) A comparison of three delivery methods of chlorhexidine in handicapped children. I: effects on plaque, gingivitis and tooth staining. Journal of Periodontal Research 58: 451–5.

Frederick FJ, Stewart MD (1982) Effectiveness of transtympanic neurectomy in management of sialoorrhea occurring in mentally retarded patients. Journal of Otolaryngology 11(4): 289–92.

Garliner D (1981) Myofunctional Therapy. Presented at the first European Congress for Myofunctional Therapy, 30 October to 1 November, Munich.

Gisel EG (1994) Oral motor skills following sensori-motor intervention in children with severe spastic cerebral palsy. Dysphagia 9(3): 180–92.

Griffiths J, Lewis D (2002) Guidelines for the oral care of patients who are dependent, dysphagic or critically ill. Journal of Disability and Oral Health 3(1): 30–3.

Haberfellner H, Gisel EG, Schwartz ST (1999) Oral-motor control and mobility in children with cerebral palsy and a moderate eating impairment. Developmental Medicine and Child Neurology 6–7.

Haberfellner H, Rossiwall B (1977) Treatment of oral sensor-motor disorders in cerebral palsied children: preliminary report. Developmental Medicine and Child Neurology 19: 350–2.

Hagg M, Larsson B (2004) Effects of motor and sensory stimulation in stroke patients with long lasting dysphagia. Dysphagia 19: 219–30.

Hallett KB, Lucas JO, Johnston T, et al. (1995). Dental health of children with cerebral palsy following sialodochoplasty. Special Care in Dentistry 15(6): 234–8.

Heine RG, Catto-Smith AG, Reddihough DS (1996) Effect of antreflux medication on salivary drooling in children with cerebral palsy. Developmental Medicine and Child Neurology 38: 1030–6.

Hilton JM, Fitzgerald DA, Cooper DM (1999) Respiratory morbidity of hospitalized children with Trisomy 21. Journal of Paediatrics and Child Health 35(4): 383–6.

Hohoff A, Ehmer U (1999) Short-term and long-term results after early treatment with Castillo Morales Stimulating Plate. J Orofacial Orthopedics 60: 2–12.

Johnson H, King J, Reddihough DS (2001) Children with sialorrhoea in the absence of neurological abnormalities. Child: Care, Health and Development 27(6): 591–602.

Johnson H, Reid S, Hazard K, et al. (2004) Effectiveness of the Innsbruck Sensori-motor Activator and Regulator in improving saliva control in children with cerebral palsy. Developmental Medicine and Child Neurology 46: 39–45.

Jongerius PH, Joosten F, Hoogen FJA, et al. (2003) The treatment of drooling by ultrasound-guided intraglandular injections of botulinum toxin type A into the salivary glands. Laryngoscope 113(1): 107–11.

Jordan K (1979) Rehabilitation of the patient with dysphagia. Ear, Nose and Throat Journal 58: 86–7.

Kapila YV, Dodds WJ, Helm JF, et al. (1984) Relationship between swallow rate and salivary flow. Digestive Diseases and Sciences 29(6): 528–33.

Kenny D, Casas MJ, Mc Pherson KA (1989) Correlation of ultrasound imaging of oral swallow with ventilatory alterations in cerebral palsied and normal children: Preliminary observations. Dysphagia 4: 112–17.

King P (2000) Poor oral health more than a sore tooth problem OR the dentists role in rehabilitation. Australian Dysphagia Newsletter, December: 1–3.

Koheil R, Sochaniwskyj A, Bablich K, et al. (1983) Biofeedback and behavioural techniques applied to remediation of drooling: An update. Paper presented at the 6th Annual Conference on Rehabilitation Engineering, San Diego, California.

Koheil R, Sochaniwskyj AE, Bablich K, et al. (1987) Biofeedback techniques and behaviour modification in the conservative remediation of drooling by children with cerebral palsy. Developmental Medicine and Child Neurology 29(1): 19–26.

Lagerlöf F, Dawes C (1984) The volume of saliva in the mouth before and after swallowing. Journal of Dental Research 63(5): 618–21.

Lancioi GE, Brouwer JA, Coninx F (1994) Automatic cueing to reduce drooling: a long-term follow up with two mentally handicapped persons. Journal of Behavioural Therapy and Experimental Psychiatry 25(2): 149–52.

Langmore SE (2001) Endoscopic Evaluation and Treatment of Swallowing Disorders. New York: Thieme Medical Publishers.

Langmore SE, Schatz K, Olsen N (1988) Fiberoptic endoscopic examination of swallowing safety: a new procedure. Dysphagia 2: 216–19.

Langmore SE, Skarupski KA, Park PS, et al. (2002) Predictors of aspiration pneumonia in nursing home residents. Dysphagia 17: 298–307.

Langmore SE, Terpenning MS, Schork A, et al. (1998) Predictors of aspiration pneumonia: how important is dysphagia? Dysphagia 13(2): 69–81.

Lash AA (2001) Sjögren's syndrome: pathogenesis, diagnosis, and treatment. Nurse Practitioner 26: 53–8.

Lear CS, Flanagan JB, Morres CFA (1965) The frequency of deglution in man. Archives of Oral Biology 10: 83–99.

Lespargot A, Langevin M, Muller S, et al. (1993) Swallowing disturbances associated with drooling in cerebral-palsied children. Developmental Medicine and Child Neurology 35: 298–304.

Levitt S (1966) Proprioceptive neuromuscular facilitation techniques in cerebral palsy. Physiotherapy 52(2): 46–51.

Limbrock GJ, Fischer-Brandies H, Avalle C (1991) Castillo-Morales' orofacial therapy: treatment of 67 children with Down syndrome. Developmental Medicine and Child Neurology 33(4): 296–303.

Logemann JA (1998) Evaluation and Treatment of Swallowing Disorders (2nd edn). Austin TX: Pro-ed.

Loiselle C (1979) Rood-based programme for decreasing pre-feeding behaviours. Canadian Journal of Occupational Therapy 46(3): 93–8.

Morris SE, Dunn Klein M (2000) Pre-Feeding Skills: A Comprehensive Resource for Mealtime Development (2nd edn). Austin, Texas: Pro-ed.

Murray J, Langmore SE, Ginsberg S, et al. (1996) The significance of accumulated oropharyngeal secretions and swallowing frequency in predicting aspiration. Dysphagia 11(2): 99–103.

Nelson CA, De Benabib RM (1991) Sensory preparation of the oral-motor area. In Langley MB, Lombardino LJ (eds) Neurodevelopmental Strategies for Managing Disorders in Children with Severe Motor Dysfunction. Austin,Texas: Pro-ed, pp. 131–58.

Perry A, Reilly S, Bloomberg K, et al. (2002) An analysis of needs for people with a disability who have complex communication needs. Melbourne: La Trobe University.

Porta M, Gamba M, Bertacchi G, et al. (2001) Treatment of sialorrhea with ultrasound guided botulinum toxin A injection in patients with neurological disorders. Journal of Neurology, Neurosurgery and Psychiatry 70(4): 538–40.

Rapp D (1980) Drool control: long-term follow-up. Developmental Medicine and Child Neurology 22(4): 448–53.

Reddihough D, Johnson H, Staples M, et al. (1990) Use of benzhexol hydrochloride to control drooling of children with cerebral palsy. Developmental Medicine and Child Neurology 32(11): 985–9.

Robbins J (1987) Swallowing in ALS and motor neuron disease. Neurology Clinics 5: 213–29.

Rudney JD, Larson CJ (1995) The prediction of saliva swallowing frequency in humans from estimates of salivary flow rate and the volume of saliva swallowed. Archives of Oral Biology 40(6): 507–12.

Scannapieco FA (1999) Role of oral bacteria in respiratory infection. Journal of Periodontal Research 70: 793–802.

Selley WG (1977) Dental help for stroke patients. British Dental Journal 143(12): 409–12.

Selley WG, Flack FC, Ellis RE, et al. (1989a) Respiratory patterns associated with swallowing: Part 1. The normal adult pattern and changes with age. Age and Ageing 18(3): 168–72.

Selley WG, Flack FC, Ellis RE, et al. (1989b) Respiratory patterns associated with swallowing: Part 2. Neurologically impaired dysphagic patients. Age and Ageing 18(3): 173–6.

Sheppard JJ, Burke L, Leone AM, et al. (2003) Frequency of saliva swallowing in children before and after feeding. American Speech-Language-Hearing Association Convention, Chicago, November.

Shirley WP, Hill JS, Woolley AL, et al. (2003) Success and complications of four duct ligation for sialorrhea. Journal of Paediatric Otorhinolaryngology 67(1): 1–6.

Smithhard DG, O'Neill PA, England RE, et al. (1997) The natural history of dysphagia in stroke. Dysphagia 12: 188–93.

Sochaniwskyj AD, Koheil RM, Bablich K, et al. (1986) Oral motor functioning, frequency of swallowing and drooling in normal children and in children with cerebral palsy. Archives of Physical Medicine and Rehabilitation 67: 866–74.

Sonies BC, Wang C, Sapper D (1996) Assessment of hyoid movement during swallowing by the use of ultrasound duplex-doppler imaging. Dysphagia 11(2): 162.

Suskind DL, Tilton A (2002) Clinical study of botulinum – a toxin in the treatment of sialorrhea in children with cerebral palsy. Laryngoscope 112(1): 73–81.

Symonds RP (2001) Radiotherapy. British Medical Journal 323: 1107–10.

Tahmassebi JF, Curzon ME (2003) The cause of drooling in children with cerebral palsy– hypersalivation or swallowing defect? International Journal of Paediatric Dentistry 13(2): 106–11.

Takahashi K, Groher ME, Micchi K (1994) Symmetry and reproducability of swallowing sounds. Dysphagia 9: 168–73.

Terpenning MS, Taylor GW, Lopatin DE, et al. (2001) Aspiration pneumonia: dental and oral risk factors in an older veteran population. Journal of the American Geriatrics Society 49(5): 557–63.

Thomas-Stonell N, Greenberg J (1988) Three treatment approaches and clinical factors in the reduction of drooling. Dysphagia 3(2): 73–8.

Uppal HS, De R, D'Souza AR, et al. (2003) Bilateral submandibular duct relocation for drooling: an evaluation of results for the Birmingham Children's Hospital. European Archives of Oto-Rhino-Laryngology 260(1): 48–51.

Van de Heyning PH, Marquet JF, Creten WL (1980) Drooling in children with cerebral palsy. Acta Oto-Rhino-Laryngologica Belgica 34(6): 691–705.

Vandenplas Y (1997) Asthma and gastroesophageal reflux. Journal of Pediatric Gastroenterology and Nutrition 24: 89–99.

Wake MA, Hesketh K, Allen MA (1999) Parental beliefs about teething: A survey of Australian parents. Journal of Paediatric Child Health 35: 446–9.

Walmsley AD (1997) The electric toothbrush: a review. British Dental Journal 182(6): 209–18.

Watanabe S, Dawes C (1988) A comparison of the effects of tasting and chewing foods on the flow rate of whole saliva in man. Archives of Oral Biology 33(10): 761–4.

Watanabe S, Dawes C (1990) Salivary flow rates and salivary film thickness in five-year-old children. Journal of Dental Research 69(5): 1150–3.

Wells R (2000) Bonfire of love. Exceptional Parent 30: 40–4.

Wilkie TF, Brody GS (1977) The surgical treatment of drooling: a ten-year review. Journal of Plastic and Reconstructive Surgery 59(6): 791–8.

Wong V, Sun JG, Wong W (2001) Traditional Chinese medicine (tongue acupuncture) in children with drooling problems. Pediatric Neurology 25(1): 47–54.

Zeppetella G (1999) Nebulized scopolamine in the management of oral dribbling: three case reports. Journal of Pain and Symptom Management 17(4): 293–5.

APPENDIX 6.1: SALIVA CONTROL ASSESSMENT FORM

Date: /   /
Name: _____
Form completed by: _____
                         _____
                         _____

1. Communication skills:
   - ❑ No problems
   - ❑ Some speech which is functional
   - ❑ Uses speech to get message across but with difficulty
   - ❑ Has difficulty making some sounds in words
   - ❑ Has no speech

2. Walking
   - ❑ No difficulty
   - ❑ Has some difficulty but walks independently without an aid
   - ❑ Needs a walking aid
   - ❑ Uses a wheelchair all or most of the time

3. Head position
   - ❑ Can hold head up without difficulty
   - ❑ Tends to sit with head down mostly

4. Is the mouth always open?
   - ❑ Yes   ❑ No   ❑ Unsure

5. Lips
   - ❑ Can hold lips together easily and for a long time
   - ❑ Can hold lips together with ease for a limited time
   - ❑ Can hold lips with effort for a limited time
   - ❑ Can bring lips together only briefly
   - ❑ Unable to bring lips together

6. Can s/he pucker lips (as in a kiss)?
   - ❑ Yes   ❑ No   ❑ Unsure

7. Does s/he push the tongue out when swallows?
   - ❑ Yes   ❑ No   ❑ Unsure

8. Straw
   - ❑ Can use a straw easily
   - ❑ Has difficulty using a straw
   - ❑ Cannot use a straw

9. Eating/drinking
   - ❑ Can eat whole hard foods that are difficult to chew
   - ❑ Eats a wide range of foods

❑ Needs to have food cut into small pieces
❑ Food needs to be mashed/pureed
❑ Drinks need to be thickened
❑ Has food through a tube (nasogastric/gastrostomy)

10. Is s/he a messy eater?
❑ Yes ❑ No ❑ Unsure

11. Can s/he swallow saliva when asked to?
❑ Yes ❑ No ❑ Attempts ❑ Unsure

12. How frequent do you notice a swallow?
❑ Once a minute ❑ Several times a minute ❑ Occasionally
❑ Only when ❑ Only when I ask him/her ❑ Unsure
   eating, drinking to swallow

13. Does s/he notice saliva on lips/chin (perhaps tries to wipe chin)?
❑ Yes ❑ No ❑ Unsure

14. General health
Does s/he have asthma?
❑ Yes ❑ No ❑ Unsure
Does s/he have frequently blocked or runny nose?
❑ Yes ❑ No ❑ Unsure
Does s/he have bouts of pneumonia?
❑ Yes ❑ No ❑ Unsure

15. Are there any difficulties with teeth cleaning?
❑ Yes ❑ No ❑ Unsure

16. Has there been a recent dental check?
❑ Yes ❑ No ❑ Unsure
❑ IF YES, who?

17. Are there any problems with bleeding gums or decayed teeth?
❑ Yes ❑ No ❑ Unsure

Thank you for completing this questionnaire.

APPENDIX 6.2: DROOLING MEASURES FORM

Date: / /
Name of child: _____
Form completed by: _____
Relationship to child: _____

1. Is your child currently on medication to reduce drooling? (*please tick*)
❑ No ❑ Yes

If yes, please give name and amount taken during the last week:

_____

_____

2. Has your child been well over the past week? (*please tick*)
   ❑ No   ❑ Yes
   If no, please give details of illness: _____

_____

3. Rating scale. Please discuss these with anyone who knows your child well and circle the number which best reflects the severity and frequency of drooling over the past week:
   Frequency

   1 No drooling – dry
   2 Occasional drooling – not every day
   3 Frequent drooling – every day but not all day
   4 Constant drooling – always wet

   Severity

   1 Dry – never drools
   2 Mild – only the lips are wet
   3 Moderate – wet on the lips and the chin
   4 Severe – drools to the extent the clothes &/or objects get wet
   5 Profuse – clothing, hands and objects become very wet

4. On an average day over the past week when your child is at home:
   Number of bib changes per day: _____
   Number of clothes changes per day: _____

For the questions 5-14, please draw a circle around the number between 1 and 10 that indicates the extent to which each question about drooling has affected you over the past week.

For example:
   How much do television advertisements annoy you?

   ☺ Not at all   [1 2 3 4 5 6 7 8 (9) 10] Heaps   ☹

5. How offensive was the smell of the saliva?

   No smell   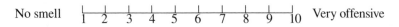   Very offensive

6. How much of a problem has there been with skin rashes on the chin and around mouth?

   No rash   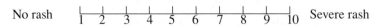   Severe rash

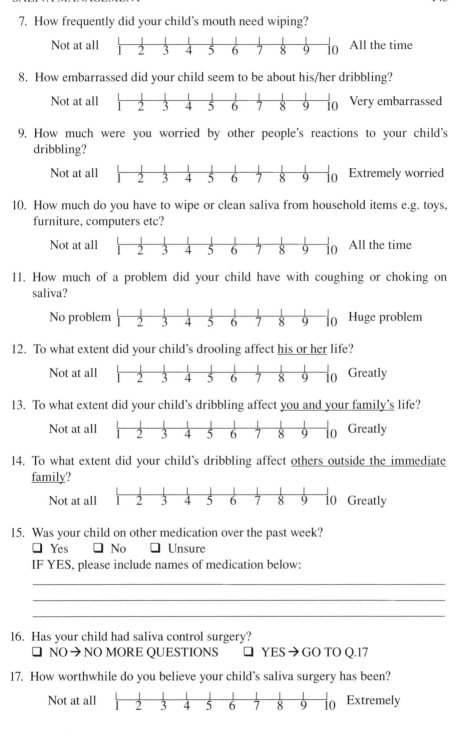

7. How frequently did your child's mouth need wiping?

Not at all   1 2 3 4 5 6 7 8 9 10   All the time

8. How embarrassed did your child seem to be about his/her dribbling?

Not at all   1 2 3 4 5 6 7 8 9 10   Very embarrassed

9. How much were you worried by other people's reactions to your child's dribbling?

Not at all   1 2 3 4 5 6 7 8 9 10   Extremely worried

10. How much do you have to wipe or clean saliva from household items e.g. toys, furniture, computers etc?

Not at all   1 2 3 4 5 6 7 8 9 10   All the time

11. How much of a problem did your child have with coughing or choking on saliva?

No problem   1 2 3 4 5 6 7 8 9 10   Huge problem

12. To what extent did your child's drooling affect <u>his or her</u> life?

Not at all   1 2 3 4 5 6 7 8 9 10   Greatly

13. To what extent did your child's dribbling affect <u>you and your family's</u> life?

Not at all   1 2 3 4 5 6 7 8 9 10   Greatly

14. To what extent did your child's dribbling affect <u>others outside the immediate family</u>?

Not at all   1 2 3 4 5 6 7 8 9 10   Greatly

15. Was your child on other medication over the past week?
 ❑ Yes   ❑ No   ❑ Unsure
 IF YES, please include names of medication below:

_____

_____

_____

16. Has your child had saliva control surgery?
 ❑ NO → NO MORE QUESTIONS   ❑ YES → GO TO Q.17

17. How worthwhile do you believe your child's saliva surgery has been?

Not at all   1 2 3 4 5 6 7 8 9 10   Extremely

18. How likely would you be to recommend this surgery to other families in the same circumstances?

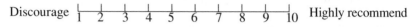

Discourage   1   2   3   4   5   6   7   8   9   10   Highly recommend

Comments:

Thank you for completing this questionnaire.

Part II Assessment of Swallowing Disorders

7 Clinical Assessment, Cervical Auscultation and Pulse Oximetry

JULIE CICHERO

Why is it important to look at non-imaging assessments of dysphagia? Primarily, because these are our first 'ports of call'. Non-imaging assessments provide information about the swallowing function that can be accessed at the bedside or in an office setting. The results can also be gathered quickly. In extended care settings, educational settings or rural settings, non-imaging techniques are often the only tools available for dysphagia assessment. It could also be argued that we gain the best understanding of our patients' everyday swallowing function from non-imaging assessments because they are carried out using real foods and fluids and in an atmosphere where we usually eat. However, there is still a need for imaging studies. Such studies indisputably provide us with covert information, particularly about pharyngeal stage function (see Chapter 8). However, we must all be skilled in non-imaging studies, for it is from here that we begin to make our hypotheses.

The best known, and most widely taught non-imaging technique is the 'clinical' or 'bedside' evaluation of dysphagia. With a solid understanding of this assessment, we gain a baseline level of a person's functional swallowing ability. We are able to examine oromotor function as it relates to swallowing and begin to make decisions as to the person's suitability for oral or non-oral feeding, of which there are many permutations. In addition, it allows us to determine which other assessments may be necessary to fully diagnose and treat the problem.

When used in isolation, the clinical assessment of dysphagia has come under attack due to its poor ability to characterize the pharyngeal phase of the swallow. The oral stage of swallowing is reasonably overt. With a thorough motor and sensory assessment of oral structure, we should be able to diagnose the majority of oral stage disorders. The pharyngeal phase of the swallow is by nature covert and it is therefore more difficult to characterize its physiology using non-imaging methods. The clinical assessment has been reported in the literature to have a poor ability to characterize the pharyngeal stage of the swallow. It credits clinicians with an ability to detect only 40% to 60% of those who aspirate (Splaingard et al., 1988; DePippo et al., 1992; Linden et al., 1993; Groher, 1994; Ruf and Stevens, 1995). Because of its poor ability to characterize the pharyngeal phase of the swallow, the clinical examination has been deemed a 'screening technique', rather than a 'diagnostic tool'. Logemann (1998) defines a

Dysphagia: Foundation, Theory and Practice. Edited by J. Cichero and B. Murdoch
© 2006 John Wiley & Sons, Ltd.

screening procedure as one where the presence or absence of a *symptom* is indicated (for example the presence or absence of aspiration). A diagnostic tool on the other hand is one where the physiology is elucidated (for example, reduced tongue-base retraction or reduced laryngeal closure). What is lost in the translation of this very black-and-white view is a large amount of additional information that is gained from a clinical examination. Information such as level of alertness, the person's ability to make decisions, self-feeding skills, and sensory awareness. There is an inexhaustive list of behaviour that the clinician can observe. Factors such as these will have a huge bearing on the potential for swallowing rehabilitation and eventual outcome.

Recently two other non-imaging assessments have received literature and clinical attention. These include cervical auscultation and pulse oximetry. Used in isolation, these techniques provide some new information about the dysphagic person's ability to swallow. Used in conjunction with the clinical examination, these tools provide powerful screening assessments as they tap into other modalities (e.g. hearing) and physiologically based information such as the inter-relationship between swallowing and respiration (see also Chapter 4). It is acknowledged that the assessments described in this chapter are screening assessments according to Logemann's definitions. However, it is through tools such as these that we can:

- begin to characterize dysphagia;
- make judgements as to the severity of the dysphagia;
- refer for diagnostic procedures that are specifically tailored to each individual because of our skill with these non-imaging assessments; and
- monitor patients on a regular basis using dietary foods and fluids.

This chapter will describe the clinical examination of dysphagia, cervical auscultation and pulse oximetry. In each case there will be a discussion of the theory and then the clinical application of the technique. The clinical examination is described in detail first. Cervical auscultation and pulse oximetry are seen as adjuncts to the clinical examination. The way in which these assessments could influence imaging studies is also discussed.

CLINICAL ASSESSMENT OF DYSPHAGIA

The clinical assessment of dysphagia affords the clinician an opportunity to look at the overall swallowing function of an individual in context. This technique is faithfully taught to all speech pathology students for this very reason. The clinical examination can be divided into eight phases. These are:

1. background history;
2. immediate observations;
3. communication and cognition;
4. clinical oropharyngeal assessment;
5. oral trial assessment;

6. referral for other assessments;
7. overall impression including diagnosis;
8. management.

PHASE 1 – BACKGROUND HISTORY

It is imperative that a thorough background history be taken. There are many other facets of information that the clinician should gather in order to adequately diagnose and treat patients. The clinician should take the time to review the following broad areas:

• medical diagnosis;
• nutritional status and immediate nutritional needs;
• current medical status;
• previous speech pathology involvement; and
• client-specific information.

Medical diagnosis

The medical diagnosis should be noted to see if any predictions about likely swallowing dysfunction can be anticipated. For example, in an individual who presents with a right-sided stroke one might expect to find a left facial droop, and reduced awareness of pooled material in the left buccal cavity. The diagnosis can give the clinician a small mental checklist to see if the medical diagnosis matches the clinical presentation. In the case of a progressive neurological disease, knowledge of the disease presentation and general course also allows the clinician to predict the severity of the swallowing disorder.

Conversely clinical presentation may also alert the speech pathologist to other underlying medical conditions that have yet to be diagnosed. For example, an individual is referred with a diagnosis of left cortical stroke, yet on presentation apart from the obvious facial palsy the individual has tears on the right lower eyelid and is unable to close the right eye. These symptoms suggest that there is lower motor neurone involvement. Perhaps the individual has upper *and* lower motor neurone disorders, or perhaps the facial weakness was misdiagnosed as a cortical stroke. Our knowledge of neuroanatomy allows us to make further inquiries. By using our problem-solving skills we are able to obtain an accurate diagnosis and therefore a more tailored treatment plan.

Back to the patient who has presented with what seems to be upper and lower motor neurone signs. Under these circumstances it would be prudent to see if there were other clinical manifestations of stroke – e.g. weakness of the right arm or leg. It may also be prudent to check whether the individual has experienced any change in their hearing function. We know that the facial (VII) and vestibulochochelar nerves (VIII) share a pathway through the internal acoustic meatus. Damage to both nerves suggests a lesion or assault that would fit with a lower motor neurone presentation, particularly if the patient complained of hearing loss. An accurate diagnosis at the outset allows the clinician to tailor a treatment plan. This is why a general 'cookbook' or recipe approach to dysphagia is ill advised.

Any co-occuring infections or other illnesses should also be noted for the safety of both patient and practitioner. For example, if a dysphagic patient presents with a head injury and also hepatitis B, this requires the speech pathologist to use universal precautions for communicable diseases. Similarly immunosuppressed patients should not be treated by speech pathologists who are themselves unwell. The clinician who continues to work while unwell risks infecting immunosuppressed patients and could be placing them in a life-threatening situation.

Nutritional status and immediate nutritional needs

The speech pathologist should be aware of the individual's current and premorbid diet. Care should be taken when individuals are noted as 'nil oral' to find out whether the 'nil oral' status is because of pending speech pathology assessment or required for a pending medical procedure (e.g. surgery requiring general anaesthesia). Nil oral patients should be viewed for the length of time that they have been without oral or supplemental intake. The presence of an intravenous drip should also be noted. Nil oral patients presenting with an intravenous drip, nasogastric tube, PEG (percutaneous endoscopic gastrostomy), or total parenteral nutrition (TPN) have some means of hydration and nutrition. Nil oral patients presenting without assisted hydration at a minimum, require immediate attention to see whether they can safely meet their hydration needs orally. At the end of the clinical assessment the speech pathologist must be in a position to indicate how nutritional needs will be met – either orally, non-orally, or a combination of both (see also Chapter 5).

Current medical status

Information on current medical status could be gathered from the medical chart, nursing staff, or the individual's carer. Current level of alertness is important to ascertain whether it is a good time to complete the physical clinical examination of swallowing function. Respiratory status should also be noted – is there a current chest infection? Does the medical chart report abnormal breath sounds such as crackles or wheezes? Is there evidence of altered respiratory rate such as bradypnea (abnormal slowness of breathing) or hyperpnea (abnormally fast rate of breathing), or dyspnea (laboured or difficult breathing)? Changes to respiration may affect the person's ability to swallow safely. For example, individuals with chronic obstructive pulmonary disease (COPD) not only have problems maintaining usual respiration patterns due to chronic lung disease but also suffer from fatigue of respiratory muscles (Martin-Harris, 2000). When we swallow, we close and protect the airway during bolus transport through the pharynx and we stop breathing. In respiratory compromised patients, the effort in maintaining respiration may make swallowing an extraordinarily difficult task.

Does the individual have a fever? This may be indicative of an infection. As a point of reference normal temperature is in the range of 35.8 °C to 37.2 °C. A low-grade fever is defined as 37.5 °C to 38.0 °C and a high grade fever as 38.8 °C and higher. Individuals in a feverish state should be closely monitored as swallowing function during the fever state may be different from when the temperature is normal. Note should also be taken if there has been a history of recurrent pneumonia or chest infections. Note also that high temperatures may be caused by conditions other than poor chest status (e.g. urinary tract infection). Liaison with medical staff is imperative in interpreting clinical signs.

A list of current medications should also be reviewed. There are some medications that are known to have adverse effects on swallowing function. Medications that cause dryness of the oral, nasal or pharyngeal mucosae can make it difficult to initiate a swallow (see Chapter 9). Other medications may produce side effects simulating extrapyramidal symptoms (see Chapter 9). The speech pathologist should also review the method by which medications are being administered (tablet, capsule, liquid, etc.). Individuals with severe dysphagia may be unable to take medication in a tablet or capsule format and may require the pharmacist to see if there is an alternative method of administration. Also note that some capsules or tablets have special enteric coatings to ensure that they do not disperse before they reach the stomach. Placing these medications in a spoonful of thickened fluids may assist the patient in swallowing the medication but reduces the effect of the medication if it disperses throughout the pharynx and oesophagus rather than in the stomach. If in doubt, always consult medical team members such as the pharmacist, doctor and nursing staff.

Previous speech pathology intervention

As part of any thorough background review, evidence of previous speech pathology intervention should also be sought. Knowledge of previous clinical reports or imaging studies such as videofluoroscopy affords the clinician a baseline of swallowing function.

Client-specific information

It is important to remember that no two individuals are the same. We each have unique biographical, cultural and religious backgrounds, educational and vocational backgrounds and behaviours. This information should direct how we interact with and provide information to our patients. For example, in providing explanations for a swallowing assessment and how it is carried out one should be aware of the patient's educational and vocational background. The explanation afforded a person with tertiary qualifications should be quite different from the explanation offered to an individual with little schooling. Cultural differences may be highlighted when it comes to discussions of the patient's goals. For example, the patient's goal may be to resume eating the premorbid diet. In Western cultures, texture-modified diets are prepared on a Western model (for example, pureed lamb, mashed potatoes, vitamized vegetables and milk desserts). For example, for individuals of Asian, European or Middle Eastern cultures, the Western texture modified diets offered may be unappealing to the point that they might cause a reluctance to eat, which then slows down recovery. This is another example of why it is important that each dysphagic individual be seen as unique, and treated as such.

In addition to the above information, some general information should be gathered from the individual with dysphagia or their next of kin or carer. Questions for the individual with dysphagia and/or their next of kin are:

- When did the swallowing problem begin?
- How long has the problem has been in existence?
- Was it an immediate or gradual onset?
- Is there pain associated with swallowing and if so where?
- Has there been a change to the length of time needed to consume a meal?
- Has there been a change in the type of foods or liquids consumed?
- Has there been a change to the sensations of smell and/or taste?

Once the background information has been obtained, the individual should be observed.

PHASE 2 – IMMEDIATE OBSERVATIONS

On greeting the patient, the clinician is able to gain much valuable information, which will assist with the actual assessment and help plan treatment. A number of areas need to be reviewed. These are:

- Is the patient alert and able to participate in an oromotor assessment and a swallowing evaluation?
- Is the patient cooperative and if not is it only transitory?
- Is the patient agitated? This aspect will influence all future mealtime events.
- Is the patient able to sit upright independently, or does he or she need support to sit upright?

    - How many people are required to have the person in the optimum position for safe swallowing?
    - Are lifting machines required to move the person to the best position for safe swallowing?

- Note the presence of an intravenous line, nasogastric tube, PEG, TPN or central line, or tracheostomy tube.
- If there is a tracheostomy tube *in situ* what size is it?

    - Is the tube cuffed/uncuffed, fenestrated/unfenestrated?
    - If suctioning is required, how often is it required?
    - Does the individual require oxygen via mask/nasal prongs?

- Is the patient ambulant?
- Is the patient prone to fatigue easily?

    - Fatigue in other aspects of care could serve as a potential indicator for fatigue during swallowing.

- Is the person aware that he or she has a swallowing problem?
- Does the person 'look healthy', or does the person seem underweight?
- Note should be taken of any shortness of breath and respiratory rate, particularly if the individual presents with a primary respiratory diagnosis.

The relationship between swallowing and respiration has been outlined in detail in Chapter 4, which includes normal respiratory rates that can be used as a reference. As noted in Chapter 4, if the resting respiratory rate is abnormal, the individual is automatically at an increased risk of aspiration. It is normal for there to be a small increase (approximately 10%) in respiratory rate after swallowing, however this rapidly returns to normal in a non-dysphagic individual (Hirst et al., 2002).

PHASE 3 – COMMUNICATION AND COGNITION

The clinician should gain information on whether the person is oriented to person, place and time. Comprehension ability should be noted, and the need for hearing aids should also be established. Expressive abilities and intelligibility should also be noted. Voice quality should also be subjectively noted (particularly for the parameters of wetness, hoarseness, breathiness or harshness). Visual ability should also be established. For example, the need for eye glasses or any disturbances in visuoperceptual skills such as those that might be found after a stroke (e.g. left neglect in the case of a right hemisphere stroke) should be noted and taken into account during assessment and treatment. Logemann et al. (1999) provide excellent descriptions of behavioural variables, gross motor function and oromotor variables that may affect swallowing in their screening procedure for oropharyngeal dysphagia.

PHASE 4 – CLINICAL OROPHARYNGEAL ASSESSMENT OF DYSPHAGIA

Prior to commencing any physical examination of the individual, the speech pathologist should ensure adherence to workplace occupational health and safety guidelines. These may include, but are not limited to, up-to-date immunization of the speech pathologist (e.g. hepatitis B), handwashing before and after assessment, the use of gloves during physical examination of the patient, and if directed the use of gowns or protective eye wear during assessment. Disposal of contaminated materials such as gloves or tongue depressors should be carried out responsibly in the manner dictated by the workplace.

The oropharyngeal assessment of dysphagia can be broken into the following sub-areas:

- inspection of the oral cavity and oropharynx;
- saliva management;
- cranial nerve assessment; and
- ability to protect the airway.

Inspection of the oral cavity and oropharynx

The clinician should be aware of any abnormalities of structures at rest within the oral cavity. Any blisters, lesions or growths should be noted and reported. Symmetry of any blisters should also be noted. For example, blisters only on the left buccal surface in a patient with a right hemisphere stroke may be indicative of the patient biting the left buccal region during eating and point to poor intraoral sensory perception for the affected side. Moisture within the oral cavity should be noted. Extensive dryness of the mouth makes it difficult to initiate a swallow, as does the presence of thick mucus (Miller, 1992). Oral hygiene should also be examined. Evidence of food debris in the buccal sulcii should be noted and removed. It should be noted whether patients care for their own oral hygiene or are reliant on carers. Langmore et al. (1998) noted that the best predictors for pneumonia were dependency for feeding, dependency for oral care, number of decayed teeth, tube feeding, more than one medical diagnosis, number of medications and smoking. In conjunction with this the state of the person's dentition should also be examined. Tooth pain should be noted, with referral made to a dental professional. Tooth pain can affect the person's tolerance of chewing. Halitosis can be caused by – but is not limited to – decaying food that has been pooled in the buccal sulcii, or even in a pharyngeal pouch. The need for dentures should be noted. There is research to suggest that poor oral hygiene may be a risk factor for respiratory tract infections, particularly for elderly institutionalized individuals. The mechanism for this includes aspiration of oral pathogens carried on saliva or food/fluid particles (Langmore et al., 1998).

Saliva management

The issue of saliva management has been thoroughly examined in Chapter 6. The clinician should note patients' awareness of their secretions. Poor awareness may be indicated by drooling or pooling of saliva within the oral cavity. It should also be noted whether the patient wipes the mouth with a hand or tissue in an attempt to control saliva management. A patient's ability to swallow his or her own secretions should also observed, particularly whether this is a spontaneous action or requires prompting by a carer to swallow pooled material. Frequency of throat clearing after swallowing of secretions should also be noted. Note that throat clearing is a protective mechanism. A gurgling vocal quality after swallowing of secretions may indicate pooled material in the pharynx.

Cranial nerve assessment

Assessment of the cranial nerves involved in chewing and swallowing affords the clinician information about the strength, speed and accuracy of movement of oral and pharyngeal structures and also provides information about sensory level of functioning. The clinician should also note symmetry or asymmetry of movement or loss of sensation. Cranial nerves V, VII, IX, X, XI and XII are most commonly assessed for swallowing function. These nerves and their function in swallowing has been discussed in detail in Chapter 1. Table 7.1 suggests clinical assessments of the cranial nerves involved in swallowing.

Table 7.1 Suggested clinical assessment of the cranial nerves associated with swallowing – Observe strength, speed, range and symmetry of movement and fatigue

Cranial nerve or swallow-respiratory skill	Suggested clinical assessment tasks
V Trigeminal	• Ask the person to clench their teeth or 'bite together' – the masseter and temporalis muscles can be palpated and felt to contract. • The clinician could also place their hand under the person's closed jaw and ask the person to open the jaw while the clinician's hand provides resistance. This provides information about the strength of the jaw for chewing.
VII Facial	Sensory • Taste can be assessed using solutions of sugar (sweet), salt (salt), vinegar (sour) or onion juice (bitter) (see Chapter 13). Motor • Observe frowning, open and close eyes. • Ask patient to open and close mouth, smile, mouth the sounds 'ooo' then 'eee'. • Puff up their cheeks with air and hold to observe labial strength and velopharyngeal sufficiency .

IX Glossopharyngeal and X vagus	• Observation of palatal movement as the patient says 'ahh'.
	   ○ If functioning normally, the soft palate should rise symmetrically and the uvula should move backwards in the midline.
	   ○ If there is asymmetry and the soft palate is sagging, the uvula will deviate towards the normal side as there is insufficient muscle tension from the affected side to hold it in the mid-line.
	• The gag reflex should be elicited using a tongue depressor walking along and touching each of (a) the posterior surface of the tongue, (b) the tonsilar region and (c) soft palate.
	   ○ If no response is elicited from the soft palate the clinician may wish to touch the posterior pharyngeal wall to see if a response can be elicited.
	   ○ The gag reflex should be tested on both sides (see text for normal variations).

(Continued)

Table 7.1 (*Continued*)

Cranial nerve or swallow-respiratory skill	Suggested clinical assessment tasks

	• Ask the individual to phonate (e.g. 'ahhhh') and listen to phonatory quality.
	 • Ask the person to cough.
	   ○ This gives an indication of (a) ability to follow a command, (b) ability to perform a voluntary cough, (c) the strength of the cough.
	   ○ Observe also any reflexive coughs as these may be different in strength to voluntary coughs.
	 • Ask the patient to perform a 'dry swallow' (i.e. swallow the saliva in their mouth).

XII Hypoglossal	• The tongue should be observed at rest for evidence of atrophy or fasiculations.
	   ○ Atrophy or fasiculations are associated with LMN lesions.
	 • The tongue should also be observed in movement.
	   ○ Ask the patient to poke the tongue out, point up towards the nose, down towards the chin, protrude to the left and the right, and then move in a circular motion as if licking the lips.
	   ○ For patients where an apraxia appears to be present the clinician may, for example, try giving a cue that 'there is something on your top lip, can you lick it off?' Often an automatic response is more easily generated than a response to a specific command.
	 • Ask the patient to use their tongue to push against a tongue depressor stick, or patient to poke tongue against the inside of their cheek while the clinician resists the movement from the external cheek (check strength of movement).
	 • Note clarity of articulation and presence of dysarthria.
	   ○ A fully functioning tongue is important for clear, intelligible speech.

Airway protection	• Ask the patient to voluntarily hold their breath for the count of two.
	   ○ This gives an indication of voluntary control over breath holding.
	   ○ Note that the apnoeic period may still be triggered reflexively during a swallow even if the individual cannot voluntarily hold their breath.

Cranial nerve V – trigeminal nerve

This nerve has both motor and sensory components. It provides general sensation for the anterior two-thirds of the tongue, and is motor to the masticatory muscles, and the floor of the mouth.

Cranial nerve VII – facial nerve

The facial nerve is both sensory and motor. It provides sensory information in the form of taste from the anterior two-thirds of the tongue via the chorda tympani. The facial nerve is motor to the following muscles: orbicularis oculi and oris, zygomatic, buccinator, platysma, stylohyoid, and stapedius.

Note that in a lesion involving upper motor neurones (UMN) only the muscles of the lower face are paralysed due to bilateral corticonuclear fibres supplying the upper face. In the case of lower motor neurone involvement (LMN) there will be complete involvement of all facial muscles on the affected side including an inability to close the affected eye, and tears on the lower eyelid of the affected eye. Apart from important neurological information gained from this assessment which will help to ascertain the cause of the swallowing problem, this assessment also provides information about the person's ability to keep the bolus within the oral cavity.

Cranial nerve IX – glossopharyngeal nerve and cranial nerve X – vagus nerve

Cranial nerves IX and X are examined together and, therefore, will be discussed together. The glossopharyngeal nerve is both sensory and motor. It is responsible for taste for the posterior one third of the tongue and sensation of the soft palate. It is motor to stylopharyngeus, the otic ganglion, and partial to the middle/inferior pharyngeal constrictor. It also supplies the parotid salivary gland. The glossopharyngeal nerve is responsible for elevation of the pharynx and larynx and contributes to pharyngeal constriction. The vagus nerve is possibly the most important nerve for swallowing function. The vagus nerve has both sensory and motor functions. It is sensory to the pharynx, larynx and viscera. It is motor to the inferior, middle and superior pharyngeal constrictors, levator veli palatini, uvular, cricothyroid, thyroarytenoid, cricoarytenoids, transverse and oblique arytenoids, and oesophagus. It is responsible for palatal elevation and depression, laryngeal movement, pharyngeal constriction and cricopharyngeal movement.

Traditionally the gag reflex is also assessed. A sluggish or absent gag reflex provides information about level of sensation in that region. Its presence is not indicative of swallowing safety. The purpose of the gag reflex is to protect the pharynx from foreign bodies. It is designed to expel vomit and refluxed material from below and foreign bodies such as an overly large bolus or the tongue depressor anteriorly. As such it works in the completely opposite way to a normal swallow, which is designed to propel the bolus through the pharynx. Oropharyngeal movements during the retching have been described in Chapter 4.

There is much confusion surrounding the gag reflex, not the least of which comes from the medical fraternity (Smithard and Spriggs, 2003). Many referrals suggest that swallowing is occurring safely because of an intact gag reflex. This assumption is often made regardless of how uncoordinated the swallow may actually be.

The assumption may be based on the sensory aspect of the reflex – if the swallow is incomplete and there is pooled material in the pharynx post swallow it is assumed that the gag reflex will be elicited and remove the material from the pharynx. The presence or absence of the gag reflex may be indicative of sensation in that region but one cannot assume that a gag reflex will be triggered in the event of pooled material in the pharynx. Neurology shows us that sensation for the soft palate, which is where the gag reflex is elicited, is mediated via the glossopharyngeal nerve, whereas sensation for the pharynx and larynx, which are where pooled material may accumulate after the swallow, is mediated via the vagus nerve. While these two nerves work in harmony the fact that one is working is not predictive that the other is also working. It is also very important to note that there is a large degree of variability in the gag reflex in healthy non-dysphagic adults. Logemann (1995) reports that approximately 40% of non-dysphagic men and 10% of non-dysphagic women do not have a gag reflex (Smithard and Spriggs, 2003).

The vagus nerve can also be assessed by asking the person to phonate. The quality of phonation gives information about vocal fold function. If the phonation sounds 'wet' or 'gurgling' it may indicate that there are secretions or pooled material over the surface of the cords or in the laryngeal vestibule. Dysphonia may also indicate inability to coordinate vocal fold closure. The length of time an individual can phonate for may also give an indication of their ability to control their respiratory system.

Warms and Richards (2000) investigated the correlation between wet vocal quality and prediction of pooled material in the larynx/trachea as indicative of aspiration or penetration. Their results indicated that such a correlation could not be made. The authors advocated that wet voice could be used as one of a cluster of clinical signs that is indicative of aspiration or penetration but used in isolation was not a reliable indicator of these events. They also stated that presence of wet voice could be more indicative of gross risk of aspiration of all materials (i.e. saliva and secretions in addition to ingested foods or fluids). The cough reflex is also routinely assessed (mediated via the vagus nerve). Physiology of the cough reflex was discussed in Chapter 4.

The patient should also be asked to perform a 'dry swallow' (or to swallow the saliva in their mouth). Again, this gives an indication of the person's ability to follow a command, and an opportunity to observe and palpate the action of the swallow. Clinicians should watch the laryngeal region, and also span their fingers out placing the index finger on the subject's hyoid bone, the middle finger on the thyroid cartilage and the ring finger on the cricoid cartilage. This palpation should be very gentle so as not to impede the mechanics of the swallowing process. The clinician should also take note of any delay in initiating the swallow.

Cranial nerve XII – hypoglossal nerve

The hypoglossal nerve is motor. It supplies the superior longitundinal, inferior longitudinal, transverse, vertical, genioglossus, hypoglossus and styloglossus muscles. It is responsible for all tongue movement as well as some involvement in the elevation of the hyoid bone (via the geniohyoid muscle). Table 7.1 gives suggestions for assessment. Note that, if lesions to the tongue are LMN origin, the tongue will deviate to the side of the lesion. However, if the lesion is UMN in origin, the tongue will deviate to the side opposite the lesion (i.e. the contralateral side). This is because of bilateral corticonuclear fibres to the hypoglossal nucleus. Reviewing movement of the tongue gives the clinician an indication of the person's possibilities in successful oral manipulation of the bolus and projection of the bolus in a controlled fashion to the posterior of the oropharynx. It also provides information about the person's ability to use the tongue to clear the buccal sulcii and teeth of remaining food post swallow.

Ability to protect the airway

There are several mechanisms that contribute to airway protection during swallowing, including deglutition apnoea, coughing and throat clearing. During the swallow is it important that respiration ceases and that a period of apnoea occurs. Swallow-respiratory coordination, including deglutition apnoea, is discussed in detail in Chapter 4. We can also protect the airway through throat clearing and coughing, both reflexive and voluntary. Suggested assessments of airway protection are included in Table 7.1. Voluntary control over respiration is a good indicator of the person's ability to use the system in a controlled manner. It may have implications for the use of swallowing manoeuvres such as the supraglottic swallow during treatment. Observations of reflexive throat clearing and coughing should be made, in addition to frequency of these events, and whether there is anything in particular that precipitates them (e.g. whether there is a build up of secretions, etc.). The strength of these reflexes in removing laryngeal material should also be noted. The patient should also be asked to clear their throat and to cough, to give an indication of voluntary control and also the strength of the reflexes. Any differences in strength between the reflexive coughing and throat clearing and voluntary cough or throat clearing should also be noted, as these may have implications for oral trials.

PHASE 5 – ORAL TRIALS

Up to this point we have looked at the swallowing mechanism. It is now time to look at the swallowing mechanism in action as used for its biological purpose of ingesting foods and fluids which are necessary for hydration and nutrition.

Suitability for oral trials

Not all individuals are suitable for oral trials. In order to be suitable to trial oral intake the following conditions should be met. The individual should:

- Be conscious and alert.
- Be able to be positioned optimally for eating and drinking.

- Show some ability to protect the airway, i.e. presence of a dry swallow, ability to cough or clear the throat, or have been observed to swallow *reflexively*, cough or clear the throat.
- Have sufficient stamina for the trial, i.e. the individual should not be so fatigued that he or she will fall asleep during the assessment.
- In the case of a tracheostomy assessment there should be medical assistance (e.g. physiotherapist, nursing staff) to suction the patient. In the event that the speech pathologist has been trained in suctioning, the speech pathologist should ensure that support is available if required.

Individual workplaces may provide further circumstances than those listed above. If these conditions are met, then the clinician may proceed with a trial of food or fluid. A quick note about positioning. It is generally accepted that the patient should be seated or supported in a position that is as upright as possible (i.e. 70° to 90°). One reported difference to this recommendation is in the case of individuals with poor hip/trunk stability, such as those with developmental disability. Dorsey (2002), found that by stabilizing the trunk using reclined supported postures of approximately 60° to 35°, individuals could artificially move their centre of gravity to the upper chest. Stability in the hip and lower trunk region using the supported reclined postures gave the individuals greater control over their upper body, which lead to improved stability of the jaw and mouth. The result was a reduced incidence of aspiration in this group. This may not be appropriate for all individuals but should be considered as an option where trunk stability is poor.

The oral trials

Oral trials are also referred to as mealtime observations or even the bedside examination. Once the individual has been deemed suitable for oral trials the clinician has to decide on what type of bolus/es to assess and the quantity.

It is common practice to err on the side of caution and start with a consistency that the individual can manage easily. For this reason, many clinicians commence with pudding or thickened fluids. Once it has been established that the thicker, more cohesive boluses can be managed safely, then trials of reducing cohesiveness are usually undertaken, finishing with the most volatile – thin fluids. Thin fluids are considered volatile because they are highly fracturable and demand considerable oral and pharyngeal control and coordination to ensure that they are swallowed safely. Alternatively, clinicians may choose to assess swallowing ability for thin fluids first as this is the most normal liquid for individuals to drink; working in graduations of thickness to arrive at a safe swallowing consistency. Certainly, during imaging studies (e.g. videofluoroscopy) it is a good idea to start with thin fluids because it gives the clinician the opportunity to assess this consistency without concern for previously pooled thickened fluids making interpretation of swallowing safety difficult (see Chapter 8). Swallowing safety for fluids is usually assessed first to establish how hydration needs will be met. Following this, solids may then be assessed. Again the clinician may choose to start with solids that do not require a lot of chewing and progress to solids that require considerable masticatory strength.

While there is reasonable cause for concern over large quantities being aspirated, it is also important to establish swallowing safety in an everyday context. It would be reasonable to assess pudding consistency or very viscous thick fluids using a teaspoon, because a teaspoon would be the way a healthy individual would ingest this type of bolus (see also Chapter 3). Quantities smaller than a teaspoon may be difficult to form into a cohesive bolus. For example, it is easier to organize the swallowing of a spoonful of peas than a single pea. The less viscous the bolus (i.e. the thinner the fluid) the more debate there is over the 'correct' amount to be used to assess the patient. Research tells us that the average mouthful of thin fluids swallowed by a male is 25 ml and by a female is 20 ml (Adnerhill et al., 1989). Yet it seems common practice that individuals are offered a spoonful (5 ml) of fluid to assess swallowing function in the clinical examination. In videofluoroscopy procedures even smaller quantities are advocated (2 ml to 5 ml). Swallowing of small amounts can be assessed purely by looking at saliva swallows, given that the average saliva bolus is only 1 ml to 2 ml. To approximate the normal ingestion of a liquid bolus something closer to the 10 ml to 20 ml range is recommended. Note also that, for individuals with sensory loss, a larger bolus may be required to trigger its presence within the oral cavity. A smaller bolus may not be sufficient to alert the brain stem to its presence, and the individual has a higher likelihood of aspiration in this event. Also note that some individuals may not have sufficient oral motor control for a large volume, with the bolus escaping prematurely and increasing risk of aspiration. Both large and small mouthfuls should be considered in assessment.

During oral trials both the oral and pharyngeal stages of the swallow should be monitored. The areas that should be investigated during oral trials are as follows:

- Ability to open the mouth to accept the bolus.
- Ability to close the mouth to contain the bolus within the oral cavity.
- Ability to chew the bolus if mastication is required.
- Evidence of primitive oral reflexes (e.g. bite reflex when the spoon is placed in or near the oral cavity).
- Ability to control the bolus orally using lips, cheeks and tongue and to form a cohesive bolus that is suitable to swallow.
- Document whether there is prompt or delayed swallow reflex initiation.
- Document the presence or absence of laryngeal elevation, and if present the extent of excursion.
- Note whether the oral and pharyngeal phases appear to be coordinated.
- Note whether the patient is able to coordinate swallowing and respiration (i.e. is there an apnoeic period, and is the apnoeic period sufficient for the time required to move the bolus and any residue through the pharynx?).
- Note any changes in phonation after swallowing. If phonation sounds gurgly or wet, the clinician may ask the patient to cough and then swallow to see if the vocal quality changes.

- Note any instances of reflexive coughing after swallowing.
- A healthy swallow is very fast. Gauge the amount of time spent in the oral phase and the pharyngeal phase. In healthy individuals each phase should be approximately one second in duration (Logemann, 1998).
- The clinician should check for oral residue after swallowing in the buccal sulcii, particularly noting any asymmetry.

  - If there is oral residue evident, note whether it is cleared spontaneously or requires the clinician to direct that it be cleared. Note the perceived efficiency of clearing pooled material.

Performance in each of these areas should be noted for each swallow tested. Care should also be taken with noting patient fatigue as some quantities or consistencies may result in higher fatigue levels. It is important to note these as they have an impact on swallowing management.

PHASE 6 – REFERRAL FOR OTHER ASSESSMENTS

As noted at the beginning of this chapter, the clinical examination is not the only assessment device available. It is imperative that we are able to carry out a thorough clinical examination in order to decide whether further assessments are required and, if so, which ones. Clinicians also need to be familiar with the applications, limitations and patient suitability for other assessment procedures. Referral for other assessments should be made on the basis of the *additional information* that these assessments will provide. This is an important point. Patients need to be selected on an individual basis for need of further assessment. Referral for further assessments is usually to provide further information about the *pharyngeal phase* of the swallow. The oral phase of the swallow is usually well quantified with a thorough clinical examination. It is not always possible, however, to infer what is happening in the pharyngeal phase of the swallow. In this instance, imaging assessments where the pharynx can be visualized are usually recommended (see Chapter 8).

PHASE 7 – OVERALL IMPRESSION

This phase of the assessment requires integration of all information gathered to date. The clinician should bear in mind the medical diagnosis of the patient, the clinical features that were observed before the assessment began, the individual's ability to communicate and to understand directions or explanations, suitability for oral trials and, if carried out, the results of oral trials. The clinician will also have made a decision about whether further instrumental assessments are required. Using all of this information the clinician should be in a position to determine the severity of the dysphagia and the prognosis. Dysphagia is usually classified as mild, moderate or severe. An alternative scale sees swallowing classified as normal, possible swallowing impairment, probable swallowing impairment or definite swallowing impairment (Mann et al., 2000). One of the key factors to determining degree of swallowing impairment is safety, and with that the degree of risk for aspiration and/or choking. The degree of risk then dictates the management and treatment plan. In some cases, it may not be until after instrumental procedures are completed that the diagnosis and management plan can be formulated.

PHASE 8 – MANAGEMENT PLAN

Treatment and management of adults with swallowing disorders are discussed in detail in Chapters 11 and 12. Cues for the problem-solving process in individual management plans are:

• Is it safe for the person to commence an oral diet?

  – What type of diet? Are there any restrictions?
  – Can the person feed himself or herself independently or is supervision/assistance required?
  – Are there any positioning issues?

• Is it safe for the person to take medications orally?

  – Prompt for review of how medications are administered.
  – Are there medications that are suspected of exacerbating the dysphagia?

• Are there special instructions for staff/carers to cease oral feeding and request a review by the speech pathologist?
• Which treatment/s are suitable for this case?
• Are there oral hygiene issues?

Once these issues have been dealt with, the clinician will be in a better position to determine treatment modes. At the completion of the assessment, the clinician should communicate the results of the assessment to the medical team, the patient and carer or family. The clinician should also decide whether referrals for instrumental procedures are warranted (see also Chapter 8).

OTHER NON-IMAGING ASSESSMENTS OF DYSPHAGIA

As noted earlier, the clinical assessment of dysphagia is the first assessment used by the speech pathologist to establish whether the individual has dysphagia. In order to enhance the reliability of the clinical assessment, two other screening tools may be used as adjuncts. These are:

• cervical auscultation; and
• pulse oximetry.

ADJUNCTS TO THE CLINICAL EXAMINATION OF DYSPHAGIA – CERVICAL AUSCULTATION

HISTORY AND DEFINITION

Cervical auscultation (CA) is an assessment of the sounds of swallowing and swallowing-related respiration. It comes from 'cervical' pertaining to the cervical region and 'auscultation' meaning to listen to movement. Auscultation is not a new concept. Colleagues in cardiac and respiratory medicine have been using it for centuries to begin the investigative process of determining normal from abnormal heart and lung sounds. Auscultation of deglutitory sounds has been reported in literature as far back as 1905 (Logan et al., 1967). Through the medical profession, CA was given voice in 1967 with Logan et al.'s and Mackowiak et al.'s work. The doctors were investigating the sounds associated with physiologic actions frequently used in medical diagnosis at the time. Using a tie-clip microphone and a spectrogram drum, the researchers recorded the spectrograms of:

- cough;
- swallow;
- forced respiration; and
- vocalization.

It was evident that each of the physiological actions produced a characteristic spectrogram – each one distinguishable from the other. The researchers also discovered that the spectrograms of swallowing sounds changed depending on the quantity and type of bolus being swallowed. They stated that the technique of listening to physiological sounds for diagnostic purposes showed great potential and should be considered as a valued assessment of normal and altered swallowing function.

Speech pathology interest in the field did not commence, however, until the late 1980s (Hamlet et al., 1988). Since that time research has been published on:

- methods of detecting swallowing sounds;
- what the sounds might mean;
- whether swallowing sounds are symmetrical;
- the acoustic characteristics of healthy swallowing sounds; and
- swallow-related respiratory sounds.

The use of sounds as a diagnostic medium is hardly new. The medical profession has been using physiological sounds to assess and monitor cardiac and respiratory function for centuries. Advancement in technology has allowed greater scope for in-depth physiological assessment; however, assessments most commonly commence with a perceptual acoustic assessment.

THE CAUSE OF SWALLOWING SOUNDS

One of the main criticisms of CA is that the cause of the sounds is unknown. If we don't know what causes the sounds, what use are they in diagnostics? There are many theories on the cause of swallowing sounds, the most recent provided by Cichero and Murdoch (1998), which will be expanded upon here. Depending on the literature, there are two or three distinct swallowing sounds. Cichero and Murdoch (1998) believe that there are two true swallowing sounds, and one swallow-related respiratory sound that occurs almost immediately after the swallow. The cause of swallowing sounds is easier to understand if the oral and pharyngeal systems are viewed as a series of mechanical and hydraulic actions caused by the movements of anatomical pumps and valves.

THE OROPHARYNX: A SERIES OF PUMPS AND VALVES

The orophayngeal anatomy can be viewed as a series of pumps and valves. Valves would include the labial valve (lips), linguapalatal valve, nasopharyngeal (soft palate), oropharyngeal valve (formed by the tongue and the soft palate), laryngeal valve, upper oesophageal valve (between pharynx and oesophagus), and oesophagastric valve (between oesophagus and stomach). These are structures that open and close. The lips need to be shut to contain the bolus within the oral cavity. The tongue must contact with the hard palate to move the bolus posteriorly. The soft palate intermittently contacts with the posterior surface of the tongue during bolus preparation. The tongue helps to seal the oral cavity from the pharyngeal cavity during the swallow. The larynx is valved in a variety of ways including intrinsically via arytenoid closure of the vocal folds and extrinsically by closure of the epiglottis over the laryngeal vestibule. Cricopharyngeus opens to allow the bolus into the oesophagus and the valve at the distal end of the oesophagus allows the bolus to pass from the oesophagus into the stomach. Failure of any of these valves will have repercussions for swallowing. The valves can be seen as part of the mechanical component to swallowing.

A number of pumps are used during swallowing. These can be seen as having a hydraulic action. Pennington and Kreutsch (1990) disclosed four pumps, these being the oral pump, the pharyngeal pump, the oesophageal pump and the respiratory pump. No formal explanation is offered but it can be extrapolated that the oral pump pertains to the tongue. Its piston-like action acts to expel the bolus from the oral cavity. The pharyngeal pump refers to the pharyngeal clearing wave of vertical shortening and horizontal contractions as the bolus is moved briskly through the pharynx. Once the upper oesophageal valve has been opened the oesophageal pump can move the bolus through this structure using peristaltic actions. The respiratory pump is included because of the anatomical configuration of the pharynx. In a unique 'biological time-share' the pharynx is the shared medium for swallowing, respiration and phonation. In a simplistic explanation the respiratory pump must shut down during swallowing and then recommence after swallowing in order to maintain its safe functioning. Problems occur when there is debris left in the mutual structure of the pharynx, or if the respiratory pump is not safely disabled, or if its mechanism is ill-protected during the swallow (see also Chapter 4). Once viewed in this manner, the explanation of what causes swallowing sounds is simpler.

THE FIRST SWALLOWING SOUND

Using principles from heart and lung sound propagation and vocal tract acoustics, Cichero and Murdoch (1998) proposed that the first swallowing sound is caused by the following actions: closure of the laryngeal valve, in conjunction with the tongue (lingual pump) delivering the bolus to the posterior pharyngeal wall. These actions set the pharynx into vibration, causing it to emit a sound. McKaig (2002) established, using 55 subjects and videofluoroscopy synchronized with cervical sound, that the first swallowing sound occurs when the bolus is visualized at the base of the tongue. In agreement with the hypothesis put forward above, he states that the first sound is likely to be generated by actions causing the bolus to be transferred into the hypopharynx. There is then a small hiatus between the first and second swallowing sound. This hiatus can last for approximately 20 ms to 60 ms (McKaig, 2002). In some individuals, however, the hiatus is so small as to be almost obscured. This is an apparent normal variation.

THE SECOND SWALLOWING SOUND

Cichero and Murdoch (1998) suggested that the bolus passes relatively quietly through the pharynx, until a second disturbance causes further vibration of the vocal tract. The authors suggest that the second sound is caused by the following actions: the mechanical movement of opening of cricopharyngeus in combination with the pharyngeal clearing wave combine to cause further vibration, which generates the second swallowing sound. The turbulence created by the bolus itself may also contribute to the sounds of swallowing. McKaig (2002) using analysis of synchronized videofluoroscopy and cervical sounds concurs that the second sound coincides with full cricopharyngeal opening, allowing the bolus to flow into the oesophagus.

THE GLOTTAL RELEASE SOUND

The presence of three audible sounds associated with swallowing has been documented since the inception of the technique in 1967. There is some debate, however, as to whether the final sound, the so-called 'third swallowing sound', is in fact a *swallowing* sound, or merely a sound that accompanies the true swallowing sounds. Mackowiak et al. (1967) stated that this final sound follows the other two swallowing sounds after a delay of 300–400 ms. Cichero and Murdoch (1998) postulated that the final sound is most likely to be the result of 'unvalving' of the respiratory system. It causes minor vibration through the opening pharyngeal pathway due to mechanical movement of the epiglottis, aryepiglottic folds, arytenoid cartilages and true vocal fold movement. These movements are responsible for a short puff of air being released from the larynx resulting from apnoea during the swallowing event. Again using synchronized videofluoroscopy with cervical sounds, McKaig (2002) showed that the final sound occurs with, but may not be exclusive to, opening of the glottis, release of trapped subglottal air, separation of the pharyngeal walls, return of the epiglottis to neutral and the reinitiation of tidal breathing. The sound of air being released is quite distinctive and it is for this reason that some authors have dubbed this sound the 'glottal release sound' (Cichero and Murdoch, 2003). Given the explanation above, it should be clear, then, that the glottal release sound follows the swallowing sounds but is not in itself a swallowing sound. It is more closely aligned with respiratory sounds.

ACOUSTIC CHARACTERISTICS OF SWALLOWING SOUNDS

Healthy non-dysphagic individuals

Swallowing sounds are highly individual. In much the same way that we have individualized voiceprints so swallowing sounds are also quite idiosyncratic. In a healthy non-dysphagic individual, swallowing sounds are short, measuring approximately 0.4 s. They have a fairly stable intensity of 43 dB and an average frequency of 2200 Hz (Cichero and Murdoch, 2002a). Interestingly the frequency range for healthy swallowing sounds is the same as for the vowel /i/ in 'heed'. Note the configuration of the tongue and oral structures when this vowel is made, and notice that it is the gesture one makes when getting ready to initiate a swallow. Descriptively, normal swallowing sounds are short, sharp and crisp. Evidence of the so-called 'double clunk' of the first two swallow sounds may be audible. It is equally the case, though, that the swallowing sounds happen in such quick succession that they may be blurred and appear as one sound.

Normal variations in swallowing sounds

Swallowing sounds change depending on the age of the person swallowing, what is swallowed, and the quantity that is swallowed. As noted above, swallowing sounds are very fast. When measured using acoustic anlaysis software, it has been demonstrated that swallowing sounds become longer as we get older. The differences are statistically significant; however, it would be with extensive exposure to a range of normal swallowing sounds that the clinician would be able to appreciate the differences perceptually. The changes in the duration of swallowing sounds as individuals age are presented in Table 7.2. Note also the physiological evidence referred to in Chapter 2, which shows that swallowing becomes slower as we age.

Table 7.2 Swallowing sound duration: Variation by age

One year[*]	18–35 years[**]	36–59 years[**]	60+ years[**]
0.12 s	0.37 s	0.48 s	0.52 s

[*]Willett (2002), [**]Cichero and Murdoch (2002).

Swallowing sounds become shorter as the bolus volume increases. The duration of a swallowing sound of a 5 ml bolus is 0.46 s, whereas the duration of the swallowing sound from a 10/15 ml bolus is 0.4 s (Cichero and Murdoch, 2003). These results are statistically significant, although would be difficult to perceive via listening alone. Swallowing sounds get shorter and lower pitched as the fluid gets thicker. The average duration of a swallow of thin fluids is 0.4 s, however the average duration of a swallow of thick fluids is 0.34 s – these differences are perceptually obvious even to the naive listener. The differences as a result of bolus viscosity can be explained as follows. Remember first that swallowing sounds are caused by putting the pharynx and surrounding structures into vibration. As an analogy, if one were to take a crystal vase and drop a cup of water into it, the highly fracturable liquid would rush against the sides of the vase and cause it to vibrate and emit a sound. The lack of cohesion of the volatile liquid bolus such as water means that it when dropped into the vase will cause turbulence before settling. Take the same crystal vase and this time drop a cup of yoghurt into it. The yoghurt will still put the vase into vibration but the yoghurt is a more cohesive substance. Its internal makeup will mean that the sound will be dampened and absorbed, hence the vase will vibrate for a shorter period of time. In addition, the sound-absorbing qualities of the yoghurt will lower the pitch of the vibration. Consequently, a more viscous bolus produces a shorter, lower pitched sound than a thin liquid bolus. A similar argument could also be made for solid boluses. Once again, these are transformed into a cohesive bolus by the process of mastication and the addition of saliva. A cohesive bolus will provide a shorter sound than a fracturable bolus.

Dysphagic individuals

There are very few studies into the acoustic characteristics of dysphagic individuals. There has been some attempt to discriminate between dysphagic individuals who aspirate/penetrate (aspirators), and dysphagic individuals who do not aspirate/penetrate (dysphagics). Both groups have longer swallowing sounds than healthy individuals (dysphagic individuals – 0.92 s; aspirating individuals – 0.6 s). Both groups have somewhat softer swallowing sounds than healthy individuals. Both groups tend to have higher pitched swallowing sounds than healthy individuals.

THE BIG PICTURE – THE SWALLOW-RESPIRATORY CYCLE

Until this point swallowing sounds have been viewed as isolated events. The act of swallowing, the pharyngeal phase, does not occur in isolation. Taken out of context it is easy to see why an assessment based purely on swallowing sounds might cause some to be concerned. There are other elements that need to be considered: the oral preparatory phase, the oral phase, and very importantly swallow-respiratory coordination. In other words, we need to consider what happens either side of the swallow.

Before the swallow

Before the swallow:

- the bolus is delivered to the mouth;
- the oral preparatory phase occurs;
- the oral phase occurs.

In healthy individuals the clinician may hear the sounds of respiration, mastication if the bolus requires chewing, sounds associated with the tongue contouring to manipulate the bolus, and perhaps fluid being transferred into the oral cavity. In dysphagic individuals, in addition to the sounds mentioned above, clinicians may hear wheezing, altered respirations (stridor, breathing through fluid), or grunting. Oropharyngeal transit time can be calculated from the pre-swallow phase. This would be the time from when the bolus enters the oral cavity until the swallowing sound is heard. For healthy individuals the average oropharyngeal transit time for thin liquids is 1.6 s, and is longer for more viscous fluids (1.9 s). Both dysphagic (4.6 s) and aspirating individuals (1.97 s) have longer oropharyngeal transit times than healthy individuals.

During the swallow

The following events occur:

- swallow reflex initiation;
- the pharyngeal phase of the swallow;
- the sound of the swallow;
- respiration has ceased.

The acoustic characteristics of healthy non-dysphagic swallows, dysphagic non-aspirating swallows, and dysphagic aspirating swallows have been described in detail above.

Immediately after the swallow

Immediately after the swallow:

- the oral and pharyngeal system is returning to rest;
- the airway reopens causing the glottal release sound.

In healthy individuals, this sound is short at approximately 0.2 s in duration. It is also softer than the swallowing sound at 38 dB. It is audible as a short sharp puff of air immediately after the swallow but before tidal respirations recommence. In dysphagic individuals the glottal release sound may be absent or very soft. When the glottal release sound is audible in the aspiration group it is often violently explosive. Both aspirating (0.53 s) and dysphagic (0.74 s) individuals have longer glottal release sounds than healthy individuals. A delay in the glottal release sound probably indicates that the airway has been closed for a longer time.

After the swallow or glottal release

After the swallow has been completed tidal breathing recommences. In healthy individuals, tidal respirations should recommence immediately after the glottal release sound. In dysphagic or aspirating individuals post swallow sounds may include coughing, throat clearing, bubbling or gurgling, 'wet' sounding respirations, stridorous breathing, wheezing, or an increased respiratory rate.

Total swallow cycle time is a useful measure of swallowing safety and efficiency. In healthy individuals the time for the whole swallowing cycle to occur (i.e. from when the bolus touches the lips until tidal respirations recommence post swallow) is very swift (2.47 s). In dysphagic and aspirating groups the picture is quite different. In general dysphagic individuals have slow oropharyngeal transit times, slow swallowing sounds, and a small delay to resuming normal rhythmic tidal respirations (9.94 s). Aspirating individuals have been found to have patterns similar to the above with a large delay to resumption of normal rhythmic tidal respirations (12.23 s). Aspirating individuals have also been found to have oropharyngeal transit times and swallowing sound times that are longer than the healthy group but shorter than the dysphagic group. However, the post-swallow time that it takes them to resume normal rhythmic tidal respirations always far exceeds that of the healthy and dysphagic groups.

TOOLS OF THE TRADE – LISTENING TO SWALLOWING SOUNDS AND SWALLOW-RELATED RESPIRATORY SOUNDS

'Auscultation' is the act of listening and is used in the medical profession to refer to the act of listening to sounds made by internal organs. The swallow-respiratory cycle makes sounds and is audible with the aid of a listening device. Listening devices include a stethoscope and a microphone. The vibrations made during swallowing and respiration can also be detected using an accelerometer. Each of these devices and its clinical applicability is described below. In clinical practice a stethoscope is most commonly used due to cost and ease of portability. A microphone is also portable when coupled to a tape recorder. An accelerometer is the least likely to be used in the clinical environment, reserved more for research purposes. Both microphone and accelerometer can be plugged into:

- a computer;
- a tape recorder;
- the audio channel of a video recorder (for example during videofluoroscopy); and
- the audio channel of a handicam camera.

The stethoscope

The stethoscope was invented in 1816 by Dr Rene Laennec. He created a cylinder from a pile of papers and placed his ear at one end and the other end on the patient's chest. Finding that this made the sound louder than if he had placed his ear directly on the patient's chest (as was the norm), it inspired him to create a wooden version (Abdulla, 2001). The name 'stethoscope' comes from the Greek *stethos* meaning chest, and *scopien* the Latin for 'to view'. The stethoscope has long been used by the medical fraternity for the clinical assessment of cardiac and respiratory systems. Even in these fields, however, it would appear that its use has waned with the advent of more sophisticated diagnostic tools. Weitz and Mangione (2000) caution, however, that bedside skills such as auscultation should be part of the formal armamentarium for initial investigations. They describe auscultation as an 'essential filter' that allows the practitioner to determine the best path for further diagnostic investigations. Without this filter there is the possibility that patients will undergo a battery of tests when realistically they may have only needed one or two if properly screened using the stethoscope. Too many instrumental assessments are likely to raise the costs of care and may be time consuming (Weitz and Mangione, 2000).

Composition of the stethoscope

The stethoscope comprises a headset – i.e. earpieces (binaurals – one earpiece per ear), connected to tubing, which connects to the 'chestpiece'. In better quality stethoscopes it is possible to adjust the angle of the earpieces so that the eartips follow the typical anatomy of the ear. The eartips should, therefore, face forward (towards the nose) as they are inserted into the ear so that sound can follow the passage of the ear canal.

The headset is usually metal and descends to meet at a junction like the letter 'Y' to the tubing, which connects the headset to the chestpiece. The tubing is usually made of either latex or plastic tubing. Latex-free tubing is likely to have more longevity than the latex variety. It is imperative that this tubing remains free from holes, as the sound is transmitted from the chestpiece via this tubing to the earpieces. Holes in the tubing allow the sound to escape, thereby making the sound softer and possibly changing the quality of what is heard. It is important that, when not in use, the stethoscope tubing should not directly touch the skin (such as the skin around the neck). The oils naturally occurring in the skin can, over time, cause perforations to occur in the tubing. It is also important that the tubing does not touch clothing or bed linen during auscultation, as the sound of these items rubbing against the tubing can be heard, thereby distorting the sound of interest. The tubing may be single or double lumen. This simply means that there may be one tube (single lumen) or two tubes, one inside the other (double lumen).

The chestpiece in most stethoscopes is made up of a bell and a diaphragm. The bell is shaped like a bell and allows a dome-shaped air-filled space to be formed when placed on the skin. The bell is best used to hear low frequency sounds, such as those below approximately 1,500 Hz. Breath sounds and heart sounds usually fall into this low frequency range (Hamlet et al., 1994). The diaphragm is found on the other side of the bell. It has a flat surface and is best used for the auscultation of high frequency sounds. The clinician selects either the bell-mode or the diaphragm-mode. This is done by holding the chestpiece stem in one hand and rotating the chestpiece with the other. On close inspection, in the centre of both the bell and diaphragm chestpieces there is a hole. If using the bell mode, the hole in the centre of the bell should be open. When the bell is placed on the patient the sound is directed through the hole, up the tubing to the earpieces. When the hole is open in the bell, it is closed on the diaphragm. To listen using the diaphragm, the clinician turns the chestpiece so that the hole is open on the diaphragm side, and then applies the diaphragm side to the patient's skin surface.

There are many different types of stethoscopes – e.g. adult and paediatric (and neonate) stethoscopes. The most distinguishing features of these are the size of the chestpieces. The chestpiece of the neonate stethoscope (bell diameter approximately 20 mm, diaphragm approximately 30 mm) is noticeably smaller than that of the adult chestpiece (bell diameter approximately 35 mm, diaphragm diameter approximately 45 mm). Some stethoscopes are simply made of better quality materials and hence are better at conducting sound; not surprisingly these are the more expensive ones. Some stethoscopes are designed for cardiac use and provide superior acoustics due to their design. There are also electronic stethoscopes where it is possible to record the audio signal and download it onto a computer.

Hamlet et al. (1994) investigated six popular stethoscopes to see:

- whether the frequency response of the stethoscope is suitable for use in the auscultation of swallowing sounds; and
- whether any of the stethoscopes investigated provided particularly favourable use for cervical auscultation of swallowing.

The authors found that stethoscopes are suitable for use in cervical auscultation of swallowing, being capable of faithfully transmitting sounds within the frequency range of swallowing sounds (up to 3,000 Hz). The authors draw attention to an important feature of stethoscopes – their ability to transmit sound at both high and low frequencies without distortion. Richardson and Moody (2000) and Kuhn (1995) noted that, for all stethoscopes, the tubing and chestpieces themselves affect the transmission of sounds and the selective filtering of the sounds. Variables that can affect what is eventually heard at the ears include: 'the length, thickness and bore of the tubing, the size and shape of the bell or diaphragm, and the material of the diaphragm' (Richardson and Moody, 2000: 795). Stethoscopes used for cervical auscultation of swallowing should be of good quality that fulfil the aim of faithfully transmitting sounds in frequency ranges important for the swallowing-respiratory cycle (i.e. approximately 500 Hz and approximately 2,000–3,000 Hz). In my clinical experience, I have found stethoscopes typically used in cardiology to be excellent for use in cervical auscultation and that the bell mode provides the cleanest acoustics for listening to swallow-respiratory sounds. The following information has been adapted from Richardson and Moody's (2000) statements to physicians about optimizing auscultation in a clinical examination:

- Use a quiet and comfortable place for assessment.
- Ensure a light but good seal between the chestpiece and patient's skin surface.

- Ensure that the earpieces are inserted correctly and have a proper airtight fit (when correctly applied it should sound as though you are 'under water'). There is a significant loss in energy resulting from air leaks.
- Reduce external noise.
- Ensure optimal placement for cervical auscultation (i.e. midline or lateral border of the trachea immediately inferior to the cricoid cartilage).
- Use universal precautions to guard against cross-contamination between patients and clinicians by using an alcohol wipe to cleanse chestpiece and eartips between patient and clinician use.

Positioning the stethoscope for cervical auscultation – sound generation

A theoretical framework has been presented above to outline the causes of sounds in the swallow-respiratory cycle. It is important to refer back to the cause of swallow-respiratory sounds to determine where the best place is to put the stethoscope. Note first of all that 'sound is a form of energy resulting from oscillation of pressure level' (Richardson and Moody, 2000: 792). The energy must then be transmitted through structures so that they are loud enough, and at a frequency range that can be heard. Cichero and Murdoch (1998) have suggested that the bolus, vibrations in the pharynx, oesophagus and trachea, together with opening and closing of the laryngeal valve and upper oesophageal valve are variously responsible for the sounds heard during the swallow-respiratory cycle. It is suggested that swallow-respiratory sounds are propagated down the pharynx, following the direction of bolus flow. This assumption is based on the idea that during speech, sound waves travel up the vocal tract to be expelled at the mouth (Davies et al., 1993), whereas for swallowing it is assumed that sound follows the bolus downstream towards the oesophagus. In much the same way that it is easier to be heard when shouting with the wind than against it, it was assumed that any acoustic unit to detect swallowing sounds should be placed downstream of the point of origin of the sound source. Note also that a lateral placement in the region of the thyroid cartilage may accentuate the carotid pulse, making it harder to distinguish the swallowing sound. In addition, a lateral cervical placement risks auscultation over the stenocleidomastoid muscle, which may dampen the swallowing sounds.

Takahashi et al. (1994) investigated 24 cervical sites in order to determine the best site of placement for a standardized CA assessment. In confirmation of the theory outlined above, they found that placing the acoustic detector unit (microphone) above the level of the thyroid cartilage yielded inferior results to those taken from sites below the level of the thyroid cartilage. Takahashi et al. (1994) found the optimal sites of placement to be (in order from most to least favourable):

1. The area over the lateral border of the trachea, immediately inferior to the cricoid cartilage (optimal site).
2. Centre of the cricoid cartilage.
3. Mid-point between the site over the centre of the cricoid cartilage and a site immediately superior to the jugular notch.

Cichero and Murdoch (2002b) concur with Takahashi et al.'s (1994) findings and also found that midline placement on the trachea immediately below the cricoid cartilage was an acceptable site of placement. Hiiemae (1994) challenged the traditional site of placement on the cervical region by using the external auditory meatus to record swallowing sounds. The author claimed that the benefits of using this site were:

- stable placement;
- reduced probability of recording skin noise; and
- reduced likelihood of recording muscle contraction noise.

There are, however, some problems with using the external acoustic meatus to record swallowing sounds as it assumes normal Eustachian tube function. Abnormal Eustachian tube function may distort the signal. Moreover, noise from the temperomandibular joint may provide additional extraneous noise. For these reasons, the cervical site of placement appears to be optimal.

In clinical practice, the site used varies marginally from patient to patient. For some patients sounds are best heard from the midline position below the cricoid; for others it is a more lateral placement on the trachea immediately below the cricoid cartilage that provides the clearest sounds. As a general rule, if tidal breath sounds can be clearly distinguished in the area immediately below the cricoid, whether midline or lateral, then this position will be best for auscultating swallow-respiratory sounds.

The microphone

Microphones, despite their variety (contact, gradient and cavity), need no particular introduction. Zenner et al. (1995) reported that microphones pick up a broad spectrum of sound, taking in the sounds of muscle, fluid movement and breath exchange. Microphones can be attached to the skin surface using tape to keep them in place. They can be connected to a tape recorder, minidisk recorder, computer, the audio channel of a video recorder or the audio channel of a handicam. These options allow the clinician to record and preserve the acoustic signal in isolation, or in conjunction with a visual image (as in the case of the video recorder and handicam recorder). A gradient microphone is reported to be the most suitable for use in cervical auscultation. These microphones have a flat frequency response over a broad frequency range, meaning that they will reliably transmit frequency information from the source of interest without attenuating parts of it. The disadvantage of any microphone is that it is likely to pick up not only the signal of interest but also any other ambient noise. This makes it difficult to filter the 'wanted acoustic signal' from the unwanted. Of the different types of microphone available, the gradient microphones are reported to provide reasonably good rejection of the unwanted noise elements. They are also light in weight, making them highly suitable for CA use. The key to good use of the microphone to record CA sounds while minimizing background noise is to ensure a good seal between the microphone and the skin surface. The best system is one where there is a relatively unbroken chain between the sound source and the listening/recording device. In this respect the stethoscope and the microphone have nearly identical requirements.

The accelerometer

The accelerometer transduces body movement at the skin surface and turns it into a proportional acoustic signal. The vibrations picked up at the skin surface are transformed into an acoustic signal. These vibrations may be the result of sound or vibration generated within the body (Kuhn, 1995; Zenner et al., 1995). Accelerometers have been popular acoustic detector units for use in CA studies due to their flat frequency response over a large frequency range. For swallowing sounds, the device should transmit sounds equally well throughout the range from 0–8 kHz, without distortion of the signal. Accelerometers are also very good at picking up only the signal of interest due to their proximity to the sound source. One does not encounter the problem of picking up extraneous background noise when these devices are used. Unfortunately, this same feature also means that has more difficulty picking up an acoustic signal where there is a large amount of subcutaneous tissue between the point where the sound is generated and the accelerometer (Takahashi et al., 1994). For this reason, it may be difficult to auscultate or record CA sounds from obese individuals. Accelerometers are also considerably more expensive than microphones.

USING CERVICAL AUSCULTATION AS AN ADJUNCT TO THE CLINICAL EXAMINATION

Cervical auscultation should be viewed as an adjunct screening tool. Clinicians use an additional medium, that of sound, to enhance their understanding of the patient's presentation. Even in cardiac auscultation, the benefits of auscultation relate directly to:

- the training of the auscultator;
- their experience in having heard a range of sounds so as to develop an internal yardstick; and
- knowledge of possible sounds that might be heard (Richardson and Moody, 2000).

Note that there is a saying, attributed to Dr Merrill Sosman, which relates to radiology but is equally relevant to auscultation: 'We only see what we look for, we recognize only what we know' (Richardson and Moody, 2000). The astute clinician uses information from the auscultation to *augment* the information that has been gathered during the clinical examination. Table 7.3 provides a guide to incorporating cervical auscultation with the clinical examination of swallowing. The following acoustic features can be observed during cervical auscultation:

Table 7.3 Clinical assessment of dysphagia plus cervical auscultation

- Standard oromotor assessment
  CN V: jaw strength, speed and range of movement
    VII: upper face, lower face
  IX, X: soft palate function, gag reflex, phonation, cough, dry swallow
    XII: tongue strength, speed and range of movement

- Observe respirations 'at rest'
  (normal adult = 16-20 breaths per minute or ~ one and a half per 5 s)
    ○ Listen to respiratory sounds via stethoscope
    ○ If sounds wet/gurgly ask pt. to cough/swallow/clear throat – > any change to respiratory quality?

- Traditional clinical assessment – swallow trials
    ○ Judge oral transit time.
    ○ Estimate delay to swallow initiation.
    ○ Feel range of laryngeal excursion.
    ○ Hypothesize competence of pharyngeal phase.

- Auscultate
    ○ (If having trouble getting good sounds start at the sternal notch in the mid line. Once you have good breath sounds, move up and slightly laterally.) Optimal position lateral border of the trachea immediately inferior to the cricoid cartilage.

Observations and scoring during auscultation

Respiration at rest	Pre-swallow	Swallow	Glottal release	Post-swallow	Post trial respiration
0	Tidal respiration.	Crisp. Clear.	Present or absent	Tidal respirations.	0
1	Breathing throughout oral phase.	Quick. Loud. Coordinated.		Gurgling. Bubbling. Stridor.	1
2	Quality of sounds.			Coughing/ clearing.	2
3	Audible tongue pumping, etc	Dissociated. Dull. Constricted. Drawn-out. Choking.		Increased respiratory rate. Crackles.	3

- Implement manoeuvres/techniques and re-assess sounds during manoeuvre.
- Trial a different consistency.
- With each change observe changes to respirations and swallowing cycle.

Scale for judgement of abnormality of respiration (Morton et al., 2002)
0 = No abnormality (regular, calm, controlled respiration).
1 = Mild abnormality (regular, fast and shallow respiration).
2 = Moderate abnormality (irregular, fast and shallow respiration).
3 = Severe (irregular, fast and deep respirations).

- presence of pharyngeal swallow events (Lefton-Greif and Loughlin, 1996);
- number of sucks per swallow (Lefton-Greif and Loughlin, 1996) or number of swallows per mouthful;
- sound of bolus transit (Lefton-Greif and Loughlin, 1996);
- estimates of the time for oral phase preparation and the initiation of the reflex stage (Lefton-Greif and Loughlin, 1996);
- bubbling sounds overlying respiration (Comrie and Helm, 1997);
- wet respirations;
- coughing, clearing and stridor (possibly elicited from penetration or aspiration of the bolus into the larynx) (Comrie and Helm, 1997);
- 'hard swallows'(Comrie and Helm, 1997);
- chirping noises (Comrie and Helm, 1997);
- gasps (Comrie and Helm, 1997);
- coughing or choking;
- coordination of swallowing and breathing (rhythmic or arrhythmic);
- apnoea (no breathing) or tachypnea (fast breathing rate).

ADVANTAGES AND LIMITATIONS OF CERVICAL AUSCULTATION

There are a number of advantages to using cervical auscultation as an adjunct to the clinical assessment of swallowing. With proper training it is easy to use and inexpensive. It has the advantage of using real food and permits the assessment to be conducted where meals are normally eaten – thus removing the 'test situation' so often seen during the instrumental assessments. In the hands of an experienced clinician, the use of cervical auscultation will allow the clinician to ask patient-specific questions of the videofluoroscopy assessment. Clinicians also have the advantage of being able to monitor swallowing throughout an entire meal period. This technique highlights the importance of the coordination between respiration and swallowing. Aberrations of the normal swallow-respiratory cycle (see Chapter 4) can be discerned by the experienced clinician. Gasping after the swallow likewise indicates that there is swallow-respiratory incoordination that potentially places the person at risk of aspiration. This insight into swallow-respiratory coordination is one of the advantages of this technique not easily matched by others.

There are of course well-documented disadvantages too, one being that we do not know what causes the sounds. Cichero and Murdoch (1998) have put forward a theoretical view of the cause of swallowing sounds; however, this theory has thus far neither been proved nor disproved. Further research is needed to verify the physiological cause of the sounds. We should take heart from the fact that physicians commonly use observations of cardiac and respiratory sounds to direct further investigations more effectively. Medical research has enabled physicians to tie specific cardiac and respiratory sounds to physiological events. For cervical auscultation of swallowing sounds it is not a case of whether this will happen, but when.

Using stethoscopy or auscultation via an amplified microphone, the clinician's hearing abilities must be excellent. Similarly, training and experience are necessary

Table 7.4 Agreement values when cervical auscultation is used as part of a clinical assessment battery

Agreement values	Clinical checklist without CA (%)	Clinical checklist with CA (%)
Sensitivity	85	89
Specificity	82	83
Positive predictive value	79	81
Negative predictive value	87	91

to benefit fully from auscultation. Cervical auscultation has a sensitivity of 84% – 87% (Zenner et al., 1995; Eicher et al., 1994) and a specificity of between 71% (Zenner et al., 1995) and 78% (Eicher et al., 1994) for detecting aspiration. CA used as an adjunct to the clinical examination provides more accurate prediction of aspiration as verified on videofluoroscopy than when the clinician exam is used in isolation (Eicher et al., 1994). These results are shown in Table 7.4.

It is worthwhile at this point to review the meaning of the terms, sensitivity, specificity, positive and negative predictive values.

Sensitivity refers to the percentage of a population showing a characteristic (e.g. aspiration) on the gold-standard assessment as compared with that predicted using the new assessment. For example, eight patients are shown to aspirate on videofluoroscopy and eight patients are identified as aspirating using CA. This gives a sensitivity rating of 100%. Note, however, that the eight patients identified as aspirating using CA may not be the same eight identified as aspirating on videofluoroscopy. The question then becomes 'of the ones that did aspirate on videofluoroscopy, how many were correctly predicted to be aspirators using CA?' The answer to this question gives the positive predictive value of the technique. Returning to the example, of the eight patients identified as aspirators using CA – it turned out that only five of them were true aspirators confirmed using videofluoroscopy. Thus, although CA in this example is highly sensitive (8/8 or 100%), its positive predictive value is not as good (5/8 or 62.5%).

Specificity refers to the percentage of the population *not exhibiting* a particular characteristic (e.g. aspiration) on the gold-standard assessment who are also predicted not to have that characteristic when assessed using the new assessment. So, for example, six patients are found *not* to be aspirating on videofluoroscopy, whereas only four are predicted *not* to be aspirating when assessed using CA. This gives a specificity rating of 66.6%. Once again, it is important to ask, of the ones that were predicted *not* to be aspirating using CA, how many did we get right when compared with the gold-standard? If three of the four were correctly identified, this gives a *negative predictive value* for the technique. From this discussion it should be apparent that a tool can have excellent sensitivity and specificity records, but abysmal positive and negative predictive values. All four aspects should be reviewed when validation studies are reported.

Shaw et al. (2004) used a multidisciplinary approach, with physiotherapists listening to swallowing sounds using the diaphragm of a stethoscope over the bronchus. They listened prior to, during, and for 15 s after oral intake. The researchers reported that risk of aspiration was accurately detected in 87% of cases and 88% of individuals not aspirating were also correctly identified. Of 105 individuals, the researchers found that one diet would have failed to have been adjusted and that 17 would have unnecessarily been adjusted.

Stroud et al. (2002) investigated inter-rater and intra-rater reliability of CA for the detection of aspiration in patients with dysphagia. They found a sensitivity of 86%, but a specificity of 56%. The authors agreed that clinicians were able to detect genuine occurrences of aspiration very accurately when it truly occurred. However, they concluded that speech pathologists were more likely to overpredict aspiration. Unfortunately, the researchers investigated the clinician's ability to determine whether aspiration had occurred from swallowing sounds isolated from all other clinical cues (including that of respiration). Apart from the fact that the test data were significantly skewed, the design of the study completely negates the underlying concept that CA is an *adjunct*, not a tool to be used in isolation. In addition, it draws solely on the swallowing sound, rather than taking it in context with pre-swallow and post-swallow events. Stroud et al. (2002) also found that the clinicians showed a positive predictive value of 31% and a negative predictive value of 94%. Although all of the clinicians accurately discerned the aspiration sounds, they also identified other sounds as aspiration sounds when they were not aspiration sounds. This is why the positive predictive value is so low. The negative predictive value is very good. This means that the clinicians were very good at accurately determining aspiration had *not* taken place. This is in itself very valuable. The absence of aspiration can be just as important as its presence. Interestingly, Stroud et al. (2002) also found that some individual clinicians had remarkably high intra-rater reliability. That is they were very consistent with their analysis of the sounds, meaning that guesswork was unlikely and that they were using their own internal criteria to determine aspiration from non-aspiration sounds (Stroud et al., 2002). However, Leslie et al. (2004) reported pockets of good, but mainly poor, intra-rater reliability and poor inter-rater reliability. Note, however, that videofluorsocopy and endoscospy also have poor inter-rater reliability (see Chapter 8). In contrast, Richardson and Moody (2000) have reported that physicians who played a musical instrument were better at auscultation, as were those who used audio training tapes. These findings suggest that we do not all share the same propensity for using auscultation, and that some clinicians may need additional training to be able to reliably use the technique.

PULSE OXIMETRY

We do not consciously remember to breathe. Our body regulates this process automatically, providing adults with approximately 16 to 20 breaths per minute. When the normal cycle of breathing is interrupted, for example by lack of oxygen or airway obstruction, the respiratory system automatically compensates. Depth of respiration may increase or the rate of respiration may become faster. When aspiration occurs, a foreign body is introduced into the respiratory system, albeit usually quite high in the system (the trachea). This will lead to a ventilation-perfusion mismatch and consequently oxygen desaturation of arterial blood. This oxygen desaturation can be measured using a pulse oximeter (Collins and Bakheit, 1997). It is logical that the aspiration of a bolus (food, liquid or saliva) that is sufficient to alter the usual respiratory pattern will have a follow-on effect on arterial blood oxygenation. If there is insufficient air coming in, there is insufficient oxygenation occurring, which means that less oxygen will be circulating in the blood. This is the basic premise behind pulse oximetry when used as an adjunct during a dysphagia screening assessment. If the patient's oxygen saturation levels fall during oral trials, the assumption is made that aspiration is likely to have occurred. This is also why it is deemed a screening assessment, as it is unable to determine why aspiration occurred, to enable visualization of the pharyngeal region, or to indicate whether the suspected aspiration occurred before, during, or after the swallow.

Pulse oximetry is a non-invasive continuous measure of arterial oxygenation using a probe attached to a pulsating vascular bed (i.e. finger, toe or ear lobe). Red and infrared light are passed though the finger, toe or ear lobe (one releases light waves, the other reads them). With an increase in oxygen circulating in the blood, the colour of the blood changes. The oximeter measures amount of light absorbed by blood in the tissue. Normal oxygen saturation (SpO_2) readings are in the region of 95% to 100%. Readings of less than 90% are suggestive of significant problems. In using pulse oximetry during swallowing trials, it is important to take a baseline before assessment commences so that there is a platform for comparison. Zaidi et al. (1995) suggest that measurement should occur over a 2 minute interval. A fall from a baseline of greater than 2% is generally agreed upon for the SpO_2, the results to be indicative of aspiration (Collins and Bakheit, 1997; Smith et al., 2000). A more conservative figure of a fall of 4% or more could be advocated to take into consideration calibration idiosyncrasies (Sellars et al., 1999). Zaidi et al. (1995) investigated oxygen saturation levels after swallowing 10 ml of water in two control groups (one group of young and fit individuals, the other a group of inpatients matched for age and sex) and a group of acute stroke patients. The investigators found that normal variability in the control groups was 3.02% (this being the mean from the young fit group of 2.7% and the inpatient matched group of 3.28%). Zaidi et al. (1995) therefore determined that aspiration was likely to have occurred only if SpO_2 saturation levels had dropped by more than 3.28%, which equated with the inpatient matched group. They found that the time taken for the stroke patients to achieve maximum fall in saturation was on average 5.31 s, but ranged from 5 to 120 s (i.e. up to 2 minutes). They also found that recovery of saturation had occurred within one minute. The fall in oxygen saturation was statistically related to an independent assessment of aspiration by a speech pathologist although the assessment by the speech pathologist was delayed by 24 hours from the pulse oximetry trial. Physiotherapy colleagues have suggested monitoring oxygen saturation changes for up to 20 minutes after oral trials.

PULSE OXIMETRY AND THE DYSPHAGIC POPULATION – THE EVIDENCE

Pulse oximetry is based on the hypothesis that when aspiration occurs individuals will, for a short time, have a reduction in oxygenated blood flow. Pulse oximetry can measure the oxygenation levels in the blood. There are a number of researchers who have investigated this hypothesis in the dysphagic population to determine whether there is any evidence for using pulse oximetry as a screening tool for aspiration. Sherman et al. (1999) investigated pulse oximetry in 46 dysphagic individuals who underwent simultaneous modified barium swallow (MBS). Firstly, the data confirmed a statistically significant association between oxygen desaturation and swallowing abnormalities. Their findings can be summarized as follows: as concurrently assessed using videofluoroscopy, individuals who did not penetrate or who did penetrate but immediately cleared the bolus did *not* demonstrate significant oxygen desaturation. However, oxygen saturation declined significantly following aspiration or uncleared penetration. The researchers monitored O_2 saturation for 3 minutes after the videofluoroscopy to see if there was any evidence of delayed aspiration (i.e. from pooled material in the pharynx). They did not, however, measure the duration of desaturation that was associated with aspiration or uncleared penetrated material. Smith et al. (2000) concur that pulse oximetry can be reliably used to identify aspiration. Smith et al. (2000) also used videofluoroscopy as the concurrent comparison assessment tool. The authors found that the technique was not sensitive enough to determine aspiration from penetration, with a drop in oxygen saturation occurring whether aspiration or penetration had occurred. They found that a combination of the bedside swallowing assessment plus pulse oximetry for the prediction of aspiration ±penetration gave a sensitivity of 86%, but a positive predictive value of 95%. Thus the combined assessment method was very likely to detect individuals who were either aspirating or penetrating the bolus.

There have been some interesting differences in the cases for and against pulse oximetry, which appear to be associated with the comparison tool. Some researchers have used concurrent videofluoroscopy with pulse oximetry; others have opted to use fibreoptic endoscopic evaluation of swallowing (FEES) (see Chapter 8). Both techniques are valid forms of identifying physiological deficits in the pharyngeal phase of swallowing. In a study by Leder (2000), the presence of aspiration did not significantly affect SpO_2 values. This was regardless of whether supplemental oxygen was supplied. Leder (2000) also recorded changes in heart rate and blood pressure during the FEES assessment. Interestingly he found that there was a consistent pattern of both higher heart rate and higher blood pressure values that occurred during the FEES assessment and for a 5-minute period post FEES. What is questionable here is whether the FEES procedure itself causes these physiological changes that could in fact mask the effect of what would otherwise happen, namely oxygen desaturation when aspiration occurs. A study that directly compares FEES plus pulse oximetry with videofluoroscopy plus pulse oximetry is important in eludicating whether there is a real effect based on assessment procedure.

Colodny (2001) in some respects concurs with Leder's (2000) findings that individuals with dysphagia do not necessarily desaturate *while* aspirating. Following normal physiology, one wouldn't expect them to. When healthy people swallow, there is a small period of apnoea while the swallow occurs. Colodny (2001) reported that SpO_2 levels are stable when healthy, non-dysphagic individuals eat or drink. Thus, the small apnoeic period during swallowing is short enough that gas exchange is not significantly interrupted. On the other hand, when a person aspirates, the person can't breathe for a period of time. Carbon dioxide levels and hydrogen ions continue to increase until the person can 'catch their breath'. It takes time (some milliseconds to seconds) for carbon dioxide levels to increase and for the 'less oxygenated blood' to reach the peripheral arteries in the fingers, toes or ear lobes where it can be recorded by the pulse oximeter. Thus pulse oximetry will *not* show a drop *at the exact moment* that aspiration occurs, but after a small delay. It provides evidence, *after the fact* that the respiratory system for some reason ceased to function effectively.

Again using FEES as the comparison tool, Colodny (2001) found that pulse oximetry is better used to record respiratory system status. Her data show that individuals with normal swallowing have the least compromised respiratory system, followed in order by penetrators, liquid aspirators and solid aspirators. She suggests that individuals with dysphagia have difficulty coordinating swallowing and respiration and this is made apparent during a pulse oximetry screen. There are, for example, individuals who may have quite a long apnoeic period in order to protect their airway. This period, however, will interfere with gas exchange and could conceivably cause a drop in SpO_2. Colodny (2001) reported that normal individuals had stable SpO_2 levels before, during and after feeding, whereas stroke and dementia patients showed a drop in SpO_2 levels during the feeding phase. Note that this is just a record of SpO_2 during feeding and does not take into account whether these people aspirated while they were feeding. Colodny's data showed that all aspiration groups (solids and liquids) had higher SpO_2 levels after feeding. Unfortunately no sensitivity, specificity, positive or negative predictive values are reported, however. Colodny's (2000) earlier study is reinforced by the 2001 study.

A small study by Tamura et al. (1999) provides support for the concept that pulse oximetry is more of a vehicle to measure swallow-respiratory abilities than episodes of aspiration. This group of researchers investigated the effect of oral feeding in the sitting position on a small group of severely disabled persons, measured using pulse oximetry, pulse rate and respiratory rate. Their hypothesis was that the sitting posture recommended during feeding could produce a great strain on severely disabled people. This strain may be evident in physiological measures such as arterial oxygen saturation, pulse rate and respiratory rate. Sitting is a posture in which the body must support and maintain a substantial portion of its own weight. Together with standing, sitting is an antigravitational posture. Tamura et al. (1999) found that feeding in an upright position was associated with a reduction in SpO_2 and an increase in pulse rate. These changes sometimes continued after feeding but were not evident when subjects were seated in the upright position without feeding. In some of the case studies, episodes of reduced SpO_2 were associated with rapid and laboured breathing and increased pulse rate. These can be seen as compensatory attempts by the body to improve oxygen saturation levels and thus gas exchange levels. The authors made two significant points.

First, they found that oral feeding in the upright position (an antigravitational posture) places a significant burden on the cardiopulmonary system of some severely disabled people. This is an important finding. Further research needs to be carried out to determine the best posture for individuals who have difficulty supporting themselves to eat. Difficulty holding trunk support inevitably affects the shoulder girdle and continues upwards through the neck to the jaw. The effort the individual needs to maintain stability may be at the expense of a stability of the oral and pharyngeal structures so necessary for the coordination of safe swallowing. The assumption that an upright position is best may not necessarily be true for all individuals. The angle of the body that provides best trunk support may also be the best angle for safe swallowing.

Secondly, Tamura et al. (1999) note that severely disabled individuals have a greater metabolic demand, but a lower physiologic reserve. Thus while they desperately need the calories that food and liquids provide to meet their metabolic demands, the physical demands of taking food occur at the expense of their cardiopulmonary system. Tamura et al. (1999) reported frequent episodes of apnoea in the group of severely disabled people studied even when feeding was not occurring. The pulse oximetry data documented in this study were coupled with changes in respiratory and pulse rates, which compensated for changes in blood oxygenation. This physiological correction mechanism lends support to Colodny's (2001) claim that pulse oximetry provides a marker of respiratory status rather than a tool for recording episodes of aspiration.

CONSIDERATIONS FOR USING THE TECHNIQUE

The pulse oximetry technique has a number of factors that will affect accurate readings of arterial oxygenation. These include: circulation status, temperature, evidence of peripheral vascular disease (e.g. diabetes or Raynaud's disease), movement artefact, extraneous environmental light, and skin pigmentation – including nail varnish (Collins and Bakheit, 1997; Colodny, 2001). There is also the suggestion that if the person is hemiplegic, the non-paretic hand be used for placement of the probe (Collins and Bakheit, 1997).

Note also that there are some peculiarities in interpreting drops in oxygen saturation levels (Sherman et al., 1999). The oxygen dissociation curve has a sigmoid profile. For example, a patient with a baseline SpO_2 of 92% will desaturate with a greater measurable decline than a person with a baseline measure of 99%. These differences are related to oxygen partial pressures. Pulse oximetry is not the tool of choice for measuring oxygen partial pressures. Due to this limitation, individuals with high baselines (95% to 100%) may not demonstrate a significant desaturation during aspiration, although their partial pressures may decline. Partial pressures are best assessed using arterial sampling (blood tests taken over time). Continuous blood sampling in the dysphagic population, however, is not feasible (Sherman et al., 1999).

CLINICAL APPLICATION IN PRACTICE

The literature supports use of pulse oximetry to document respiratory function during swallowing. It will not, however, necessarily respond purely to an aspiration episode. This is why the evidence is somewhat confusing. Individuals who penetrate but do not aspirate may also show declines in SpO_2. It doesn't matter so much whether material is aspirated or penetrated, the key is whether the gas exchange has been interrupted. It is a change in oxygen saturation levels, which is mediated by gas exchange in the lungs that is recorded by pulse oximetry. Note that aspiration is not the 'be-all and end-all' of diagnosis. It is important to identify what has caused aspiration, how often it occurs, and what, if anything, can be done by either compensation or rehabilitation to alleviate the cause. It is equally important to determine whether the respiratory system can cope with impaired swallowing. With this in mind, pulse oximetry may be well placed to be used in conjunction with bedside evaluation to identify individuals who require further instrumental assessments. For example, individuals who do not show any clinical indicators of aspiration but demonstrate desaturation could be referred for further radiological investigations (Sherman et al., 1999). Those who do not show clinical signs of aspiration and also have a normal pulse oximetry reading during oral trials are potentially at a lower risk than individuals with abnormal pulse oximetry recordings on a background of an uneventful clinical examination (Sherman et al., 1999).

PHARYNGEAL MANOMETRY AND ELECTROMYOGRAPHY

Other non-imaging assessments that may add information about swallowing function include *pharyngeal manometry* and *electromyography*. These techniques are not commonly used in clinical practice, however. Pharyngeal manometry is an invasive assessment using solid-state transducers at strategic places within the pharynx to assess the pressure dynamics of the pharynx and upper oesophageal sphincter during swallowing. Sensors are usually placed at:

- the base of the tongue;
- level of the upper oesophageal sphincter; and
- cervical oesophagus (Logemann, 1994).

Pharyngeal manometry is usually performed by a gastroenterologist. Manofluorography (i.e. simultaneous manometry and fluoroscopy) is used predominantly for research purposes. Manometric measures may include: pharyngeal contraction pressure, pharyngeal contraction duration, upper oesophageal sphincter relaxation and the duration of its relaxation, and UES coordination (Bulow et al., 1999). Pharyngeal manometry is frequently used where gastroesophageal reflux is anticipated.

Electromyography (EMG) measures functioning at the level of skeletal muscle. It can be used in either an invasive or non-invasive regime. The non-invasive technique uses electrodes attached to the skin surface over the muscle/s of interest (sEMG). The floor-of-mouth muscles are often evaluated in this manner. The disadvantage of this technique is that placement must be accurate to provide reliable information about the muscles of interest. There are numerous overlapping muscles at the floor of the mouth, making it difficult to judge which particular muscle is generating the response. The invasive method uses hooked wire electrodes placed directly into the muscle of interest. While more accurate, this technique is obviously more invasive and consequently not often used clinically. Therapeutic uses of sEMG are detailed in Chapter 12.

SUMMARY

The clinical assessment of swallowing disorders is a thorough and involved assessment of function. It takes swallowing ability in context, using real foods and fluids. Clinicians must integrate their knowledge of anatomy, neuroanatomy, physiology, medicine, communication, and idiosyncratic variables such as the individual's educational, vocational and cultural background to arrive at a diagnosis and treatment plan specific to each individual. It is possible to start with a basic framework, which is what the section above is seen to offer. The direction of each assessment, however, is dictated by each client and that client's unique set of circumstances. The information provided above explains why the various facets of the assessment are important.

The clinical assessment of dysphagia can be further enhanced by using other techniques. As noted above, cervical auscultation uses assessment of swallowing and swallow-respiratory sounds, whereas pulse oximetry uses information about blood oxygenation to alert the clinician to respiratory side effects of swallowing. Cervical auscultation and pulse oximetry should be used in conjunction with the clinical assessment to provide the clinician with further information that will assist in decision-making for suitability for oral intake, treatment options and overall management. At the completion of all clinical assessments, the clinician should decide whether further diagnostic assessments are required. These are discussed in detail in Chapter 8.

REFERENCES

Abdulla R-I (2001) The history of the stethoscope. Pediatric Cardiology 22: 371–2.
Adnerhill I, Ekberg O, Groher ME (1989) Determining normal bolus size for thin fluids. Dysphagia 4: 1–3.

Bulow M, Olsson R, Ekberg O (1999) Videomanometric analysis of supraglottic swallow, effortful swallow, and chin tuck in healthy volunteers. Dysphagia 14: 67–72.

Cichero JAY, Murdoch BE (1998) The physiologic cause of swallowing sounds: Answers from heart sounds and vocal tract acoustics. Dysphagia 13: 39–52.

Cichero JAY, Murdoch BE (2002a) Acoustic signature of the normal swallow: Characterisation by age, gender and bolus volume. Annals of Otology, Rhinology and Laryngology 111(7/1): 623–32.

Cichero JAY, Murdoch BE. (2002b) Detection of swallowing sounds: methodology reviewed. Dysphagia 17(1): 40–9.

Cichero JAY, Murdoch (2003). What happens after the swallow? Introducing the glottal release sound. Journal of Medical Speech-Language Pathology 11(1): 31–41.

Collins MJ, Bakheit AMO (1997) Does pulse oximetry reliably detect aspiration in dysphagic stroke patients? Stroke 28(9): 1773–5.

Colodny N. (2001) Effects of age, gender, disease, and multisystem involvement on oxygen saturation levels in dysphagic persons. Dysphagia 16: 48–57.

Comrie JD, Helm JM (1997) Common feeding problems in the intensive care nursery: maturation, organization, evaluation, and management strategies. Seminars in Speech and Language 18(3): 239–59.

Davies POAL, McGowan RS, Shadle CH (1993) Practical flow duct acoustics applied to the vocal tract. In IR Titze (ed.) Vocal Fold Physiology: Frontiers in Basic Science. San Diego: Singular Publishing Group.

DePippo KL, Holas MA, Reding MJ (1992) Validation of the 3-oz water swallow test for aspiration following stroke. Archives of Neurology 49: 1259–61.

Dorsey LD (2002) Effects of reclined supported postures on management of dysphagic adults with severe developmental disabilities (Abstract). Dysphagia 17(2): 180.

Eicher PS, Mano CJ, Fox CA, et al. (1994) Impact of cervical auscultation on accuracy of clinical evaluation in predicting penetration or aspiration in a pediatric population. Minute – Second Workshop on Cervical Auscultation, McLean, Virginia.

Groher ME (1994) The detection of aspiration and videofluorscopy (editorial). Dysphagia 9(3): 147–8.

Hamlet S, Nelson R, Patterson R (1988) Sounds of swallowing (abstract). Journal of the Acoustic Society of America 83 (supp. 1): s23.

Hamlet S, Penney DG, Formolo J (1994) Stethoscope acoustics and cervical auscultation of swallowing. Dysphagia 9: 63–8.

Hiiemae K (1994) The sounds of swallowing: a preliminary methodological investigation. Minute – Second Workshop on Cervical Auscultation, McLean, Virginia.

Hirst LJ, Ford GA, Gibson J, Wilson JA (2002) Swallow-induced alterations in breathing in normal older people. Dysphagia 17: 152–61.

Kuhn PM (1995) A review of sensing devices for cervical auscultation. Minute – Third Meeting on Cervical Auscultation, Virginia, McLean.

Langmore SE, Terpenning MS, Schork A, et al. (1998) Predictors of aspiration pneumonia: how important is dysphagia? Dysphagia 13: 69–81.

Leder SB (2000) Use of aterial oxygen saturation, heart rate, and blood pressure as indirect objective physiologic markers to predict aspiration. Dysphagia 15: 201–5.

Lefton-Greif MA, Loughlin GM (1996) Specialized studies in pediatric dysphagia. Seminars in Speech and Language 17(4): 311–29.

Leslie P, Drinnan MJ, Finn P, et al. (2004) Reliability and validity of cervical auscultation: a controlled comparison using videofluoroscopy. Dysphagia 19: 231–40.

Linden P, Kuhlemeier KV, Patterson C (1993) The probability of correctly predicting sub-glottic penetration from clinical observations. Dysphagia 8: 170–9.

Logan WJ, Kavanagh JF, Wornall AW (1967) Sonic correlates of human deglutition. Journal of Applied Physiology 23(2): 279–84.

Logemann JA (1994) Non-imaging techniques for the study of swallowing. Acta Oto-Rhino-Laryngologica Belgica 48: 139–42.

Logemann JA (1995) Dysphagia: evaluation and treatment. Folia Phoniatrica et Logopedica 47: 140–64.

Logemann JA (1998) Evaluation and Treatment of Swallowing Disorders (2nd edn). Austin TX: Pro-ed.

Logemann JA, Veis S, Colangelo L (1999) A screening procedure for oropharyngeal dysphagia. Dysphagia 14: 44–51.

Mackowiak RC, Brenman HS, Friedman MHF (1967) Acoustic profile of deglutition. Proceedings of the Society for Experimental Biology and Medicine 125: 1149–52.

Mann G, Hankey GJ, Cameron D (2000) Swallowing disorders following acute stroke: Prevalence and diagnostic accuracy. Cerebrovascular Diseases 10: 380–6.

Martin-Harris B (2000) Optimal patterns of care in patients with chronic obstructive pulmonary disease. Seminars in Speech and Language 21(4): 311–21.

McKaig TN (2002) Personal communication. Paper presented at the Eleventh Annual Dysphagia Research Society Meeting, Miami, Florida, October 3–5.

Miller RM (1992) Clinical examination for dysphagia. In Groher ME (ed.) Dysphagia: Diagnosis and Management (2nd edn). Boston: Butterworth-Heinemann, pp. 143–62.

Morton R, Minford J, Ellis R, et al. (2002) Aspiration with dysphagia: the interaction between oropharyngeal and respiratory impairments. Dysphagia 17: 192–6.

Pennington GR, Kreutsch JA (1990) Swallowing disorders: assessment and rehabilitation. British Journal of Hospital Medicine 44: 17–22.

Richardson TR, Moody JM (2000) Bedside cardiac examination: constancy in a sea of change. Current Problems in Cardiology 25(11): 785–825.

Ruf JM, Stevens JH (1995) Accuracy of bedside versus videofluoroscopy swallowing evaluation (Abstract). Dysphagia 10: 63.

Sellars C, Dunnet C, Carter R (1998) A preliminary comparison of videofluoroscopy of swallow and pulse oximetry in the identification of aspiration in dysphagic patients. Dysphagia 13: 82–6.

Shaw JL, Sharpe S, Dyson SE, et al. (2004) Bronchial auscultation: an effective adjunct to speech and language therapy assessment when detecting dysphagia and aspiration? Dysphagia 19: 211–18.

Sherman B, Nisenboum JM, Jesberger BL, et al. (1999) Assessment of dysphagia with the use of pulse oximetry. Dysphagia 14: 152–6.

Smith HA, Lee SA, O'Neill PA, et al. (2000) The combination of bedside swallowing assessment and oxygen saturation monitoring of swallowing in acute stroke: a safe and humane screening tool. Age and Ageing 29: 495–9.

Smithard DG, Spriggs D (2003) No gag, no food (research letter). Age and Ageing 32: 674.

Splaingard ML, Hutchins B, Sulton LD, et al. (1988) Aspiration in rehabilitation patients: videofluoroscopy vs. bedside clinical assessment. Archives of Physical Medicine and Rehabilitation 69: 637–40.

Stroud AE, Lawrie BW, Wiles CM (2002) Inter- and intra-rater reliability of cervical auscultation to detect aspiration in patients with dysphagia. Clinical Rehabilitation 16(6): 640–5.

DYSPHAGIA: FOUNDATION, THEORY AND PRACTICE

Takahashi K, Groher ME, Michi K-I (1994) Methodology for detecting swallowing sounds.
Dysphagia 9: 54–62.
Tamura F, Shishikura J, Mukai Y, et al. (1999) Arterial oxygen saturation in severely disabled
people: Effect of oral feeding in the sitting position. Dysphagia 14: 204–11.
Warms T, Richards J (2000) 'Wet voice' as a predictor of penetration and aspiration in
oropharyngeal dysphagia. Dysphagia 15: 84–8.
Weitz HH, Mangione S (2000) In defense of the stethoscope and the bedside. American
Journal of Medicine 108: 669–71.
Willett S (2002) Cervical auscultation: objective evaluation of the swallow in normally
developing 12-month-olds. Unpublished thesis for the Bachelor of Speech Pathology (hon-
ours) degree, University of Queensland.
Zaidi NH, Smith HA, King SC, et al. (1995) Oxygen desaturation on swallowing as a potential marker of aspiration in acute stroke. Age and Ageing 24(4): 267–70.
Zenner PM, Losinski DS, Mills RH (1995) Using cervical auscultation in the clinical
dysphagia examination in long-term care. Dysphagia 10: 27–31.

8 Imaging Assessments

JULIE CICHERO and SUSAN LANGMORE

INTRODUCTION

The previous chapter discussed the most common non-imaging assessments of dysphagia. This chapter focuses on imaging assessments of dysphagia, i.e. those assessments where a visual image is generated. The best known and most widely used imaging assessments used by speech pathologists are videofluoroscopy, otherwise known as the modified barium swallow (MBS), and fibreoptic endoscopic evaluation of swallowing (FEES). Both techniques aim to provide the clinician with detailed information about the anatomical structures involved in swallowing ('the what') and the physiology of the oropharyngeal swallow ('the why').

'Most of our impressions about the world and our memories of it are based on sight' (Kandel and Wurtz, 2000: 492). Our reliance on imaging techniques for elucidating swallowing pathophysiology should, therefore, come as no surprise. There are multiple visual areas in the brain and at least two major interacting neural pathways. These pathways are responsible for our perception of depth, form, motion and colour, which are all required for accurate interpretation of both x-ray and endoscopic images (Kandel and Wurtz, 2000). Both MBS and FEES purport to be 'objective measures' but this is only true of the image itself. The *interpretation* of the data, whether it is video x-ray or video endoscopy, comes back to the fallible human. This is perhaps one of the reasons why reasonably poor interrater and intrarater reliability is reported for fluoroscopy studies (Scott et al., 1998; Stoeckli et al., 2003). The assessments detailed in this chapter also fall under the banner of 'diagnostic assessments' rather than 'screening assessments'. Screening tools identify the presence or absence of a problem. They may be able to identify that an individual is aspirating but will not be able to say 'why' the aspiration is occurring. A diagnostic tool on the other hand details the 'why'. This chapter will detail the theory and application of the MBS with an emphasis on clinically relevant assessment regimes. A discussion of radiation safety is also included. The theory and practical application of FEES is also discussed, in addition to its relative advantages and limitations. To this point, the MBS and FEES have been viewed as 'either/or' assessments. What is becoming increasingly relevant is that both assessments provide unique information about the pharyngeal stage of the swallow in particular. The information they provide is complementary rather than exclusionary. There may indeed be some patients where one

Dysphagia: Foundation, Theory and Practice. Edited by J. Cichero and B. Murdoch
© 2006 John Wiley & Sons, Ltd.

technique would be preferable to the other due to the presenting signs and symptoms, and vice versa. A brief review of ultrasound and nuclear scintigraphy, also imaging techniques, is included at the end of the chapter for the sake of completeness.

THE MODIFIED BARIUM SWALLOW OR VIDEOFLUOROSCOPY

The modified barium swallow (MBS) or videofluoscopy is arguably the best known and most widely used imaging assessment for dysphagia. It was pioneered by Professor Jeri Logemann and she has done much to introduce and refine the technique. Aside from information about the anatomy and physiology of the oropharyngeal swallow, the MBS offers information about the effectiveness of therapeutic techniques (see Chapter 12) and also compensatory strategies and approaches (see Chapter 11). It allows us to determine oral and pharyngeal transit times with good accuracy. In addition, it allows the clinician to ascertain the relative functioning of the various 'valves' within the oropharyngeal system. The MBS affords the astute clinician the ability to detect aspiration when it occurs and the evidence needed to postulate why it might have occurred. The amount aspirated may also be guessed. For example, the amount aspirated may be noted as minimal, moderate or severe (Palmer et al., 1993).

WHEN TO REFER

An MBS procedure should be considered when orophayngeal dysphagia is suspected as part of the clinical examination but the nature of the problem has not been accurately identified, or when the problem is amenable to therapeutic intervention. For example, the clinician may be aware that laryngeal excursion is suboptimal and that the patient has a delayed weak cough after swallowing; however, the clinical examination cannot provide evidence of the physiological cause of these events. In this example, a delayed cough after swallowing may be due to post-swallow aspiration from material pooled in:

- the valleculae;
- the pyriform sinuses; or
- both.

Hence, the underlying problem is reduced bolus clearance. Modified barium swallow may also be useful to rule out aspiration associated with eating and/or drinking as a cause of respiratory disease, chronic cough or hoarseness that cannot be otherwise explained (Feinberg, 1993). Feinberg (1993) also advocates use of the MBS to assist in the diagnosis of individuals with unexplained weight loss – particularly the elderly or chronically ill patient. The MBS may also be useful in ascertaining the severity of dysphagia or providing more information to patients, their families or even their physicians. It provides objective information about the pharyngeal phase of the swallow. Whenever aspiration is suspected from clinical observations (e.g. temperature spikes coupled with deteriorating chest condition, with or without reduced consumption of food or fluids, and with or without wet, gurgly vocal quality) an MBS is most likely to elucidate the reason why aspiration, or suspected aspiration is occurring. This information then allows the clinician to try compensatory manoeuvres or different dietary textures or fluids. Note, however, that an MBS procedure should only be considered if the results of the assessment are likely to change the way the clinician manages the case. There is little reason to expose a patient to ionizing radiation if the management of the patient is not going to change. Individuals undergoing palliative care may fall into this category. The MBS procedure is suitable for both adults and children. With appropriate seating equipment, most individuals could undergo an MBS procedure should the need arise.

Paediatric considerations

In addition to the signs and symptoms listed above indicating that an MBS is necessary, the following specific information should also be considered for paediatric clients:

- an increase in congestion during and after feeds;
- poor weight gain or weight loss;
- primitive oral reflexes; and
- oxygen desaturation during meals.

THE MBS TEAM

The MBS team is relatively large. The patient should be the centre of the team. All patients recommended for an MBS require a written referral by a medical officer. The patient is supported by the speech pathologist(s), radiographer, radiologist, nurse, parent or carer, or other professionals (e.g. gastroenterologist, or ear, nose and throat specialist).

The speech pathologist has a number of tasks or roles to undertake during the MBS. He or she is responsible for:

- explaining the procedure to the client;
- testing food and fluid consistencies; and
- applying different therapeutic techniques or compensatory strategies, as appropriate for the individual.

In conjunction with other members of the team, the speech pathologist will identify the symptoms (for example, wet vocal quality post swallow, perceptions of delayed swallow reflex or reduced hyolaryngeal excursion) and anatomical or physiological causes of dysphagia. Symptoms are gathered from the clinical examination and patient interview. It is for this reason that the clinical assessment of dysphagia should always precede the radiological assessment. Using the information gathered from the MBS procedure, the speech pathologist will decide upon the safety of oral feeding and will plan appropriate dysphagia management. The speech pathologist should be involved in recording the procedure and reporting the results and recommendations to all team members.

The radiologist is a medical practitioner specializing in radiation medicine. The radiologist has expertise in making a medical diagnosis and in the identification of anatomical abnormalities, masses and structural deviations. A radiographer produces high quality images of organs, limbs and other parts of the body, which allow the radiologist to diagnose disorders and assess injuries. In the case of the MBS, the images are of the oral cavity and pharynx and often the oesophagus. The radiographer may be instrumental in positioning the patient, moving the imaging equipment and adjusting the equipment to ensure that high quality images are produced with the minimum amount of radiation exposure required. Nursing staff provide care to the patient such as suctioning, assistance with correct positioning of the patient and connection or disconnection of oxygen or feeds (e.g. nasogastric feeds). Other individuals may also assist with moving and positioning the patient for the procedure.

Modified barium swallow procedural practices vary from institution to institution. In many institutions it is common for the radiologist and speech pathologist to be present for the duration of the MBS procedure – from administration through to interpretation. At some facilities, the procedures may vary such that the speech pathologist and the radiographer conduct the actual MBS procedure, with the captured images then interpreted by the speech pathologist and the radiologist after the procedure. In most cases the speech pathologist generates a written report, as does the radiologist. The radiologist's report will detail all phases of swallowing (oral, pharyngeal and oesophageal), whereas the speech pathologist will comment on the oral and pharyngeal phases of swallowing.

THE PROCEDURE

Equipment

Investigation of oropharyngeal function is best achieved using 'moving x-rays' or rapid filming to capture the dynamics of the swallow. Examples of these include videofluoroscopy and cineradiography. Although cineradiography produces better quality images, it requires more processing units (x-ray generator, cine camera, cine film processing units, etc.) and radiation exposure rates are 5–10 times higher than fluoroscopic exposure rates (Mahesh et al., 2003). Consequently videofluoroscopy units are more commonly used. Most recently digital video formats have allowed even higher resolution than standard videotape procedures. In addition digital formats offer reduced radiation doses with pulsed fluoroscopy (Mahesh et al., 2003). Unfortunately, the digital imaging equipment sometimes captures fewer than 30 frames per second, which is unacceptable for a swallow study (see below). Often swallowing studies are conducted with a tilt-table fluoroscope tilted into an upright position. The x-ray tube is located under the table top. The patient stands or sits between the upright table and the fluoroscope. The fluoroscope can be moved up and down, and to an extent laterally, to focus on different portions of the individual's anatomy (e.g. oral cavity or oesophagus). The x-rays are projected from the x-ray tube and pass through the patient to the fluoroscope. Passing through the person, the intensity of the x-rays reduces. For example, thin or low-density areas of the body allow a high degree of x-ray penetration and cause a bright video image. Thicker, denser areas tend to absorb x-rays and produce an image that is not as bright. The change in the intensity of the x-rays exiting the patient is projected into the image intensifier, which is housed behind the fluoroscope. The intensifier converts the image into a visual form and this image is then fed to a video camera, where the image can be viewed via a monitor and/or recorded (Beck and Gayler, 1990). 'The oropharyngeal swallow is quicker than the eye' (Dodds et al., 1990: 956). Consequently a frame rate of 30/s is required for adequate dynamic images, with the eye blurring sequential images together to give the impression of a continuous image (Beck and Gayler, 1990). Capturing images at this rate also allows for frame-by-frame analysis and slow-motion playback. The ability to play images back is important. Only part of the image can be selected as the focus of attention; the remainder, even transiently, is relegated to the background. In reviewing images, different portions of the swallow can be viewed as a focus, allowing the clinician to detail all phases of swallowing with some accuracy.

Preparation for the procedure

The client should be well informed about the procedure. The client should know what the clinician is hoping to achieve from the procedure and also that the procedure involves ionizing radiation. Patients do not usually have to fast before an MBS procedure. They should understand that they will be asked to consume barium impregnated foods or fluids, which may make the foods and fluids taste chalky. Please note that the patient should also be informed that barium is not absorbed and as such is passed through the system. As a result, patients may notice that their stools are white in colour after the procedure, and this is simply the barium being passed out of the system. If the person is able to tolerate thin fluids safely, they should be encouraged to drink water to help move the barium through the gastrointestinal system and prevent constipation. Note also that the radiologist should decide on the type of contrast agent to be used (i.e. the agent added to the foods or fluids to make them radioopaque). For example, for individuals with suspected tissue perforation, certain types of contrast agent are contraindicated (e.g. barium sulfate suspension). Another type of contrast agent, gastrograffin, may be used where tissue perforation is suspected. However, this is contraindicated for individuals at risk of aspiration as it can cause pulmonary oedema (Speech Pathology Australia, 2004). There are a number of different contrast agents available, and the clinician should be guided by the radiologist for the best contrast agent to be used for individuals undergoing an MBS procedure. The patient should be aware of the likely amount of foods/fluids they will try and the procedures that are in place in case of emergency. Emergency suctioning may be required if large amounts of barium are aspirated, or if a piece of solid food becomes lodged in the larynx or trachea. Fortunately, emergencies are relatively rare.

Paediatric considerations

In addition to the information outlined above, parents/carers of children undergoing an MBS should, whenever possible, be given an opportunity to familiarize themselves and their children with the radiology suite. It may assist the procedure for the parents/carers to bring in the child's own spoon/cup/plate, and for the feeding technique to be practised prior to the procedure. The procedure should be scheduled for a time when the child is usually awake (i.e. not a morning or afternoon sleep time). It may also be of benefit for children to be fasted prior to the procedure to ensure that they are hungry and thus more likely to take the foods/fluids offered. Ideally children should be able to manage their own secretions and also be at a stage where they can tolerate fingers or toys in their mouth. In addition they should also be able to tolerate 3–4 consecutive small spoonfuls of fluids or puree. These skills should assist in providing the best possible set of circumstances for a successful MBS. Children's attention spans and cooperation are typically short and the clinician, radiographer and radiologist must bear this in mind with a paediatric swallowing study (Kramer, 1989).

Anatomical structures

The image should focus on the lips anteriorly, the hard palate superiorly, the pharyngeal wall posteriorly, the trachea (to the level of the bifurcation of the airway) and the oesophagus inferiorly. The mandible can be clearly visualized as can the soft palate. The base of the skull and cervical spine can also be viewed. The hyoid bone, epiglottis and vocal folds can be visualized. The nasopharynx extends from the base of the skull to the superior surface of the soft palate. The oropharynx extends from the pharyngeal aspect of the palate superiorly to the base of tongue or pit of valleculae and the hyoid bone inferiorly. The hypopharynx extends from the valleculae to the level of cricopharyngeus.

Other structures that may be viewed include cervical osteophytes and pharyngeal pouch or Zenker's diverticulum. An osteophyte is a bony outgrowth. In the case of a cervical osteophyte, it is a bony outgrowth of one or more of the cervical vertebrae. Cervical osteophytes are common in elderly patients and are often associated with dysphagia as they cause the cervical spine to bulge into the pharyngeal space. This causes a structural narrowing of the pharynx and/or compression of the oesophagus and larynx. This compression contributes to dysphagia, mainly for solids. Pharyngeal or oesophageal obstruction is the most frequent complaint of individuals with cervical osteophytes (Maiuri et al., 2002). If the osteophytes are particularly large, they may also cause dyspnea (shortness of breath). In extreme cases the respiratory distress caused by the osteophytes may be relieved via tracheostomy (Maiuri et al., 2002; Aronowitz and Cobarrubias, 2003). Maiuri et al. (2002) reported that CT or MRI are the best techniques for determining the size and status of the osteophytes. Osteophytes can be managed by altering the patient's diet or alternatively, by surgical removal of the osteophytes. The removal of the bony growth alleviates the dysphagia and the dyspnea, however, it can also result in long-term spinal instability (Maiuri et al., 2002).

A pharyngeal pouch (also known as a Zenker's diverticula) is an outpouching of pharyngeal mucosa through Killian's triangle. Killian's triangle is the anatomical region found posteriorly between the oblique and horizontal fibres of the cricopharyngeal muscle (Jones, 2003b). The diverticulum or pouch is thought to be formed by a combination of muscular incoordination while swallowing and higher than normal cricopharyngeal tone (Van Eeden et al., 1999). The walls of the pharynx are progressively weakened by this combination until the walls 'give' and a pouch forms. The pouch is capable of holding food, which the patient may then regurgitate at a later stage. If the pouch becomes too full it may spill over into the larynx and result in recurrent aspiration pneumonia. Pouches may be attended to medically using a surgical approach (e.g. suspension, inversion or excision of the pouch, often coupled with cricophayngeal myotomy) or surgical stapling of the pouch (Ong et al., 1999; Van Eeden et al., 1999).

Dodds et al. (1990) noted that mucosal webs may be seen on the anterior wall of the cervical oesophagus – these are apparently a normal variation. It is likewise normal to find small amounts of residual barium coating the valleculae after swallowing (Dodds et al., 1990). In some institutions, the radiologist will also complete an examination of the oesophagus during an MBS procedure. Screening for oesophageal disorders such as:

- strictures or obstructive rings;
- abnormal motor function;
- oesophageal reflux; or
- oesophageal neoplasm may occur (Dodds et al., 1990).

Views used

The view that the radiologist or radiographer uses will determine the detail of the various structures seen during the procedure. Typically the views used during an MBS procedure are the lateral view (see Figures 8.1 and 8.2) and the antero-posterior (AP) view. Both views aim to show the oral cavity and the pharynx to the level of cervical oesophagus. The image should be held steady such that the oral cavity and pharynx are fully in view during the procedure. The radiographer or radiologist may choose to follow the bolus down into the oesophagus after the oral and pharyngeal phases have been thoroughly examined. The lateral view shows the individual in profile. It is possible to see the person accept the bolus into the oral cavity and process the bolus using the teeth and tongue. It is also possible to see movement of the soft plate in the lateral view. The movements of hyolaryngeal excursion and epiglottic inversion are well distinguished. Opening of the upper oesphageal sphincter (UES) is also able to be visualized. When the tongue propels the bolus into the pharynx it is tempting to suggest that the image portrays the posterior pharyngeal wall moving in to meet the base of tongue. However, one must recall that the x-ray is a two-dimensional medium. As noted in Chapter 4, the

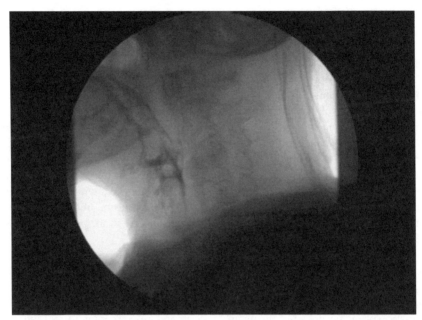

Figure 8.1   Lateral view of the posterior portion of the oral cavity and pharynx. There is barium coating of the oral and pharyngeal structures. The cervical spine can be viewed at the right of the radiograph. Reproduced by permission of Kay PENTAX

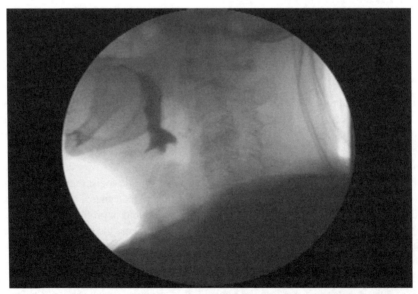

Figure 8.2   Lateral radiograph. The bolus has traversed the angle of the mandible and progressed into the pharynx to the level of valleculae. Reproduced by permission of Kay PENTAX

left and right pharyngeal walls *medialize* and meet the posterior moving base of tongue. The x-ray gives the illusion that it is the posterior pharyngeal wall moving, when in fact it is a medialization of the left and right pharyngeal walls. Also in the lateral view, it is possible to delineate the larynx and to identify the vocal folds and the trachea. Some radiologists use a 'lateral oblique view' (15° to 20°), which allows a better view of the individual left and right valleculae and pyrifom sinuses than the traditional lateral view (Dodds et al., 1990). In this position the individual retains their head in a lateral plane and shifts their shoulders such that the shoulder closest to the image intensifier is positioned further back, giving the shoulders the 'oblique arrangement'. This posture ensures that the shoulders do not block the x-ray view of the pharyngeal region.

The AP view shows individuals as though they are looking directly into the camera. This view is particularly good for identifying chewing, symmetry of movement and pooling. For example, it is possible to see whether the individual has residue that remains in one or both valleculae or pyriform sinuses. This information is not afforded in the lateral view, as the paired valleculae or pyriform sinuses are transposed one over the top of the other in the lateral view. The AP view is also useful for evaluating vocal fold approximation during phonation. A typical MBS procedure would start with the client in a lateral or lateral oblique position, with progression to the AP view as required.

Commencing the examination

Wherever possible, the patient should be seated in their usual position for eating/drinking. This may not always be possible and depends upon, the patient's posture and also the equipment available in the radiology suite. The fluoroscopy table, which is normally horizontal, is rotated so that it assumes a vertical orientation. Many radiology suites use the footplate of the table as a platform for the patient to stand/sit on for the MBS procedure. The footplate is moveable and if the patient is unable to stand, but has adequate balance and stability, the footplate can be moved along the table such that the patient can sit on the ledge-like footplate. This system is not optimal for individuals without adequate balance or stability (e.g. stroke, head injury, conditions with an associated hemiparesis). Given that the distance between the X-ray tube (under the table) and the fluoroscope is quite narrow, a narrow plastic chair may be used for the patient to sit, or even a narrow-width wheelchair (such as those found on airplanes). There are specialty x-ray chairs that have been developed also. These have been specially designed to meet the narrow space requirements of the x-ray equipment configuration and are adjustable to meet the posturing needs of the individual patient. For paediatric patients, chairs such as the MAMA chair or radiolucent tumbleform seats may be used (Kramer, 1989; Arvedson and Brodsky, 2002).

Foods and fluids tested

The foods and fluids tested during the MBS procedure will vary from workplace to workplace. They will also vary depending upon the reason for requesting the MBS, the clinical hypothesis and the patient's performance during the procedure (e.g. fatigue, aspiration, uncooperative behaviour). Each MBS examination should be tailored to the individual. An MBS procedure may include trials of different levels of thickness of fluids (thin, nectar thick, half or honey thick and pudding thick) and may also include trials of food textures (biscuit, bread, jelly and marshmallow). In order for foods and fluids to be 'seen' during the x-ray, a radiopaque substance called barium is added to the foods and fluids.

Foods and fluids should mirror normal day-to-day eating wherever possible. The addition of barium to foods and liquids changes the internal make up of the foods and fluids. For example, barium is a solid and increases the weight to substances to which it is added. Chapter 3 provides a detailed discussion about changes that occur to fluids when barium is added to them. Ideally only sufficient barium should be added to the fluids to ensure that they are radiopaque. Barium has been used in the cooking of biscuits, bread and marshmallows so that taste is minimally affected and normal food texture is retained. It is not ideal to coat biscuits and bread in a barium liquid as it presents a mixed consistency (liquid and solid). Foods with mixed consistency are often harder for dysphagic individuals to control, and may predispose them to further difficulties that may not be present if only a solid texture was used. Many fluoroscopy suites keep barium pills; if not, it is possible to obtain empty capsules from pharmacy departments and place barium powder inside the capsules to observe how the individual manages in swallowing medications. Some elderly individuals have great difficulty swallowing tablets and this method may enable the clinician to observe their attempts and work on strategies to help make the process easier for them.

Ideally the patient should test two to three swallows of each type of food or fluid consistency of interest. A single swallow of a given consistency may not give a representative view of how the individual copes with that consistency. There is a tendency to provide small amounts of fluids under the assumption that, if the fluid is in fact aspirated, only a small amount will be aspirated. However, bearing in mind anatomy and physiology, we know that the average mouthful an individual will swallow is approximately 20 ml. Thus a dessert spoon or tablespoon amount would better assess this volume than a 1, 3 or 5 ml bolus. Smaller bolus volumes may be useful for determining how the individual manages saliva swallows; however, these small amounts should not be used as indicators for how the individual would swallow at meal times. In the event that the individual has reduced sensory awareness, the small volume may serve only to slip under the 'sensory radar' and actually set the patient up to aspirate, the very thing we are trying to avoid. A more normal sized bolus may provide sufficient sensory cues to allow the oral and pharyngeal mechanisms to show a true indication of how they cope with a 'normal bolus'. Palmer et al. (1993: 211) have produced a standard sequence for videofluoroscopy procedures:

- Lateral projection:

  - swallow 5 ml of thick liquid from a spoon;
  - drink thick liquid from a cup (1 swallow);

  – swallow 5ml thin fluid from a spoon;
  – drink thin liquid from a cup (1 swallow);
  – modifications and other liquids as appropriate;
  – chew and swallow approximately 1 teaspoon of puree, or marshmallow;
  – chew and swallow approximately 1 teaspoon of solids (e.g. biscuit or bread);
  – modifications and other foods as appropriate.

• Antero-posterior position:

  – observe patient vocal fold movement as they phonate (e.g. /ahh/);
  – take thin liquid from a cup, hold and then swallow;
  – modifications or other foods as appropriate;
  – additional swallows of thin liquid as needed for imaging the oesophagus.

Note, that the 1 ml, 3 ml and 5 ml boluses are most likely to be suitable for paediatric clients given their smaller oral cavity for containment of the bolus.

   It is best to start the x-ray 'on time' when the patient is ready to commence swallowing. It is not ideal to provide patients with a bolus and ask them to hold it in the oral cavity until told to swallow. This kind of scenario will predispose the patient with a poor ability to hold the bolus in the oral cavity to aspirate before the swallow. In addition, as noted in Chapter 4, there is a specific sequence of events that is initiated when a bolus approaches and enters the oral cavity and this governs the inter-relationship between swallowing and respiration. By asking an individual to 'hold the bolus till I tell you to swallow', we upset this natural sequence of events, again potentially causing the already compromised individual to miss-time their swallow-respiratory coordination. The clinician may choose to include one such request for the patient to hold the bolus specifically to determine the patient's degree of volitional control, as this may be useful information when determining rehabilitation strategies. However, it is advisable to commence the study with the patient's more usual pattern.

Paediatric considerations

Paediatric clients are our least predictable clients. It may be possible to inject small amounts of barium into the children's mouth or buccal cavities if children are unwilling or unable to take the barium for themselves. The clinician should be prepared to forgo the procedure rather than pursue a procedure where the child is clearly upset. In an agitated state the child is most unlikely to produce swallowing activities that are indicative of everyday feeding. Consequently it may not be possible to perform the ideal MBS with every child. It may be that the clinician must decide on the most important questions to be answered for this particular child at this particular time. When time is of the essence, the questions asked might include:

• Is swallowing influenced by the amount?
• Is swallowing influenced by the texture?
• Is there a delay in swallowing on any consistency?
• Is swallowing ability influenced by fatigue (e.g. at the end of the meal)?

Contraindications

Modified barium swallow is contraindicated when the individual in question has a depressed level of consciousness or even a fluctuating level of alertness. For safety reasons, individuals with a depressed level of consciousness should not attempt oral intake of any form. Similarly, a fluctuating level of alertness would limit the generalizability of the results to the mealtime setting. Individuals who are unable to be positioned for an MBS are unsuitable for the procedure, as are individuals who are uncooperative. The space between the x-ray tube and fluoroscope is quite narrow – often only the width that is able to accommodate an airline wheelchair. Obese individuals may simply not fit in the prescribed space limitations. Without the aid of specially designed MBS chairs, individuals with a severe hemiparesis and poor sitting or standing balance may not be able to be positioned to safely undergo the procedure. Individuals with movement disorders, or those with dementia or cognitive impairment, may be difficult to assess and the findings of the examination may be limited; hence these groups are only assessed where the need to determine swallowing safety is very great. Individuals who are medically unstable are also often unsuitable for MBS assessment. It is in the best interest of patients to wait until their medical condition has stabilized before putting them through a radiological investigation, particularly if the medical condition is an influencing factor in their dysphagia. Individuals who have already undergone a number of diagnostic or therapeutic radiological procedures may need to have good reason to undergo further radiation exposure. For this reason it is important that the speech pathologist use good judgement in requesting repeat MBS procedures. In Australia, the Australian Radiation Protection and Nuclear Safety Agency provides guidelines for dose limits per year for:

- patients;
- individuals involved in biomedical research; and
- those who are occupationally exposed to radiation.

Assessment of the upper oesophageal sphincter (UES) and reflux

The MBS can be used by the speech pathologist to provide information about the integrity of the upper oesophageal sphincter (UES). As noted in Chapter 4, poor hyolaryngeal elevation contributes markedly to insufficient opening of the UES due to the pulley-like system that operates between these areas. Evidence of poor UES function can be seen by:

- small amounts of the bolus passing through the UES even when the bolus size increases; and
- material pooled primarily in the pyriform sinuses post swallow.

Thickening of the UES may also be noticeable. The UES anatomically marks the end of the speech pathologist's assessment of dysphagia. The radiologist will probably assess the integrity of the oesophageal phase of swallowing to complete the clinical diagnosis. The motility of the oesophagus (i.e. peristalsis) is radiologically assessed in the horizontal position (Jones, 2003a). In the vertical position, gravity assists with emptying. Assessment of oesophageal dysphagia or dysfunction should be interpreted by the radiologist. A gastroenterologist treats oesophageal dysphagia. Note, however, that a poorly functioning oesophagus can have an impact on swallowing safety. For example, an individual with poor oesophageal function may have delayed oesophageal emptying into the stomach. The oesophagus is a tube of finite length. Once the tube is full and with insufficient emptying from below, physics deems the bolus will move back up, i.e. the material will be refluxed. Note this is termed 'oesophageal reflux' and material can also be refluxed from the stomach back up into the oesophagus (i.e. gastroesophageal reflux). When the bolus moves back up it can go through the UES and into the pyriform sinuses. So imagine now that the bolus has passed into the oesophagus, the oesophagus is too full to accommodate any further material and is not emptying at a sufficient rate to receive any further material. The bolus pushes back up through the UES into the pyriform sinuses. By this stage the swallow has been completed and the person has recommenced tidal breathing. Recall that the pyriform sinuses are the chutes on either sides of the larynx. They are the channels through which the bolus passes and they end at the UES. This material that has pooled in the pyriform sinuses is now in a prime location to be inhaled into the larynx with each respiration, leading to aspiration after the swallow. The importance of this information is that the individual may present with an aspiration pneumonia; however, it may well be from dysphagia of *oesophageal* origin that is impacting on the pharynx and larynx *after* the swallow. The MBS will provide the most information about both pharyngeal and oesophageal functioning in this type of scenario. Reflux may be demonstrated most frequently when the patient is turned from the prone to the supine position (Jones, 2003a).

Discontinuing the procedure

The MBS procedure may be discontinued at any time, however it is not necessarily discontinued if an episode of aspiration occurs. An aspiration event affords the clinician an opportunity to determine why aspiration is occurring and propose an intervention. The intervention may be a modification in head or body positioning, the introduction of a swallowing manoeuvre or a change in the texture of the food or thickness of the fluids offered (further details of these compensatory mechanisms are described in detail in Chapter 11). The clinician can review the physiology and determine the most appropriate compensatory technique (position, manoeuvre, change to diet texture or viscosity) and trial their hypothesis in the radiology suite to see if the modification does indeed prevent or minimize the aspiration. The clinician should be very much aware of this dual role of the MBS. It is intended to diagnose and describe the anatomy and physiology of the oropharyngeal swallow. However, it is also intended to be used for therapeutic purposes to provide an account of whether compensatory strategies are, in fact, effective. Palmer et al. (1993) suggested that the MBS should be discontinued under the following circumstances:

- airway obstruction;
- laryngospasm;
- bronchospasm;
- 'occlusion or impaction of the foodway';
- aspiration of acidic material;
- total absence of laryngeal protection; or
- where there is evidence of a tracheoesophageal fistula with free flowing of fluid into the trachea (Palmer et al., 1993).

REPORTING AND INTERPRETING THE MBS

The reporting and interpretation of MBS procedures is a multi-stage process. The clinician needs to be able to make 'online' judgements during the procedure to determine which fluid and food consistencies to test and which compensatory positions or manoeuvres to test (if any). Much of this information will be preempted from the clinical assessment. Following the procedure, the clinician may also be afforded the time to review the video recording or CD image of the MBS to look at the events of the swallow in more detail. This gives the advantage of slow motion replay. The clinician may find it beneficial to have a 'worksheet' and then use the worksheet to write the MBS report.

In the initial phase of reviewing the tape it is useful to think of viewing the swallow as one might a car crash or a scene of devastation. In viewing a car crash, for example, the eye is drawn, darting, to various areas of the image – those with the most damage for instance. In the case of the swallow, the eye is often drawn directly to the larynx and the trachea – these being the most vulnerable areas. The clinician is mindful not to miss an aspiration episode. At the initial stages of viewing the video this is a good place to start. The worksheet concept would look to addressing questions such as:

- What was the damage?
- Where did it happen?
- When did it happen?
- How bad was the damage?
- What caused the damage?
- Was there a response?

Critical areas to look at when reviewing a videofluoroscopy are:

- Ability to protect airway (penetration/aspiration) (hyolaryngeal region).
- UES (does the bolus enter the oesophagus?).
- Where was the swallow triggered from? (Anatomical site.)
- Pharyngeal and oral *residue.*
- Pharyngeal region abnormalities (transport – shortening of the pharyngeal musculature).
- Oral region abnormalities (transport – tongue function).
- Oesophageal region abnormalities (does it stay there and does it clear?)

The clinician should then put the pieces together slowly. This does not necessarily mean that a linear, anterior-to-posterior, superior-to-inferior system should be used. The clinician might focus on the larynx during the first few runs, then focus on hyolaryngeal excursion, then tongue function (oral stage and end oral stage), then UES function, and finally soft palate function and lip movement. The order of events (e.g. oral to pharyngeal to oesophageal) is not important while compiling information on the worksheet. At this stage the clinician is gathering information. It is suggested that in the initial phase of reviewing the tape, the clinician should follow the movement of the bolus. In a normal swallow everything happens very quickly. The bolus is processed in the oral cavity and the tongue deftly moves the bolus from the oral cavity into the pharynx. Hyolaryngeal excursion occurs, and also epiglottic deflection, with the bolus being progressed through the pharynx aided by the constrictors. The UES opens and the bolus passes through the UES into the oesophagus. The UES closes, and the bolus continues on its way inferiorly to the stomach, and the hyolaryngeal region returns to rest. This all happens in approximately 2 s in a normal swallow (detailed discussion in Chapter 1). Abnormal events may include:

- pooling of material in the oral cavity, pharynx proper, valleculae, pyriform sinuses or in structures such as a pharyngeal pouch;
- aspiration and/or penetration; and
- oesophageal transport abnormalities.

Once abnormal events have been noted, the clinician can turn their attention to the biomechanics of swallowing. These are the moving structures at work within the oral cavity and pharynx. Useful questions to ask when interpreting a videofluoroscopic assessment of swallowing function are:

- What is the hyolaryngeal excursion like?
- How efficient is the epiglottic inversion?
- How effective is UES opening?
- Is the pharyngeal shortening and constriction adequate?
- How efficient are the actions of the tongue in ejecting the bolus from the oral cavity and propelling it into the pharynx?
- Are the lips closed and the soft palate raised during the swallow? (a closed system will create a vacuum and draw the bolus down)
- Was there aspiration/penetration?
- Was there pooling post swallow?
- Did the UES open? (Did it open enough?)
- Was there adequate strength in the pharynx?
- What was the base of tongue to pharyngeal wall action like?
- Did the bolus enter the pharynx prematurely?
- What was the tongue function like orally?
- What was bolus control like orally?
- Did the material stay in the oesophagus?

- Did the oesophageal function look okay? (Refer to radiologist for details.)
- Did the patient react to any abnormality of function (e.g. cough with aspiration)?
- How many swallows did it take to clear the bolus?
- If aspiration occurred what was the response of the patient to the aspiration event?

  - Did the patient clear the aspirate spontaneously and how effective was the clearance?
  - Did the patient require prompting by the speech pathologist to clear the aspirate?

Once the symptoms have been identified, the clinician can then set about linking the symptom (what was seen) with the physiological abnormality. Huckabee and Pelletier (1999) have documented a ready reference of symptoms and their likely physiological causes. They strongly advocate that clinicians should tie symptoms to physiological cause. For example, if the symptom is 'pooling in the valleculae after the swallow', the possible physiological explanations for this include:

- inadequate base of tongue-to-pharyngeal-wall contact;
- inadequate epiglottic deflection leading to post-swallow pooling;
- inadequate hyolaryngeal excursion; and/or
- pharyngeal weakness.

It is imperative that symptoms be tied to physiology if rehabilitation of the swallow is to occur. The clinician must treat the cause of the problem, not the symptom, if there is to be lasting relief from dysphagia.

If aspiration occurs, the clinician should make note of *when* it occurs? Is it before, during, or after the swallow and what is the magnitude of the response? Feinberg (1993) reported that it is common for relatively healthy people to react violently to penetration or minor aspiration, whereas individuals with gross aspiration may show a weakened response. Feinberg (1993) cites older individuals as having reduced afferent airway receptors, causing them not to react until the material has entered the distal end of the trachea, or even the main bronchi. Reduced sensation and a weak response to aspiration mediated by ageing is an excellent recipe for increasing the likelihood of aspiration (see also Chapter 2).

Once the worksheet information has been collected, the clinician can write a succinct report. Unlike the worksheet, the report should clearly follow the natural progression of the bolus from the oral cavity to the pharynx and then the oesophagus. The clinician should succinctly report the results of the assessment in the context of the background information and clinical assessment of swallowing. Likewise, the recommendations at the end of the report should integrate all information from the patient's background and also the MBS results to propose a plan that is suitable for the individual's needs. Any special instructions to staff or carers should be included in the report. For example, staff should be requested to contact the speech pathologist if the patient appears unable to cope with the textures or diets recommended. Cues for this may be a reduction in overall diet and fluid consumption, a sudden deterioration in chest status and/or temperature spikes. Requests for supervised feeding, the use of special utensils, or swallowing techniques should be included in the report. Cues for the type of information that should be included in an MBS report are:

- Background information (social and medical).
- Results of clinical examination of swallowing:

    - general observations;
    - oromotor assessment;
    - food/fluid trials.

- Reason for requesting the MBS.
- MBS results:

    - views used during the procedure;
    - consistencies tested;
    - results for the oral and pharyngeal stages of swallowing (with the radiologist reporting the oesophageal phase);
    - any strategies tested (e.g. chin tuck, supraglottic swallow);
    - overall impression and diagnosis, including severity.

- Recommendations:

    - diets (liquids and solids, which may include non-oral methods of nutrition, e.g. nasogastric tube, percutaneous endoscopic gastrostomy (PEG), or combinations of oral and non-oral methods of nutrition);
    - recommended feeding position (e.g. upright, supported reclined – see also Chapter 11);
    - instructions to staff or carers;
    - any other referrals to medical or allied health staff.

Paediatric considerations

In the interpretation of the paediatric MBS study, the clinician must be familiar with normal paediatric anatomy, growth and swallowing function (see Chapters 2, 13, 14). Moreover, the clinician must take into account the child's developmental age as well as their chronological age (this is particularly important for premature infants).

RADIATION SAFETY ISSUES

Protecting the patient

The radiation dose delivered to the patient is determined by the radiographer or radiologist, the machine used and the individual needs of the patient. Factors such as:

- the patient's size or the body part being imaged;
- the density and location of the body part;

- the x-ray dose rate;
- the level of magnification used;
- the x-ray field size; and
- the fluoro 'on time'.

All contribute to the amount of radiation the patient will be exposed to during an MBS (Beck and Gayler, 1990). Patients who are pregnant should not be assessed. Females of child-bearing age should have a lead apron wrapped around them at waist level to reduce accidental or refracted irradiation of the pelvic region. Children should wear a lead apron from their waist down. In order to minimize the effects of radiation, the amount of time the patient is exposed to x-rays (i.e. fluoro 'on time') should be kept to a minimum. Beck and Gayler (1990) recommend that initial diagnostic studies should rarely exceed 2 minutes of x-ray 'on time'. However, they acknowledge that trials of multiple consistencies, differing head or body positions, and swallowing manoeuvres may add additional time to the average procedure. Palmer et al. (1993) have reported longer times of over 4 minutes for their population of individuals with dysphagia of neurological origin and Crawley et al. (2004) reported a median screening time of 3.7 minutes (range 2.5 to 4.3) in a heterogeneous population. As noted above, the patient should lead the investigation in so far as the patient should be given the bolus roughly as the x-ray equipment is turned on. This is preferable to the patient taking and holding the food or fluid in the oral cavity and possibly swallowing it before the image can be captured. 'Panning' or moving the image intensifier to follow the barium bolus should be minimized. Although panning may be required for the oesophageal phase of the study, it should not be used during evaluation of the oropharyngeal phase (Mahesh et al., 2003). Practising any manoeuvres prior to the MBS assessment will also minimize radiation exposure time in that patients are not being taught these manoeuvres while they are being radiated.

Studies investigating the dose given to the patient during an MBS show that the radiological procedure provides low radiation risks. Crawley et al. (2004) found that the effective dose rate to the patient in an MBS procedure was 0.85 mSv (range 0.76 mSv to 1.3 mSv). Overall radiation risks associated with MBS were judged to be 1 in 16,000. The organ receiving the greatest dose rate was the thyroid, with an equivalent dose rate of 13.9 (12.3 mSv to 20.7 mSv). In contrast to the MBS, the barium swallow was reported to have an average screening time of 104 s, but a dose area product of 6.6 Gycm² to 6.8 Gycm² which is twice that of the MBS (3.5 Gycm²) (Crawley et al., 2004). The reason given for higher dose rate during barium studies was the use of spot images. Spot images are not often recorded for MBS procedures. The annual effective dose rate for the general public has been reported as 1 mSv per year (Chan et al., 2002).

Protecting the clinician

The speech pathologist should wear a lead apron throughout the MBS procedure to protect them from radiation exposure. The lead apron covers the trunk of the body.

In addition a thyroid protector may also be worn. Some radiological suites also offer lead impregnated gloves and glasses (to protect the lens of the eye). Beck and Gayler (1990) have advocated that lead glasses are more appropriate for radiological procedures where the dose rate is considerably higher than during an MBS procedure (e.g. cardiovascular procedures). Many suites have a lead-impregnated shielded area from where one can view the procedure, but it is not possible to assist with the procedure from this vantage point.

The concept of reducing x-ray 'on time' also assists the operator. The less time the patient is being irradiated, the less time the clinician is in an environment where they could be exposed to radiation. Clinicians should also carefully consider where they stand during an MBS procedure. As the x-rays pass through the patient they scatter to surrounding areas. Positions behind the patient or in line with the patient provide opportunity for increased radiation exposure due to x-ray scatter reflected from the patient. A position in front of the patient (i.e. near the image intensifier) provides a physically safe position (Mahesh et al., 2003). In addition, sheer distance from the patient also affords protection as scatter dose rate reduces with distance (Beck and Gayler, 1990). A distance of 30 cm from the patient's neck provides a mean dose of 33.68 µSv. At 60 cm it is reduced to 8.42 µSv and at 100 cm it is 3.03 µSv. The distance from the hand to the neck of the patient during feeding is approximately 30 cm, and the position of the body of the feeder from the patient is 60 cm.

Radiation monitoring badges may also be available from the radiology department, depending upon the policies and procedures of the individual workplace. These devices measure a cumulative exposure to ionizing radiation. In many cases it is more appropriate that they are worn by individuals who routinely work in radiology suites (e.g. radiographers). The annual dose limit for Australia can be found at www.arpansa.gov.au. This website contains the recommendations for limiting exposure to ionizing radiation (1995) and the national standard for limiting occupational exposure to ionizing radiation (2002). Chan et al. (2002) have reported that an annual dose limit of 20 mSv, and that based on their findings a radiology worker could perform 2,583 MBS studies per year and still not exceed dose limits. Crawley et al. (2004) report that in doing 50 MBS studies per year, the operator would incur an annual radiation dose of 0.6 mSv to the body, 1 mSv for eyes, and 1.8 mSv for the extremities, against legal doses of 20 mSv (body), 150 mSv (eyes) and 500 mSv (extremities).

RELIABILITY AND TRAINING

As noted in the introduction, the MBS procedure provides objective images that are then interpreted by clinicians. Both training and the ability to discuss the results with others have been found to improve the reliability of the results. Logemann et al. (2000) found that even a 4-hour training period produced an improvement in identification of radiographic anatomy and also swallowing disorders in clinicians with an average of three years' work experience. There are no published studies to document the number of hours of training a new graduate clinician requires in order to accurately identify anatomy radiographically and correctly interpret the results of the MBS examination.

Agreement with MBS ratings has been found to be higher when clinicians are given definitions of parameters to be rated, such as that used in the penetration-aspiration scale (Rosenbek et al., 1996). Stoeckli et al. (2003) found that of all the parameters that were rated, only the presence of aspiration was reliably reported in their study that included experienced speech pathologists from nine different international swallowing centres. Parameters such as: efficiency of lip closure, tongue movement, palatal movement, amount of residue etc., showed poor inter-rater reliability. The authors concluded that consensus of definitions for the parameters observed during an MBS would significantly improve inter-rater reliability. Further to this, Scott et al. (1998) have found that agreement between raters improves when ratings are made after group discussions, and that levels of agreement are lowest when individuals work alone. The researchers found that ratings for semi-solid boluses were better than for liquid boluses.

Other factors found to affect reliability of performance also included image quality. Hyper-illumination of body images makes it difficult to discern anatomical boundaries. Kandel and Wurtz (2000) noted that edges are very important to the perceptual organization of our visual fields, so bright margins at body extremities, for example around the lips, will distort the clinician's view of these structures. Strong technical skill provided by the radiographer or radiologist will assist in minimizing variability due to image quality. The task complexity associated with reviewing and interpreting an MBS examination has also been perceived to influence clinician judgements (Scott et al., 1998). In line with the suggestion to provide parameter definitions is the suggestion that the number of parameters to be interpreted be kept to the most salient ones. Once again, individual experience will determine the possible data set of 'the most salient parameters' for investigation.

The issue of rater reliability also draws the question of training undergraduate students. Wooi et al. (2001) conducted a study with undergraduate speech pathology students, providing them with 5 hours of structured sessions for interpretation of MBS studies, and assessment via worksheets. They concluded that upon completion of the sessions, the students would still have needed access to senior or supervising staff for competence in interpretation of MBS studies, with the suggestion that accredited postgraduate courses should be made available to new graduates. The University of Minnesota offers an opportunity to practise identification and evaluation of videofluoroscopic swallowing images using the Web (http://www.d.umn. edu/csd/video/swallowing.htm). The CD-ROM *The Dynamic Swallow* developed by Scholten and Russell at Flinders University (Australia) is a multimedia package including diagrams, animations and videos of swallowing. It is available through *Clear Vision* (South Australia) or http://www.fusion.com.au/tds/.

ADVANTAGES AND LIMITATIONS

All assessment techniques present with advantages and limitations and the MBS is no exception. Although the MBS procedure aims to provide objective data, the quality of the image will depend upon the operator's skill in reducing or eliminating image noise, receptor blur and motion blur in addition to producing optimum contrast and image sharpness. Once the image has been acquired the interpretation requires the skills of human beings. Our interpretation can hardly be described as 'objective'. It clearly depends upon skill and experience in both conducting the procedure and interpreting the results. Martin-Harris et al. (2000) purport that the MBS positively affects clinical practice by providing referral to other specialists after the procedure, adjustment of dietary textures, and identification of strategies to improve patient safety. This being said the advantages and limitations of the procedure are detailed below.

Advantages

- The procedure provides views of the oral, pharyngeal and oesophageal structures and phases of swallowing.
- One is able to assess the duration of each of the oral, pharyngeal and oesophageal stages of swallowing.
- The procedure provides information about the safety of different food and fluid textures/viscosities and the ability of the individual to use compensatory techniques or therapeutic manoeuvres (see Chapters 11 and 12).
- Images are recorded to allow later review and analysis and to allow a comparison of function over time.

Limitations

- The procedure involves the use of ionizing radiation (radiation dose rates are understandably limited each year). Radiation is an issue to both the patient and the operator (including the speech pathologist). For the same reason, frequent test repetition is inappropriate.
- The procedure does not use regular dietary foods and fluids. The barium may affect the taste and/or the texture of the foods/fluids and does not provide a true example of how the individual manages dietary foods and fluids (see also Chapter 3).
- The MBS provides a 'test' or artificial situation that may not be representative of normal function. Due to time limitations of the procedure (because of radiation safety considerations), the time required for some patients to eat may be underestimated and fatigue might also be less obvious.
- The MBS focuses on motor function, but is unable to directly analyse the sensory function of the oropharyngeal system.
- There are difficulties in the accessibility and availability of the procedure, particularly in rural and remote areas. In the future these difficulties may be somewhat alleviated by telehealth medicine.
- The procedure is necessarily costly due to the equipment, resources and staff required to perform the procedure.

- Difficulties with patient size (e.g. obesity) or stability (e.g. hemiparesis) may mean that certain individuals cannot be accommodated with an MBS procedure.

MODIFIED BARIUM SWALLOW VERSUS BARIUM SWALLOW

The MBS should not be confused with the barium swallow. The barium swallow is also a radiological imaging technique that assesses swallowing function. Its focus is on the structural competence of the oesophagus, with only a scan of the oropharynx. It requires the patient to swallow large amounts of liquid barium rapidly (over 50 ml). It is used as a diagnostic tool for the oesophagus and aims to indicate whether there is a problem with the structure or functioning of the oesophagus. It usually involves a radiographer and/or a radiologist. The speech pathologist is not usually involved in a barium swallow, however, may be called in to examine the oropharyngeal swallow if it becomes apparent during the barium swallow that the patient is experiencing difficulties in the oral or pharyngeal phases. The MBS on the other hand has its primary focus on the oral and pharyngeal phases of swallowing, with a scan of the oesophagus. It is more than a diagnostic procedure as it also affords the opportunity to commence treatment planning and to see if the treatment works. If a patient with oropharyngeal dysphagia is inadvertently referred for a barium swallow, considerable aspiration may occur before the trial can be aborted. The consequences of massive aspiration can cause major medical complications requiring acute care hospitalization (Pennington, 1993).

FIBREOPTIC ENDOSCOPIC EVALUATION OF SWALLOWING (FEES)

The endoscopic evaluation of swallowing is another visual procedure that affords the clinician a different visual perspective. Rather than the two-dimensional, black-and-white image of shadows and lines afforded by x-ray, the clinician can take advantage of a direct view of structures from a horizontal plane affording what appears to be a colour image. (Of course, the view is really two-dimensional.) This being said, both the MBS and endoscopic evaluation of swallowing are complementary rather than one being superior to the other. Each technique offers the clinician a different perspective, and the clinician's choice as to which imaging technique to use should be patient driven. The original purpose of the endoscopic evaluation of swallowing was the provision of an assessment when fluoroscopy could not be done. It has since become a standard assessment of swallowing in the United States and sometimes the preferred assessment tool. Its use in other countries, such as Australia, is also growing steadily.

The FEES procedure, with its inception in 1988 (Langmore et al., 1988), affords the clinician:

- an assessment of the anatomy and physiology of many of the structures associated with swallowing;
- an assessment of swallowing ability for food, liquid and secretions; and
- an assessment of the patient's response to therapeutic interventions (Langmore, 2004).

Fibreoptic endoscopic evaluation of swallowing was given a copyright to distinguish this procedure from (a) a standard ENT laryngology examination used to diagnose medical pathology and (b) a screening tool to detect aspiration (Langmore, 2003).

EQUIPMENT AND ACCREDITATION

A laryngoscope, a light source, chip camera, videotape or digital recorder and a monitor are the equipment requirements for performing endoscopic evaluation of swallowing. The chip camera converts the image seen to a video signal allowing the image to be viewed on a monitor and recorded onto a video recorder (Murray, 2001). The diameter of the portion of the endoscope that is inserted into the nares is very small, at approximately 3 mm to 4 mm for adults and 2.2 mm diameter for children. It is possible to pan the tip of the endoscope to a 90° field of view, using the angulation lever on the handset of the endoscope. Detailed information regarding the mechanics of the endoscope and the technique for handling the tool can be found in Langmore's (2001) text *Endoscopic Evaluation and Treatment of Swallowing Disorders.* Nasal anaesthetic (gel or ointment) may be applied to the nares to allow the scope to be passed comfortably; however, if the anaesthesia reaches the pharyneal tissue it may disrupt sensory perceptions required for swallowing and adversely affect the swallowing examination. For this reason also, anaesthetic spray should not be used, as its coverage of the mucosa cannot be well controlled. Nasal decongestants have also been advocated to increase the size of the nares, which makes passing the scope more comfortable. However, medical orders for both anaesthetics and decongestants may be required (Langmore, 2004).

Infection control is very important in using endoscopy. Universal precautions prior to, during and after the examination are required (hand washing, use of gloves, disposal of gloves etc.). The endoscope also requires disinfection after each examination. Ear, nose and throat or otolaryngology specialists can provide advice on proper disinfection of the endoscopy equipment. Endosheaths may be used but still require disinfection of the endoscope. These are single-use disposable sleeves that fit over the flexible tube of the endoscope. (available from Vision Science in the US and Global Scientific in Australia).

Not surprisingly, for a clinician to use endoscopy to assess swallowing function, dedicated training is required. There are a few different clinical models for performing endoscopic swallow studies. At the most conservative end, the procedure is carried out jointly by an ENT specialist and the speech pathologist. Both provide specialist knowledge from their relevant fields of expertise and this type of examination will provide the most detailed evaluation possible. It is not always possible or practicable to have an ENT specialist present for the entire duration of the swallowing assessment, however. In this event, the ENT specialist may pass the scope and provide a quick investigation of the larynx and pharynx for medical pathology. At the completion of this stage, the ENT specialist may leave the speech pathologist to take over the scoping and complete the swallowing evaluation independently. There is also a model that has speech pathologists trained with due accreditation to perform the endoscopic evaluation of swallowing independently. In this model, the speech pathologist passes the endoscope and performs the examination independently. If the procedure is recorded, an ENT may view the tape at a later date and comment on the presence or absence of anatomical disease. There is some controversy about speech pathologists' use of endoscopic evaluation of swallowing. Some speech pathologists are concerned about:

- whether it is within the scope of practice for the speech pathologist to perform the procedure;
- whether endoscopy is sensitive enough to the physiology of swallowing; and
- the comfort levels of the patient during the procedure (Hiss and Postma, 2003).

Ear, nose and throat specialists have also expressed concern regarding:

- whether speech pathologists will work outside their area of expertise and attempt to diagnose medical pathology; and
- whether medical pathology may be missed because an ENT is not present in some models of service delivery (Hiss and Postma, 2003).

Hiss and Postma (2003) reported that speech pathologists with expertise in dysphagia, who have appropriate and specialized training in endoscopy are qualified to use the procedure for assessing swallowing function, and related functions of structures within the upper aerodigestive tract. The model chosen (ENT + speech pathologist or speech pathologist only) will be determined by the skills and accreditation of the speech pathologist, availability of medical specialists, and institutional or licensure requirements. Clinicians who plan to be the endoscopist require training in the technique and skill of passing the endoscope safely, with minimal patient discomfort, and in such a manner as to obtain an optimal view. Clinical knowledge about normal and abnormal swallowing and appropriate therapeutic interventions, as viewed endoscopically is needed by all clinicians, whether or not they are the endoscopists. In all cases, development of written policies, including management of adverse reactions is strongly advocated prior to implementing the endoscopic evaluation of swallowing.

ANATOMICAL STRUCTURES AND VIEWS

Endoscopy allows the clinician to view directly the velum, the structures of the oropharynx, the hypopharynx, the larynx and the entrance to the trachea. The clinician can also visualize pooling of secretions in the hypopharynx. Tissue oedema and erythema (redness) can also be seen, as well as any other mucosal abnormality. Altered anatomy can be easily appreciated for its impact on swallowing.

PHYSIOLOGY

Fibreoptic endoscopic evaluation of swallowing provides the clinician with physiological information about speech (i.e. soft palate, vocal fold movement), non-speech tasks (e.g. airway protection and cough) and swallowing movements. Endoscopic evaluations provide information regarding the pharyngeal phase of swallowing, aspiration and risk of aspiration. They also afford the clinician more information about swallow-respiratory coordination. Premature spillage into the hypopharynx can be visualized and the path of the bolus can be seen clearly. Tongue base retraction, velopharyngeal closure, and epiglottic inversion can be viewed endoscopically just as the swallow begins. After the swallow, the epiglottis can be visualized as it returns to rest.

In a normal swallow, the view during the height of the swallow is interrupted. With the tip of the endoscope just above the epiglottis, the pharyngeal walls are seen as they begin to medialize and the base of tongue begins to move towards the pharyngeal walls. As the lateral pharyngeal walls medialize, and the epiglottis begins to invert, the closure of the airspace will produce a momentary 'white out' where the view is obscured by light being reflected back to the endoscope (Langmore, 2004). This 'white out' period usually lasts approximately half a second. Where the white out period is shorter than this or absent altogether, it indicates that airway closure was incomplete.

A view of airway closure at the onset of the swallow can also be visualized endoscopically. Investigation has shown that the order of events for the swallow may vary slightly from person to person, but they are generally consistent within the same person (Van Daele et al., 2005). With the scope positioned behind the epiglottis (over the laryngeal surface about half way down the epiglottis), the first structural movement to be seen is from the arytenoids as they medialize and then tilt forward towards the base of the epiglottis. Soon after this movement begins, the epiglottis begins to retroflex. It is at this point that the hyoid elevation and anterior movement begin. The vocal folds are the last layer of airway closure to be executed: they do not close until approximately half a second after the arytenoids have begun their medial movement. Glottic closure may not be seen at all endoscopically since white out may occlude the view before it occurs. This order of airway closure is very different from that for breath-holding and has many implications for teaching patients strategies for protecting their airway during swallowing.

Sensation can be assessed formally using the fibreoptic endoscopic evaluation of swallowing with sensory testing (FEEST), which is outlined below. Informally, sensation can also be tested from the patient's response to various features of the endoscopic examination. Indications of sensory status are the response of the patient to the following (adapted from Langmore, 2004):

- Presence of the scope in the nose, and pharynx.
- Stimulation of salivary flow.
- Reaction of the patient to post-swallow residue in the pharynx.
- Reaction to premature spillage of the bolus into the pharynx prior to a swallow reflex being generated.

- Reaction to any material (food, liquid, saliva) in the laryngeal vestibule.
- Reaction to aspiration.
- Reaction to direct touch (i.e. touching of the endoscope onto the pharyngeal or laryngeal structures).

THE PROCEDURE

If the patient is bedbound, the procedure should be done with the clinician standing on one side of the bed and the monitor on the other. The endoscope straddles the bed and the examiner holds the endoscope to his/her nose in a 'fishing pole' posture. If the patient can come to the clinic, he/she is generally seated facing the monitor while the examiner stands to his/her side so that he/she can also view the monitor. A table will usually be placed in front of the patient so he/she can eat the food in front of him/her.

The scope is passed through the left or right nasal passage, generally hugging the floor of the nares and following its contours to exit over the soft palate. The nasal septum and especially the turbinates, should be avoided as this is likely to cause discomfort (Murray, 2001). For individuals who are nervous, lifting the chin and asking the individual to phonate or hum as been suggested (Crary and Groher, 1999). A lubricating gel or even water on the sheath of the endoscope can be used to lubricate the scope in order to minimize patient discomfort while the scope is being placed into position. Once *in situ* the clinician should take care to 'anchor' the scope by using their finger to pinch the scope against the nose. This minimizes unnecessary movement and discomfort. The clinician should stay well away from the base of tongue and lateral pharyngeal walls at the level of the nasopharynx as this will probably trigger the gag reflex. From time to time, the examiner will need to dip down closer to the vocal folds to get a good look at the infra-larynx, but then return to the 'home position' before the next swallow.

THE FEES PROCEDURE

The FEES examination consists of an assessment of functional integrity of the muscles required for swallowing during non-swallowing tasks, followed by an assessment of swallowing, concluding with therapeutic interventions. The full, revised FEES protocol is included in the appendix to this chapter. Observed and inferred findings from the FEES examination are documented in Table 8.1.

Part I of the FEES procedure: assessment of anatomy and structural movement – non-swallowing tasks

In Part I of the FEES examination, the velum, pharynx, larynx, and base of tongue are assessed for structural integrity and movement. The examination generally commences with an assessment of velar and lateral pharyngeal wall movement to close the velopharyngeal (VP) port. Movement of these structures can be viewed while the

Table 8.1 Salient findings with endoscopy and fluorosocpy (usually inferred from adequacy of bolus flow)

Finding	Directly observed MBS	Directly FEES	Inferred MBS	Inferred FEES
Poor *oral* bolus control (out of mouth)	✓	✓		
Premature entry of the bolus into the pharynx	✓	✓		
Pre-swallow aspiration	✓	✓		
Post-swallow aspiration	✓	✓		
Residue in the valleculae	✓	✓		
Residue in the pyriform sinuses	✓	✓		
Residue in the laryngeal vestibule			✓	✓
Reduced pharyngeal contraction			✓	✓
Reduced laryngeal elevation	✓			✓
Reduced epiglottic inversion	✓	✓		
Reduced glottic closure		✓	✓	
Reduced VP closure		✓	✓	
Reduced upper oesophageal sphincter opening	✓			✓
Reduced sensation/ response to sensory stimuli		✓	✓	

Source: adapted from Crary and Groher (1999) and expanded.

individual hums, produces nasal and oral phonemes, and oral and nasal sentences. A swallow will also activate the VP port and complete closure should be observed. Once the VP port has been assessed, the scope can be advanced to provide a view of the oropharynx. The clinician can now view the symmetry and bulk of the base of the tongue. Speech tasks, such as the American pronunciation of the post-vocalic 'l' as in 'ball', provide a view of tongue-base retraction (Langmore, 2004). Examinations of the pharynx may include requesting the individual to phonate in a high strained voice. When phonating this way, the pharyngeal walls should move towards each other. Failure to do so may indicate weakness of the pharyngeal walls (Crary and Groher, 1999). The patient can also be asked to glide up in pitch until strained to demonstrate movement of the pharyngeal constrictors and laryngeal elevation. The scope may be advanced slightly further still to afford the clinician a view of the pharynx, larynx and the tracheal opening. Asking the individual to 'sniff' will afford a view of vocal fold abduction associated with voluntary airway opening. To view opening and closing of the glottis, the clinician may ask the patient to perform the following: 'sniff – say /eeee/ – sniff – say /eee/' (Crary and Groher, 1999). Sustained phonation of /eee/, and repeated and fast repetitions of /heee/ may also provide information regarding symmetry, completeness, precision and speed of vocal fold movement during phonation. Putting the vocal folds through the extremes of abduction and abduction in the 'sniff – eee' procedure will probably cause weak vocal folds to fatigue and hence may highlight subtle vocal fold paresis or paralysis (Mercati and Rieder, 2003). Observation of a forced breath hold should show the glottis tightly closed by the true vocal folds, false vocal folds, and arytenoids. Can the individual sustain a breath hold to a count of five or seven? If not, then voluntary breath-holding manoeuvres such as the supraglottic swallow (see Chapters 11 and 12) may not be useful therapeutically (Langmore, 2004). Patients can also be asked to cough or clear the throat in order that the clinician can view the adequacy of these actions.

Throughout the entire time when the patient is asked to perform the non-swallowing tasks, the examiner will be observing the anatomy within the region of interest. Anatomy can greatly affect swallowing behaviour. Missing or altered structures, oedema, intrusion of foreign bodies such as a feeding tube or tumour, or even normal anatomical variants can be the primary underlying reason why a patient can swallow successfully or not. Anatomy is needed to support structural movement and it directs the bolus through the hypopharynx. Endoscopy is a superior tool to appreciate this fact.

Management of secretions can be successfully assessed during an endoscopic assessment. Passing of the scope should stimulate salivary flow and spontaneous swallows. If secretions are visible in the pharynx, the clinician should evaluate the extent of secretions, where they occur and whether they are transient or lasting. Note also that it is normal for there to be some small accumulations of saliva in the pyriform sinuses, however, these should be spontaneously swallowed (see Chapter 3). It is not normal for there to be secretions in the laryngeal vestibule or excessive secretions in the pharynx. In fact the accumulation of secretions in the laryngeal vestibule has been found to predict aspiration of food or fluids (Murray et al., 1996).

Part II of the FEES procedure: direct assessment of swallowing

In Part II of the FEES examination, swallowing is directly assessed. A range of bolus types can be given, with the advantage that real foods and fluids are used. The clinician could start with the current diet and fluids to evaluate current function. In a FEES examination, issues relating to the taste, texture, viscosity and density of barium, which are critical for the MBS procedure (see also Chapter 3), are not of concern. The clinician does have to be mindful of the colour of the substances chosen. Purple, blue, green and orange food/fluid colourings are generally easier to perceive (see Figures 8.3 and 8.4). Grape juice and pureed apricots are naturally occurring colourants that may be useful for FEES examinations. Spillage can be accomplished with any thin liquid, but detection of aspiration of thin liquids requires a substance that is highly visible and leaves a more permanent trail behind. Barium liquid or milk dyed green or blue, are good choices as they leave a coating behind in their path and aspiration is easily detected. As with the clinical examination and the MBS, varying volumes, taste, temperature, and textures can be assessed. The bolus volumes and number of different textures assessed will be patient specific.

For a standard examination, the clinician may allow the patient to self-pace quantities of foods and fluids tested. This will allow the clinician to determine what normally happens at meal times. After this has been observed, the clinician may alter

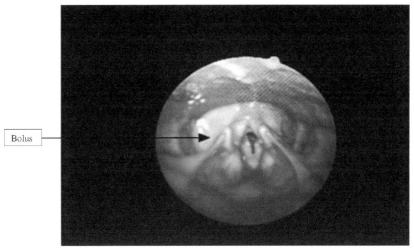

Figure 8.3 Endoscopic image of the pharynx and larynx viewed from above. The green dyed bolus has traversed the aryepiglottic fold and is also visible in the pyriform sinus. A portion of the vocal folds is open. Reproduced by permission of Kay PENTAX

bolus size, rate of delivery and different bolus textures and viscosities. As abnormal swallow behaviour is detected, the examiner brings his knowledge of dysphagia and skills in clinical decision making to the examination so that the problem can be well understood and appropriate interventions can be tested.

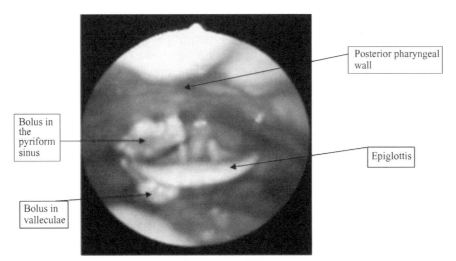

Figure 8.4 Endoscopic view of the pharynx. The epiglottis and pharyngeal walls are visible. The arytenoids appear to be adducted. The green dyed bolus is visible in both the valleculae and the pyriform sinus. Reproduced by permission of Kay PENTAX

For individuals with a severe dysphagia, the clinician should perform a controlled and conservative examination. In this event, the clinician would control the textures, viscosities, bolus size and rate of delivery. The clinician may also choose to administer coloured ice chips (e.g. green to increase visualization). These have the advantage of providing a cold stimulus that may enhance sensory feedback and assist swallowing initiation. The ice chip protocol may be particularly useful for individuals who are non-oral as these individuals frequently have a dry mouth, which makes it difficult to initiate a swallow (Langmore, 2004). An ice chip is a relatively benign bolus to test the patient's ability to swallow without risking complications of aspiration.

It is also possible to put food colouring into a nasogastric feed and scope the patient after a bolus feed to see if there is visual evidence of refluxed material. In addition, with individuals who have a tracheostomy, the clinician may view the larynx from inferior by placing the scope into the stoma and positioning it to look at the vocal folds and larynx from below. This technique will only be effective when the tracheostomy tube has been removed (e.g. during changing of the tube for hygiene or sizing requirements), as the tube would occlude the view of the cords.

Part III of the FEES procedure: therapeutic intervention

After swallowing ability has been assessed, the examiner needs to address any problems that have been identified. The nature of the swallowing problem and other patient variables determine which therapeutic intervention should be tried; compensatory or rehabilitative. Any of the compensatory interventions that can be tried in fluoroscopy can also be tried under endoscopy to determine if they are effective in making the swallow safer or more effective. The clinician can teach the patient to use double swallows or alternative manoeuvres to reduce post-swallow pharyngeal residue and the effect on residue can be assessed immediately. An advantage of endoscopy is that there is more time to try a variety of postures, manoeuvres, or bolus alterations than would be possible in the fluoroscopic suite.

Moreover, if there is time, endoscopy can also be used as a biofeedback tool to make patients aware of their problems or to teach them new strategies. With immediate visual feedback paired with the ongoing swallowing activity, patients learn quickly what works and what does not. Biofeedback is a very powerful method of learning or re-learning behaviour and the clinician can use this tool to teach a manoeuvre or just to emphasize a point. For example, if the clinician sees residue in the pharynx, it may be worth asking patients if they can feel any residue. If they do not feel the residue, they may benefit from them directly seeing the residue on the monitor. This strategy is especially valuable with the patient who is a silent aspirator. Principles of biofeedback are discussed in Chapter 12. Swallowing compensation and rehabilitation are discussed in detail in Chapters 11 and 12.

IDENTIFICATION OF FINDINGS AND INTERPRETATION OF RESULTS

After the FEES examination is over, the clinician needs to review the examination, summarize the findings, interpret the results in terms of the underlying anatomical or physiologic problem, make a prognosis, and make recommendations for management. The report will differ from a fluoroscopy report in some ways, but the impressions section should be very similar. The following is a list of common findings obtained from a FEES or an MBS examination.

- Poor oral control/awareness leading to spillage into the hypopharynx during the oral stage.
- Spillage of the bolus after the oral stage has been completed, or delayed initiation of the swallow:

  - duration of spillage time;
  - the last point the bolus touched before a swallow was triggered.

- Aspiration before the onset of the swallow.
- Aspiration during the swallow (during white out):

  - observed from residue after the air space returns;
  - incomplete bolus clearance; rate severity and the following locations: base of tongue, valleculae, lateral channels, pyriforms, laryngeal rim (specify where);
  - aspiration after the swallow;
  - oesophageal-pharyngeal reflux;

- Sensory awareness and motor response of the patient to abnormal findings above.

The pattern of abnormality can be summarized as an underlying problem with one or more of the following:

- oral control, manipulation of the bolus;
- timely initiation of the swallow;
- airway protection and velopharyngeal valving;
- bolus driving/ clearing forces (tongue, pharynx).

PRECAUTIONS/CONTRAINDICATIONS

Langmore (2004) reported that FEES has an excellent safety record, with no known serious complications arising from the procedure. There are some specific potential events that the clinician should be aware of, however. Where a topical anaesthetic is used for the nasal cavity to ease the discomfort associated with endoscope insertion, the clinician should be mindful of allergic reactions to the anaesthetic. Given that a scope is placed transnasally during the procedure, nosebleed is a potential complication. Anxious individuals may have a vasovagal response to the procedure and faint during the examination. To alleviate possible fainting episodes, the examination should be calm, with the examiner confident and reassuring. The clinician may also wish to ascertain whether the patient has a history of fainting or if they have any acute cardiac conditions, in which case heart rate or blood pressure may need to be monitored.

Laryngospasm is another potential complication, fortunately rarely seen. Laryngospasm is an exaggerated laryngeal adductor response. It is a protective reflex and a response to sudden or unexpected stimulus that is perceived as noxious. It is most commonly associated with gastroesophageal reflux (acid), aspiration, drowning and following general anaesthesia (e.g. during extubation). Prevention of laryngospasm can be afforded by a cautious examination – the larynx should not be purposely or forcefully touched. In the event that it does occur, the patient should be calmed, and the spasm will subside. Forceful blowing of air at the mouth may also break the spasm.

ADVANTAGES AND LIMITATIONS

The advantages of the FEES technique are:

• portability;
• reduced cost in comparison with fluoroscopy;
• the ability to use real foods and fluids;
• the ease of repeat procedures;
• ability to directly assess the larynx and secretion management; and
• use in an extended therapy session.

In addition, it has the large benefit of not requiring radiation. This means that re-peat procedures can be performed as often as the patient will tolerate it. Also, be-cause of the lack of radiation issues, it can be used to good effect as a biofeedback tool.

There are a few limitations to the technique. Firstly, it is a limitation that the view of the larynx is obscured by the medializing pharyngeal walls and epiglottic inversion during the critical period of the swallow. It is not possible to see material enter the larynx when this 'white out' view occurs. Evidence of aspiration is often assumed from residue or coating in areas where there should not be coating (i.e. subglottic shelf of the trachea), or staining of the vocal folds, etc. Thus the clinician is left to infer from secondary observations, rather than seeing the primary event. Fortunately, 90% or more of all aspiration events occur before or after the swallow (Smith, et al., 1999), thus endoscopy is well equipped to detect the majority of aspi-ration events. In addition, the use of barium liquid will leave a coating behind so that the evidence of aspiration is usually visible. Table 8.2 provides information regard-ing common causes of aspiration as related to the timing of the aspiration episode (before, during or after the swallow).

Secondly, it is not possible to provide information about the oesophageal phase from the endoscopic evaluation. It may be possible to infer an oesophageal problem if material is seen to re-enter the hypopharynx after the swallow has been completed (i.e. reflux). Further oesophageal assessments would then be required. There are also some queries as to whether the endoscopic examination still provides an assess-ment situation that is truly representative of normal eating. Patients have described the procedure as anything from mildly to moderately uncomfortable (Leder et al., 1997).

Table 8.2 Common causes of aspiration as related to timing of aspiration episode

Timing of aspiration	Common causes of aspiration	Percentage occurrence of aspiration events[1]
Prior to swallowing	Failure of glossopalatal seal with premature leakage from mouth and entry into open larynx. Reduced sensory awareness of the bolus.	24%–25% prior to swallow
During swallowing	Late/ delayed airway closure. Reduced laryngeal elevation (hyoid, cricothyroid, epiglottis). Poor laryngeal closure (arytenoids/true vocal cords). Incomplete epiglottic tilt – anatomical cause.	6–8% during swallow
After swallowing	Overflow of retained bolus. Late emptying of a pouch or diverticulum. Regurgitation from oesophagus GER.	67% after the swallow

[1]Smith et al. (1999).

Source: adapted from Jones, 2003c: 69.

FORMAL SENSORY THRESHOLD TESTING (FEEST)

A variation of the endoscopic evaluation of swallowing is the addition of formal sensory threshold testing (FEEST). In this mode, the endoscope is passed as usual; however, there is the facility for a calibrated puff of air to be delivered to the pharyngeal and laryngeal structures. The air puff is delivered for 50 ms duration (Aviv, 2000). The body's response to different levels of air pressure provides the clinician with objective information regarding sensory integrity of the area assessed. The calibrated puff of air is delivered to the aryepiglottic folds and individuals with normal sensation will produce a laryngeal adduction reflex (like a 'blink' of the vocal folds). The puff of air stimulates receptors in the laryngeal mucosa that are carried by the afferent nerve fibres of the superior laryngeal nerve to the brain stem. From the brain stem, the efferent signal is carried via the recurrent laryngeal nerve to the vocal folds, causing them to momentarily adduct. While the FEEST procedure directly assesses the ability of a mechanical stimulus to excite the laryngeal adductor reflex, the laryngeal mucosa is also sensitive to chemical and taste stimulants. Because there is presumed to be high overlap within the laryngeal areas of these different receptors, clinicians generalize the findings of the sensory test to the patient's ability to handle food and liquid safely – i.e., to protect the airway. Further research as to the validity of this impression remains to be done.

Setzen et al. (2003) suggested that normal sensation is triggered at pressures below 4 mmHg. Moderate deficits in sensation occur if a response does not occur until the range of 4–6 mmHg. Severe deficits in sensation are detected when the response does not occur when the calibrated puff exceeds 6 mmHg. Information regarding sensory loss may provide useful information for patients at risk of aspiration because the laryngeal adductor reflex (LAR) provides a measure of airway protection. An age-related change in laryngopharyngeal sensation has been reported (Aviv et al., 1994). Aviv also reported that patients after cerebrovascular accident with abnormally high thresholds for activating the LAR were significantly more likely to get aspiration pneumonia (Aviv et al., 1997). Abnormal laryngopharyngeal sensation is associated with dysphagia and aspiration. Where the laryngopharyngeal adductor reflex is absent, individuals are more likely to penetrate and aspirate on both puree and liquid consistencies (Aviv et al., 2002). Nearly all individuals with severe pharyngeal motor dysfunction in addition to laryngopharyngeal sensory dysfunction aspirate (Setzen et al., 2003). A combination of poor motor function and poor sensory function significantly increases the odds of aspiration occurring. Aviv et al. (2002) found that when the pharyngeal motor response was intact, individuals tolerated puree consistencies well, regardless of the integrity of the sensory system. However, an intact pharyngeal motor system in combination with a severe laryngopharyngeal sensory deficit will result in penetration/aspiration of thin liquids. These studies serve to highlight the importance of both the sensory system and the motor system in the assessment and treatment of dysphagia.

COMPARISON BETWEEN FLUOROSCOPY AND ENDOSCOPY

RELIABILITY AND VALIDITY

Several investigators have sought to examine the relative merits of fluoroscopy over endoscopy (Bastian, 1991; Wu et al., 1997). Langmore et al. (1991) reported very high rates of agreement for endoscopy to ascertain tracheal aspiration, laryngeal penetration and pharyngeal residue. They concluded that FEES proved to be a sensitive tool for identifying abnormal findings, including aspiration. Similarly high results were also reported by Wu et al. (1997) for pooling in the pharynx, laryngeal penetration and tracheal aspiration. Leder et al. (1998) reported agreement on 96% of subjects based on MBS and FEES assessments. It has also been noted that endoscopy is able to identify laryngeal penetration which has been misidentified as residue using fluoroscopy (Langmore, 2004). In summary, neither procedure is 100% accurate. For this reason, we agree with Doggett et al. (2002), Hiss and Postma (2003), and Rao et al. (2003) that neither fluoroscopy nor the FEES procedure should be labelled as the 'gold standard' unless they are compared to a less sensitive procedure such as a clinical examination.

The best reports of clinician reliability for interpretation of videofluoroscopy studies have been related to Rosenbek's eight-point penetration/aspiration scale (Rosenbek et al., 1996; see also Chapter 16). This is a multidimensional scale examining depth of bolus invasion into the airway and the patient's response to the bolus. It has also been applied to endoscopy with good effect, showing high interrater reliability (Colodny, 2002). Colodny (2002) notes, however, that FEES shows superiority in the diagnosis of penetration relative to aspiration but may not be as reliable as MBS in

Table 8.3 Penetration-Aspiration Scale Multidimensional depth of airway invasion and residue, single-digit scoring system for the Penetration-Aspiration Scale (Robbins, Coyle, Rosenbek, Roecker and Wood, 1999)

Category	Score	Description
No penetration or aspiration	1	Contrast does not enter the airway
P E N E T R A T I O N	2	Contrast enters the airway, remains above the cords, no residue
	3	Contrast remains above vocal folds, visible residue remains
	4	Contrast contacts vocal folds, no residue
	5	Contrast contacts vocal folds, visible residue remains
A S P I R A T I O N	6	Contrast passes glottis, no sub-glottic residue visible
	7	Contrast passes glottis, visible sub-glottic residue despite patient's response
	8	Contrast passes glottis, visible sub-glottic residue, absent patient response

determining the degree of aspiration (scale points 6, 7, and 8). The scale is shown in Table 8.3. FEES is, however, accurate in distinguishing penetration from aspiration (Colodny, 2002). As noted in Table 8.1, both endoscopy and MBS provide the clinician with observed findings and inferred findings. The observed endoscopic findings have been reported to provide the best correlations between fluoroscopic findings and endoscopic findings. Inferred endoscopic findings have been reported to have a weak relationship with videofluoroscopy findings (Crary and Baron, 1997).

DECISION MAKING – WHICH IMAGING TECHNIQUE SHOULD THE CLINICIAN USE?

When choosing which examination to use, the clinician must decide on the reason for doing the examination and the view that will provide them with the most useful data for that particular patient. If the patient presents with an unknown medical aetiology, then a fluoroscopic evaluation of swallowing will provide a comprehensive view of the entire physiology of the swallow (oral, pharyngeal and oesophageal phases) and may be more likely to identify the problem. Fluoroscopy is also the tool of choice for views of the oral phase and oesophageal phase. Complaints that may be related to cricopharyngeal function (e.g. globus or reflux) may also be better viewed using x-ray. Fibre- endoscopic evaluation of swallowing may be the preferred assessment for practical reasons such as eliminating radiation exposure, inability to move the patient to radiology, and difficulties with correctly positioning the patient for fluoroscopy. Clinically the endoscopic evaluation may be preferable when the clinician wishes to view the larynx, or view evidence of swallow-respiratory coordination. Secretion management is also best visualized using endoscopy. As noted above, laryngopharyngeal sensation can also be assessed endoscopically and is not afforded fluoroscopically. Langmore (2004) suggests that if the first examination (either endoscopy or fluoroscopy) fails to provide answers to the clinical questions, then the other procedure should be employed.

ENDOSCOPY AND THE PAEDIATRIC POPULATION

Note also that endoscopy is applicable to the paediatric population and also individuals with severe disability. The clinician should be mindful to explain the procedure as carefully as possible at a level that the patient can comprehend. Active participation in the procedure where possible and having some degree of control during the procedure (e.g. assisting in choosing food or cup) have both been found to enhance patient compliance and comfort (Migliore et al., 1999). Migliore et al. (1999) provided a useful discussion of ways to ensure an examination that is successful both for the information that it provides as well as the comfort of the patient with special needs. Leder et al. (2000) investigated a small paediatric sample (n = 7; aged 11 days to 20 years) with both videofluoroscopy and FEES assessments. They found 100% agreement in a blinded diagnostic result and also subsequent feeding recommendations. Thompson (2003) used sensory assessment in a paediatric population and found that children with a high laryngopharyngeal sensory threshold had higher incidence of recurrent pneumonia. In addition, children with gastroesophageal reflux (GER) had higher laryngopharyngeal sensory thresholds than children without reflux. Responses to calibrations of greater than 4.5 mmHg were associated with laryngeal penetration/aspiration, pooled hypopharyngeal secretions, and a history of pneumonia, neurological disease and GER.

The MBS and endoscopy provide the two most commonly used instrumental assessments for evaluating swallowing function. Two other instrumental techniques have been reported in the literature: ultrasound and nuclear scintigraphy. They are not often used clinically and are included in this chapter for the sake of completeness.

ULTRASOUND

Ultrasound is a technique that visualizes the oral cavity and hypopharynx during swallowing, using a transducer placed submentally below the chin to obtain an image. Ultrasound is defined as 'the imaging of deep structures of the body by recording the echoes of pulses of 1–10 megahertz ultrasound reflected by tissue planes where there is a change in density' (Dorland, 1982: 703). Sonies et al. (2003) reported a sound wave range of 1–40 MHz for medical imaging. Any commercial ultrasound real-time sector or phased-array system can be used, and the equipment and necessary expertise are available in most hospitals and radiology services. The information is transmitted to a monitor where the image is updated many times per second. The image represents a single 2D plane at any one time, although multiple views can be used (e.g. Saggital, coronal or transverse views). The physics of sound travel proves a limitation to the ultrasound technique. While sounds travel well through fluids and soft tissues, it does not travel well through fat, due to its complex tissue structure. This limits the type of client with whom ultrasound swallowing assessment can be used.

Ultrasound can be used to evaluate the salivary glands, the tongue, soft palate and floor of the mouth (Sonies et al., 2003). In addition, no contrast agents are required for ultrasound assessments of swallowing. The procedure is safe and comfortable for the patient and, like FEES, repeated studies can be done at will. Patients can be studied when awake or asleep (Sonies et al., 2003). By way of swallowing applications, ultrasound can be used to assess the oral preparation phase and oropharyngeal transport phase of swallowing, including epiglottic deflection. Infants can be evaluated suckling or bottle feeding, which may be useful in comparing function in these two scenarios. Similarly, comparison between nutritive and non-nutritive sucking can also be afforded using ultrasound. Tongue-to-hyoid approximation can be viewed and the movement of the pharyngeal walls can also be visualized. Movement of the vocal folds can be ascertained for symmetry, and residue in the valleculae or vestibule can also be determined. However, another limitation of the technique is that sound will not pass through bone or air. It will be completely reflected (Benson and Tuchman, 1994). Therefore, the trachea cannot be visualized as it is an air-filled space and thus ultrasound is unable to detect penetration or aspiration of contents into the trachea. It can, however, detect pooling of secretions and residue in the valleculae (Sonies et al., 2003). These factors limit its use in characterization of the pharyngeal phase of the swallow; however, the oral cavity is well visualized during ultrasound. One disadvantage, however, is that the hard palate, because it is a bony structure, cannot be visualized, making it difficult to judge glossopalatal function and adequacy. Ultrasound of swallowing is conducted by an experienced speech pathologist and an ultrasound technician.

NUCLEAR SCINTIGRAPHY

Nuclear scintigraphy uses radionuclide scanning during the ingestion of a radioactive bolus (usually Technetium-99m) to track the bolus as it passes from the oropharynx to the oesophagus (Sonies and Baum, 1988; Silver et al., 1991; Sonies, 1991; Silver and Van Nostrand, 1994). The radiopharmaceutical is not absorbed after ingestion, nor does it become attached to the gastrointestinal mucosa (Benson and Tuchman, 1994). Scintigraphy is an expensive, dynamic assessment of swallowing, requiring a gamma scintillation camera, a low-energy collimater and a dedicated computer (Sonies and Baum, 1988). Nuclear scintigraphy is conducted by a medical officer trained in nuclear medicine imaging techniques.

It is predominantly a research tool and for the most part has been used in the assessment of gastrointestinal reflux (Silver et al., 1991). Measures such as pharyngeal transit time, number of swallows required to clear pharyngeal residue and regurgitation can be obtained. Although scintigraphy is said to offer precise quantification of bolus volume in any area at a particular time or over time (Humphreys et al., 1987; Hamlet et al., 1989) there is much debate in the literature as to the tool's ability to detect and quantify aspiration (Sonies and Baum, 1988; Benson and Tuchman, 1994). Silver et al. (1991) and Silver and Van Nostrand (1994) describe that during an assessment of oropharyngeal swallowing using nuclear scintigraphy, the patient is required to ingest approximately 100 cc of a fluid treated with the radionuclide. The technique requires the patient to remain stationary throughout the assessment. Dynamic images are acquired as the patient swallows the entire 100 cc solution (not piecemeal). Static images are then acquired after the patient has rinsed the oral cavity and ingested a further 50 ml of water to clear the oesophagus. Antero-posterior images are captured at set times post ingestion (e.g., 3, 5 and 24 hours after the assessment).

It should also be noted that nuclear scintigraphy provides a digitized configuration of the flow of the bolus, not a representation of the person's anatomy (Sonies and Baum, 1988; Sonies, 1991; Benson and Tuchman, 1994). It does have certain advantages, these being (a) that radiation exposure is greatly reduced, and (b) the amount of liquid aspirated and rate of clearance from the pulmonary system is measurable in a semi-quantitative manner. There are, however, certain disadvantages that raise serious questions about its practical viability as an assessment of dysphagia.

- It is not possible to image in the lateral plane. Imaging in the AP plane means that the trachea cannot be distinguished from the oesophagus – negating the possibility of diagnosing laryngotracheal aspiration.
- The patient is required to remain perfectly still and to swallow without coughing or spilling the liquid.
- There is poor image resolution when compared to the MBS.
- The technique requires expensive equipment, and increased time demands are made on the patient and medical radiation staff for repeated imaging throughout the day.
- Few allowances are made for differing body density measurements and attenuation of body tissue.

SUMMARY

The discussions above highlight the complimentary use of imaging techniques for dysphagia assessment. The techniques described in this chapter provide the clinician with additional information with which to guide clinical management of the patient. The chapter highlighted the inherent difficulties in each of the assessment tools, showing that there is no one tool that is perfect for every dysphagia assessment. Finally, further research remains to be done to determine minimum training requirements for competency in carrying out and interpreting the procedures described in this chapter.

REFERENCES

Aronowitz P, Cobarrubias F (2003) Anterior cervical osteophytes causing airway compromise. New England Journal of Medicine 349: 26.

Arvedson JC, Brodsky L (2002) Pediatric Swallowing and Feeding: Assessment and Management (2nd edn). Albany NY: Singular Publishing.

Aviv JE (2000) Clinical assessment of pharyngolaryngeal sensitivity. American Journal of Medicine 105(Supp 4A): 68S–72S.

Aviv JE, Martin JH, Jones ME, et al. (1994). Age-related changes in pharyngeal and supraglottic sensation. Annals of Otology Rhinology and Laryngology 103: 749–52.

Aviv JE, Sacco RL, Thomson J, et al. (1997) Silent laryngopharyngeal sensory deficits after stroke. Annals of Otology, Rhinology and Laryngology 106(2): 87–93.

Aviv JE, Spitzer J, Cohen M, et al. (2002) Laryngeal adductor reflux and pharyngeal squeeze as predictors of laryngeal penetration and aspiration. Laryngoscope 112(2): 338–41.

Bastian RW (1991) Videoendoscopic evaluation of patients with dysphagia: an adjunct to the modified barium swallow. Otolaryngology – Head and Neck Surgery 104: 339–50.

Beck TJ, Gayler BW (1990) Image quality and radiation levels in videofluoroscopy for swallowing studies: A review. Dysphagia 5: 118–28.

Benson JE, Tuchman D (1994) Other diagnostic tests used for evaluation of swallowing disorders. In Tuchman DN, Walter RS (eds) Disorders of Feeding and Swallowing in Infants and Children. San Diego: Singular Publishing Group.

Chan CB, Chan LK, Lam HS (2002) Scattered radiation level during videofluoroscopy for swallowing study. Clinical Radiology 57: 614–16.

Colodny N (2002) Interjudge and intrajudge reliabilities in fibreoptic endoscopic evaluation of swallowing (FEES) using the Penetration-Aspiration Scale: a replication study. Dysphagia 17: 308–15.

Crary MA, Baron J (1997) Endoscopic and fluoroscopic evaluations of swallowing: Comparison of observed and inferred findings. Dysphagia 2: 108.

Crary M, Groher M (1999) Endoscopic evaluation of swallow function. Paper presented at Neurogenic Dysphagia, Australian dysphagia seminar, Sydney, September.

Crawley MT, Savage P, Oakley F (2004) Patient and operator dose during fluoroscopic examination of swallow mechanism. British Journal of Radiology 77 (920): 654–6.

Dodds WJ, Stewart ED, Logemann JA (1990) Physiology and radiology of the normal oral and pharyngeal phases of swallowing. American Journal of Roentgenology 154: 953–63.

Doggett DL, Turkelson C.M, Coates V (2002) Recent developments in diagnosis and intervention for aspiration and dysphagia in stroke and other neuromuscular disorders. Current Atherosclerosis Reports 4: 311–18.

Dorland's Pocket Medical Dictionary (1982) 23rd edn. Philadelphia: WB Saunders Company.

230   DYSPHAGIA: FOUNDATION, THEORY AND PRACTICE

Feinberg MJ (1993) Radiographic techniques and interpretation of abnormal swallowing in adults and elderly patients. Dysphagia 8: 356–8.

Hamlet SL, Muz J, Patterson R, et al. (1989) Pharyngeal transit time: assessment with videofluoroscopy and scintigraphic techniques. Dysphagia 4: 4–7.

Hiss SG, Postma GN (2003) Endoscopic evaluation of swallowing. Laryngoscope 113 (8): 1386–93.

Huckabee ML, Pelletier CA (1999) Management of Adult Neurogenic Dysphagia. San Diego: Singular Publishing Group.

Humphreys B, Mathog R, Rosen R, et al. (1987) Videofluoroscopic and scintigraphic analysis of dysphagia in the head and neck cancer patient. Laryngoscope 97: 25–32.

Jones B (2003a) The tailored examination. In Jones B (ed.) Normal and Abnormal Swallowing: Imaging in Diagnosis and Therapy (2nd edn). New York: Springer, pp. 35–53.

Jones B (2003b) Common structural lesions. In B Jones (ed.) Normal and Abnormal Swallowing: Imaging in Diagnosis and Therapy (2nd edn) (pp. 103–18). Springer: New York.

Jones B (2003c) Interpreting the study. In B Jones (ed.) Normal and Abnormal Swallowing: Imaging in Diagnosis and Therapy (2nd edn). New York: Springer, pp. 55–82.

Kandel ER, Wurtz RH (2000) Constructing the visual image. In Kandel ER, Schwartz JH, Jessell TM (eds) Principles of Neural Science (4th edn). New York: McGraw-Hill.

Kramer SS (1989) Radiologic examination of the swallowing impaired child. Dysphagia 3: 117–25.

Langmore SE (2001) (ed.) Endoscopic Evaluation and Treatment of Swallowing Disorders. New York: Thieme.

Langmore SE (2003) Evaluation of oropharyngeal dysphagia: which diagnostic tool is superior? Current Opinion in Otolaryngology and Head and Neck Surgery 11: 485–9.

Langmore S (2004) Fibreoptic Endoscopic Evaluation of Swallowing®: An Introduction. March 15–16. Melbourne, Australia.

Langmore SE, Schatz K, Olson N (1988) Fiberoptic endoscopic examination of swallowing safety: a new procedure. Dysphagia 2: 216–19.

Langmore SE, Schatz K, Olson N (1991) Endoscopic and videofluoroscopic evaluations of swallowing and aspiration. Annals of Otology Rhinology and Laryngology 100: 678–81.

Leder SB, Ross DA, Briskin KB, et al. (1997) A prospective, double-blind, randomized study on the use of a topical anesthetic, vaso-constrictor, and placebo during transnasal flexible fibreoptic endoscopy. Journal of Speech and Hearing Research 40: 1352–7.

Leder S, Sasaki CT, Burrell MI (1998) Fibreoptic endoscopic evaluation of dysphagia to identify silent aspiration. Dysphagia 13: 19–21.

Logemann JA, Lazarus CL, Phillips Keeley S et al. (2000) Effectiveness of four hours of education in interpretation of radiographic studies. Dysphagia 15: 180–3.

Mahesh M, Gayler BW, Beck TJ (2003) Radiation in videorecorded fluoroscopy. In B Jones (ed.) Normal and Abnormal Swallowing: Imaging in Diagnosis and Therapy (2nd edn). New York: Springer, pp. 1–9.

Maiuri F, Stella L, Sardo L, et al. (2002) Dysphagia and dyspnea due to anterior cervical osteophyte. Archives of Orthopaedic Trauma and Surgery 122: 245–7.

Martin-Harris B, Logemann JA, Schleicher M, et al. (2000) Clinical utility of the modified barium swallow. Dysphagia 15: 136–41.

Merati AL, Rieder AA (2003) Normal endoscopic anatomy of the pharynx and larynx. American Journal of Medicine 115(3A): 10S–14S.

Migliore LE, Scoopo FJ, Robey KL (1999) Fireoptic examination of swallowing in children and young adults with severe developmental disability. American Journal of Speech-Language Pathology 8(4): 303–8.

Murray J (2001) Endoscopic mechanics and technique. In SE Langmore (ed.) Endoscopic Evaluation and Treatment of Swallowing Disorders. Thieme: New York.

Murray J, Langmore SE, Ginsberg S, et al. (1996) The significance of accumulated oropharyngeal secretions and swallowing frequency in predicting aspiration. Dysphagia 11: 99–103.

Ong C, Elton P, Mitchell D (1999) Pharyngeal pouch endoscopic stapling – are postoperative barium swallow radiographs of any value? Journal of Laryngology and Otology 113: 233–6.

Palmer JB, Kuhlemeier KV, Tippet DC, et al. (1993) A protocol for the videofluorographic swallowing study. Dysphagia 8: 209–14.

Pennington GR (1993) Severe complications following a 'barium swallow' investigation for dysphagia. Medical Journal of Australia 159: 764–5.

Rao N, Brady SL, Chaudhuri G, et al. (2003) Gold-standard? Analysis of the videofluoroscopic and fiberoptic endoscopic swallow examinations. Journal of Applied Research 3(1): 1–8.

Robbins JA, Coyle J, Rosenbek J, et al. (1999) Differentiation of normal and abnormal airway protection during swallowing using the Penetration-Aspiration Scale. Dysphagia 14(4): 228–32.

Rosenbek JC, Robbins J-A, Roecker EB, et al. (1996) A penetration-aspiration scale. Dysphagia 11: 93–8.

Scott A, Perry A, Bench J (1998) A study of interrater reliability when using videofluoroscopy as an assessment of swallowing. Dysphagia 13: 223–7.

Setzen M, Cohen MA, Perlman PW, et al. (2003) The association between laryngopharyngeal sensory deficits, pharyngeal motor function and the prevalence of aspiration with thin liquids. Otolaryngology, Head and Neck Surgery 128(1): 99–102.

Speech Pathology Australia (2004) Dysphagia: Modified Barium Swallow. Position Paper. Melbourne: Speech Pathology Australia.

Silver KH, Van Nostrand D (1994) The use of scintigraphy in the management of patients with pulmonary aspiration. Dysphagia 9: 107–15.

Silver KH, Van Nostrand D, Kuhlemeier K, et al. (1991) Scintigraphy for the detection and quantification of subglottic aspiration: Preliminary observations. Archives of Physical Medicine and Rehabilitation 72: 902–10.

Smith CH, Logemann JA, Colangelo LA, et al. (1999) Incidence and patient characteristics associated with silent aspiration in the acute care setting. Dysphagia 14: 1–7.

Sonies BC (1991) Instrumental procedures for dysphagia diagnosis. Seminars in Speech and Language 12(3): 185–97.

Sonies BC, Baum BJ (1988) Evaluation of swallowing pathophysiology. Otolaryngologic Clinics of North America 21(4): 637–48.

Sonies BC, Chi-Fishman G, Miller JL (2003) Ultrasound imaging and swallowing. In Jones B (ed.) Normal and Abnormal Swallowing: Imaging in Diagnosis and Therapy (2nd edn). New York: Springer, pp. 119–38.

Stoeckli SJ, Huisman TAGM, Burkhardt S, et al. (2003) Interrater reliability of videofluoroscopic swallow evaluation. Dysphagia 18: 53–7.

Thompson D (2003) Laryngopharyngeal sensory testing and assessment of airway protection in pediatric patients. The American Journal of Medicine 115(3A): 166–8S.

Van Daele D, McCulloch T, Palmer P, et al. (2005) Timing of glottic closure during swallowing: a combined electromyographic and endoscopic analysis. Annals of Otology, Rhinology and Laryngology 114(6): 478–87.

Van Eeden S, Lloyd V, Tranter R (1999) Comparison of the endoscopic stapling technique with more established procedures for pharyngeal pouches: results and patient satisfaction survey. Journal of Laryngology and Otology 113: 237–40.

Wooi M, Scott A, Perry A (2001) Teaching speech pathology students the interpretation of videofluoroscopic swallow studies. Dysphagia 16(1): 32–9.

Wu C-H, Hsiao T-Y, Chen J-C, et al. (1997) Evaluation of swallowing safety with fiberoptic endoscope: Comparison with videofluoroscopic technique. Laryngoscope 107(5): 396–401.

APPENDIX 8.1: THE FEES PROTOCOL, REVISED

FEES® EXAMINATION PROTOCOL
Susan E. Langmore, Ph.D. (2004)

Patient Name:_____Date:_____
Examiner:_____

I. ANATOMIC-PHYSIOLOGIC ASSESSMENT
  A. Velopharyngeal Closure
    Task: Say "ee", "ss", other oral sounds; alternate oral & nasal sounds ("duh-nuh")Task: Dry swallow
    Optional task: Swallow liquids and look for nasal leakage
  B. Appearance of Hypopharynx and Larynx at Rest
    Scan around entire HP to note symmetry and abnormalities that impact swallowing and might require referral to otolaryngology or other specialty.
    Optional task: Hold your breath and blow out cheeks forcefully (pyriform sinuses)
  C. Handling of Secretions and Swallow Frequency
    Observe amount and location of secretions and frequency of dry swallows over a period of at least 2 minutes.
    Task: If no spontaneous swallowing noted, cue the patient to swallow
    Go to Ice Chip Protocol if secretions in laryngeal vestibule or if no ability to swallow saliva.
  D. Base of Tongue & Pharyngeal Muscles
    1. Base of Tongue:
    Task: Say "earl, ball, call" or other post-vocalic – 'l' words
    2. Pharyngeal Wall Medialization
    Task: Screech; hold a high pitched, strained 'ee'
    (Task: see laryngeal elevation task below)
  E. Laryngeal Function
    1. Respiration
    Observe larynx during rest breathing (respiratory rate; adduction/abduction)
    Tasks: Sniff, pant, or alternate "ee" with light inhalation (abduction)
    Phonation
    Task: Hold "ee" (glottic closure)
    Task: Repeat "hee-hee-hee" 5-7 times (symmetry, precision)
    Elevation
    Glide upward in pitch until strained; hold it (pharyngeal walls also recruited)
    Airway Protection
    Task: Hold your breath lightly (true vocal folds)
    Task: Hold your breath very tightly (ventricular folds; arytenoids)
    Task: Hold your breath to the count of 7
    Optional: Cough, clear throat, Valsalva maneuver
  F. Sensory Testing
    Note response to presence of scope
    Optional task: Lightly touch tongue, pharyngeal walls, epiglottis, AE folds
    Optional task: Perform formal sensory testing with air pulse stimulator
    **Note: Additional information about sensation will be obtained in Part II and formal testing can be deferred until the end of the examination if desired.

II. SWALLOWING OF FOOD & LIQUID. All foods/liquids dyed green or blue with food coloring.

Consistencies to try will vary depending on patient needs and problems observed. Suggested consistencies to try:

- Ice chips – usually 1/3 to 1/2 teaspoon, dyed green
- Thin liquids – milk, juice, formula. Milk or other light-colored thin liquid is recommended for visibility. Barium liquid is excellent to detect aspiration, but retract the scope to prevent gunking during the swallow.
- Thick liquids – nectar or honey consistency; milkshakes
- Puree
- Semi-solid food – mashed potato, banana, pasta
- Soft solid food (requires some chewing) – bread & cheese, soft cookie, casserole, meat loaf, vegetables
- Hard, chewy, crunchy food – meat, raw fruit, green salad
- Mixed consistencies – soup with food bits, cereal with milk

Amounts/Bolus Sizes

If measured bolus sizes are given, a rule of thumb that applies to many patients is to increase the bolus size with each presentation until penetration or aspiration is seen. When that occurs, repeat the same bolus size to determine if this pattern is consistent. If penetration/aspiration occurs again, do not continue with that bolus amount. The following progression of bolus volumes are suggested:

<5 cc if pt is medically fragile and/or pulmonary clearance is poor
5 cc (1 teaspoon)
10 cc
15 cc (1 tablespoon)
20 cc (heaping tablespoon, delivered)
Single swallow from cup or straw – monitored
Single swallow from cup or straw – self-presented
Free consecutive swallows – self-presented
Feed self food at own rate

The FEES[R] Ice Chip Protocol
Part I: Emphasize anatomy, secretions, laryngeal competence, sensation
    - Note spontaneous swallows, cued swallow
Part II: Deliver ice chips
    - Note effect on swallowing, effect on secretions, cough if aspirated

Part III Aetiologies and Treatment of Adults with Swallowing Disorders

9 Conditions Commonly Associated with Dysphagia

JULIE CICHERO

CAUSES OF SWALLOWING IMPAIRMENT

Dysphagia is now recognised as a disease. It is also a symptom that is associated with many different types of disorders and diseases. It is not possible to arrange the causes of swallowing impairment into neat groups and classifications because of the extensive overlap among and between those disorders. Impairments fall into the broad classifications of conditions associated with:

- stroke;
- neurological medicine;
- burns;
- palliative medicine;
- infectious diseases;
- gastroenterology;
- trauma;
- respiratory medicine;
- surgery;
- general medicine;
- psychiatric medicine;
- tracheostomy; and
- medications.

The overlap will become clear as the various disorders are described. Normal ageing also impairs a variety of neural and muscular processes; however, ageing in and of itself does not cause dysphagia. Age-related changes that occur with swallowing were detailed in Chapter 2. Note, however, that the ageing process may exacerbate a dysphagia caused by a disease. This chapter provides detailed medical information pertaining to the various causes of swallowing impairment. There are tables throughout the chapter to highlight the specific swallowing characteristics associated with different disorders. Mealtimes are a social event, and the inability to participate affects our mental wellbeing (Nguyen et al., 2005). Where appropriate the nutritional and psychological effects of dysphagia are also discussed. It is also noteworthy that the WHO also recognise dysphagia as a disability.

Dysphagia: Foundation, Theory and Practice. Edited by J. Cichero and B. Murdoch
© 2006 John Wiley & Sons, Ltd.

STROKE

Stroke, also referred to as a cerebrovascular accident (CVA), has an annual incidence of 280 in 100,000. Stroke is characterized by a sudden onset and signs and symptoms that are focal and last longer than 24 hours. Transient ischaemic attacks (TIA) on the other hand, usually resolve within an hour, and have an annual incidence of approximately 35 in 100,000 (Counihan, 2004). Strokes are classified as either *ischaemic* or *haemorrhagic*. Ischaemic strokes account for 85% of all strokes and are often caused by emboli. Intracerebral haemorrhage is usually caused by rupture of a deep penetrating artery within the brain and is often related to hypertension (Counihan, 2004). Haemorrhage may also arise from the rupture of a cerebral aneurysm of arteriovenous malformation (AVM). Computerized tomography scanning, rather than clinical assessment, differentiates between ischaemic and haemorrhagic strokes. Forty per cent of individuals who have an ischaemic stroke are likely to die within the first 30 days (Macleod and Mumford, 2004). Intracranial haemorrhages account for 15% of all strokes. If severe, the individual may be comatose; if mild there may be focal neurological deficits that are usually indistinguishable from cerebral infarction. The prognosis for haemorrhagic stroke is that 30% to 50% will die within the first 30 days (Macleod and Mumford, 2004). Lacunar strokes are another type of stroke. These are small deep infarctions involving a penetrating branch of a large cerebral artery. These types of stroke are usually associated with chronic hypertension, with the most common clinical symptom being pure motor hemiparesis (Counihan, 2004). Strokes can be unilateral, bilateral, singular or multiple.

Stroke most commonly affects individuals over 50 years of age (Macleod and Mumford, 2004). The neurological signs of stroke include: hemiplegia, hemianopia, aphasia (if left hemisphere involvement), visuospatial disorder (if the right hemisphere is involved), agnosia (visual, auditory, olfactory, etc., depending on site of lesion), unilateral neglect, and apraxia (limb, oral, speech). Impulsivity may also be a feature. Complications from stroke include: dysphagia, aspiration, shoulder subluxation, deep-vein thrombosis, hemiparesis, pneumonia, depression, apathy, fatigue and emotional lability. Emotional lability is an increase in the frequency of crying or laughing, often starting with little or no warning. It is a frequent presentation in acute stroke and reduces over the following month to 6 months.

Ischaemic strokes where dysphagia has been implicated include among the clinical manifestations those that involve:

- the vertebral arteries, and posterior inferior cerebellar arteries; and
- the basilar artery.

Strokes involving these arterial systems may contribute to dysphagia by the effects on the lateral medulla, the brain stem, cerebellum, internal capsule and pons. Lesions to non-capsular pathways such as the hypothalamus, the limbic system and basal ganglia, frontal cortex and corticobulbar tracts may result in dysphagia (Gordon et al., 1987). Where the vertebral arteries or posterior inferio-cerebellar arteries are affected, in addition to dysphagia, the individual may present with ipsilateral facial sensory loss and contralateral loss of temperature or pain sensation, in addition to other clinical signs. Basilar artery occlusion causes massive brain stem dysfunction and is often fatal. If the medulla is spared, the individual may present with 'locked-in syndrome'. In this condition, individuals are quadriplegic and can only communicate by means of eye movement (Counihan, 2004). Brin and Younger (1988) reported that factors that adversely affect prognosis in the first week post stroke also increase the risk of aspiration.

Oropharyngeal dysphagia occurs in up to a third of patients presenting with unilateral hemiplegic stroke (Hamdy et al., 1997). Paciaroni et al. (2004) reported that 34.7% of 406 patients with stroke presented with dysphagia. Dysphagia was also found to be more frequent in individuals with haemorrhagic stroke. Dysphagia was also significantly related to the outcomes of death and disability. Five-year mortality rates of approximately 20% have been reported to be related to aspiration pneumonia (Iwamoto et al., 2005). Recent research indicates that swallowing has representation on the motor and premotor cortexes of both hemispheres, but displays interhemispheric asymmetry that is independent of handedness (Hamdy and Rothwell, 1988; Hamdy et al., 1996). This means that for some people the right hemisphere is 'dominant' for swallowing while for others it is the left, irrespective of their dominant hand. This may well explain why two individuals may have a stroke in the same region, and one will present with dysphagia, whereas the other may not. Paciaroni et al. (2004) found that lesion size rather than lesion location was most important in dysphagia presentation. Anterior lesions and subcortical periventricular white matter sites are more associated with risk of aspiration than posterior sites or lesions to the subcortical grey matter structures (Daniels and Foundas, 1999). In cortical stroke, the middle cerebral artery is most likely to be responsible for dysphagia (Paciaroni et al., 2004). The most common dysphagic symptoms secondary to stroke include:

- delayed or absent swallow reflex;
- decreased control of the tongue;
- reduced pharyngeal contraction; and
- reduced hyolaryngeal excursion (Veis and Logemann, 1985; Gordon et al., 1987; Logemann, 1996).

These symptoms usually occur in combination. The symptoms contribute to post-stroke aspiration in 40% of cases (Gordon et al., 1987). Nilsson et al. (1996) reported that in the initial stages of recovery, pharyngeal function was more disturbed than oral function. Smithard et al. (1997) have noted that swallowing function fluctuates over time. For example, although many swallowing problems resolve over the first week, within a 6-month period 6% to 8% of the population will have persistent problems, with 2% to 3% developing swallowing problems 6 months post onset.

CORTICAL AND SUBCORTICAL STROKES AND DYSPHAGIA

Higher incidences of aspiration have been noted in individuals following a right-sided stroke (Horner, 1988; Robbins et al., 1993). Robbins and Levine (1988) broadly differentiated right- and left-sided stroke dysphagia. They found that individuals post right-sided stroke had more pharyngeal stage difficulties, whereas the left-sided group experienced more difficulties in the oral phase (often motility related). Left-sided strokes may also feature apraxia. Apraxia is an inability to perform skilled acts of movements that cannot be accounted for by weakness, sensory loss, inco-ordination, inattention and perceptual or comprehension impairment (Carota et al., 2003). In swallowing apraxia, there is difficulty initiating the swallow, sometimes with searching movements of the tongue prior to swallow initiation (Logemann, 1998). The differences for dysphagia between left- and right-hemispheric strokes are small and most probably due to the fact that swallowing is mediated by both cerebral hemispheres with descending input to the medulla. Recent research shows that recovery of swallowing after stroke is associated with increased pharyngeal representation in the unaffected hemisphere (Hamdy et al., 1998). This suggests cortical plasticity with reorganization of the intact hemisphere during recovery of swallowing function. Individuals presenting with a subcortical stroke (for example, a stroke affecting the basal ganglia) may demonstrate delays in the oral and pharyn-geal phases of swallowing due to the affects of the subcortical structures on motor as well as sensory pathways to and from the cortex. (Logemann, 1998).

BRAIN STEM STROKES AND DYSPHAGIA

The brain stem can be affected by stroke in the medullary region or the pontine region. The medullary region houses the nuclei critical to swallowing coordination and organization (nucleus of the tractus solitarious and the nucleus ambiguous). These nuclei receive the incoming sensory information and plan the motor response. A stroke in this region may result in near normal oral control but significant difficul-ties in the organization of the pharyngeal phase of the swallow (Logemann, 1998). With the pharyngeal phase affected, deficits are seen in bolus propulsion through the pharynx, reduction in hyolaryngeal excursion and consequently pooling in the pharynx after the swallow (valleculae and pyriform sinuses). Movement of the vo-cal folds may also be affected due to its nerve supply. Patients may spontaneously apply manoeuvres such as the effortful swallow in an attempt to move the bolus out of the oral cavity and through the pharynx. Clinicians should also be aware that the respiratory centres are housed in this medullary region. Lack of swallow-respiratory coordination could well be anticipated. Logemann (1998) reported that dysphagia is quite severe in the first 1 to 2 weeks after a medullary stroke. Often patients are reported to have a functional swallow at 3 weeks after the stroke; however, for those where dysphagia remains, the recovery period may be up to 6 months after the stroke.

Pontine strokes, which are also in the brain stem, but higher than the medulla, may cause spasticity of the pharyngeal musculature. The spasticity will affect the promptness of triggering a swallow reflex, and efficiency in moving the bolus through the pharynx. Consequently, pharyngeal stage pooling will also be a feature of these strokes. Logemann (1998) reported that recovery of swallowing function

Table 9.1 Dysphagia characteristics associated with stroke

CVA type	Oropharygeal presentations	Other
Cortical		
Left	• Maybe 'swallowing apraxia'	• Dys/aphasia
	• Oral stage disorders	• Dysarthria
Right	• Pharyngeal stage disorder	• Verbose
		• Hemi-inattention
		• ↓attention
		• ↓new learning
Subcortical	• Oral phase disorder	
(Basal ganglia)	• Pharyngeal phase disorder	
Brainstem	• Delayed swallow reflex	
Medulla (lower brainstem)		
	• Pharyngeal phase dysfunction	
Pontine	• Slow recovery	• Muscle spasticity (pharynx)
Multiple strokes	• More significant problems	
	• + slow oral transit	
	• Severe delays in triggering swallow reflex	
	• ↓ability to protect airway	
	• ↓laryngeal excursion	
	• ↑likelihood of residue in pharynx post swallow	

after a pontine stroke is often slow and difficult. Treatment should focus on reducing muscle tone prior to swallowing therapy. A summary of the presenting post-stroke dysphagia characteristics can be seen in Table 9.1.

NUTRITION AND STROKE

There are a number of factors specifically associated with stroke that will affect nutritional status. After acute stroke, the prevalence of malnutrition has been reported to increase from about 16% on admission to between 22% and 35% at 2 weeks. Factors contributing to difficulty eating and nutritional deficits post stroke are the following (adapted from Finestone and Greene-Finestone, 2003):

• dysphagia;
• factors affecting ability to self-feed (e.g. paralysis, apraxia, perceptual deficits);
• cognitive changes affecting behaviour (attention, concentration, eating too fast or too slowly, forgetting to swallow, inappropriately long chewing time);
• visual neglect;
• disturbance of sensory function;
• depression;
• agnosis.

One of the difficulties with providing adequate nutrition to the stroke population, and many others, is compliance with the texture-modified diet. Perry (2004) has described a reduced energy intake that is associated with modified diets. Six months after a stroke, individuals with dysphagia and communication impairment presented with significant energy and protein deficits, high levels of eating-related disability and nutritional risk. Research is also under way to ensure that the texture-modified diets are nutrient dense, flavoursome and appealing. Risk of dehydration is also high amongst stroke survivors. There is a compliance issue with thickened fluids. In a very small study, Garon et al. (1997) found that if individuals known to aspirate were given access to unlimited water in addition to thickened fluids, their daily combined hydration input was better than if only thickened fluids were provided. Neither group presented with adverse respiratory conditions during the trial or for 30 days after the trial. Interestingly the group that received the combination of thickened fluids and water were discharged earlier than the individuals who received only thickened fluids. Note also that fluid requirements need to take into account the individual's age, disease, medical treatment and conditions associated with body fluid loss (e.g. drooling, fever, diarrhoea, vomiting, etc.). Perry (2004) reported a high incidence (80%) of non-oral feeding in the first week after the stroke where communication impairment was also implicated. This gradually decreased to about 11% remaining non-oral 6 months after the stroke. Independence in feeding reached a high of only 39% 6 months after the stroke, with 50% of the population requiring continued assistance.

CLINICAL INFERENCES

The clinician needs to be aware of the confounding problem of fatigue associated with stroke. It is reported in up to 70% of patients, even a considerable time after stroke (Carota et al., 2003). Fatigue and depression can have an impact on cognitive, physical and social functioning, which will affect their success with rehabilitation. Note that, with right-sided stroke, the following additional features need to be taken into account:

• impulsivity;
• verbosity;
• left-sided neglect; and
• cognitive impairment such as poor attention and concentration.

Impulsivity during eating may be observed as the patient continually fills the oral cavity without necessarily swallowing the previous bolus. Verbosity may become problematic at meal times due to the inclination to continue speaking while attempting to chew the bolus and/or swallow. This pattern then places them at higher risk of aspiration. Left neglect may increase the likelihood of left-sided oral cavity pooling which the patient may not be aware of. Impaired cognitive skills (poor attention or concentration) may affect any individual with stroke, regardless of side of lesion. Cognitive deficits make it difficult or even impossible for the patient to learn compensatory manoeuvres or strategies. Consequently, it may not be feasible to teach stroke patients with poor cognitive skills compensatory manoeuvres as they may not action them with each and every swallow. As noted above, individuals with left-sided stroke may present with apraxia (swallowing apraxia or oral apraxia). Patients with swallowing apraxia tend to do better if able to self-feed, rather than with verbal commands to swallow (Logemann, 1998).

It is also important for the clinician to be aware that most stroke patients with dysphagia will rarely perceive that they have a swallowing problem (Parker et al., 2004). Individuals with a good awareness of the clinical indicators of dysphagia (e.g. wet voice, post-swallow cough, etc.) tend to consume smaller quantities than individuals without that awareness (6 ml rather than 10 ml) and drink at a slower speed (1 ml/s rather than 5 ml/s). Patients with a poor awareness of the clinical indicators of dysphagia are more likely to present with complications even several months post stroke (Parker et al., 2004).

NEUROLOGICAL MEDICINE

CRANIAL NERVE LESIONS

Macleod and Mumford (2004) have identified a number of cranial nerve lesions that may precipitate dysphagia. The ones most salient to swallowing are included in Table 9.2. Cranial nerve deficits may arise from compression of the cranial nerves, poor vascular supply or from inflammation. Dysphagia is most likely to be affected by compression or inflammation of the cranial nerves.

Compression

Acoustic neuromas that spread from the internal auditory meatus may involve compression of the facial (VII) and trigeminal (V) nerves. Note also that deafness is likely due to involvement of the auditory nerve (VIII). The reader is referred to Chapter 1 for the specific functions of these nerves. In brief, these nerves are critical for the oral preparatory phase of swallowing and the sensation of taste. The potential for dysphagia will be affected by the degree of nerve compression.

Inflammation

Bell's palsy is an example of a benign isolated lower motor neurone facial weakness. Its cause is unknown and all facial muscles on the side affected by the inflammation are affected. It may be associated with changes to perception of taste, dysarthria, and slow oral preparation of food, depending on the individual's compensatory abilities. Individuals will need to be aware of the potential for pocketing of food in the lateral sulcus of the side affected. The person may also encounter injury to the buccal mucosa during mastication. In the region of 60% to 80% of patients with Bell's palsy recover completely, especially if the palsy is incomplete. A palsy that does not begin

Table 9.2 Cranial nerve lesions that have implications for swallowing

Cranial nerve	Site of damage or disease	Implication for swallowing
CNI – olfactory	• Local damage to nasal mucosa (smoking, nasal obstruction from infection or polyps). • Olfactor nerve damage – head injury = bilateral loss, subfrontal meningioma (unilateral loss). Note olfactory N damage is rare.	Reduced ability to smell foods and fluids and reduced appreciation of flavour. May impact upon hunger levels and amount of oral intake.
CN V – trigeminal	• Lower two divisions – tumour in the nasopharynx. • All three divisions – pontine lesions (e.g. tumour, haemorrhage, infarct).	Impairments relating to mastication.
CN VII – facial	• Unilateral, LMN facial weakness – idiopathic (Bell's palsy); Herpes zoster; diabetes mellitus; sarcoidosis; Lyme disease; fracture of the petrous temporal bone; acoustic neuroma; middle ear infection; large parotid gland; benign or malignant tumours. • Bilateral LMN facial weakness – Guillain-Baree syndrome; myasthenia gravis; myopathy (especially myotnic dystrophy); Lyme disease. • UMN facial weakness – contralateral hemisphere stroke or tumour; multiple sclerosis.	Impairment relating to abilty to retain food within the oral cavity (e.g. deficient lip seal). Possibility of food pocketing in the buccal cavities.
CN IX	• Tumour or vascular lesion of the medulla. • Acoustic neuroma. • Syringobulbia. • Motor neurone disease. • Demyelination. • Lesions of the jugular foramen. • Lesions of the retropharyngeal or retroparotic space (e.g. nasopharyngeal carcinoma).	Cranial nerves IX and X together may show impairments related to the soft palate, pharynx, and larynx. Ability to seal the nasal cavity during swallowing may be affected, poor pharyngeal clearance may result and poor airway protection may ensue.
CN X	• Tumour or vascular lesion of the medulla. • Syringobulbia. • MND. • Demyelination. • Basal meningitis. • Tumour in or surgery to the chest affecting the recurrent laryngeal nerve.	

Cranial nerve	Site of damage or disease	Implication for swallowing
CN XII	• Brainstem tumours. • Vascular damage. • Basal meningitis. • Tumours of the base of skull. • Carotid dissection following carotid endarterectomy. • Motor neurone disease (in this case the lesion is bilateral LMN).	Deficits relating to tongue function are implicated. For example, ability to contain and control the bolus within the oral cavity, and to initiate the swallow reflex.

Source: adapted from Macleod and Mumford (2004).

to recover in the first 8 weeks shows a poorer prognosis. Age is also an adverse prognostic indicator (Bateman, 1992).

BULBAR AND PSEUDOBULBAR PALSY

Briefly, upper motor neurone lesions refer to lesions that have interrupted the neural pathway above the anterior horn cell (e.g. motor pathways in the cerebral cortex, internal capsule, cerebral peduncles, brain stem or spinal cord). Muscle wasting is slight or absent, and spasticity is often a feature. Lower motor neurone lesions interrupt either motor cranial nerves or spinal nerves and cause muscle wasting, reduced or absent reflexes and sometimes fasciculations (Talley and O'Connor, 2001). Deficits of the lower motor neurones can result in dysarthria, dysphagia, choking and hoarseness. Bulbar palsy may be a feature of a tumour in the medulla, myasthenia gravis, syringobulbia and of inflammation of the basal meninges (e.g. tuberculosis meningitis, sarcoidosis) and others (Macleod and Mumford, 2004). Tongue involvement in a bulbar palsy will show signs of muscle wasting and possibly fasciculations. Facial musculature on the affected side is weak, including eyelid closure. This is a critical distinguishing factor between lower and upper motor neurone palsies. The muscles of the forehead have bilateral cortical innervation, which explains why the upper part of the face is spared in upper motor neurone lesions. Where lower motor neurones are affected, disorders of taste, lacrimation and salivation may occur (Bateman, 1992). Upper motor neurone lesions will show affected facial musculature, but relative sparing of eyelid closure on the affected side. Pseudobulbar palsy on the other hand is caused by *bilateral* upper motor neurone lesions and is characterized by stiff, slow tongue movement without tongue wasting, nasality of voice, brisk jaw jerk and emotional lability. It may be a feature of stroke, motor neurone disease and multiple sclerosis (Macleod and Mumford, 2004).

MYASTHENIA GRAVIS

Myasthenia gravis is a neuromuscular disorder and autoimmune disease characterized by weakness and fatiguability of the voluntary muscles. It has a prevalence of

10 in 100,000 (Macleod and Mumford, 2004). Weakness is exacerbated by effort and improved by rest. The condition may be worsened by extremes of temperature, viral or other infections and even excitement (Griggs, 2004a).

Myasthenia gravis affects, in order of decreasing frequency, the ocular, bulbar, neck, limb girdle, distal limb and trunk muscles (Hillman and Bishop, 2004). Patients complain of weakness, double vision, drooping eyelids, dysphonia, and dysphagia that worsens as the day progresses (Haider-Ali et al., 1998; Macleod and Mumford, 2004). Loss of facial expression, jaw drop, nasal regurgitation of fluids, choking on foods and secretions, dysarthria and nasal sounding speech have also been reported to be symptoms associated with myasthenia gravis (Griggs, 2004b). In an acute presentation dysphagia should be managed immediately. If respiratory function has been affected, the clinician should be cognizant of the impact of impaired respiration on swallowing and vice versa (see also Chapter 4). Ventilatory failure is attributed to involvement of the diaphragm and intercostals muscles (Haider-Ali et al., 1998). Upper oesophageal sphincter resting pressure is generally lower in individuals with myasthenia gravis (Haider-Ali et al., 1998). One of the drugs used to treat myasthenia gravis (pyridostigmine) has a side effect of increasing salivary secretions. If the individual presents with dysphagia, the clinician should be aware of this side effect and assist the patient in management of salivary secretions (see Chapter 6). Note also that compensatory strategies are recommended as rehabilitation exercises may serve only to exacerbate fatigue. On videofluoroscopy assessment, the clinician may choose to examine the patient initially, then have them eat 'off-line' for 15-20 minutes and then re-assess radiographically to view the effects of fatigue on swallowing (Logemann, 1998).

GUILLAIN-BARRE SYNDROME

Guillain-Barre syndrome is the most common acute neuropathy, affecting 2 per 100,000, with peaks in adolescence and the elderly (Hillman and Bishop, 2004; Macleod and Mumford, 2004). It begins a few days after an acute infection by an antibody-mediated attack on the peripheral nerves (Hillman and Bishop, 2004). Weakness may progress rapidly to complete flaccid quadriparesis with involvement of the respiratory muscles and cranial nerves. Some patients may have a prolonged period of paralysis requiring ventilation. Respiratory difficulties, dysphagia and autonomic dysregulation can be life threatening (Griggs, 2004a). Two-thirds will eventually recover completely, most within 6 months. In addition, 70% of patients are at their worst by 2 weeks (Hillman and Bishop, 2004). However, mortality occurs in approximately 8% of cases via respiratory failure or pulmonary embolism (Macleod and Mumford, 2004). Permanent disabling weakness or severe neurological deficits occur in approximately 5% to 10% of patients (Hillman and Bishop, 2004). Radiographic assessment of swallowing in the acute exacerbation phase is reported to show generalized weakness of the oral and pharyngeal musculature affecting the oral and pharyngeal phases of swallowing (Logemann, 1998). Respiratory support should be stable before commencing swallowing therapy. Resistance and a range of motion exercises have been recommended to improve swallowing function. Manoeuvres or techniques that affect respiratory control (e.g. the supraglottic swallow) should be avoided until the individual has recovered sufficiently to be able to safely manage these manoeuvres.

MULTIPLE SCLEROSIS

Multiple sclerosis (MS) is an inflammatory condition affecting the myelin sheath of the central nervous system, but not peripheral neurones (Macleod and Mumford, 2004). It involves autoimmune-mediated inflammatory demyelination and axonal injury (Griggs, 2004c). There is a prevalence of 110 in 100,000 in the UK. It is a disease of young adults with two-thirds of those affected being female (Macleod and Mumford, 2004). The condition may

- present as a benign disease; or
- a remitting and relapsing condition; or
- show 'inexorable progression' from outset.

A combination of genetic predisposition and environmental factors in early life seem to be important in its aetiology (Griggs, 2004c; Macleod and Mumford, 2004). Symptoms can arise from any part of the central nervous system; however, there is a typical presentation of the disease. Griggs (2004c) reported that in younger individuals the disease starts with focal neurological symptoms, often of the optic nerves, pyramidal tracts, posterior columns, cerebellum, central vestibular system or medial longitudinal fasiculus. In older individuals the pattern is different, with progressive myelopathy, axial instability and bladder impairment. The majority of patients have resolution of their initial symptoms. Clinical features of MS include:

- *optic nerve features*: optic neuritis, optic atrophy;
- *brain stem features*: diplopia, internuclear opthalmoplegia, sensory loss of face (CN V), facial weakness (CN VII), slurred speech, difficulty swallowing;
- *cerebellar features*: slurred speech, unsteady gait, nystagmus;
- *spinal cord features*: monoparesis, paraparesis, quadriparesis, sensory loss, bladder and bowel dysfunction, sexual dysfunction;
- *paroxysmal features*: trigeminal neuralgia, paroxysmal motor and sensory symptoms; and
- *cerebral hemisphere features*: euphoria, confusion, dementia (Macleod and Mumford, 2004).

Dysphagia is a frequent presentation in MS and, like the disease itself, the swallowing problems may also be relapsing and remitting (Jones, 2003a). There is a vast degree of variation in the presentation of swallowing disorders in this population due to the diversity of the extent and focus of demyelization. Pharyngeal stage disorders are the most common presentations of dysphagia in individuals with MS (delayed pharyngeal reflex initiation and reduced pharyngeal wall contraction). Oral phase disorders are reportedly less common (Logemann, 1998).

Cases of dysphagia need to be examined and treated on a case-by-case basis, remembering the relapsing and remitting nature of the disease. Sensory treatment may be employed to good effect to improve the triggering of the swallow reflex (Logemann, 1998; see also Chapter 12).

BURNS

There are three separate varieties of burns that can have an impact on swallowing function:

- thermal smoke and fire burns;
- thermal food and fluid burns; and
- caustic burns.

These will be expanded upon briefly below. The circumstances of the burn will also provide the clinician with additional features to consider. For example:

- explosions may be associated with fractures and intra-abdominal bleeding;
- burning wood, chemicals and plastic may produce cyanide-type poisoning and other gases causing pneumotitis;
- burns in an enclosed space may suggest a need for carbon monoxide poisoning to be considered (Hillman and Bishop, 2004).

THERMAL SMOKE AND FIRE BURNS

Individuals can sustain thermal burns in explosions, house, car and bush fires. Inhalation injury can result from thermal burns. It is defined as injury to the epithelial lining of the lower tracheobronchial tree and lower airway. It is present in approximately 20% to 30% of patients treated in burns units (Muehlberger et al., 1998; Hillman and Bishop, 2004). The most immediate danger from inhalation injury is upper airway obstruction caused by oedema. Depending on the site of the injury the facial and cervical skin and muscles may also be affected by burns, leading to reduced range of motion of the facial muscles and laryngeal strap muscles. Exposure to fire and smoke can cause 'singed facial hair, singed nasal vibrissae, facial burns, oral and/nasal soot, cough, carbonaceous sputum and swallowing difficulties' (Muehlberger et al., 1998: 1004). Injury to the pharynx may include supraglottic and/or subglottic oedema. Pooled secretions may also be found in the posterior portion of the glottis and interarytenoid space. When supraglottic structures are affected there may be particles evident on endoscopy assessment, in addition to oedema and impaired mucous production of the upper airway. When subglottic structures are affected there may be bronchial obstruction and the toxic gases may affect the alveoli with subsequent necrosis and ulceration (Muehlbeger et al., 1998).

Individuals in this population are often treated with intubation to ensure a patent airway. However, complications with endotracheal intubation in this population include: granuloma formation, vocal fold paralysis, bleeding, laryngeal chrondomalacia and tracheoesophageal fistula (Muehlberger et al., 1998). Muehlberger et al. (1998) suggested that fibreoptic laryngoscopy should be part of the routine examination of burns victims to aid in determining whether endotracheal intubation is warranted, due to its superior ability to visualize the airway. While lateral still x-rays may help to diagnose a severely oedematous epiglottis, it is not considered sufficient to evaluate less severe inhalation injuries (Muehlberger et al., 1998). Elevated carboxyhaemoglobin levels may also be found in individuals who have sustained an inhalation injury. It is important to note that pulse oximetry will not be accurate, as the oximeter will read the carboxyhaemoglobin as normal oxyhaemoglobin (Muehlberger et al., 1998).

The speech pathologist's role in the burns unit is to establish communication, assess and treat swallowing disorders, assess and treat vocal cord dysfunction, and assist in the reduction of scar formation of facial and oral musculature. In addition to the inhalation injury outlined above, individuals who have suffered a burns injury may also suffer from pain on swallowing (odynophagia). Other factors to be considered in the burns population include: general physical weakness, pulmonary hypertension with tachypnea, oral and facial skin grafts and/or scar formation, multiple surgeries, medications, difficulty with positioning, damage to the central nervous system due to hypoxia, and hypermetabolism with caloric push (Snyder and Ubben, 2003). Snyder and Ubben (2003) conducted a study to determine how often speech pathology intervention occurred in the burns unit. They found that the number of speech pathologists was limited despite burns victims requiring alternative or augmentative communication (often due to tracheostomy), oromotor intervention (facial expression and articulation, resonance and voice projection), treatment of swallowing and therapy for cognitive-linguistic disturbances due to hypoxia.

The impact of the cognitive-linguistic deficits was often related to poor memory and verbal problem-solving skills, difficulties with self-care and safety. The authors suggested that increased referrals to speech pathology rather than aggressive pulmonary care in isolation may be a more cost-effective treatment regime for burns patients. Ward et al. (2001) found, in a retrospective study, that the average duration of hospitalization for a group of 30 burns patients was 84 days, with speech pathology intervention for roughly half that time. Individuals often experienced a period of 30 days between admission and their first safe oral intake, probably due to their unstable medical condition. By discharge, the majority of burns patients were found to be managing thin fluids, with all taking a diet and most taking a 'normal' diet (Ward et al., 2001). Ward et al. (2001) found that the patient's medical status, acute surgical requirements, wound debridement, medications (corticosteroids and antibiotics), oedema and tracheostomy all prolonged the inactivity of the muscles required for swallowing. Compensatory strategies were most often employed to treat this population, with adjustment to foods and fluids the most likely course of treatment.

CAUSTIC BURNS

Individuals may sustain caustic burns by accidentally or willingly (suicide attempts) swallowing caustic and acidic agents (detergents, bleaches or other substances containing alkalis or acids). When caustic substances are ingested, the upper airway and larynx will work to drive the fluid out. Consequently the most profound damage occurs in the pharynx and to the epiglottis. The vocal folds are usually preserved (Chen et al., 2003). The degree of damage to the aerodigestive system will depend on the type of substance swallowed and the amount. In some instances not only the oral and pharyngeal regions are affected, but the oesophagus is affected also. Shikowitz et al. (1996) detailed four phases of recovery from caustic burns. The acute phase occurs over the first 4–7 days and includes vascular thrombosis, inflammation, bacterial infiltration, cell death and the formation of necrotic tissue. The middle phase finds the necrotic tissue starting to ulcerate. This is the point when the oesophageal walls are reportedly at their weakest (Shikowitz et al., 1996). The latent phase occurs during weeks 2–4, and finds the beginning of granulation tissue formation. During the latent phase there is also a high risk of circulatory collapse and pulmonary necrosis. The chronic phase shows scar tissue formation, the potential for abscesses, oesophageal strictures and gastric obstruction. Where the oesophagus has been irrevocably affected, a piece of the colon or jejunum may be used to bypass the oesophagus. Some individuals may be left with a permanent jejunostomy.

A jejunostomy is where nutrition is delivered directly into the jejunum. Over time, the jejunal site may become odorous due to a combination of fermenting food and gastric secretions (Chen et al., 2003). Chen et al. (2003) reported a procedure using a free jejunal flap to reconstruct the oesophagus. The new segment allows for the mouth and stomach to be physically connected, while simultaneously protecting the airway. Food and fluids are passed into the buccogingival sulcus, where the opening of the flap is situated. The patient is taught to blow up the cheek to open the inlet and increase intraoral pressure. The graft then runs external to the mandible, following the path of where the oesophagus would be. This new type of surgery allows individuals to continue to eat and drink orally without the complications of aspiration and phobia about choking. Saliva production continues to occur, and must either be swallowed or expectorated. If there is severe damage to the supralgottic structures, aspiration may continue to occur, possibly leading to recurrent pneumonia.

Shikotwitz et al. (1996) reported the following features of dysphagia associated with caustic burns: reduced tongue base retraction, reduced pharyngeal wall movement, reduced laryngeal elevation and reduced laryngeal closure. They also reported a latency of approximately 6 months for dysphagia recovery. The team best equipped to treat an individual with caustic burns consisted of an otolaryngologist, thoracic surgeon, radiologist, psychiatrist and speech pathologist.

THERMAL FOOD AND FLUID BURNS

Goto et al. (2002) reported that thermal burns to the oral cavity from swallowing hot fluids are fairly common and usually do not result in serious injuries. The reason for this may be due to the fact that the teeth and oral tissues are very good at dissipating heat (Longman and Pearson, 1987). In addition, hot foods tend to be consumed at lower temperatures than hot fluids. Thermal burns to the pharyngeal and laryngeal region due to swallowing hot foods/liquids is rare and most often found in the paediatric population with foods or drinks being heated in a microwave (Goto et al., 2002). Damage to the epiglottis is a common consequence, even where the mouth and pharynx appear to only be mildly scalded. Damage to the supraglottic region may include red, oedematous and white-coloured aryepiglottic folds, arytenoids and false vocal folds and swollen epiglottis (Goto et al., 2002). Patients with laryngeal burns may require a tracheostomy. There is also the risk of pneumonia. Goto et al. (2002) recommend examination using a flexible endoscope to visualize the supraglottic region or failing that a lateral x-ray of the region (see Chapter 8 regarding endoscopy and x-ray assessment).

PALLIATIVE MEDICINE

MOTOR NEURONE DISEASE

Motor neurone disease (MND) has a prevalence of 6 in 1,000 and an annual incidence of 2 in 100,000. MND is rare in individuals under the age of 50 years. It is also known as amyotrophic lateral sclerosis (ALS). It is a disease of the peripheral nerves and neuromuscular junction with degeneration of upper and lower motor neurones. The cause of the disease is not known and the median survival time is approximately 3 years from symptom onset, with a worse prognosis if bulbar signs are present (Macleod and Mumford, 2004). Bulbar involvement, limb weakness and respiratory involvement are associated with MND. Motor neurone disease starts with painless, progressive weakness, and moves to muscle wasting and fasciculation. Dysarthric speech, dysphagia, choking, nasal regurgitation, hoarse voice and 'bovine cough' are all features of the MND client. Pseudobulbar palsy affects both the oral and pharyngeal muscles, with slowness or stiffness of the tongue and weakness of the pharyngeal musculature. LMN involvement causes wasted fasciculation of the tongue, 'bovine cough' and weakness of the pharyngeal and laryngeal muscles. Involvement of the tongue affects the individual's ability to prepare the bolus adequately, and to control the bolus within the oral cavity. Thermal stimulation may be beneficial (Logemann, 1998, see also Chapter 12). Involvement of the pharyngeal musculature predisposes the individual to pooling of material in the pharynx post swallow. This material may be aspirated if not adequately cleared with subsequent swallows. Involvement of the neck muscles may require head support and correct positioning for safe feeding. Adjustment in dietary textures and fluid thickness may allow the individual with MND to continue to consume foods and fluids orally.

Placement of a non-oral feeding tube may prolong life, with the individual choosing to take some foods and fluids orally for quality of life reasons. The patient's choice in this matter is crucial. Rehabilitation exercises may exacerbate fatigue. Once the laryngeal and laryngeal suspensory muscles become involved protection of the airway becomes more difficult, or even impossible. From a respiratory perspective, the involvement of the intercostals muscles and diaphragm often leads to respiratory failure by muscle paralysis (Griggs, 2004a). Wasting and fasciculation of the intercostals muscles may occur. Hadjikoutis et al. (2000) reported an abnormal swallow-respiratory pattern in individuals with MND. Rather than the normal pattern of exhalation after the swallow, individuals with MND are more likely to inhale post swallow. They also present with a prolonged swallow apnoea period and multiple swallows per bolus. Inhalation after the swallow has been highlighted as a red flag for potential aspiration risk, particularly if there is residue in the pharynx post swallow. Hadjikoutis et al. (2000) found that in a 12–18 month follow-up of individuals with MND that this abnormal swallow-respiratory pattern did not predict chest infections, coughing or choking episodes during meals or survival rate.

With MND there is preservation of eye movement, sensation and sphincter control. Higher cognitive function is usually preserved; however, there is a subset of MND patients who may present with some degree of frontal dementia, which may precede the onset of MND (Macleod and Mumford, 2004). Motor neurone disease can affect the corticobulbar tracts (as described above), the corticospinal tracts or both (Logemann, 1998). Individuals, who present with predominantly corticospinal tract presentation, may not experience dysphagia until late in the disease process, whereas individuals with a more corticobulbar involvement will have dysphagia as part of their initial presentation. Interestingly, individuals with corticospinal tract involvement present with dysphagia characterized by reduced movement of the soft palate and reduced pharyngeal wall contraction. In addition, their initial presentation may just be slowly progressive unplanned weight loss (Logemann, 1998).

Patients with MND may be treated with tricyclic antidepressants. Riluzole has also been used in the treatment of MND to slow disease progression. However, the drug has the following side effects: 'nausea, vomiting, somnolence, headache, dizziness, vertigo, abdominal pain, circumoral paraesthesia, alterations to liver function tests and neutropenia' (Macloed and Mumford, 2004: 948). Medications may also be used in an attempt to dry oral secretions; however, they must be used carefully with individuals with respiratory involvement as these same medications make respiratory secretions thicker and more difficult to clear (Geis et al., 2004).

PARKINSON'S DISEASE

Parkinson's disease is a neurodegenerative disease affecting dopaminergic neurones of the extrapyramidal system causing:

- disturbance of the control of movement and posture;
- abnormalities of cognition and mood; and
- disturbance of the autonomic nervous system.

Parkinson's disease has a prevalence of 150 in 100,000 and annual incidence of 20 in 100,000 in the UK (Macleod and Mumford, 2004). Parkinson's disease rarely presents in individuals under 50 years of age and probably occurs equally in both sexes (Macleod and Mumford, 2004). The actual cause of Parkinson's disease is unknown, however there seems to be an interaction between genetics and environmental factors. Interestingly, it is one of the few conditions that are less common in cigarette smokers (Macleod and Mumford, 2004). The median duration from diagnosis to death is roughly 15 years, with many patients dying *with* their Parkinson's disease rather than dying *of* their Parkinson's disease (Macleod and Mumford, 2004: 925).

Diagnosis of Parkinson's disease is made if there is:

- rigidity, tremor and bradykinesia;
- abnormalities are restricted to the extrapyramidal system;
- there is no other obvious cause; and
- there is a good response to L-dopa medication (Macleod and Mumford, 2004).

There are also a number of secondary features of the disease, which include:

- masked facial expression;
- dysphagia;
- hypophonia/palilalia;
- stooped posture; and
- festinating gait and 'start hesitation'.

There are also autonomic deficits relating primarily to continence, alterations to behaviour, depression, dementia and sensory complaints (aching, numbness, tingling) (Macleod and Mumford, 2004).

Dysphagia associated with Parkinson's disease reflects the impairment of volitional and autonomic movement due to bradykinesia and rigidity. Dysphagia has been reported in half of the presentations of Parkinson's disease, with drooling in up to three-quarters of those who present with the disease (Johnston et al., 1995; Jones, 2003a; Geis et al., 2004). Individuals with Parkinson's disease do not salivate more than healthy elders, the problem is related to poor oral function, causing pooling in the oral cavity (Johnston et al., 1995). Dysarthria is a common feature of Parkinson's disease because of involvement of the lips, tongue and soft palate. There is reduced vocal fold adduction, weak, breathy voice and limited respiratory support (Geis et al., 2004). The Lee Silverman Voice Treatment (LSVT®) programme is used in the treatment of dysarthria in individuals with Parkinson's disease to improve vocal intensity, but has also been used to good effect in the treatment of dysphagia (Sharkawi et al., 2002). Sharkawi et al. (2002) reported improved oral tongue and tongue base activity during the oral and pharyngeal phases of swallowing and increased vocal intensity after using the LSVT programme. Improved oral transit time and a reduction in post-swallow oral residue were also determined from pre- and post-treatment videofluorscopy assessments.

The primary predictors of dysphagia in Parkinson's disease are:

- duration of the disease;
- severity of the disease; and
- tremor and speech disturbances (Geis et al., 2004).

Dysphagia tends to be multifactorial and its presentation will depend upon degree of cognitive involvement, extrapyramidal and autonomic impairment, and psychological state. Impairment in mastication and oral preparation are the most common presentations of dysphagia in individuals with Parkinson's disease, with difficulty for solids reported more frequently than for liquids (Johnston et al., 1995; Volonte et al., 2002; Jones, 2003a). Bradykinesia is linked to impairment of tongue functioning and oral motility problems, including piecemeal deglutition, oral residue and premature loss of the bolus from the oral cavity into the pharynx. Impairment of pharyngeal motility may cause pooling of material in the pharynx after swallowing, which is an aspiration risk factor. Aspiration is not an early feature of the disease. However, timely education regarding clinical signs of aspiration and education regarding dietary modification should be considered by the speech pathologist in preparation for disease progression. The oesophageal phase may also be affected with presentation of delayed oeosphageal transport, oesophageal stasis, reflux and tertiary oesophageal contractions (Johnston et al., 1995; Geis et al., 2004). Note that poor distensibility of the oesophagus has particularly been noted in individuals with Parkinson's disease who also present with dysphagia. Individuals with Parkinson's disease present with postural instability and a predisposition to falls. Liaison with a physiotherapist to ensure adequate positioning and stability for eating and drinking is recommended (see also Chapter 11).

Logemann (1998) reported that rehabilitation exercises aimed at the lips, tongue and improvement of laryngeal elevation are appropriate for individuals with Parkinson's disease. In the early stages of the disease, manoeuvres such as the supraglottic swallow may be appropriate to assist in reducing the likelihood of aspiration. Note, however that end-stage Parkinson's' disease may also include dementia. This will severely limit the types of treatments the speech pathologist is able to offer, and much dysphagia treatment may eventually consist of dietary modifications. Weight loss is a common but poorly understood presentation of Parkinson's disease (Pfeiffer, 2003).

The most common medication for the treatment of advanced Parkinson's disease is carbidopa/levodopa (Sinemet). L-dopa aims to improve the movement disorder. Individuals may also be placed on antidepressants, which may improve nutrition by enhancing mood and appetite (Johnston et al., 1995). Individuals should be given an opportunity to adjust to their medication to determine any medication effects on swallowing ability (Logemann, 1998). The majority of studies that assess the effect of L-dopa on swallowing individuals with Parkinson's disease noted an improvement by reducing oral and pharyngeal impairment but also by enhancing upper extremity function (Buckholz, 1987; Johnston et al., 1995). Note also that concurrent gastroparesis can cause erratic absorption of drugs used to treat Parkinson's disease (Pfeiffer, 2003).

PROGRESSIVE SUPRANUCLEAR PALSY

Progressive supranuclear palsy is a type of degenerative disease affecting multiple systems as well as the extrapyramidal system (Pakalnis et al., 1992; Macleod and Mumford, 2004). It involves the frontal cortex and connections to basal ganglia and brain stem. The disease results in dementia, supranuclear gaze palsy, axial rigidity and pseudobulbar palsy (Macleod and Mumford, 2004). It is also known as Steel-Richardson Olszewski syndrome. Progressive supranuclear palsy presents with a more rapid decline than Parkinson's disease, and dysphagia is a common feature of this syndrome (Jones, 2003a). Both oral and pharyngeal phase deficits have been reported in this group, although they are less likely to present with the lingual tremor that is common in individuals with Parkinson's disease, despite the existence of extrapyramidal disorder (Jones, 2003a).

ALZHEIMER'S DISEASE

Alzheimer's disease is a chronic progressive dementia. It is another neurodegenerative disorder associated with dysphagia. It is associated with the formation of neurofibrillary plaques and tangles, and 'senile' plaques of the cerebral cortex and hippocampus (Macleod and Mumford, 2004). One in 20 individuals over the age of 65 and one in five over the age of 80 years are reported to present with Alzheimer's disease (Macleod and Mumford). As the disease progresses, oropharyngeal dysphagia becomes evident, and may or may not include an eventual inability to swallow (Eggenberger et al., 2004). Apraxia for feeding has been described in individuals with Alzheimer's disease, making it difficult to initiate the oral phase of the swallow (Logemann, 1998). The individuals may also exhibit an agnosia for food, giving little reason to swallow the foods/fluids in their mouth (Logemann, 1998). Significant delays in oral preparation and delays between swallow may be encountered (e.g. 3–4 minutes to initiate a swallow) (Logemann, 1998). There are some physiological changes to the swallowing mechanism that also occur with Alzheimer's disease (e.g. reduced oral phase efficiency, delayed swallow reflex initiation, reduced laryngeal excursion and pharyngeal weakness abnormalities), but the overwhelming problem may be in getting sufficient foods and fluids into individuals with Alzheimer's disease because of the length of time it takes to feed them. The problem then becomes one of nutrition and hydration with the ethical issues surrounding long-term non-oral feeding coming to the fore. Techniques to enhance oral sensation may initially be useful in promoting a more prompt swallow reflex. However, the clinician needs to be aware that there will come a time when the patient no longer benefits from treatment, and that swallowing therapy should at that point be terminated (Logemann, 1998).

In the diseases outlined above, the end stage for many may be the provision of non-oral feeding. In some cases individuals may continue to take some foods and fluids orally for quality of life, but receive the majority of their nutrition via non-oral means. Non-oral feeding can be used therapeutically for individuals with stroke or head injury, where the non-oral feeding is usually a temporary measure, with the aim of tipping the balance back towards total oral nutrition, where possible. In the palliative care population there are incredible moral dilemmas about the provision of artificial nutrition and hydration. The patient's family may be guilt-ridden for not placing non-oral feeding tubes in individuals in the final stages of a palliative disorder. Eggenberger et al. (2004) note, however, that tubefeeding is a passive process and is really nothing like the social function provided by eating and drinking. In addition, the researchers note that there is scientific evidence that supports the notion that foregoing artificial hydration and nutrition actually decreases a dying patient's suffering. Death from dehydration is reported to be a pain-free and peaceful process (Eggenberger et al., 2004). It is, nonetheless, a difficult ethical and moral issue to deal with both for the speech pathologist and also for the family and carers of the patient. The speech pathologist will often be the one to decide when oral feeding is no longer safe or sufficient to meet nutrition and hydration needs. For individuals with a palliative condition, the patient's wishes must be kept uppermost. Information about enteral and parenteral nutrition is supplied below to enhance the knowledge of the speech pathologist. The dietitian is responsible for the prescription of enteral and parenteral regimes.

ENTERAL AND PARENTERAL NUTRITION

Nutritional support is often considered for individuals who have lost more than 10% of their body weight, whose body mass index is less than 20, or if malnutrition is suspected. Close coordination with a dietitian is extremely important, as speech pathologists do not have sufficient training to advise on nutritional support. Where nutrition needs to be provided non-orally, it can be provided enterally (directly into the gastrointestinal tract) or parenterally (intravenously). If intestinal function is adequate, enteral nutrition should be used as the preferred option. Note that some patients may require non-oral nutrition as their sole source of nutrition if their dysphagia is very severe. Other dysphagic individuals may be able to cope with a combination of oral and non-oral feeding. Each individual is different, and only the clinician, the patient and the dietitian, with medical support, will be able to determine the optimum method of providing nutrition.

ENTERAL NUTRITION

There are two main types of enteral nutrition used in individuals with dysphagia: the nasogastric tube and the gastrostomy tube. The nasogastric tube is a lubricated fine-bore plastic tube that is inserted through the nares and passed gently down the oesophagus to the stomach. Medical and nursing staff are responsible for placement of the tube to ensure that it is correctly positioned (i.e. in the stomach and not in the lungs). Fine-bore tubes can be left *in situ* for two weeks. After this time, if swallowing has not improved, more permanent methods of non-oral feeding need to be considered. Large-bore tubes are not appropriate for enteral feeding for more than 7 days due to nasal discomfort, oesophagitis and peptic stricture (Davies and Rampton, 2004).

Longer term non-oral feeding can be afforded via a gastrostomy tube. The gastrostomy tube may be placed via standard surgery aided by radiology, or via percutaneous endoscopic surgery (PEG). Enteral feeds can be administered continuously or taken at night only. When progressing dysphagic individuals towards an oral diet it may be possible to speak with the dietitian about night feeds to allow the individual to experience the sensation of hunger during the day, and thus be more inclined to test oral intake.

The speech pathologist should be made aware of some complications of enteral feeding. These include:

- diarrhoea;
- pulmonary aspiration (from a dislodged tube that finds it way to the pharynx or if rapid feed administration is refluxed);
- inflammation of the nose or oesophagus; and
- metabolic problems.

Note also that there a better outcome (i.e. reduced mortality) is associated with NGT feeding in individuals with acute stroke, in the first few days after stroke and extending to 2 to 3 weeks post stroke (FOOD Trial Collaboration, 2005). In individuals with acute stroke, the decision to provide gastrostomy feeding should be reserved until after 3 weeks unless the individual is unable to tolerate nasogastric tubefeeding. The FOOD Trial Collaboration (2005) found that individuals who had a PEG placed in preference to an NGT were more likely to be institutionalized, with a higher dependency for care.

PARENTERAL NUTRITION

Parenteral nutrition is a complex means of delivering nutrition to the patient and requires a specialized team (clinicians, nurses, pharmacists and dietitians). As noted above, the intravenous method of delivering nutrition is reserved for individuals where gastrointestinal function is so severely impaired that they would be unable to absorb sufficient nutrients enterally. When appropriate for use, parenteral nutrition is delivered slowly into a large central vein where it is diluted with blood. Provided that the site does not become infected, it is possible that the line may be left *in situ* for a period of months (Davies and Rampton, 2004).

Complications of parenteral nutrition include:

- local trauma;
- air embolism;
- fluid infusion into the mediastinum or pleural cavity;
- thrombosis of the vein;
- infection; and
- metabolic problems (Davies and Rampton, 2004).

INFECTIOUS DISEASES

POLIOMYELITIS (POLIO) AND POST-POLIO

Poliomyelitis (polio) is an enteroviral infection that destroys anterior horn cells of the spinal cord and motor neurone cell bodies in the bulbar nuclei (Gillespie,

Sonnex et al., 2004). It has also been reported to affect the reticular formation and hypothalamic nuclei. The virus gains access through the oral or nasal cavity, with individuals experiencing flu-like symptoms, or being asymptomatic. In less than 2% of people affected, individuals go on to develop involvement of the central nervous system. In those affected, the virus invades and kills spinal or bulbar lower motor neurones, causing paralysis. Respiratory or bulbar paralysis may be dominant features, resulting in dysphagia, dysarthria and dysphonia (Gillespie, Sonnex et al., 2004). There may be some residual paralysis or paresis after recovery from the acute phase. There is neuronal plasticity in that new axons may sprout from surviving neighbouring motor axons. Although it is rarely diagnosed now, because there is an active international vaccination campaign underway to eradicate the virus, it was prevalent in the 1940s and 1950s.

Post-polio syndrome is reported to affect between 25% and 90% of people previously affected by polio. Post-polio syndrome occurs 20 to 30 years after the initial polio infection. It is characterized by fatigue, progressive weakness of both affected and previously unaffected muscles, and pain. It is reported to occur more frequently at times of physical or emotional stress. In addition, it is more likely to affect people who were:

- infected with polio when they were older than 10 years;
- on a ventilator; or
- if their initial polio infection was quite extensive.

Treatment of post-polio syndrome must be provided on a case-by-case basis due to the variations that are found in presentation. Treatment should address maintenance of the airway and optimization of voice quality, in addition to treatment of any residual dysphagia. Swallowing problems may include pharyngeal wall weakness, reduced tongue base retraction and reduced laryngeal excursion (Logemann, 1998). This combination of deficits generally leads to aspiration after the swallow from material pooled in the pharynx post swallow. Logemann (1998) reported that exercises aimed at increasing muscle strength, may actually cause muscle fatigue (see also Chapter 12). Consequently, treatment by compensation may be better suited to this population (see Chapter 11). The progression of post-polio syndrome, by way of progressive muscular decline is reported to be slow.

HUMAN IMMUNODEFICIENCY VIRUS AND AIDS

Human immunodeficiency virus has been reported to have originated in 'simian immunodeficiency virus' found in chimpanzees in central Africa (Gillespie, Brodsky et al., 2004). It is a retrovirus and is widespread throughout the world with 10 different subtypes having been identified. The main consequence of the infection is the reduction in T-helper lymphocytes, which causes severe immunosuppression. It is the manifestations of this immunosuppression that result in acquired immunodeficiency syndrome (AIDS) (Gillespie, Brodsky et al., 2004). AIDS is part of the final stage of an infection associated with HIV. It is defined as 'the life-threatening diseases caused by HIV' (Gillespie, Brodsky et al., 2004: 170). AIDS patients may present with Karposi's sarcoma, pneumonia, fever, malaise, tiredness, loss of weight, dysphagia and more.

Nervous system complications are most often found in individuals with untreated HIV (Gillespie, Brodsky et al., 2004). They range from mild cognitive disorders to serious central nervous system infections. Encephalopathy and dementia related to HIV may produce problems with coordination, short-term memory deficits, preservation of alertness in relation to cognitive loss, emotional lability, ataxia, aphasia, global cognitive deterioration, and relative mutism. This list is not exhaustive. Individuals who develop primary central nervous system lymphoma may present with confusion, memory loss, hemiparesis, aphasia and cranial nerve palsies. Progressive dementia, stroke, meningitis, and facial lesions have also been recognized as neurological manifestations of AIDS (Macleod and Mumford, 2004; Hillman and Bishop, 2004).

Dysphagia in AIDS is often related to the oesophagus and may result from inflammation, ulceration, strictures, masses (e.g. Karposi's sarcoma, lymphoma) and/or oesophageal motility problems (Meux and Wall, 2004). Infectious, inflammatory and myoplastic processes have been reported in the pharynx as well as the oesophagus, although oesophageal dysphagia has been estimated to affect nearly half of all individuals presenting with AIDS (Halvorsen et al., 2003; Meux and Wall, 2004). The patient may present with pain on swallowing (odynophagia), dysphonia and/or hoarseness. Pain on swallowing is often related to opportunistic infection with the Herpes Simplex virus and can lead to painful swallowing and mouth ulcers. Candida infection is another opportunistic infection and is the most common cause of oesophagitis in AIDS patients. Patients present with the symptoms of dysphagia, odynophagia and nausea (Meux and Wall, 2004; Gillespie, Brodsky et al., 2004). In addition, individuals with oesophageal cadidasis often present with oral candidasis. The condition is usually managed with oral anti-*Candida* agents.

In a small study of the swallowing abilities of individuals with AIDS, Halvorsen et al. (2003) reported that their group of 17 demonstrated abnormalities in the oral, pharyngeal and oesophageal phases of swallowing, with aspiration occurring in eight of the 17 and silent aspiration a common finding in those that aspirated. The oral phase of the swallow was found to be affected by disorders related to manipulation and transport of the bolus. The pharyngeal phase deficits were related to a reduction in laryngeal excursion, pooling in the pharynx and aspiration (Halvorsen et al., 2003).

CLINICAL IMPLICATIONS

Medical specialists will define treatment regimes for individuals with AIDS. The clinician will need to consider communication deficits in individuals with AIDS in addition to any dysphagia, recognizing that treatment will predominantly be compensatory and related to posture and dietary management. The presence of cognitive deterioration significantly reduces the individual's ability to learn new information. Consequently, the potential for dysphagia rehabilitation may be limited.

Moreover, many of the compensatory exercises may also be contraindicated, particularly if they need to be implemented with every swallow. For example, if the individual cannot remember the sequence of events to perform a safe supraglottic swallow for *every* mouthful of food or fluid, teaching them the technique may prove to do more harm than good. Case-by-case decision making is needed. Good oral hygiene is also important to reduce the likelihood of individuals with pharyngeal stage disorders aspirating bacteria laden microflora. The clinician will need to ensure that their own health is good, so as not to bring an infection to the AIDS patients. In the immunosupressed patient, even the most seemingly benign everyday infections can potentially be life threatening.

GASTROENTEROLOGY

Although the expertise of the speech pathologist in dysphagia management is related to the oral and pharyngeal phases of swallowing, knowledge of the oesophageal phase and its disorders is important. The clinician needs to be aware that oeosophageal disorders can adversely impact on the pharynx post swallow. Reflux (prandial or gastric), that enters the pharynx post swallow and dwells in the pharynx, is at risk of being drawn into the airway with inspiratory airflow. The pharynx and larynx may also be damaged by the acidic nature of *gastric* reflux, causing pain on swallowing. As individuals age, the likelihood of them experiencing oesophageal disorders increases (see Chapter 2). Consequently, older individuals are more at risk of oesophageal disorders and reflux related pharyngeal complications. This section provides information relating to: gastroesophageal reflux, laryngopharyngeal reflux, oesophageal motility disorders, and foreign body ingestion. While specialists in gastroenterology will be responsible for treatment of oesophageal disorders, the speech pathologist may be called upon to provide a differential diagnosis to rule out concomitant oropharyngeal dysphagia.

GASTROESOPHAGEAL REFLUX (GER)

This condition often occurs when the lower oesophageal sphincter (LES) fails to keep food in the stomach and backflow of food occurs into the oesophagus. Gastroesophageal reflux is a clinical term that is applied when the reflux is excessive and causes tissue damage (oesophagitis) and/or clinical symptoms (e.g. Heartburn) (Koufman et al., 2002). Reflux may also be caused by oesophageal dysmotility, and prolonged oesophageal acid clearance. It is extremely common, affecting roughly 30% of the population, particularly in affluent societies (Davies and Rampton, 2004). Additional causes of GER include:

- hiatus hernia;
- obesity;
- drugs: non-steroidal anti-inflammatory drugs (NSAIDS), antidepressants, anti-cholingergics, and calcium-channel blockers.

Gastro-oesophageal reflux is usually prevented by:

- the LES and its resting tone;
- acute angle of entry of the oesophagus into the stomach;
- compression of the intra-abdominal segment of the oesophagus by intra-abdominal pressure;
- diaphragmatic hiatus; and
- neutralization of any acid reflux by swallowed saliva (which equates to approximately 1 litre/day) (Davies and Rampton, 2004).

The vagus nerve provides the main parasympathetic supply to the oesophagus and its action is to cause increased contractility and reduced sphincter tone. There are also sympathetic supplies throughout the oesophagus, which have the opposite effect (Davies and Rampton, 2004).

Symptoms of GER

Individuals may complain of a burning sensation, which is often worse at night time. This is because the person is in the supine position and backflow occurs more readily in this position. Individuals may also complain of burning in the pharynx and coughing or gagging after the swallow. It may be possible to see redness of the arytenoids cartilages via endoscopy. Gastric contents are highly acidic and 'burn' tissue, hence the redness seen. Discomfort due to reflux may also limit the amount of oral intake, which will have an effect on overall health and wellbeing. A reduction in lower oesophageal pressure may be caused by fatty foods, alcohol, smoking, drugs (see Table 9.3), and pregnancy. Smoking also causes increased gastric acid secretion, which will effectively increase the amount of acid available in a reflux susceptible individual.

Gastroesophageal reflux and hiatus hernia, Barrett's oesophagus and oesophageal adenocarcinoma

Gastroesophageal reflux has also been linked to hiatus hernia, Barrett's oesophagus and oesophageal adenocarcinoma. A hiatus hernia occurs when part of the stomach is present in the chest. Not all patients with GER have a hiatus hernia and not all patients with a hiatus hernia have GER. However, it has been reported that the larger the hiatus hernia, generally the more likely the compliance of the lower oesophageal sphincter is negatively affected (Davies and Rampton, 2004). Suggestions for management of reflux are provided in Table 9.3.

In individuals with Barrett's oesophagus, there are changes to the normal epithelium that lines the distal oesophagus. The epithelial tissue undergoes metaplastic change such that it predisposes the individual to oesophageal carcinoma. The condition is exacerbated by GER. Barrett's oesophagus is an acquired condition, and it is likely caused by the body's response to excessive reflux of caustic gastric material.

Table 9.3 Management of gastroesophageal reflux

Treatment format	
General advice	• Avoid stooping. • Elevate bed-head by 10–15 cm. • Stop smoking. • Avoid causative drugs (e.g. NSAIDS, antidepressants, anticholingergics, calcium-channel blockers).
Diet	• Reduce weight. • Avoid fatty and spicy foods. • Avoid late-night meals. • Avoid alcohol. • Avoid hot drinks (especially tea and coffee). • Avoid large meals.
Medical treatment	• Antacids.
Surgery or laparoscopy	• Antireflux operation: fundoplication.

Source: Davies and Rampton, 2004.

Primary carcinoma of the oesophagus is usually the result of (a) Barrett's oesophagus (adenocarcinoma) and (b) squamous cell carcinoma associated with environmental carcinogens (Davies and Rampton, 2004). Squamous cell carcinoma is strongly associated with smoking, alcohol and dietary factors.

Gastroesophageal reflux and asthma

Given that the vagus nerve is the common innervation for both the lungs and the oesophagus, it should not be surprising that many patients with asthma also have GER. In addition, reflux may contribute to respiratory symptoms that are clinically indistinguishable from asthma (Canning and Mazzone, 2003). Note that airway nociceptors triggered by noxious stimuli such as acid, ethanol, capsaicin and cigarette smoke terminate in the nucleus of tractus solitarius. Note that some oesophageal sensory nerves also terminate in this area, and this may be part of the reason for the link between the two disorders (Canning and Mazzone, 2003). Khoshoo et al. (2003) reported that the provision of anti-reflux medications in patients with both GER and asthma lead to a reduced requirement for asthma medications. The relationship between the two disorders is, however, quite complex and the subject of continued research.

Laryngopharyngeal reflux

Laryngopharyngeal reflux (LPR) is a new distinction that is being made from GER and describes retrograde propulsion of stomach acid to the level of the pharynx and larynx. It has also been termed extraoesophageal reflux. The main distinguishing factor of LPR from GER is that patients with LPR are predominantly upright and daytime refluxers (Koufman et al., 2002; Belafsky, 2003; Lewin et al., 2003).

Table 9.4 Characteristic signs and symptoms that differentiate gastroesophageal reflux from laryngopharyngeal reflux (Lenderking et al., 2003)

Sign or symptom	Gastroesophageal reflux (GER)	Laryngopharyngeal reflux (LPR)
Heartburn	+++	+
Acid regurgitation	+++	+++
Epigastric pain	+	Not usually
Oesophageal dysmotility	+++	++
Dysphagia	+	++
Asthma	+	+
Hoarseness	Not usually	+++
Chronic cough	Not usually	+++
Globus sensation	Not usually	+++
Acid pH	pH < 4 lower oesophagus	pH < 5 upper oesophagus and pharynx
Inflammation and oedema		Laryngopharyngeal region
Position attack triggered in	Supine position	Upright position
Site of dysfunction	Lower oesophagus sphincter	Upper and lower oesophageal sphincter

One of the cardinal symptoms of GER is heartburn, however this is not the case for LPR. Table 9.4 provides a comparison of characteristic signs and symptoms of GER and LPR.

The primary defect in LPR is believed to be dysfunction of the upper oesophageal sphincter. It has been linked as a potential predisposing factor for laryngeal carcinoma, leukoplakia, laryngeal stenosis and aspiration pneumonia. It is intermittent or 'chronic-intermittent' and individuals may exhibit the following clinical symptoms: hoarseness, chronic cough, throat clearing and sore throat, dysphagia, globus, and vocal cord granulomas. Less common manifestations include: buccal burning, halitosis, otalgia, stridor and abnormality or loss of taste (Lenderking et al., 2003). Note these same symptoms may also be caused by rhinitis, asthma and laryngeal cancer. Note also that there appears to be laryngopharyngeal sensory deficits in individuals with LPR and this appears to predispose them to dysphagia (Aviv et al., 2000). Research is continuing into LPR, as some degree of 'normal' pharyngeal reflux is common in healthy, non-dysphagic individuals. However, there are many things to be determined including the extent of that normal range and the optimal method of its quantification (Richardson et al., 2004).

CLINICAL IMPLICATIONS

The speech pathologist should be aware that up to half of patients with laryngeal and voice disorders have reflux (Koufman et al., 2002). In addition, dysphagia is a very real risk for patients with GER and LPR, although it is more often associated with LPR (Lenderking et al., 2003). Aspiration of refluxed material is very damaging to the respiratory system due to its acidity. The oesophagus is better equipped to deal with reflux due to its extrinsic and intrinsic epithelial defence mechanisms (Koufman et al., 2002). As few as three episodes of LPR in a week can cause significant laryngeal damage. Treatment depends on the severity of the symptoms. It is recommended that a gastroenterologist and an ENT specialist provide medical care for the patient with LPR. Medical treatment often includes twice-daily dosing of protein pump inhibitors for a period of at least 6 months (Koufman et al., 2001). Quality of life concerns from individuals with LPR are predominantly related to social functioning. The conditions that cause them the most psychological distress include: voice problems, chronic cough, swallowing disorders and throat clearing. These negatively impact on their self-esteem and their relationships, and heighten fatigue, frustration, and stress levels (Lenderking et al., 2003). The clinician will need to bear these quality-of-life issues in mind when planning treatment.

OESOPHAGEAL DISORDERS

Patients experiencing more difficulty with solids than with fluids may suggest a mechanical cause of dysphagia. Mechanical oesophageal disorders include: oesophagitis, peptic stricture, carcinoma, and foreign body ingestion. Motility disorders of the oesophagus include achalasia and spasm.

Mechanical oesophageal disorders

Benign oesophageal strictures are often caused by acid. It is a consequence of prolonged and severe reflux (Davies and Rampton, 2004). Individuals with oesophageal strictures often present with dysphagia and weight loss. The speech pathologist may be involved in ruling out oropharyngeal dysphagia. Oesophageal dysphagia will be treated by a gastroenterologist. Oesophageal cancer has been described in the section above. Another cause of mechanical obstruction of the oesophagus is the ingestion of foreign bodies. A number of small non-food items may be swallowed by individuals (often children, the disabled or the psychologically disturbed). When the foreign bodies do not pass through into the stomach they may lodge at the cricopharyngeal level or in the distal oesophagus. If impaction occurs, it often results in dysphagia, frequently with chest pain. If left untreated the foreign body may perforate the wall of the oesophagus. Ulug et al. (2003) described an unusual case of 'foreign body sensation' that was caused by subluxation of the corniculate cartilage. The corniculate cartilages lie above the arytenoids in the posterior region of the aryepiglottic folds. There is a great degree of variability in their presence in the general population. In the case reported, the corniculate cartilage had subluxed (been dislocated) and was lying in direct contact with the posterior pharyngeal wall on abduction of the folds. The condition was diagnosed using endoscopy and the authors suspected that corniculate cartilage subluxation is perhaps more common than reported in the literature and often being misdiagnosed.

Oesophageal motility disorders

Achalasia and oesophageal spasm may contribute to dysphagia and associated chest pain. In achalasia there is a loss of oesophageal peristalsis and the lower oesophageal sphincter fails to relax after the swallow. The most common signs of achalasia may be malnutrition and pulmonary complications. Dysphagia may be intermittent initially. Later, more persistent dysphagia may cause nutritional deficits and weight loss (Davies and Rampton, 2004). Initially the difficulties may be relieved by drinking, but later liquids may be worse than solids. Respiratory symptoms associated with achalasia include coughing, nocturnal wheezing and chest infections. These are probably due to aspirated material that has passed back into the pharynx after swallows. 'Cricopharyngeal achalasia', distinct from oesophageal achalasia, is very rare and refers to complete failure of the cricopharyngeus to relax (Jones, 2003b). It may be diagnosed using a combination of videofluoroscopy and manometry. Failure of the cricopharyngeus to relax will result in material remaining in the pharynx, with a heightened risk of aspiration after the swallow in addition to malnutrition from insufficient supply of nutrients. A gastroenterologist will treat individuals with achalasia, often with medication or dilatation of the LES.

Oesophageal spasm is an idiopathic motility disorder (Davies and Rampton, 2004). It is characterized by intermittent, non-propulsive oesophageal contractions, sometimes with dysphagia and chest pain. Treatment is reported to be difficult. Some attacks appear to be caused by GER. Again, a gastroenterologist provides treatment.

TRAUMA

HEAD TRAUMA

Trauma to the head may be classified as 'open' or 'closed'. Open head injuries are those where the brain or meninges are exposed, whereas closed head injuries are those where the meninges are intact even though the skull may be fractured. Following trauma to the base of the skull, implicating damage to the cranial nerves or their nuclei, sensory and motor aspects of swallowing may occur. Despite the diversity of the head injury population, this group presents at risk for dysphagia due to concomitant variables:

- depressed level of consciousness;
- direct trauma to the cranial nerves, their nuclei or pyramidal pathways; and
- cognitive deficits.

The incidence of cranial nerve injury in head trauma ranges from 5% to 23% (Pilitis and Rengachary, 2001). Fortunately injuries related to the trigeminal, facial, glossopharyngeal, accessory, vagus, and hypoglossal nerves are rare. The most commonly injured cranial nerve is the olfactory nerve, with a reduction in the ability to smell affected in 5% to 10% of head injuries, being mainly related to frontal or occipital blows or fractures of the cribriform plate. Approximately 40% of individuals are reported to recover their sense of smell post head injury (Pilitsis and Rengachary, 2001).

Individuals with head injury are also at risk of pulmonary and gastrointestinal complications. Aspiration pneumonia and gastritis are typically reported complications of head injury. Risk factors for aspiration pneumonia include depressed level of consciousness, nasotracheal/nasogastric tubes, impaired swallowing and tracheostomy (Pilitsis and Rengachary, 2001). Tracheostomy and swallowing are covered later in this chapter. Individuals with severe brain injuries have heightened caloric needs secondary to metabolic responses to the injury and energy expenditure. As a result it is important to address issues that interfere with oral intake as expediently as possible (Mackay et al., 1999).

Swallowing impairment after head injury has been reported to be as high as 60% (Morgan and Mackay, 1999; Pilitsis and Rengachary, 2001). Loss of bolus control and reduced lingual movement/control are the most frequent abnormalities identified in this population (Lazarus and Logemann, 1987; Mackay et al., 1999). Prolonged oral transit, delayed initiation of the swallowing reflex and reduced pharyngeal contractions have also been reported. Individuals will often present with combinations of problems also (e.g. poor tongue control plus delayed swallow reflex initiation) (Lazarus and Logemann, 1987). The common oropharyngeal abnormalities associated with head injury are (Lazarus and Logemann, 1987; Mackay et al., 1999; Morgan and Mackay, 1999):

- abnormal oral reflexes;
- reductions in range of motion of the tongue or coordination of tongue musculature;
- reduced base of tongue strength;
- increased muscle tone of the oral musculature;
- reductions in labial strength;
- reduced soft palate function;
- delay in triggering the pharyngeal swallow;
- abnormal pharyngeal constrictor activity;
- reduced pharyngeal sensation;
- reduced laryngeal excursion.

Note also that in individuals with head injury, the incidence of aspiration is reported to be as high as 41% (Morgan and Mackay, 1999). Where oropharyngeal dysphagia is implicated, aspiration most commonly occurs during the swallow, with aspiration before the swallow being the next most common pattern. Aspiration after the swallow has been found to occur to a lesser extent (Mackay et al., 1999). Individuals are at risk of aspiration even before hospitalization, mainly from loss of consciousness resulting in an inability to protect the airway and then subsequent aspiration of gastric contents. Individuals with a severe head injury are more at risk of developing aspiration pneumonia.

Note, that not all individuals with an early onset of pneumonia have a swallowing disorder (Morgan and Mackay, 1999). The clinician should be careful not to over-interpret oropharyngeal signs. Risk factors for abnormal swallowing include:

- low admitting Glasgow Coma Score (GCS);
- severe admitting cognitive deficits;
- presence of tracheostomy; and
- ventilation time >2 weeks (Mackay et al., 1999).

Deficits in physical strength, swallowing ability and dynamic balance on acute re-habilitation admission have been found to predict the need for assistance for up to 1 year after discharge. For individuals with impaired swallowing on rehabilitation admission, 45% are reported to require continued assistance at discharge, and 15% require assistance 1 year after brain injury (Duong et al., 2004). While the treatment for mobility and self-care after brain injury are the conditions most readily consid-ered for rehabilitation, rehabilitation of the ability to eat and drink is not as obvious, yet it is critical for individuals to continue to thrive and for socialization. Individuals who have suffered a traumatic brain injury are significantly less active in social and recreational activities than individuals without a disability (Brown et al., 2003). The key contributing factors to this reduction in social participation were found to be de-pression and fatigue. The clinician should be aware of both of these features as they will have an impact on motivation and resilience for rehabilitation of swallowing.

Non-oral supplementation is often required for individuals who present with dysphagia following a head injury. Even in individuals where swallowing has been relatively preserved, 2 to 3 weeks of non-oral supplementation has been reported, in-creasing to 8 weeks non-oral supplementation in individuals with dysphagia (Mackay et al., 1999). Individuals with dysphagia, who are intubated, may take approximately one month to begin oral intake (Mackay et al., 1999).

Cognitive sequelae of head injury may also affect the ability to swallow safely. Some of the cognitive deficits encountered include problems of motor planning, integration and execution of information, and faulty judgement. The deficits may lead to inappropriate bolus sizes or food and fluid ingestion rates (Feinberg, 1993). Poor attention, concentration and reduced auditory comprehension may further re-duce safe swallowing. It has been suggested that cognitive levels affect not only the time at which an individual begins oral intake, but also an individual's ability to tolerate a full oral diet (Mackay et al., 1999). Halper et al. (1999) state that the speech pathologist should treat not only the physiology of swallowing but also the cognitive-communication and behavioural manifestations of head injury in order to achieve resolution of dysphagia. A severity scale for cognitive-communicative skills is included in Table 9.5.

DIRECT LARYNGEAL TRAUMA

It is possible for the larynx to be traumatized during intubation (e.g. endotracheal intubation) or by external trauma of the neck. In these conditions the cricoarytenoid

Table 9.5 Cognitive-communication skills severity scale (Halper et al., 1999: 493)

Severity rating	Cognition and communication features
Severe	• No functional communication is possible due to severe deficits of behaviour and cognition.
Moderately severe	• Functional communication is inconsistent. • Behavioural and cognitive problems are conspicuous.
Moderate	• Functional communication is present in simple, familiar contexts. • Behavioural and cognitive deficits interfere with accuracy and appropriateness.
Mild-to-moderate	• Generally accurate and appropriate communication occurs in everyday contexts. • Obvious errors are present in more complex contexts due to cognitive problems.
Mild	• Communicates in a full range of ordinary contexts, but with inconsistent accuracy or appropriateness due to cognitive problems.
Minimal	• Communicates in a full range of adult contexts, although subtle deficits in cognition are present.

joint may become subluxed. The patient may present with hoarseness, poor vocal fold mobility and malpositioning of the arytenoid cartilages (Ulug et al., 2003). Vocal fold mobility deficits and poor arytenoid positioning may affect the individual's ability to protect the airway during swallowing. Aspiration during the swallow is then a possibility. Careful examination, potentially using both videofluoroscopy and endoscopy may provide the clinician with information to determine an appropriate treatment plan. Team collaboration with an ENT specialist is also recommended.

RESPIRATORY

CHRONIC OBSTRUCTIVE PULMONARY DISEASE (COPD)

Chronic obstructive pulmonary disease (COPD) is an often described but poorly defined medical term applied to individuals presenting with chronic bronchitis, emphysema or a combination of both (Martin-Harris, 2000). The commonality in diagnosis is airflow obstruction. The COPD population present as a group that is implicated in underdiagnosed dysphagia (Coelho, 1987; Good-Fraturelli et al., 2000). Good-Fraturelli et al. (2000) reported that only 4% of their facility's COPD outpatients were referred for radiological assessment of swallowing, yet 85% of those referred for investigation of swallowing disorders were found to have some degree of dysphagia. Stein et al. (1990) concurred that dysphagia may be as high as 84% in patients with moderate-severe COPD who have had frequent infective exacerbations. Good-Fraturelli et al. (2000) also reported that evidence of laryngeal penetration or aspiration was observed in more than half their patients with COPD.

The nature of the dysphagic symptoms in patients with COPD predisposes them to increased risk of aspiration. Their deficits fall into three broad areas:

- abnormal *eating/swallowing behaviour* characterized by aerophagia, anxiety during mealtimes, dyspnea, hypoxia, reduced appetite, frequent expectoration of mucus, and fatigue;
- *altered mechanisms for airway protection* characterized by delayed initiation of pharyngeal swallow, delayed laryngeal closure, premature laryngeal opening, preponderance of pharyngeal residue, and diminished pulmonary defence mechanisms; and
- *impairments in swallowing efficiency* characterized by slow and effortful bolus preparation, channelling of food into the pyriform sinuses, oropharyngeal xerostomia, pharyngeal residue and slow oesophageal clearance (Martin-Harris, 2000).

Moreover, patients with COPD present with alterations in swallow-respiratory coordination (Shaker et al., 1992; Good-Fraturelli et al., 2000; Mokhlesi et al., 2002). There is a highly developed synchrony between respiration and swallowing that is crucial for the safe transit of food to the stomach. Incoordination results in a dangerously high risk of penetration and aspiration. As noted in Chapter 4, healthy individuals exhale prior to swallowing, have a period of apnoea during the swallow to protect the airway, and then recommence respiration in the expiratory phase (Selley et al., 1989). Individuals with COPD interrupt the inspiratory phase to swallow and recommence respiration in the inspiratory phase of respiration (Shaker et al., 1992). This population has been reported to have post-swallow pharyngeal residue, hence an inhalation immediately after the swallow will only serve to draw this material directly into the bronchial tree. A heightened predisposition to aspiration, in combination with an already weakened pulmonary system, places this population at serious risk for life-threatening complications. Langmore et al. (2002) reported that COPD is the second strongest predictor of aspiration pneumonia in nursing home residents. Shaker et al. (1992) have reported that swallow-respiratory coordination in the basal state of COPD is significantly different from its presentation during an acute exacerbation. Note that a recent history of smoking or COPD also shows the presentation of impaired mucocilliary clearance and a reduced cough reflex. The cough reflex is an important protective mechanism in the event of aspiration. Failing that, mucocilliary clearance would usually attempt to clear the aspirate. Note that both mechanisms are defective in individuals with COPD (Kikawada et al., 2005).

The COPD population also presents with a medley of other characteristics that affect not only their swallowing status but also their nutritional status in a vicious cycle. Martin-Harris (2000) reported that the COPD group are often malnourished and have a high metabolic rate. These patients expend a lot of energy simply in breathing. The energy needed to breath, therefore, increases their metabolic rate, and thereby increases their caloric needs. The COPD group need to eat enough to meet their heightened caloric needs, yet Martin-Harris (2000) also documented that COPD patients complain that eating is tiring. She suggested that the physiological load placed on COPD patients during eating and drinking puts further stress on an already compromised respiratory system during mealtimes. Note also that the COPD group present with xerostomia, poor dentition and purulent sputum (Martin-Harris, 2000). Harding (2002) suggested that episodes of microaspiration may predispose this group to the introduction of bacteria into the upper airway. If oral hygiene is poor, an acute exacerbation of symptoms may be triggered by microaspiration of 'bad' bacterial flora from the oral cavity.

CLINICAL IMPLICATIONS

The clinician will need to be fully aware of the interrelationship between swallowing and breathing. Individuals with COPD present with reduced swallow-respiratory co-ordination. Given a choice of breathing or swallowing, individuals choose to breathe. The clinician needs to work closely with the dietitian to ensure these individuals maintain optimal weight, considering that oral input may be limited in quantity and slow. The clinician may wish to recommend small frequent meals, ceasing oral intake when there is noticeable fatigue. In addition, attention to good oral hygiene is important to reduce the likelihood of aspirating infected oral microflora. Although it may seem logical to implement some of the airway protective manoeuvres for this population, techniques such as the supra glottic swallow are often not appropriate as they place too much stress on the respiratory system, rapidly depleting respiratory reserve.

GENERAL MEDICINE

SCLERODERMA (SYSTEMIC SCLEROSIS)

Systemic sclerosis is a multisystem syndrome causing inflammation, fibrosis and vascular damage to the skin, and internal organs. The gastrointestinal tract, lungs, heart and kidneys are most often involved. 'Scleroderma' is a descriptive word for the involvement of the skin and means 'hard skin'. It is an uncommon disease with an annual incidence reported to be 12 in 1 million (Axford, 2004). It predominantly affects females and is most common in the 30- to 50-year age bracket (Axford, 2004). Skin thickening and hardness is a characteristic feature. If scleroderma occurs on the face, the result is thickened skin that is tightly tethered to the underlying fascia and a loss of subcutaneous fat (Korn, 2004). The extent of facial scleroderma may impinge on the oral preparatory phase of swallowing. The layering of external skin may also occur internally in the form of mucosal layering, such as in the gastrointestinal tract. Oesophageal disorders have been noted, including hypomotility, severe gastroesophageal reflux, loss of lower oesophageal sphincter function and at times oesophageal strictures and ulcers (Korn, 2004). Regurgitation (i.e. oesophageal reflux) and aspiration, malabsorption and pseudo-obstruction are complications of the gastrointestinal component of systemic sclerosis. Malabsorption has been linked with bacterial overgrowth. If the gastrointestinal system has been severely affected, progressive weight loss is likely. Fatigue and malaise are common.

SJOGREN'S SYNDROME

Sjogren's syndrome is a chronic autoimmune disorder. It primarily affects the exocrine glands (eyes, mouth, respiratory system, gastrointestinal system, kidneys and skin), by destruction of the lachrymal and salivary glands. In addition, it affects the musculoskeletal system, thyroid, nervous system and blood vessels. Ninety-five per cent of individuals affected are female, and the syndrome most commonly presents between ages 30 and 50 years (Axford, 2004).

Salivary involvement is common in Sjogren's syndrome, and is usually unilateral and episodic. There is a reduction in salivary flow leading to oral dryness. Individuals with an acute exacerbation may experience lip cracking or ulceration, oral soreness, fissuring and ulceration of the tongue, atrophy of the oral mucosa, secondary candida and dental disease (Axford, 2004). These symptoms of reduced salivary involvement will have an effect on the individuals' ability to bind the bolus orally and also to initiate the swallow reflex. Try swallowing rapidly three times in a row. Now try swallowing again. Without saliva in the oral cavity, it is very difficult to initiate a swallowing reflex. Gastroesophageal reflux is also associated with salivary gland dysfunction. Xerostomia may be treated with artificial saliva, fluoride treatment and frequent dental care. Chapter 6 provides further details related to saliva management. Note also the gastrointestinal complications of Sjogren's syndrome. Mild dysphagia or chronic gastritis has been noted in individuals with this condition (Axford, 2004). Individuals presenting with Sjogren's syndrome should also be reviewed by a pharmacist to determine whether any medications they are taking have anticholinergic properties (symptoms include dry mouth and eyes) because these should be avoided where possible. Individuals with Sjogren's syndrome are also at risk of chronic bronchitis due to dryness of the tracheobronchial tree and also chronic obstructive pulmonary disease (Merkel, 2004).

SURGICAL

HEAD AND NECK SURGERY

Swallowing difficulties as a result of surgery to the head and neck region are directly related to the location and extent of the surgery. Swallowing deficits may accompany the following types of head and neck surgery: (a) partial tongue resection; (b) near total glossectomy; (c) anterior floor of mouth composite resection; (d) tonsil/base of tongue composite resection; (e) hemilaryngectomy; (f) supraglottic laryngectomy; (g) total laryngectomy; (h) pharyngeal resection, and (i) radiation therapy to the oral cavity and neck. For profiles (a) to (d) the most common sequelae are lingual and pharyngeal disorders. The extent of the resection and the nature of any reconstruction determine the severity of resulting swallowing problems. Pharyngeal stage problems may also present in laryngectomy-related cases.

Oropharyngeal swallowing disorders are frequently reported as a consequence of head and neck cancer, with dysphagia present in up to 50% of head and neck cancer survivors (Gillespie, Brodsky et al., 2004). Research shows that speech and swallowing function of surgically treated oral and oropharyngeal cancer patients does not improve progressively between one and 12 months post surgery. In fact some individuals may worsen at 6 months after surgery, although this may be related to the effects of radiation treatment (see below). In general, the level of functioning that was evident at 3 months after surgery was characteristic of these patrients' status one-year after surgery (Pauloski, et al., 1994). In addition, Ward et al. (2002) found that even three years after surgery 42% of laryngectomy and 50% of pharyngolaryngectomy patients continued to experience dysphagia requiring dietary modification. Campbell et al. (2004) reported that nearly half of non-laryngectomized individuals, experienced aspiration 5 years or more after treatment and, of those, half again showed inadequate protection of the airway. Campbell et al. (2004) also found that individuals who aspirated were likely to have had a mean weight loss of 10 kg, whereas individuals who did not aspirate had gained approximately 2 kg. Persistent weight loss in long-term head and neck cancer survivors should alert the clinician to possible aspiration (Campbell et al., 2004).

Despite the knowledge that swallowing is frequently impaired after surgical treatment for oral cancer, few investigations have defined specific effects of particular surgical interventions (Logemann et al., 1993; Pauloski et al., 1994). In addition, the various combinations of surgical procedures for head and neck subjects make them a highly heterogeneous group. There are:

- a wide range of head/neck sites;
- differences in the extent of resection, and
- differences in methods of reconstruction.

Logemann et al. (1993: 918) point out that these issues make it difficult for any 'single institution to access and study a homogenous group of patients in any single resection/reconstruction category.' This has implications for signs and symptoms of dysphagia following surgery to the head and neck. Individuals undergoing surgery of the head and neck region are truly unique. While some generalities can be made, the presentation of any dysphagia will be entirely idiosyncratic. Treatment must acknowledge the individual nature of dysphagia in the head and neck surgery population.

ORAL SURGERY – GENERAL

In general, in individuals who have undergone base of tongue resection or those who have undergone anterior tongue and floor of mouth resection, swallowing function is noted to deteriorate after surgery and show little improvement 3 months after surgery (Logemann et al., 1993). Oral and pharyngeal stage deficits are both implicated. Stachler et al. (1994) also found no significant difference in swallowing ability of anterior versus posterior surgical resections. Individuals in this group were also noted to have more difficulty swallowing viscous boluses (Logemann et al., 1993). In a review of a heterogenous group (lesions of the tongue, oropharynx and floor of mouth), Pauloski et al. (1994) found that aspiration occurred in only 3% of cases. Aspiration can occur before, during or after the swallow. For individuals who have undergone oral surgery, aspiration after the swallow (of pharyngeal residue) occurs most frequently. Treatment for oral phase disorders may include:

- range of motion exercises;
- sensory enhancement to promote the swallow reflex;
- supraglottic swallow technique or effortful swallow;
- alterations to head posture.

Treatment will need to be tailored to the individual's presenting symptoms and physiology.

Laryngeal surgery – general

Individuals who undergo a supraglottic laryngectomy are at high risk for dysphagia and aspiration post surgically. Supraglottic laryngectomy involves resection of the epiglottis and aryepiglottic folds and false vocal folds, as well as most or all of the hyoid bone. The removal of these structures robs the patient of some of the mechanical airway protection mechanisms as well as skeletal support for laryngeal suspension (Logemann et al., 1994). Post-surgically, these individuals present with difficulties relating to airway closure. Aspiration is common in at least 50% of individuals in the first month post surgery. Aspiration typically occurs during the swallow but may also occur after the swallow from post swallow pharyngeal residue (Logemann et al., 1994). Non-oral feeding or supplementation is common for at least two weeks post surgery (Logemann et al., 1994; Grobbelaar et al., 2004). Critical factors associated with recovery of swallowing function were found to be achievement of:

- airway closure at the laryngeal entrance (i.e. arytenoids to base of tongue contact); and
- movement of the tongue base to make complete contact with the medializing pharyngeal walls on swallowing.

Recommended therapy included:

- teaching the supraglottic or super-supraglottic swallow techniques;
- exercises to improve bolus propulsion;
- exercises to improve posterior base of tongue movement (e.g. Masako manoeuvre);
- exercises to improve anterior tilting of the arytenoid cartilages, and
- changes to head posture or positioning.

Swallowing difficulties have also been reported following total laryngectomy. The mechanism for this may be due to (a) formation of a pseudo-epiglottis by scar tissue at the base of the tongue, or (b) stricture from tight closure of residual pharyngeal mucosa in the case of partial pharyngectomy. In the case of pharyngolaryngectomies where a piece of jejunum is used to replace the pharynx, it is possible to

Table 9.6 Swallowing disorders associated with laryngectomy, partial laryngectomy and glossectomy

Laryngectomy
- No risk of aspiration (unless leakage via a fistula or leakage via a voice prosthesis).
- 'Pseudo epiglottis' caused during surgery can trap foods and fluids in the pharynx, preventing them from being swallowed.
- Strictures that narrow the oesophagus can cause dysphagia.
- Graft dysfunction in pharyngolaryngectomy patients.
  - Where jejunum has been used to 'replace' the portion of the pharynx removed:
    - Strictures at the top or bottom anastomoses of the graft can cause dysphagia.
    - Reverse peristalsis can occur.

Partial laryngectomy
- ↑ risk of aspiration.
  - ↓ airway protection due to loss of laryngeal structures.
- ↓ pharyngeal contraction.

Glossectomy
- ↓ bolus control and chewing.
- ↑ oral transit time.
- Premature loss of bolus into pharynx causing aspiration risk.
- ↓ base of tongue movement.
- Delayed pharyngeal swallow reflex.
- Potential for ↓ laryngeal excursion if intrinsic muscles of tongue have been resected (due to interplay between floor of mouth to hyoid connections).

have reverse peristalsis action, whereby material swallowed is then regurgitated by the persitalsitic jejunum back towards the mouth. Nutrition is compromised in this case. Aspiration is possible in individuals who have a laryngectomy in addition to a puncture to allow a voice prosthesis to be used. The puncture site houses the voice prosthesis, but also allows a communication between the respiratory system and the oesophagus. An ill-fitting voice prosthesis may allow aspiration of material into the stoma and hence the lungs. Some broad information relating to presentation of dysphagia following laryngectomy, partial laryngectomy and glossectomy can be found in Table 9.6.

Psychological sequelae to head and neck surgery

There are also psychological sequelae to head and neck surgery. Moderate to severe dysphagia complications after treatment of head and neck cancer are significantly associated with poor quality of life (Nguyen et al., 2005). Patients experience anxiety and depression related to their dysphagia. These in combination with weight loss, pain and speech deficits affect their general wellbeing. Management of the dysphagic patient following head and neck surgery requires a team approach. Individuals may require nutritional support, pain control, antidepressive medication, counselling in addition to speech and swallowing rehabilitation.

Radiation therapy and chemotherapy

Apart from surgery, radiation therapy and chemotherapy are the primary treatments used in head and neck cancer management. In combination, the surgery, and chemotherapy and radiation therapy result in a series of long-term side effects, which include xerostomia, dental decay, numbness, tissue loss, loss of taste and tissue fibrosis (Campbell et al., 2004). These factors are implicated in the development of dysphagia post therapy. Significant weight loss is a very real effect of dysphagia post radiation or chemotherapy (Grobbelaar et al., 2004). Radiotherapy is often provided after surgery and after healing of the surgical wound as it tends to devascularize tissue, making healing after surgery more difficult (Logemann, 1998). Chemotherapy is an adjunct treatment used in conjunction with radiotherapy. It is used to control regional and metastatic disease, rather than to treat the primary tumour (Logemann, 1998).

Ionizing radiation aims to reduce tumour size but has the unfortunate effect of damaging normal tissue located in the radiation field (Guchelaar et al., 1997). Oral sequelae of radiotherapy of the head and neck region will likely include damage to: the salivary glands, oral mucosa, bone, teeth, masticatory muscles and temporomandibular joints. Of these the most distressing is often xerostomia, which results in oral discomfort (fissures of the lips and tongue), decreased perception of taste, difficulty with oral functioning (chewing and speaking) and difficulty *initiating* a swallow reflex. Changes in oral microflora also results from reduced salivary flow, and this plays a part in associated increases in dental caries and periodontal disease (Guchelaar et al., 1997). Both of these factors have been implicated in the development of aspiration pneumonia (Langmore et al., 1998). Loss of salivary flow means that oesophageal pH remains elevated, and this may contribute to the development of GER (Guchelaar et al., 1997). There is a 50% to 60% reduction in salivary flow that occurs during the first week of radiation treatment. During this time the saliva becomes thick and mucoid. Mucosal alterations (i.e. mucositis) such as inflammation, atrophy and ulceration are also a common consequence of radiation therapy. Unfortunately the effects are also long lasting. Treatment for radiation-induced xerostomia may include moistening agents (chewing sugarless gum, frequent sips of water etc.), saliva substitutes (commercially available), medication to improve salivary flow (sialagogues) or surgery where the submandibular salivary gland is transferred into the submental space (Rieger et al., 2005). Often, though, the moistening agents and saliva substitute treatments only offer temporary relief. The surgical approach has shown success not only in maintaining salivary flow rate but also improving food transport efficiency through the mouth and into the pharynx (Rieger et al., 2005).

Other permanent effects of radiotherapy include trismus, fibrosis of tissues irradiated (e.g. pharynx or larynx) and potentially pharyngeal stenosis (Pauloski et al., 1994; Nguyen et al., 2005). Structures most likely to be damaged by intensive radiation and chemotherapy include the pharyngeal constrictors and the muscles of the glottis and supraglottis, resulting in dysfunction and loss of elasticity (Eisbruch et al., 2004). A reduction in laryngopharyngeal sensation has also been implicated, which plays a major role in risk for aspiration (Eisbruch et al., 2004). Cranial nerve

Table 9.7 Chemotherapy and radiation effects on swallowing

Radiotherapy	Chemotherapy

• Oedema and swelling of tissues (can affect tongue mobility and ability to retain dentures).
• Scarring and fibrosis
  ○ ↓ tongue mobility
  ○ ↓ pharyngeal contractions
  ○ ↓ laryngeal excursion.
• Xerostomia.
• Mucositis (reddened and ulcerated mucosa)
  ○ aggravated by spicy or citrus flavours
  ○ pain on swallowing
• ↓ Taste.
• Impaired jaw function (reduced mouth opening).
• Delayed pharyngeal swallow.
	• Mucositis (reddened and aggravated mucosa).
	• Pain on swallowing.
	• Nausea and vomiting reduces desire for oral intake.

Source: Lazarus (1993); Lazarus et al. (1996).

palsies have also been implicated as a complication of radiotherapy for nasopharyngeal cancer. The vagus and hypoglossal nerves are commonly affected (Nguyen et al., 2005). A summary of radiation and chemotherapy effects on swallowing are included in Table 9.7.

Cardiac surgery

Individuals who undergo cardiac surgery are also at modest risk of developing dysphagia. Ferraris et al. (2001) found that approximately 3% of patients (n = 1,042) presented with frank oropharyngeal dysphagia post cardiac surgery. The authors suggest that the prevalence figures may well be higher, as only patients who showed obvious signs of swallowing were included, meaning that silent aspirators are unlikely to have been included in the group. Individuals undergoing cardiac surgery who were most likely to develop oropharyngeal dysphagia postoperatively included:

• older individuals (e.g. 71 years versus 62 years);
• individuals with diabetes;
• individuals with renal insufficiency;
• individuals with hyperlipidemia;
• those with preoperative congestive heart failure; and
• individuals having non-coronary artery bypass procedures.

Anterior cervical spine surgery

Anterior cervical spine fusion has been used to treat infections, vascular disease, tumours and degenerative diseases of the cervical spine (Grisoli et al., 1989).

Post-operative dysphagia is reported in the literature (Stewart et al., 1995). Swallowing difficulties associated with this procedure include: impaired pharyngeal contraction in the proximity of the surgical site; reduced laryngeal closure, reduced epiglottic inversion and reduced opening of the upper oesophageal sphincter (Martin et al., 1997). Complications arising from surgery (oedema, tissue tear, haematoma, infection and deinnervation) may contribute to the development of dysphagia in this population (Buckholz et al., 1993).

PSYCHIATRIC DISORDERS

A very small group of individuals may present with fear of swallowing 'phagophobia'. This is a form of psychogenic dysphagia. Individuals present with a sensation of being unable to swallow a bolus and sometimes a fear of aspiration (Shapiro et al., 1997). Associated complaints may include a feeling of throat pressure, constriction or closure and difficulty initiating the swallow reflex. Some individuals may also describe the sensation of a foreign body in the throat (see earlier section on mechanical oesophageal disorders), which is present at rest and not aided by swallowing a bolus. Unplanned weight loss is also a symptom of this disorder. Diagnosis of phagophobia can only be made where there are normal head and neck examinations and normal videofluroscopy or endsocospy results. Individuals with this disorder often have difficulty managing stress in their lives, and the suggestion has been made that the fear of swallowing symptomatology is an attempt to channel their anxiety into the bodies. The speech pathologist may play a part in assuring the patient that there is no true dysphagia, and then consider referring the individual for psychological support.

TRACHEOSTOMY

The tracheostomy population is cause for special reference. A bedside clinical assessment is used most often in this population due to the difficulties associated with transporting or positioning them for instrumental assessments. There are entire texts devoted to the assessment and treatment of the tracheotomized patient (e.g. Dikeman and Kazandjian, 2003). This text will provide an outline of the assessment and management of the tracheotomized patient. The speech pathologist's role in tracheostomy is:

- the assessment of swallowing function;
- treatment and management of swallowing disorders;
- decannulation; and
- voice and communication.

Teamwork in this population is integral. The team involved with the tracheostomized patient may include: the speech pathologist, ENT, nursing staff, physiotherapist, and other medical specialties such as neurosurgery. This list is not exhaustive.

Tracheostomy or tracheotomy: what is it and why is it used?

A tracheo*tomy* is the *incision* that is made into the trachea through the skin and muscles of the neck. The incision is usually made between the third and fourth tracheal rings, well away from the true vocal folds to avoid damage to the larynx. A tracheo*stomy* is the creation of an opening into the trachea where the tracheal mucosa is brought into continuity with the skin (Dorlands, 1989). A tracheostomy tube is a tube made of plastic or stainless steel that is placed into the incision site to ensure that the 'opening' remains open. A relatively small portion of the tube can be seen on the external surface of the neck, with the larger portion contained within the trachea (see Figure 9.1). Once a tracheostomy tube is placed, the individual breathes in and out of the tube, not through the mouth. Similarly, coughing causes expulsion of secretions from the trache tube, not the mouth. Voice cannot be produced (see note below) as the air from the lungs that would usually cause the vocal folds to vibrate to cause speech is redirected out of the body at the level of the neck, rather than up through the cords.

Tracheostomy tubes are usually placed to:

• allow ventilation and oxygentation;
• to maintain an airway that would otherwise close;
• to eliminate airway obstruction (for example oedema that may occur after oral, pharyngeal or laryngeal surgery);
• to reduce the potential for aspiration (see cuffed versus uncuffed tubes below); and
• provide access to the airway and lungs for pulmonary toilet.

Tracheostomy tubes may be long term or short term. Long-term trache tubes are generally made of robust materials including silver, stainless steel or silicone plastic. Shorter term trache tubes may be made from PVC plastic.

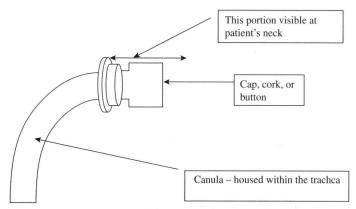

Figure 9.1   Schematic diagram of an uncuffed tracheostomy tube (note the cap/cork/button is not usually in place – see text)

The tracheostomy tube – a walking tour

The tracheostomy tube is a tube that curves gently at an angle of about 45° (see Figure 9.1). It consists of:

- an obturator;
- a cannula; and
- a cap, cork, or button.

The obturator is a device that fits inside the cannula (i.e. the tube). The surgeon uses it during the initial insertion of the trache tube into the incision. It is blunt ended and projects through the end of the trache tube that sits inside the patient's trachea. It is round ended so that during insertion it does not cause unnecessary trauma to the patient's tissue and mucosa. Once the trache tube is *in situ,* the obturator is redundant, having served its purpose to aid in the insertion process.

The *cannula* is the trache tube proper. As noted above, a small portion is visible at the patient's neck, with the majority of the tube sitting inside the trachea. The cannula is usually tied in place around the neck with a thin cloth strap. The tube holds the incision site open and fights the body's natural urge to 'heal and close the incision'. The trache tube may consist of two tubes, one inside the other. These are known as outer and inner cannulas. The outer cannula remains in the patient's trachea at all times, whereas the inner cannula can be removed for cleaning purposes. Not all trache tubes have two cannulas, with many having only one. There is a range of cannula sizes (e.g. size 4, 6 or 8). These sizes denote the size of the tube opening (the diameter). The size of the tube can be found on the flange of the trache tube at the patient's neck. The size of the trache tube is important. A large diameter tube, (e.g. size 8) takes up a lot of the available space within the trachea (another tube) whereas a smaller size tube (i.e. a size 4) takes up less space. Note also that the inner diameter of the tube is necessarily smaller than the outer diameter (e.g. inner diameter 5 mm, outer diameter of same tube 7 mm).

The cannula may be cuffed or uncuffed. The cuff is a balloon that fits around the lower portion of the trache tube. The cuff can be inflated or deflated. Figure 9.2 shows a schematic drawing of a cuffed trache tube where the cuff is inflated. When the cuff is inflated it forms a physical barrier between what is above the cuff (i.e. the larynx, pharynx etc.) and what is below it (the lungs and bronchial tree), with air passing only through the trache tube. It is like a little rubber tyre that, when inflated, should only press gently in against the walls of the trachea to seal it off from material (food, saliva, blood) that would otherwise enter it from the oral or pharyngeal regions. When the cuff is deflated, the little balloon/tyre shrinks so that air can pass *around* the trachea tube as well as through the trache tube. In addition, material from the oral or pharyngeal cavities can potentially pass down the sides of the trache tube and into the trachea and lungs. Because the cuff is inside the patient, we can't tell by looking at them whether the cuff is up or down. For this reason, the cuff is connected via a thin tube to a 'pilot balloon', which is attached to the outside of the trache tube. When the pilot balloon is inflated, the cuff inside the trachea is inflated, when the

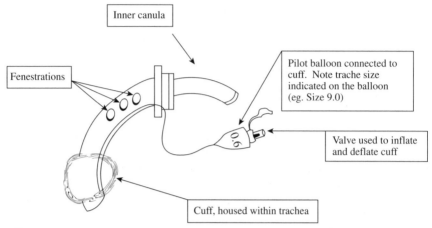

Figure 9.2   Cuffed tracheostomy tube with cuff inflated (note pilot balloon, size etc.)

pilot balloon is deflated the cuff inside the trachea is deflated. The cuff inside the trachea is inflated or deflated using the pilot balloon. There is a one-way valve on the pilot balloon to ensure that the air either stays in the cuff or is properly removed from the cuff. A syringe is typically used to inflate or deflate the pilot balloon, and hence the cuff.

There are recommendations for the amount of air that should be inserted into the cuff to ensure that it fills to the point where the cuff touches the tracheal circumference without pushing the trachea out of shape by overinflation. Overinflation may cause damage to the mucosa of the trachea and result in medical complications. The patient's treating doctor, nurse or physiotherapist should be consulted to determine the appropriate amount of air that should be placed into the pilot balloon, often using the 'minimal leak technique'. The minimal leak technique is when the cuff is inflated to the point where air cannot be passed around the trache tube, and then 1 cc to 2 cc of air is removed from the pilot to ensure that the cuff is not irritating the tracheal wall.

A cuffed trache tube may be used when it is needed for respiratory treatment or if the patient is at high risk of aspiration. The uncuffed trache tube still allows access to the lungs for suctioning; however, the patient can still 'breathe around' the trache tube as well as through the tube. Without the cuff, there is no physical barrier to prevent aspiration. There are different types of cuffs available, varying in the type of material, shape or fit (Dikeman and Kazandjian, 2003). For example, there is a foam cuff, which is quite spongy when compared with a plastic cuff. The foam cuff is less irritating on the tracheal wall when inflated than the plastic cuff. However, it is not possible to totally deflate the foam cuff as effectively as the plastic cuff.

The cannula or tube may also be fenestrated or unfenestrated. Fenestration comes from the Italian word *finestra* meaning 'window' (see also Figure 9.2). This simply means that the trache tube may (fenestrated) or may not (unfenestrated) have a hole or 'window', in the tube that sits inside the patient's trachea. When it is present the fenestration is usually in the curved portion of the tube. The hole in the trache tube allows the air to pass through the hole (fenestration) to the vocal folds above it. This promotes vocalization if the trache tube is occluded during voice production trials. There may be one large hole or multiple smaller holes that form the fenestration. The fenestration is usually in the outer cannula when there is an outer and inner cannula present. The inner cannula may or may not also be fenestrated. If it is not fenestrated, the clinician may take the inner cannula out during therapy to use the fenestration to good effect. If the inner cannula is fenestrated, care should be taken when positioning it back into the outer cannula, in order that the fenestrations on the inner and outer cannulas are aligned. If the fenestrations are not well aligned there is the possibility of granulation tissue forming over the fenestration. Generally, a patient with a fenestrated trache tube will be at low risk for aspiration.

The trache tube may also have a cap, cork, button or plug. These are interchangeable terms that do as they suggest and plug the end of the tracheostomy tube. When the plug is in place, the air from the lungs must travel up through the trachea, through the narrow space around the trache tube through the larynx and up via the pharynx, nasal and oral cavities for speech production. If the patient has an inner and outer cannula, the inner cannula should be removed before placing the plug onto the trache tube. The plug is most often used when the patient is getting ready for decannulation (i.e. removal of the tracheostomy tube). When the plug is in place, the patient can speak, using the vocal folds as the air is being passed in the usual way from the lungs up to the vocal tract. Trache tubes can also be occluded momentarily using a gloved finger. This process would allow the clinician to determine whether the patient can achieve voice, with the ability to remove the gloved finger from the end of the trache tube very quickly if the patient becomes distressed (either emotional or respiratory distress).

Humidification

There is often artificial humidification applied to the trache tube opening in the neck. A tracheal mask or thermovent may be attached to or placed over the end of the trache tube. Non-tracheostomized individuals usually breathe air that is humidified by the nose. In the tracheostomized person, the air enters directly into the pulmonary system, bypassing the nasal cavity. The humidification of air reduces the risk of drying the respiratory mucosa. By keeping secretions moist, there is a reduced risk of secretions becoming thick. Moist secretions will also be more easily cleared than viscous ones.

TRACHEOSTOMY SWALLOWING ASSESSMENT – A VARIATION ON THE STANDARD BEDSIDE EXAMINATION

Ideally the speech pathologist works as part of a team for swallowing assessment of the tracheostomized patient. Although institution-specific, usually a nurse or physiotherapist will assist during the assessment to provide suctioning. The swallowing assessment should be deferred if there is:

- reduced/fluctuating level of consciousness;
- poor respiratory status;
- poor chest condition;
- poor ability to manage secretions/spontaneous swallow; or
- an ineffective cough.

The team should be consulted to determine whether any of the above conditions apply. The speech pathologist should be aware of whether the patient requires ventilation support. Oxygen saturation monitoring may be required, or the physiotherapist may 'bag' the patient. 'Bagging' is the process of manually providing air to the pulmonary system by way of a balloon like device. Phases one to three of the bedside assessment outlined previously should be carried out. The difference between the bedside examination of a non-tracheotomized patient and one with a tracheostomy tube lies in two areas: (a) the clinician's understanding of the differences that the tracheostomy tube makes to respiration, swallowing and phonation, and (b) the actual process of assessing the tracheostomized patient.

The clinician should determine:

- the size of the trache tube;
- whether it is cuffed or uncuffed;
- fenestrated or non-fenestrated;
- outer cannula only or inner and outer cannula.

If the trache tube is cuffed, the clinician should determine from the team whether it is possible to deflate the cuff during swallowing trials. If it is possible to deflate the cuff, the clinician should deflate the cuff while the nurse or physiotherapist simultaneously suctions. This occurs prior to any oral trials to ensure that the pulmonary system is clear. The patient is then given foods or fluids to swallow. The clinician determines the best texture to start with and the amount tested. Generally small amounts of thicker substances are tested first, with the patient then suctioned to see whether any of the material has been aspirated. In order to make it easier to determine whether the material suctioned has come from the swallowing trial the material may be dyed blue. This is known as the *Modified Evans Blue Dye Test*.

The blue dye test

The blue dye test is an assessment for clients with a tracheostomy tube *in situ* only. The client is given fluid or food impregnated with an inert blue dye, obtainable upon prescription ('methylene blue') or food or fluid coloured with blue food colouring. Saliva may also be impregnated with blue dye. A blue dye is chosen as it provides a non-organic colour immediately distinguishable from blood, sputum or mucous. There have been conflicting reports of the validity of the technique (Wilson, 1992; Logemann, 1994; Thompson-Henry and Braddock, 1995). There is also some evidence that clients may experience gastric irritation from food dyes. At present there is no standardized protocol for this procedure. Speech pathologists who are not experienced in trache management are not advised to use this test without qualified supervision.

The Evans Blue Dye Test involves placing drops of blue dye on the tongue every 4 hours and the trachea is suctioned at set intervals over a 48-hour period, with the secretions monitored for evidence of a blue tinge (Belafsky et al., 2003). The efficacy of these tests will be discussed further below. The patient may be suctioned on more than one occasion during the swallowing trials. For example suctioning may occur after a few trial mouthfuls, and then again later in the assessment. The clinician should bear in mind that it is possible for material to pool in the pharynx and that there may be a time delay before the material is aspirated. For this reason it is advisable to have a delay between testing of different textures of fluids so as not to confuse the results from one consistency with another. Dikeman and Kazandjian (1995) suggested that the patient should be suctioned immediately after the trial and then at 15-minute intervals over a 1 hour period. Clinicians will then often monitor the patient for the remainder of the day. A delay of 2 hours between trials of, say, thickened fluids and thin fluids may be required to ensure, as far as possible, that the results refer only to the consistency being tested. The presence of any dye in the tracheal secretions is monitored accordingly. A 'positive test' is the presence of blue dye in the tracheal suctioning, which indicates that the bolus or secretions have entered the trachea. A 'negative test' is the absence of blue dye in the secretions suctioned. There are acknowledged problems with the technique. For example, (a) it is unclear when the person aspirated – before, during or after the swallow, or (b) why the aspiration occurred, and (c) exactly how much they aspirated. The blue dye test is also not able to provide information that will aid in swallowing re-education. The blue dye test should be viewed as *part* of the information that makes up the *total clinical examination*. Dikeman and Kazandjian (2003) also noted that blue dye could be added to nasogastric or gastrostomy feeds to provide evidence of gastrointestinal contents in tracheal secretions. This may provide evidence of reflux which would require further investigation.

During the clinical assessment of the tracheostomized patient, the patient's vocal quality and cough reflex can also be assessed. Momentary occlusion of the trache using a gloved finger, if it is medically safe to do so and tolerated by the patient, may assist the patient in producing phonation or a cough. At the conclusion of the swallowing trials, the patient's cuff should be reinflated, using the minimal leak technique of institutional recommendations. If the blue dye test is positive, the test should be terminated and another consistency tested if it is logical to do so. If a negative test occurs, the clinician may proceed with caution to larger volumes and different textures.

Efficacy of the blue dye test

The Evans Blue Dye Test and the Modified Evans Blue Dye test are used as an assessment of swallowing function in tracheostomized patients to ascertain whether there is a connection between the oral cavity and the trachea that should not be there. There have been conflicting results as to the validity of the blue dye test. Wilson (1992) investigated 20 medical and surgical patients with cuffed tracheostomy tubes in place and demonstrated that the blue dye test was valid and reliable for determining aspiration with a liquid bolus, but not for a custard consistency. The results were compared with videofluorscopy evidence of aspiration. However, Thompson-Henry and Braddock (1995), in a retrospective study of only five tracheostomy patients, found that when compared to videofluoroscopy or fibreoptic evaluation of swallowing (FEES), the blue dye test was not as accurate in detecting aspiration.

Belafsky et al. (2003) recently reported a study of 30 tracheostomy patients that overall sensitivity of the blue dye test was 82%, with a specificity of 38%. The authors found that the sensitivity of the blue dye test improved for patients receiving mechanical ventilation to be 100%, compared with 76% for individuals not receiving mechanical ventilation. However, the specificity of the blue dye test in both conditions remained poor. There were, however, some methodological issues with this research. The gold standard used in this case was FEES; however, the FEES assessment was not carried out until 24 hours after the final administration of the test bolus. It is very difficult to predict retrospectively what the patient was doing the day before. The authors themselves state that swallowing safety fluctuates significantly depending on numerous things, some of which include the time of day, the level of fatigue, mental status and patient positioning. Donzelli et al. (2001) also investigated the use of the blue dye test in determining aspiration. These investigators used the novel approach of inserting an endoscope into the tracheal opening and viewing upwards towards the vocal folds, and downwards towards the bronchial tree to visually inspect for evidence of aspiration and compare this to material suctioned from the trachea. This design is good. However, the researchers only conducted a visual inspection immediately after the bolus had been swallowed. They were disparaging of the blue dye test because the suctioning of the tracheal secretions failed to capture blue dye that had appeared above the stoma site. If the researchers had suctioned again at 30 and 60 minutes post-trial and had also visualized with each of these, the results may have been different. This aspect of repeated suctioning at regular intervals after swallow trials is important to the successful use of the technique. The authors argued that the blue dye test was better for determining frank aspiration, than trace amounts.

O'Neil-Pirozzi et al. (2003) conducted an extremely thorough assessment of the use of the blue dye test for determining aspiration in the tracheotomized population. The most interesting findings of this study were that aspiration judgements were more likely to agree when:

• a cuff was deflated than when it was inflated, or when the trache tube was cuffless; and
• a speaking valve was worn as opposed to it being unoccluded or buttoned.

There were no significant differences dependant upon the diameter of trache tube, type of trache tube (fenestrated or unfenestrated), or consistency of bolus tested (liquid, nectar liquid, puree). The authors did find pureed solids to be the consistency aspirated most frequently, followed by secretions and thin liquids and finally thick nectar liquid. O'Neil-Pirozzi et al. (2003) found that the sensitivity of the blue dye test of 79.3% and the specificity of 61.9%. The positive predictive value was 74.2% and the negative predictive value was 68.4%.

Clearly the blue dye test is not fail safe. However, in acutely unwell individuals who are often not able to be transported to or able to cope with instrumental assessment, it is an adjunct screening assessment worth doing. Some of the factors that could make use of the blue dye test more variable include: the amount of dye used, the type of dye used (e.g. blue food colouring or methylene blue, or other variations of same), frequency of suctioning after trials, and experience and skill of the person performing the suctioning of tracheal secretions.

Cuff deflation trials and decannulation – the role of the speech pathologist

As with the swallowing assessment, the speech pathologist works as part of a team during the process of cuff deflation trials and decannulation. Decannulation is the removal of the tracheostomy tube. The patient may commence cuff deflation trials when the medical team deems it safe to do so. The cuff is deflated for set periods of time that gradually increase until the patient is able to tolerate cuff deflation for 24 to 48 hours. Once this milestone has been reached, in consultation with the team, the patient may then be a candidate for having his or her tracheostomy tube removed. The cuff deflation trials are closely supervised for patient distress or inability to cope (either emotional or respiratory). Cuff deflation trials are also commenced during the day, with overnight trials the final step of achievement. Some indicators that the patient may be ready to commence cuff deflation trials are:

- adequate level of alertness;
- clear chest;
- effective cough (i.e. ability to cough up to the trache tube);
- spontaneous saliva swallows;
- infrequent oral or tracheal suctioning (as a guide, frequent suctioning would be more than once per half hour, however, the clinician should consult team members);
- no clinical evidence of aspiration.

During cuff deflation trials it is important that the patient be monitored. This is to ensure that if the patient becomes distressed the cuff can be reinflated. The amount of time the patient tolerates cuff deflation should also be recorded and the reason or reasons why the cuff was reinflated should be documented. As the cuff is deflated and the patient is suctioned, the speech pathologist should note whether the patient coughs as the cuff is deflated and the amount of secretions suctioned after deflating the cuff. Either coughing immediately after cuff deflation and/or increased secretions suctioned after cuff deflation may indicate that the patient has been pooling material above the cuff. Evidence of increasing cough, inability to cope with oral secretions, temperature spikes, increased frequency of suctioning or deterioration in chest condition all indicate that cuff deflation is not being tolerated. Cuff deflation may not be tolerated for a number of reasons. Some of these include: poor respiratory function, upper airway obstruction, a tight fitting or too large trache tube, or vocal fold dysfunction.

During cuff deflation trials the speech pathologist may also wish to see how the patient copes with temporary occlusion of the trache so that the normal pattern of breathing, swallowing and speaking is temporarily resumed. This can be done with a gloved finger placed over the tracheostomy tube opening. The patient can be asked to inhale and then attempt to speak or phonate. The speech pathologist can gather information on effort required during inhalation and voice quality while the tube is occluded. Concerns regarding vocal fold function (via voice quality) or respiratory ability with the tube occluded should be promptly referred to an ENT specialist for further investigation. Patients may also be taught to occlude their trache tube with their fingers if their cognition is adequate. For longer-term use, the tube may be corked, capped or buttoned by placing the cork over the tracheal opening. Again the patient should be monitored closely for signs of distress.

An alternative to corking the tube is to provide a speaking valve. A speaking valve is a one-way valve that is placed over the end of the trache tube in the same manner as a cork. It differs in that the patient can still take air directly into the trache tube during inhalation. The valve then closes allowing air to be directed from the lungs up through the vocal folds so that speech can be made. Patients with thick viscous secretions or those that require frequent suctioning are not candidates for speaking valves. Patients who are unable to tolerate cuff deflation trials, or whose cuff cannot be fully deflated (e.g. those patients with foam-cuffed trache tubes), are not candidates for the speaking valve. Vocal fold paralysis, unstable medical or pulmonary status or cognitive affect would also be contraindications for use of the speaking valve.

After a successful period of cuff deflation trials (24 to 48 hours), plus or minus occlusion trials, *the team* may decide to remove the trache tube (decannulation). Alternatives to decannulation include downsizing the trache tube over a period of days, or replacing the tube with a fenestrated tube. The rationale for these regimes is that the trache tube can fill somewhere between two-thirds and three-quarters of the tracheal space, leaving little space for the patient to 'breathe around' the tube when it is occluded. It also increases the likelihood of respiratory distress if the patient has an extremely narrow space to breathe through. There is also the risk of medical complications or infections with increased frequency of tube changes. Thompson-Ward et al. (1999) used a retrospective study to document the decannulation process. They found that using the 24–48 hours successful cuff deflation method was a reliable method for indicating when it was appropriate to decannulate the patient. In comparison with changing trache tubes and progressively downsizing or changing to a fenestrated tube, the patient was better off with the new 'wait and see if they tolerate it' method. Using the 24–48 hour successful cuff deflation method, the researchers found the patients had:

- fewer trache tube changes;
- fewer days with a trache tube in place (5 days fewer);
- no significant increase in recannulation.

Once the trache tube is removed, the wound is covered with a water-resistant dressing. The patient will have to place his or her hand gently over the dressing and apply pressure to ensure that the air does not escape through the stoma site when coughing, talking and swallowing. The site generally heals in 4–5 days.

SWALLOWING DIFFICULTIES ASSOCIATED WITH TRACHEOSTOMY TUBES

The clinician should be aware that there are some swallowing difficulties intimately linked with having a tracheostomy tube. These include: reduced laryngeal excursion, 'reduced pharyngeal sensation, reduced cough response, disuse atrophy of the laryngeal muscles, oesophageal compression by an inflated cuff, and loss of subglottic air pressure and glottic flow' (Donzelli et al., 2001: 1746). O'Neil-Pirozzi et al. (2003) also note that reduced glottic closure may be a feature of the tracheostomized patient. Each of the conditions listed above can affect swallowing physiology. The presence of an opening at the neck also affects the 'valve' system during swallowing such that there is 'leakage' of the system. The patient requiring ventilation support loses the ability to use the natural swallow-respiratory cycle, with a pattern of respiration being forced upon them. Other less common complications include granuloma (an abrasion at the stoma site) and tracheoesophageal fistula (where the tracheal and oesophageal walls become connected and communicate, advancing the risk for dangerous aspiration). Tracheoesophageal fistulas can be caused by overinflating the trache tube so that there is pressure on the tracheal wall, which is immediately anterior to the oesophageal wall, or a nasogastric tube that is too large and causes rubbing of the same wall. A fistula will require surgical closure.

IN BRIEF – TRACHEOSTOMY AND THE PAEDIATRIC POPULATION

Paediatric tracheostomies are more demanding than adult tracheostomies and carry higher mortality and complication rates (Midwinter et al., 2002). There has been a change in the common indications for tracheostomy in the paediatric population. Introduction of endotracheal intubation in the 1970s and 1980s and the introduction of the haemophilus influenzae type B vaccine has significantly reduced rates of acute epiglottitis and laryngotracheobronchitis, which had previously been managed by tracheostomy tube (Hadfield et al., 2003). The most common indications for paediatric tracheostomy now include prolonged ventilation due to neuromuscular or respiratory problems or subglottic stenosis. Other indicators for tracheostomy include: tracheal stenosis, respiratory papillomatosis, caustic alkali ingestion and craniofacial syndromes (Hadfield et al., 2003). Tracheostomies may also be required for physiological airway anomalies including neuromuscular disease, head or spinal cord injury or damage to the central nervous system.

Midwinter et al. (2002) reported that 65% of patients tracheostomized in their facility were less than one year of age with approximately 30% less than three months of age at the time of tracheostomy. With advances in medical management of critically sick and premature infants, their survival rates have improved, which may explain the percentage of traches in young infants. Midwinter et al. (2002) found that children who required tracheostomy for acquired subglottic stenosis frequently required a longer period of cannulation (months or years) than children who required a tracheostomy for acute upper airway infections (days or weeks). The most frequent complication for paediatric tracheostomies is granulation formation around the stoma, with children under one year of age having a higher risk of complication (Midwinter et al., 2002). The most common complication of decannulation was persistence of tracheocutaneous fistula, the incidence of which was related to the age of the child (mean age 11.5 months) and longer duration of tracheostomy (mean length 39 months).

Tracheostomy tubes for the paediatric population are by necessity smaller in size and diameter to accommodate their smaller structures. The average paediatric tubes appear to commence at 3 mm, and can extend up to 7 mm depending on the brand purchased. Like the adult tubes, paediatric tubes can be cuffed or uncuffed, fenestrated or unfenestrated and come in a range of material types. Speaking valves can also be attached to paediatric trache tubes.

One of the key differences between adult and paediatric tracheostomies and speaking valves is a method of explanation that is suitable to the child's level of development. There is a range of commercial resources available to assist the clinician in doing this. The clinician should also be aware that children may develop aversive behaviours towards speaking valves including coughing and breath holding. The behavioural element in children makes working with tracheostomy tubes in this population very challenging. Therapy needs to be highly motivational, fun, functional and family-centred. Note that there is also a correlation between tracheostomy tubes and high risk of speech and language delay or deficit (Arvedson and Brodsky, 1992). More specifically, slow development of sound acquisition, vowel production, the distinction between voiced and voiceless consonants, and excessive use of immature phonological processes have been associated with children with a history of trachestomy prior to eight months of age (Kertoy et al., 1999).

Clinical assessment of children with tracheostomy tubes should include a standard oromotor assessment, assessment of oral reflexes, and clinical feeding evaluation. Blue dye tests are also possible in this population. Intervention typically covers oral stimulation or desensitization programmes (client specific), taste programmes, oral trials and carer education sessions. Midwinter et al. (2002) describe their regime for decannulation, which begins with endoscopy to determine patency of the airway. Once this has been established to be adequate, the tracheostomy tube is reduced in size. Trache occlusion trials occur as per the adult regime, and a speaking valve could be used if the patient is suitable. Midwinter et al. (2002) then also perform endoscopy to again assess the airway immediately prior to decannulation. The trache tube is removed under general anaesthetic. The child is carefully monitored for tolerance of tube removal for 48 hours. Decannulation regimes will vary from institution to institution.

MEDICATION AND DYSPHAGIA

The speech pathologist needs to be aware of the effects of administration of certain types of medications on swallowing function, and also the way in which medications are provided to individuals with dysphagia. The speech pathologist is not expected to have expert pharmacological knowledge.

MEDICATIONS THAT CAN INDUCE DYSPHAGIA

There are four main effects of medications on swallowing function:

• those that act as CNS depressants;
• neuroleptic medications that can result in extrapyramidal symptoms;
• those that affect oesophageal disorders; and
• those that affect salivary flow.

A summary is provided in Table 9.8.

CENTRAL NERVOUS SYSTEM (CNS) EFFECTS

Medications such as tranquillizers, narcotic analgesics or barbiturates are CNS depressants. These sorts of drugs may impair the patient's level of consciousness and thereby suppress the protective reflexes necessary for swallow-respiratory co-ordination (Palmer and Carden, 2003). Antipsychotic medications (e.g. haloperidol) are often used in the treatment of dementia, and can also have a sedative effect on the CNS depending on dosage (Stanniland and Taylor, 2000). Other drugs, such as the anticholinergics, have been linked with constipation, dry mouth, possible cognitive impairment and confusion, amongst other symptoms (Stanniland and Taylor, 2000).

DRUG-INDUCED EXTRAPYRAMIDAL SYNDROMES

Neuroleptic medications can cause extrapyramidal symptoms than can affect swallowing. Neuroleptics are also known as antipsychotics and are often used in the treatment of psychosis and schizophrenia. Neuroleptic-induced Parkinsonism has been reported to occur in 12% to 45% of individuals, more commonly in the elderly (Sokoloff and Pavlakovic, 1997). It presents with the features of Parkinson's disease, including the disorders of swallowing (described earlier). Fortunately, when the medication is discontinued the condition resolves; however, resolution may take

Table 9.8 Drugs that cause dysphagia

Mechanism	Drug/drug classification
Xerostomia	Anticholinergics
	Antihypertensives
	Cardiovascular agents
	Diuretics
	Opiates
	Antipsychotics
	Antiemetics
	Antidepressents
	Muscle relaxants
	Antihistamines
Reduced lower oesophageal sphincter	Theophylline
pressure (increased reflux risk)	Nitrates
	Calcium antagonists
	Anticholinergics
	Diazepam
	Morphine
Oesophageal injury	Antibiotics
	Ascorbic acid
	Nonsteroidal anti-inflammatory drugs
	(NSAIDS) and aspirin
	Ferrous sulfate
	Prednisone
	Potassium chloride
	Quinidine
Extrapyramidal effects	Antipsychotics
	Metoclopramide
	Prochlorperazine(risperidone)

Source: Sokoloff and Pavlakovic (1997: 178).

months. There is a general consensus that atypical neuroleptics (e.g. risperidone) are less often associated with extrapyramidal side effects but this is not always the case (Sokoloff and Pavlakovic, 1997; Stewart, 2003). Again, once the medication is discontinued, the condition is eventually reversible.

Antipsychotic medications can also result in an extrapyramidal presentation known as tardive dyskinesia. This is characterized by abnormal involuntary orofacial movements (e.g. tongue protrusion or increased rate of eye blinking) and persists despite withdrawal of the antipsychotic medication (Stanniland and Taylor, 2000). The oral, pharyngeal or oesophageal phases of swallowing may all be disrupted due to the dyskinetic movement and extrapyramidal symptoms.

OESOPHAGEAL DISORDERS

There are more than 70 drugs that have been implicated in the induction of oesophageal disorders. Capsules or tablets may be delayed in their passage through the oesophagus, with direct and acute injury to the oesophagus caused by caustic coating, chemical concentration including pH, size of the tablet, etc. (Jasperson, 2000). Patients may present with pain on swallowing. Factors that contribute to drug-induced oesophageal disorders include fasting, recumbent position, reduced saliva production, not enough fluid taken with the medication, duration of direct contact of the medication with the mucosa, pre-exisiting oesophageal disease, age and polypharmacy (Jasperson, 2000). Older individuals are most at risk of drug-induced oesophagitis due to the fact that older people receive more medications (for multiple medical problems), they spend more time in a recumbent position, they produce less saliva, and may be prone to forgetting doctor's instructions on correct ingestion of the tablet/capsule (e.g. sufficient water) (Jasperson, 2000). Hyper or hypo oesophageal sphincter disorders will also predispose the individual to oeosphageal injury. Note that in the case of pharyngeal motility disorders, it is equally possible for oral medications to collect in the valleculae or pyriform sinus post swallow, causing similar local damage to the pharyngeal mucosa. Drugs that reduce lower oesophageal sphincter tone include: theophylline, calcium channel antagonists, benzodiazepines, nonsteroidal anti-inflammatory drugs (Kikawada et al., 2005).

SALIVARY FLOW

Drugs that are known to reduce salivary flow include: tricyclic antidepressants, antiparkinsonian drugs, diuretics, neuroleptics, antiemetics, antihypertensives, and antihistamines. A reduction in salivary flow allows favourable conditions for the growth of pathogenic oral microflora and an increase in dental and periodontal disease (see also section on effects of radiation and chemotherapy in this chapter).

ADMINISTRATION OF DRUGS TO INDIVIDUALS WITH DYSPHAGIA

The speech pathologist has a role in liaising with medical staff in ensuring that medications are provided safely to individuals with dysphagia. It makes little sense to provide an individual on a vitamized diet and full thick fluids with tablets, capsules, or even 'thin liquid' medications. Individuals with facial palsy may pocket the tablet in the buccal region, which may cause discomfort as the tablet dissolves, or else presents as an aspiration risk. Where there is any concern, the speech pathologist should liaise with pharmacy and medical staff to ensure the patient's safety. Note also that it may not be possible to crush some tablets as it destroys enteric coating and allows premature exposure of the contents to regions for which they are not intended (e.g. the pharynx). Some tablets may not be able to be carried in a jam bolus or thick liquid bolus for similar reasons. Inability to comply with, or poor compliance with, medications is also not in the best interests of the patient. Morita (2003) has developed a 'deglutition aid jelly' which changes 'all solid preparations into gelatinous dosage form preparations'. Caution is required, however, in that not all medications may be suitable for this type of transformation. Collaboration with a pharmacist and treating doctor is advised in all cases.

REFERENCES

Arvedson JC, Brodsky L (1992) Paediatric tracheotomy referrals to speech language pathology in a children's hospital. International Journal of Paediatric Otorhinolaryngology 23(3): 237–43.

Aviv JE, Liu H, Kaplan ST, et al. (2000) Laryngopharyngeal sensory deficits in patients with laryngopharyngeal reflux and dysphagia. Annals of Otology, Rhinology and Laryngology 109(11): 1000–6.

Axford JS (2004) Rheumatic disease. In Axford JS, O'Callaghan CA (eds) Medicine (2nd edn). Boston MA: Blackwell Science.

Bateman DE (1992) Neurology of the face: facial palsy. British Journal of Hospital Medicine 47(6): 430–1.

Belafsky PC (2003) Abnormal endoscopic pharyngeal and laryngeal findings attributable to reflux. American Journal of Medicine 115: 90–6.

Belafsky PC, Blumenfeld L, LePage A, et al. (2003) The accuracy of the modified Evan's blue dye test in predicting aspiration. Laryngoscope 113(11): 1969–72.

Brin MF, Younger D (1988) Neurologic disorders and aspiration. Otolaryngolic Clinics of North America 21(4): 691–9.

Brown M, Gordon WA, Spielman L (2003) Participation in social and recreational activity in the community by individuals with traumatic brain injury. Rehabilitation Psychology 48(4): 266–74.

Buckholz D (1987) Neurologic causes of dysphagia. Dysphagia 1: 152–6.

Buckholz D, Jones B, Ravic WJ (1993) Dysphagia following anterior cervical fusion. Dysphagia 8: 390.

Campbell BH, Spinelli K, Marbella AM, et al. (2004) Aspiration, weight loss, and quality of life in head and neck cancer survivors. Archives of Otolaryngology – Head and Neck Surgery 130(9): 1100–1103.

Canning BJ, Mazzone SB (2003) Reflex mechanisms in gastroesophageal reflux disease and asthma. American Journal of Medicine 115(3A): 45S–48S.

Carota A, Staub F, Bogousslavsky J (2003) The behaviours of the acute stroke patient. In Bogousslavsky J (ed.) Acute Stroke Treatment (2nd edn). London: Martin Dunitz.

Chen H-C, Chana J, Chang C-H, et al. (2003) A new method of subcutaneous placement of free jejunal flaps to reconstruct a diversionary conduit for swallowing in complicated pharyngoesophageal injury. Plastic and Reconstructive Surgery 112(6): 1528–33.

Coelho CA (1987) Preliminary findings on the nature of dysphagia in patients with chronic obstructive pulmonary disease. Dysphagia 2: 28–31.

Counihan TJ (2004) Cerebrovascular disease. In Andreoli TE, Carpenter CCJ, Griggs RC, Loscalzo J (eds) CECIL Essentials of Medicine (6th edn). Philadelphia: WB Saunders.

Daniels SK, Foundas AL (1999) Lesion localisation in acute stroke with risk of aspiration. Journal of Neuroimaging 9: 91–8.

Davies GR, Rampton DS (2004) Gastrointestinal disease. In Axford JS, O'Callaghan CA (eds) Medicine (2nd edn). Boston MA: Blackwell Science.

Dikeman KJ, Kazandjian MS (1995) Communication and Swallowing Management of Tracheostomized and Ventilator-Dependent Adults. San Diego CA: Singular.

Dikeman KJ, Kazandjian MS (2003) Communication and Swallowing Management of Tracheostomized and Ventilator-Dependent Adults (2nd edn). New York: Thomson, Delmar Learning.

Donzelli J, Brady S, Wesling M, et al. (2001) Simultaneous modified Evans blue dye procedure and video nasal endoscopic evaluation of the swallow. Laryngoscope 111(10): 1746–50.

Dorland's Pocket Medical Dictionary (1989) 24th edn. Philadelphia: WB Saunders.

Duong TT, Englander J, Wright J, et al. (2004) Relationship between strength, balance, and swallowing deficits and outcome after traumatic brain injury: a multicenter analysis. Archives of Physical Medicine and Rehabilitation 85: 1291–7.

Eggenberger SK, Nelms TP (2004) Artificial hydration and nutrition in advanced Alzheimer's disease: Facilitating family decision-making. Journal of Clinical Nursing 13(6): 661–7.

Eisbruch A, Schwartz M., Rasch C, et al. (2002) Dysphagia and aspiration after chemoradiotherapy for head-and-neck cancer: which anatomic structures are affected and can they be spared by IMRT? International Journal of Radiation Oncology 60(5): 1425–39.

Feinberg MJ (1993) Radiographic techniques and interpretation of abnormal swallowing in adults and elderly patients. Dysphagia 8: 356–8.

Ferraris VA, Ferraris SP, Moritzm D, et al. (2001) Oropharyngeal dysphagia after cardiac operations. Annals of Thoracic Surgery 71: 1792–6.

Finestone HM, Greene-Finestone LS (2003) Rehabilitation medicine: 2. Diagnosis of dysphagia and its nutritional management for stroke patients. Canadian Medical Association Journal 169(10): 1041–4.

FOOD Trial Collaboration (2005) Effect of timing and method of enteral tube feeding for dysphagic stroke patients (FOOD): a multicentre randomised controlled trial. Lancet 365: 764–72.

Garon BR, Engle M, Ormiston C (1997) A randomized control study to determine the effects of unlimited oral intake of water in patient with identified aspiration. Journal of Neurologic Rehabilitation 11(3): 139–48.

Geis CC, Moroz A, O'Neill BJ, et al. (2004) Stroke and neurodegenerative disorders 4. Neurodegenerative disorders. Archives of Physical Medicine and Rehabilitation 85(3): S21–S33 Supplement 1.

Gillespie MB, Brodsky MB, Day TA, et al. (2004) Swallowing-related quality of life after head and neck cancer treatment. Laryngoscope, 114(8): 1362–7.

Gillespie SH, Sonnex C, Carne C (2004) Infectious diseases. In Axford JS, O'Callaghan CA (eds) Medicine (2nd edn). Boston MA: Blackwell Science.

Good-Fratturelli MD, Curlee, RF, Holle JL (2000) Prevalence and nature of dysphagia in VA patients with COPD referred for videofluoroscopic swallow examination. Journal of Communication Disorders 33: 93–110.

Gordon C, Hewer RL, Wade DT (1987) Dysphagia in acute stroke. British Medical Journal 295: 411–14.

Goto R, Miyabe K, Mori N (2002) Thermal burn of the pharynx and larynx after swallowing hot milk. Auris, Nanus, Larynx 29: 301–3.

Griggs RC (2004a) Neuromuscular diseases: disorder of the motor neuron and plexus and peripheral nerve disease. In Andreoli TE, Carpenter CCJ, Griggs RC, et al. (eds) CECIL Essentials of Medicine (6th edn). Philadelphia PA: WB Saunders.

Griggs RC (2004b) Neuromuscular junction disease. In Andreoli TE, Carpenter CCJ, Griggs RC, et al. (eds) CECIL Essentials of Medicine (6th edn). Philadelphia PA: WB Saunders.

Griggs RC (2004c) Demyelinating and inflammatory disorders. In Andreoli TE, Carpenter CCJ, Griggs RC, et al. (eds) CECIL Essentials of Medicine (6th edn). Philadelphia PA: WB Saunders.

Grisoli F, Garziana N, Fabrizi A, et al. (1989) Anterior discectomy without fusion for treatment of cervical lateral soft disc extrusion: a follow-up of 120 cases. Neurosurgery 24(6): 853–9.

Grobbelaar EJ, Owen S, Tomance AD, et al. (2004) Nutritional challenges in head and neck cancer. Clinical Otolaryngology 29(4): 307–13.

Guchelaar HJ, Vermes A, Meerwaldt JH (1997) Radiation-induced xerostomia: Pathophysiology, clinical course and supportive treatment. Support Care Cancer 5: 281–8.

Hadfield PJ, Lloyd-Faulconbridge RV, Almeyda J, et al. (2003) The changing indications for pediatric tracheostomy. International Journal of Pediatric Otorhinolaryngology 67: 7–10.

Hadjikoutis S, Pickersgill TP, Dawson K, et al. (2000) Abnormal patterns of breathing during swallowing in neurological disorders. Brain 123(9): 1863–73.

Haider-Ali AM, Macgregor FB. Stewart M (1998) Myasthenia gravis presenting with dysphagia and post-operative ventilatory failure. Journal of Laryngology and Otology 112(12): 1194–5.

Halper AS, Cherney LR, Cichowski K, et al. (1999) Dysphagia after head trauma: the effect of cognitive-communicative impairments on functional outcomes. Journal of Head Trauma Rehabilitation 14(5): 486–96.

Halvorsen RA Jnr, Moelleken SMC, Kearney AT (2003) Videofluoroscopic evaluation of HIV/AIDS patients with swallowing dysfunction. Abdominal Imaging 28(2): 244–7.

Hamdy S, Aziz Q, Rothwell JC, et al. (1996) The cortical topography of human swallowing musculature in health and disease. Nature Medicine 2: 1217–24.

Hamdy S, Aziz Q, Rothwell JC, et al. (1997) Explaining oro-pharyngeal dysphagia after unilateral hemispheric stroke. Lancet 350: 686–92.

Hamdy S, Aziz Q, Rothwell JC, et al. (1998) Recovery of function after dysphagic stroke relates to functional reorganization in the intact motor cortex. Gastroenterology 115: 1104–12.

Hamdy S, Rothwell JC (1998) Gut feelings about recovery after stroke: the organisation and reorganisation of human swallowing motor cortex. Trends in Neuroscineces 21: 278–82.

Harding SM (2002) Oropharyngeal dysfunction in COPD patients. The need for clinical research (Editorial). Chest 121(2): 315–17.

Hillman K, Bishop G (2004) Clinical Intensive Care and Acute Medicine (2nd edn). Cambridge: Cambridge University Press.

Horner J, Massey EW, Riski JE, et al. (1988) Aspiration following stroke: clinical correlates and outcome. Neurology 38: 1359–62.

Iwamoto T, Fukuda S, Kikawada M, et al. (2005) Prognostic implications of swallowing deficits in elderly patients after initial recovery from stroke. Journals of Gerontology Series A 60(1): 120–4.

Jasperson D (2000) Drug-induced oesophageal disorders: pathogenesis, incidence, prevention and management. Drug Safety 22(3): 237–49.

Johnston BT, Li Q, Castell JA, et al. (1995) Swallowing and esophageal function in Parkinson's disease. American Journal of Gastroenterology 90(10): 1741–6.

Jones B (2003a) Aging and neurological disease. In Jones B (ed.) Normal and Abnormal Swallowing: Imaging in Diagnosis and Therapy (2nd edn). New York: Springer.

Jones B (2003b) Interpreting the study. In Jones B (ed.) Normal and Abnormal Swallowing: Imaging in Diagnosis and Therapy (2nd edn). New York: Springer.

Kertoy MK, Guest CM, Quart E, et al. (1999) Speech and phonological characteristics of individual children with a history of tracheostomy. Journal of Speech Language and Hearing Research 42(3): 621–35.

Khoshoo V, Le T, Haydel Jr RM, et al. (2003) Role of gastroesophageal reflux in older children with persistent asthma. Chest 123(4): 1008–13.

Kikawada M, Iwamoo T, Masaru T (2005) Aspiration and infection in the elderly: Epidemiology, diagnosis and management. Drugs and Ageing 22(2): 115–30.

Korn JH (2004) Systemic sclerosis (scleroderma). In Andreoli TE, Carpenter CCJ, Griggs RC, Loscalzo J (eds) CECIL Essentials of Medicine (6th edn). Philadelphia PA: WB Saunders.

Koufman JA, Aviv JE, Casiano RR, et al. (2002) Laryngopharyngeal reflux: position statement of the committee on speech, voice, and swallowing disorders of the American Academy of Otolaryngology-Head and Neck Surgery. Otolaryngology – Head and Neck Surgery 127(1): 32–5.

Langmore SE, Skarupski KA, Park PS, et al. (2002) Predictors of aspiration pneumonia in nursing home residents. Dysphagia 17: 298–307.

Langmore SE, Terpenning MS, Schork A, et al. (1998) Predictors of aspiration pneumonia: how important is dysphagia? Dysphagia 13: 69–81.

Lazarus CL (1993) Effects of radiation therapy and voluntary maneuvers on swallow functioning in head and neck cancer patients. Clinics in Communication Disorders 3(4): 11–20.

Lazarus C, Logemann J (1987) Swallowing disorders in closed head injury: diagnosis and treatment. Archives of Physical Medicine and Rehabilitation 68: 79–84.

Lazarus CL, Logemann JA, Pauloski R (1996) Swallowing disorders in head and neck cancer patients treated with radiotherapy and adjuvant chemotherapy. Laryngoscope 106: 1157–66.

Lenderking WR, Hillson E, Crawley JA, et al. (2003) The clinical characteristics and impact of laryngopharyngeal reflux disease on health-related quality of life. Value in Health 6(5): 560–5.

Lewin JS, Gillenwater AM, Garrett D, et al. (2003) Characterisation of laryngopharyngeal reflux in patients with premalignant or early carcinoma of the larynx. Cancer 97(4): 1010–14.

Logemann JA (1994) Non-imaging techniques for the study of swallowing. Acta Oto-Rhino-Laryngologica Belgica 48: 139–42.

Logemann JA (1996) Dysphagia in head and neck cancer. Paper presented at the National Dysphagia Symposium. Royal Prince Alfred Hospital, Sydney, Australia, 19–21 September.

Logemann JA (1998) Evaluation and Treatment of Swallowing Disorders (2nd edn). Austin TX: Pro-ed.

Logemann JA, Gibbons P, Rademaker AW, et al. (1994) Mechanisms of recovery of swallow after supraglottic laryngectomy. Journal of Speech and Hearing Research 37: 965–74.

Logemann JA, Roa Pauloski B, Rademaker AW, et al. (1993) Speech and swallow function after tonsil/base of tongue resection with primary closure. Journal of Speech and Hearing Research 36: 918–26.

Longman CM, Pearson GJ (1987) Variations in tooth surface temperature in the oral cavity during fluid intake. Biomaterials 8: 411–14.

Mackay LE, Morgan AS, Bernstein BA (1999) Swallowing disorders in severe brain injury: Risk factors affecting return to oral intake. Archives of Physical Medicine and Rehabilitation 80: 365–71.

Macleod M, Mumford CJ (2004) Neurological diseases. In JS Axford, CA O'Callaghan (eds) Medicine (2nd edn). Boston: Blackwell Science.

Martin RE, Neary MA, Diamant NE (1997) Dysphagia following cervical spine surgery. Dysphagia 12: 2–8.

Martin-Harris B (2000) Optimal patterns of care in patients with chronic obstructive pulmonary disease. Seminars in Speech and Language 21(4): 311–21.

Merkel PA (2004) Sjogren's syndrome. In Andreoli TE, Carpenter CCJ, Griggs RC, Loscalzo J (eds) CECIL Essentials of Medicine (6th edn). Philadelphia PA: WB Saunders.

Meux MD, Wall SD (2004) Dysphagia and AIDS. In Jones B (ed.) Normal and Abnormal Swallowing: Imaging in Diagnosis and Therapy (2nd edn). New York: Springer.

Midwinter KI, Carrie S, Bull PD (2002) Paediatric tracheostomy: Sheffield experience 1979–1999. Journal of Laryngology and Otology 116(7): 532–45.

Mokhlesi B, Logemann JA, Rademaker AW, et al. (2002) Oropharyngeal deglutition in stable COPD. Chest 121(2): 361–9.

Morgan AS, Mackay LE (1999) Causes and complications associated with swallowing disorders in traumatic brain injury. Journal of Head Trauma Rehabilitation 14(5): 454–61.

Morita T (2003) Development of deglutition aid jelly for oral administration (Abstract). Yakugaku Zasshi, The Pharmaceutical Society of Japan 8: 665–71.

Muehlberger T, Kunar D, Munster A, et al. (1998) Efficacy of fiberoptic laryngoscopy in the diagnosis of inhalation injuries. Archives of Otolaryngology – Head and Neck Surgery 124(9): 1003–7.

Nguyen NP, Frank C, Molitz CC, et al. (2005) Impact of dysphagia on quality of life after treatment of head-and-neck cancer. International Journal of Radiation Oncology Biology Physics 61(3): 772–8.

Nilsson H, Ekberg O, Olssob R, et al. (1996) Quantitative aspects of swallowing in an elderly nondysphagic population. Dysphagia 11: 180–4.

O'Neill-Pirozi TM, Lisiecki DJ, Momose KJ, et al. (2003) Simultaneous modified barium swallow and blue dye tests: a determination of the accuracy of the blue dye test aspiration findings. Dysphagia 18: 32–8.

Paciaroni M, Mazzotta G, Corea F, et al. (2004) Dysphagia following stroke. European Neurology 51(3): 162–7.

Pakalnis A, Drake ME, Huber S, et al. (1992) Central conduction time in progresive supranuclear palsy. Electromyography and Clinical Neurophysiology 32(1–2): 41–2.

Palmer JB, Carden EA (2003) The role of radiology in rehabilitation of swallowing. In Jones B (ed.) Normal and Abnormal Swallowing: Imaging in Diagnosis and Therapy (2nd edn). New York: Springer.

Parker C, Power M, Hamdy S, et al. (2004) Awareness of dysphagia by patients following stroke predicts swallowing performance. Dysphagia 19: 28–35.

Pauloski BR, Logemann JA, Rademaker AW, et al. (1994) Speech and swallowing function after oral and oropharyngeal resections: One-year follow-up. Head and Neck 16(4): 313–22.

Perry L (2004) Eating and dietary intake in communication-impaired stroke survivors: a cohort study from acute-stage hospital admission to six months post acute stroke. Clinical Nutrition 23(6): 1333–43.

Pfeiffer RF (2003) Gastrointestinal function in Parkinson's disease. Lancet – Neurology 2(2): 107–16.

Pilitsis JG, Rengachary SS (2001) Complications of head injury. Neurological Research 23(2/3): 227–36.

Richardson BE, Heywood BM, Sims S, et al. (2004) Laryngopharyngeal reflux: Trends in diagnostic interpretation criteria. Dysphagia 19: 248–55.

Rieger J, Seikaly H, Jha N, et al. (2005) Submandibular gland transfer for prevention of xerostomia after radiation therapy. Archives of Otolaryngology – Head and Neck Surgery 131(2): 140–5.

Robbins J, Levine RL (1988) Swallowing dysfunction after unilateral stroke of the cerebral cortex: Preliminary experience. Dysphagia 3: 11–17.

Robbins J, Levine RL, Maser A, et al. (1993) Swallowing after unilateral stroke of the cerebral cortex. Archives of Physical Medicine and Rehabilitation 74: 1295–300.

Selley WG, Flack FC, Ellis RE, et al. (1989) Respiratory patterns associated with swallowing: Part 1. The normal adult pattern and changes with age. Age and Ageing 18: 168–72.

Shaker R, Li Q, Ren J, et al. (1992) Coordination of deglutition and phases of respiration: effect of aging, tachypnea, bolus volume, and chronic obstructive pulmonary disease. American Journal of Physiology 263: G750–G755.

Shapiro J, Franko DL, Gagne A (1997) Phagophobia: a form of psychogenic dysphagia. Annals of Otology Rhinology and Laryngology 106(4): 286–90.

Sharkawi A, Ramig L, Logemann J, et al. (2002) Swallowing and voice effects of Lee Silverman Voice Treatment (LSVT®): a pilot study. Journal of Neurology, Neurosurgery and Psychiatry 72(1): 31–6.

Shikowitz MJ, Levy J, Villano D, et al. (1996) Speech and swallowing rehabilitation following devastating caustic ingestion: Techniques and indications for success. The Laryngoscope 106(2, supp. 78): 1–12.

Smithard DG, O'Neill PA, England RE, et al. (1997) The natural history of dysphagia following a stroke. Dysphagia 12: 188–93.

Snyder C, Ubben P (2003) Use of speech pathology services in the burn unit. Journal of Burn Care and Rehabilitation 24(4): 217–22.

Sokoloff LG, Pavlakovic R (1997) Neuroleptic-induced dysphagia. Dysphagia 12: 177–9.

Stachler RJ, Hamlet SL, Mathog RH, et al. (1994) Swallowing of bolus types by postsurgical head and neck cancer patients. Head and Neck 16(5): 413–19.

Stanniland C, Taylor D (2000) Tolerability of atypical antipsychotics. Drug Safety 22(3): 195–214.

Stein M, Williams AJ, Grossman F (1990) Cricopharyngeal dysfunction in chronic obstructive pulmonary disease. Chest 97: 347–52.

Stewart JT (2003) Dysphagia associated with risperidone therapy. Dysphagia 18: 274–5.

Stewart M, Johnson RA, Stewart I, Wilson JA (1995) Swallowing performance following anterior cervical spine surgery. British Journal of Neurosurgery 9: 605–9.

Talley NJ, O'Connor S (2001) Clinical Examination: A Systematic Guide to Physical Diagnosis (4th edn). Sydney: Maclennan & Petty.

Thompson-Henry S, Braddock B (1995) The modified Evan's blue dye procedure fails to detect aspiration in the tracheotomized patient: Five case reports. Dysphagia 10: 172–4.

Thompson-Ward E, Boots R, Frisby J, et al. (1999) Evaluating suitability for tracheostomy decannulation: A critical evaluation of two management strategies. Journal of Medical Speech-Language Pathology 7(4): 273–81.

Ulug T, Ulubil A (2003) An unusual cause of foreign-body sensation in the throat: corniculate cartilage subluxation. American Journal of Otolaryngology 24(2): 118–20.

Veiss SL, Logemann JA (1985) Swallowing disorders in persons with cerebrovascular accident. Archives of Physical Medicine and Rehabilitation 66: 372–5.

Volonte MA, Porta M, Comi G (2002) Clinical assessment of dysphagia in early phases of Parkinson's disease. Neurological Sciences 23(2): S121–2.

Ward EC, Bishop B, Frisby J, et al. (2002) Swallowing outcomes following laryngectomy and pharyngolaryngectomy. Archives of Otolaryngology Head and Neck Surgery 128: 181–6.

Ward EC, Uriarte M, Conroy A-L (2001) Duration of dysphagic symptoms and swallowing outcomes after thermal burn injury. Journal of Burn Care and Rehabilitation 22(6): 441–53.

Wilson DJ (1992) The reliability of the methylene blue test to detect aspiration in patients with a tracheostomy tube (CD-ROM). ProQuest Dissertation Abstracts Item: AAC 1348204.

10 Developmental Disability and Swallowing Disorders in Adults

JUSTINE JOAN SHEPPARD

THE POPULATION

The adult with developmental disability has a chronic disorder that may include mental and physical impairments. The onset of the disorder is prior to adulthood, 22 years old by US statute, and is often apparent at birth or in early childhood. Developmental disabilities include intellectual disability (mental retardation), serious emotional disturbance, autism, sensory impairments, traumatic brain injury, physical and health impairments, and combinations of impairment categories referred to as multiple disabilities. The level of severity must be such that there are significant, lifelong needs for support in multiple functional domains. These include self-care, communication, learning, mobility, and capacity for independent living. In the US, prevalence of developmental disability, including both paediatric and adult individuals, is estimated to be 1.2% to 1.65% of the total population (Crocker, 1989; MacFarland, 2003). Databases and classification criteria vary among nations, making it difficult to compare prevalence statistics. The difficulties were illustrated in a study of the prevalence in Finland of intellectual disability (ID), a subset of developmental disability (DD), in which the prevalence estimates of various registries were compared. The estimates ranged from 0.6% to 1.7% dependent on the methodology (Westerinen et al., 2004).

CHARACTERISTICS OF DISORDER

The prevalence of swallowing and feeding disorders is higher in developmental disability at all ages than in typical populations. It is estimated that 27% to 40% of children with cerebral palsy have dysphagia (Love et al., 1980; Waterman et al., 1992) with 85% to 90% expected to have feeding and swallowing problems at some time in their lives (Reilly et al., 1996). The prevalence of behavioural problems associated with the dysphagia may be as high as 80% (Burklow et al., 1998).

In a study of 575 adults with ID and/or DD nourished by oral feeding in residential care Sheppard and Hochman (1989) found 49% with chronic, oral and pharyngeal, swallowing and feeding disorders of sufficient severity to require individualized, daily care plans for meals and snacks. Ten per cent of this population suffered nutritional deficits and respiratory disorders associated with their dysphagia. Good nutritional

Dysphagia: Foundation, Theory and Practice.   Edited by J. Cichero and B. Murdoch
© 2006 John Wiley & Sons, Ltd.

and respiratory health was maintained for the remaining individuals with dysphagia through a team approach for prescriptive, individualized mealtime plans and ongoing monitoring. Rogers and colleagues (1994) found that, among adults with developmental disability who aspirated, 65% exhibited mealtime respiratory distress and 55% had chronic lung disease. Oral preparatory stage swallowing involvement was a poor predictor of aspiration. Aspiration was associated significantly with delayed initiation of swallowing and pharyngeal dysmotility. Kurtz, and colleagues (1998) reported on 21 individuals with I/DD and dysphagia who had been nourished by enteral tubefeeding for 6- to 61-months. Twelve of the 19 surviving Ss receive some oral feeding. Overall, there has been a substantial reduction in undernutrition and respiratory disorder.

Adults with severe and profound intellectual disability, physical and health impairments and multiple disabilities are most likely to have swallowing and feeding disorders. Swallowing and feeding disorders in this population are unique in that the paediatric disorders may persist into adulthood (Sheppard and Hochman, 1988; Sheppard, 1991; Rogers et al., 1994). The adult swallowing and feeding disorder carried over from childhood may include persistent failure to acquire functional developmental, oral preparation and self-feeding skills, and/or dysphagia associated with sensory-motor, anatomical, medical and psychiatric aetiologies. When these deficiencies persist, they are exacerbated by adult-onset swallowing disorders and by the physiological changes associated with ageing. Behavioural disorders that predispose to choking interfere with activities that involve swallowing. Furthermore, as with the normal adult, the person with developmental disability may suffer trauma, acute onset medical events, or acquired diseases, and medical conditions that are associated with dysphagia. In these instances, their chronic swallowing and feeding disorder may acquire new dimensions. Whether or not swallowing and feeding have been competent in the past, the adult onset dysphagia is managed within the constraints of the ongoing developmental disability. As in other populations, the swallowing disorder may involve eating, drinking, taking oral medications, swallowing saliva and managing the oral hygiene bolus. Swallowing and feeding disorders that are associated with I/DD and are seen less frequently in other populations include rumination, gastroesophageal reflux disease (GERD), dysphagia secondary to cervical osteophytes, foreign body ingestion and pica behaviours, choking, vomiting and recurrent aspiration syndrome.

There is a paucity of research in all areas of assessment and management of swallowing and feeding disorders in adults with developmental disability. Thus the evidence base for management is thin. Expert opinions are derived from clinical experience and may be supported by studies of children with developmental disability or from studies of adult onset disorders and normal ageing.

COMMON AETIOLOGIES

Developmental disability may originate from a variety of causes:

• hereditary disorders, e.g. inborn errors of metabolism, and gene and chromosomal abnormalities;

- alterations in embryonic development, e.g. the chromosomal aberration of Down syndrome and the prenatal effects of alcohol toxicity and congenital rubella;
- pregnancy issues and perinatal morbidity, e.g. maternal diabetes and perinatal asphyxia;
- acquired childhood diseases, e.g. central nervous system infection, cranial trauma and related mishaps; and
- childhood onset psychosis and autism.

However, developmental disabilities arising from unknown mechanisms account for substantial numbers (Crocker, 1989; Arvedson and Brodsky, 2002).

Contributing causes

Swallowing and feeding disorders are most consistently associated with neuro-motor impairments, anatomical anomalies, psychiatric conditions, and severe and profound intellectual disability. The neuromotor impairments include paralytic conditions, such as cerebral palsy and muscular dystrophy, CNS consequences of chronic seizure disorder, and disorders of muscle tone and movement associated with genetic disorders such as Down syndrome. Swallowing and feeding disorders associated with psychiatric conditions may be the result of associated behavioural changes, e.g. manic cycles, or of side effects of drug therapy (Rubin and Crocker, 1989; Rogoff, 1989; Poon, 1995). Although the current generation of anti-psychotic medications is reported to have fewer side effects, the potential for dysphagia has been reported (Stewart, 2003).

Disorders in any one or more phases of swallowing may occur from neuromo-tor or psychiatric impairments. Severe and profound intellectual disorders are most often associated with failure to achieve and maintain oral preparatory skills and difficulty compensating for gastrointestinal disorders, pulmonary disorders and de-ficiencies in oral initiation, pharyngeal or oesophageal phases of swallowing that may occur at any age. Gastroesophageal disorder has been estimated to occur in 10% to 15% of people with developmental disability. Primary, oesophageal phase dysphagia, and secondary effects on pharyngeal mucosal integrity and eating behav-iours occur often in this group (Roberts, 1989).

Effects of ageing

Swallowing and feeding competencies of adults with developmental disability and severe and profound intellectual disability have been found to deteriorate with age. In an 18-year retrospective study of adults with severe and profound intellectual dis-ability, the average age at which swallowing and feeding competencies began to dete-riorate was 33 years. Those who had the most severe swallowing disorder at the outset of the study interval began to decline at younger ages than did those with a less severe disorder or no disorder. Those who had no swallowing and feeding disorder at the outset tended to acquire oral preparatory phase deficits. Those who had swallowing and feeding disorders at the outset of the study interval demonstrated deterioration in oral preparatory skills and signs of onset or deterioration of involvement in oral initiation, pharyngeal and oesophageal phases (Sheppard, 2002). Although, the effects of chronic illness, existing disability, long-term use of medications and the physiological changes associated with ageing may be associated with these findings, further study is needed to determine the causes of early adult onset deterioration in swallowing and feeding in this population.

MANAGEMENT COMPLICATIONS

Co-occurring conditions may complicate dysphagia assessment and management and may restrict management options, decrease the likelihood of compliance with recommendations, and increase the assistance and supervision that are needed for maintaining nutrition, hydration, airway protection and ease and comfort in swallowing activities. Some of the more commonly occurring complications in developmental disability are:

• intellectual disability and its impact on ability to learn compensatory strategies and retain skills;
• communication limitations;
• postural control issues, including congenital and acquired skeletal abnormalities and conditions, and neuromuscular impairments that may interfere with postural alignment for eating and control of respiration;
• dyspraxia and associated difficulties with sensory integration, and planning and performing motor tasks;
• psychiatric and behavioural disorders, including pica, disruptive mealtime behaviours, and bipolar disorder;
• vision and hearing disorders, including acuity, perception and integration issues;
• epilepsy including the effects of seizures on eating and the side effects of medications used to manage the disorder; and
• gastrointestinal, gastroesophageal and pulmonary disorders, including constipation, rumination and chronic obstructive pulmonary disease.

In addition, side effects from long-term use of medications may cause or complicate dysphagia in this population (Rubin and Crocker, 1989; Rosenthal et al., 1994). Although any one of these management complications may be seen in the adult with acute onset dysphagia and in the normal, ageing adult, it is the frequency with which clusters of these issues occur, their severity and their onset early in life that distinguish the presentation of the adult with developmental disability.

THE CLINICIAN'S ROLE IN MANAGING THIS POPULATION

The role of the speech-language pathologist (SLP) in managing the feeding and swallowing disorders of the adult with DD is, as in other populations with chronic disorders, dependent on work site. The primary differences will be the extent to which assessment may involve collaborations with other allied health and medical specialists and the scope of the daily management programmes that may be needed. In acute care and outpatient settings, in addition to instrumental and clinical assessments, daily management plans and therapy for eating, taking oral medications, saliva management and oral hygiene may be needed. Adults with DD, admitted to hospital for acute care, may be referred to the SLP by nursing staff for guidance in managing swallowing and feeding issues during the hospitalization. Carers, who accompany the patient, may provide information on typical care-giving strategies; however, the hospitalization may involve feeding and oral hygiene in different postural alignments, with unfamiliar foods, and unfamiliar personnel. In addition, the impact of the illness on swallowing and feeding capabilities, whether resulting from general debilitation or specific dysphagia aetiology, may be substantial. Following an assessment, the SLP will be able to assist carers and staff in selecting the appropriate diet consistencies, positioning, utensils, feeding techniques and techniques for administering oral medications within the constraints of availability in hospital. The SLP will determine if there is a need for instrumented dysphagia assessment and/or for collaborative assessments by other allied health, medical or dental specialists for issues related to the dysphagia.

In residential centres, long-term healthcare facilities, and daily treatment centres, clinical dysphagia assessments may be part of an interdisciplinary nutritional management programme (NMP) involving SLP, and allied health (usually occupational therapy, physical therapy, nurse and dietitian), dental, medical nursing and residential staff. The NMP is a comprehensive care strategy that incorporates screening for onset and changes in disorder, clinical evaluation, and re-evaluation as needed, daily management of activities that involve swallowing, training to maintain skills and underlying competencies for swallowing and therapy for regaining and improving function (Sheppard, 1991; Barks and Sheppard, 2005). In addition, the NMP will include provisions for carer education and support, assistance in making long-term care decisions, and monitoring the implementation of the programme. An alternative residential care model used for this population is the physical nutritional management plan (PNMP). The PNMP is an expanded model that integrates a 24-hour positioning plan into the NMP. These integrated care models are intended to promote optimum health and wellbeing. The components of a 'nutritional management plan' are:

- medical and nursing care for monitoring and managing gastrointestinal, pulmonary and nutritional issues;
- infection control in group eating environments;
- dietary management and monitoring;
- dysphagia screening, clinical and instrumented assessments;
- periodic repeat assessments for monitoring course of the disorder;
- repeat assessments following worsening dysphagia or dysphagia incidents; including choking, nutritional deterioration, eating refusal and pneumonia;
- adaptive and other prescriptive equipment for seating, self-feeding, and dependent eating;

- eating management strategies including supervision, assistance, adaptive feeding techniques, and behavioural management;
- individualized oral hygiene plan;
- individualized plan for administration of oral medications;
- structuring eating environments for supporting effective eating behaviours and pleasant eating experiences;
- rehabilitation for maintaining functional skills and restoring skills following regression;
- training programme for clinicians, carers and family members to advance and maintain nutritional management skills;
- monitoring and quality assurance systems for assuring that mealtime environments and management of individual needs are satisfactory.

In some instances adults with DD may have guardians who are legally empowered to make their healthcare and lifestyle decisions. The guardian may be a parent or a court-appointed family member or agent. In these instances, the role of the clinician will include collaboration with the guardian, and education and support for the guardian, in making the assessment and treatment decisions.

ASSESSMENT

The assessment issues for the adult with DD differ somewhat from those in other populations. Efficient and effective assessment systems are essential for identifying the condition, monitoring its course and intervening in a timely manner. These systems are needed because of the high prevalence and incidence of feeding and swallowing disorders (Sheppard and Hochman, 1988) their persistence, their insidious onset in adulthood, their tendency to worsen with age (Sheppard, 2002), and the high prevalence and incidence of co-occurring conditions, including communication disorders. In those instances where the swallowing and feeding disorders are chronic, there are correlates of dysphagia that provide a general indication of the disorder and its severity (Sheppard et al., 1988; Rogers, et al., 1994). These include mealtime distress, nutritional failure, body mass index (BMI), the need for therapeutic diets, and respiratory illnesses. Sheppard and colleagues (1988) found that the best predictor of severity of dysphagia in this population was BMI.

SCREENING

The screening assessment is used in management of the DD population as an efficient means for identifying individuals with signs or symptoms of swallowing and feeding disorders and monitoring for changes in the characteristics and severity of the disorder. Screening strategies are especially useful in this population because of the high prevalence of reduced alertness and of limitations in the ability to communicate the onset of problems and the change in swallowing and feeding symptoms.

The relatively high prevalence of chronic and adult onset disorder and the tendency for deterioration of swallowing and feeding competencies during adulthood warrant systematic monitoring.

Screening assessments are limited to determining the need for consultation and referral. They do not identify contributing causes and typically rely on inferential clinical signs for indications of airway protection failure and oesophageal dysmotility. Some screening assessments are ordinal, functional scales in which overall levels of disorder are designated (Enderby, 1997). Alternatively, the screening assessment may consist of a task analysis and provide a numerical score as a measure of apparent severity of disorder. (Sheppard and Hochman, 1988).

Kuhn and Matson (2002) developed a screening assessment for pica and rumination, two swallowing disorders seen in I/DD. The Dysphagia Disorders Survey examines swallowing and feeding behaviours during an eating activity. It is used in conjunction with the Dysphagia Management Staging Scale, which provides a level of severity of disorder based on management needs. The two assessments, which were standardized on children and adults with developmental disability, together provide a description of the clinical presentation of the swallowing and feeding disorder, a percentile ranking of severity of disorder, and a scaled level of severity of disorder (Sheppard and Hochman, 1988).

CLINICAL DYSPHAGIA ASSESSMENT

Models for the clinical dysphagia assessment (CDA) may vary depending on established procedures at the work site. The model may be the more conventional, transdisciplinary, 'bedside' evaluation administered by an SLP. Depending on the results of the CDA, referrals are made, as needed, to collaborating specialists for medical, dental, nutritional, behavioural, or physical management assessments (Logemann, 1998). Alternately, the CDA may be a team evaluation in which two or more specialists collaborate, each evaluating their own specialty area(s) and combining their impressions and referrals into a joint statement. Referrals may result from this assessment as well. Typically the interdisciplinary team model, when used for evaluating people with developmental disability, includes an SLP as a dysphagia specialist, a dietitian, a physical management specialist, usually an occupational or physical therapist and, in some instances, a nurse (Bryan and Pressman, 1995; Barks and Sheppard, 2005).

The components of the CDA for developmental disability are similar to the professional standards for evaluation of other adult populations. However, there are special considerations for issues that have a higher prevalence in the population and warrant special attention for management of the disorder. Patients with limitations in their ability to communicate their symptoms may be using an alternative communication modality. The clinician will need to consider the special communication needs in interviewing patients and carers, assessing the problem, and providing management recommendations. A careful history, always essential to a CDA, should include nutritional and pulmonary status as well as review of neurological, orthopaedic, cardiac and gastrointestinal issues. Questions regarding past and current difficulty with eating, taking oral medications, saliva management and oral hygiene, including coughing and choking, are relevant, as are related disorders such as pica, vomiting and rumination. Medications are reviewed for side effects that may impact on the adequacy of swallowing and feeding (Pronsky, 2002).

The physical examination includes careful attention to:

• physical anomalies that may impact on postural control and maintenance of postural control for sitting;
• respiratory support for eating; and
• oral and facial structural anomalies.

The examination of stability, range and ease of movement of oral structures is made, typically, through observations of oral postural control, control of saliva, voice and articulation and examination of oral-facial (infantile) and pharyngeal reflexes. These observations provide inferential information that, in association with observations of eating, lead to hypotheses regarding the nature and severity of contributing causes (Sheppard, 1987; 1991; 1995). Finally, during observations of eating, issues related to independence and behavioural problems are important. Carers may be helpful in this regard. Oral and pharyngeal bolus management may differ in dependent, as opposed to independent, conditions. If the person is inconsistently independent both conditions should be observed. Behavioural issues in this population are complex and varied. Behavioural problems may be habitual, maladaptive patterns associated with medical conditions or medication side effects, or may be related directly to psychiatric diagnoses (Rubin and Crocker, 1989). Significant issues are:

• uncontrolled eating rates, including both excessive bolus size and excessive rate of intake;
• reduced alertness and lethargy;
• disruptive mealtime behaviours;
• anorexia, including both liquid and solid food refusal;
• apprehensiveness;
• obsessive routines; and
• non-compliance with eating restrictions and swallowing strategies.

INSTRUMENTED ASSESSMENT

The instrumented assessment is used to supplement the findings of the CDA when there are clinical indications of oral initiation, pharyngeal or oesophageal deficiencies, and delineation of these deficiencies is needed to determine the management needs (Marquis and Pressman, 1995). The individual's potential for tolerance of the procedure, the capabilities of the assessment site for managing the particular needs of the individual, as well as the particular questions that are being asked, are considered when selecting the assessment type and site, and making the referral.

Special considerations for administering these assessments are associated, primarily, with special needs of the population for communication, positioning for the assessment, and behavioural management. Adaptations for the modified barium swallow (MBS) may include doing the study in the patient's own seating equipment, use of an adaptive collar to stabilize head and neck during the study, mixing barium with food to enhance acceptability and facilitate patient cooperation, and oesophageal follow-through to screen for oesophageal motility issues that may be contributing. The oesophageal follow-through may be used for detection of intraoesophageal reflux and intraoesophageal stasis as differentiated from GERD (Zarate et al., 2001). Marquis and Pressman (1995) discussed these issues with reference to MBS assessment of children with developmental disability. Migliore et al. (1999) discussed the use of fibreoptic endoscopic evaluation of swallowing (FEES) and fibreoptic evaluation of swallowing and sensory testing (FEESST) for this population. They describe the advantages in using FEES and FEESST for direct physical examination of pharyngeal structures. They commented on the benefits of examining swallowing with preferred foods in the seating equipment that is typically used for eating, and the opportunity for more extended observation of oral and pharyngeal function. They noted the difficulties of maintaining compliant behaviours during testing as well. The capability of FEES for determining adequacy of oral initiation of swallow and pharyngeal control for saliva swallowing, for detecting the oedema and erythema of pharyngeal mucosa that are associated with acid reflux into the pharynx, for observing acid and non-acid reflux into the pharynx directly during eating and for examining the integrity of pharyngeal structures render it a useful procedure that compliments rather than substitutes for the MBS.

SCHEDULES FOR REPEAT ASSESSMENTS

The accepted professional practice for repeating screenings, and CDAs depends on the potential for nutritional and respiratory consequences of the disorder, the complexity of management needs, and the short-term expectations for change in condition. Generally the more severe and less stable the condition, the shorter the reassessment cycle. For individuals who are at risk for onset of swallowing and feeding disorder, and have reduced capability for self-report of symptoms, the duration of the cycle depends on the age of the individual and potential risk for nutritional and respiratory complications. Typically, instrumented and other medical evaluations are repeated when there is a deterioration of the swallowing disorder, nutritional condition or respiratory health. Re-evaluation may also be triggered by a pneumonia or choking episode that required assistance, such as the Heimlich manoeuvre, to resolve.

TREATMENT

The treatment programme for this population consists of

- management plans for daily activities that involve swallowing;
- incidental/situational strategies for maintaining the adequacy of, and improving, skills and behaviours; and
- indirect and direct therapy for improving underlying competencies for swallowing or the swallowing and feeding function.

As with assessment, treatment may be provided by an interdisciplinary team. When this occurs, each member of the team provides services as prescribed by the inter-disciplinary plan (Barks and Sheppard, 2005). Alternatively, the SLP, as dysphagia specialist provides the primary services for the feeding and swallowing disorder and refers as needed for collaborative management consultations.

MANAGING DAILY ACTIVITIES

Management of daily activities involves planning for supportive environments for eating, oral hygiene and taking oral medications, and selecting strategies to manage the particular characteristics of the individual's swallowing and feeding disorder. The aims of this two-pronged approach are to (a) protect the health and safety of the individual, (b) provide optimum quality of this life experience, (c) provide for the least restrictive life-style, and (d) support maximum independence in all aspects of the swallowing activities. As in other populations, SLPs educate the patient and/ or the guardian in those aspects of daily swallowing activity that relate to health, safety and quality of life, and advise and support them as they make the treatment decisions that are compatible with their own values and will best accomplish the aims of the programme. An individualized plan may be needed for eating, oral hygiene, and oral medications. For the purposes of this chapter, the focus will be on eating.

THE EATING ENVIRONMENT

There is a high prevalence of behavioural instability in this population associated with the primary neurological and psychiatric disorders and sensory impairments. Reduced attending skills, auditory and visual acuity and perception deficiencies, reduced skills for integration of sensory information, and reduced capabilities for motor performance limit the tolerance for haphazard environmental structures and events. For example, radio or television or other acoustic distractions may increase the difficulty in attending to, and performing the eating task and interfere with com-municative interactions. When feeding and swallowing skills are vulnerable, careful consideration should be given to the acoustic and visual distractions in the eating area, the supervision and assistance, the level of extraneous activity, and the fa-miliarity of personnel, environment, equipment and routines. The general rule is to reduce the complexity of the eating task, e.g. provide easier foods or increased supervision and assistance, when environmental stresses are increased.

THE INDIVIDUAL MEALTIME PLAN

Individual considerations for eating that are specific to the needs of the individual are often referred to as the individual mealtime plan (IMP). The IMP may include stipulations for aspects of the meal, beginning with the time interval just prior to eating and ending with the interval following eating. Snacks should conform to the stipulations for the meal. In all aspects of the IMP, the SLP may provide transdisciplinary care or may participate with team members of an interdisciplinary dysphagia team.

Pre-eating interval

The purpose of structuring the pre-eating interval is to facilitate optimum performance during eating. These are readiness activities. The IMP may include a rest period, putting on or removing orthotics, such as splints or braces, an oral or facial stimulation routine, and routine washing of hands and face.

Positioning/seating

Correct seating for eating is important for facilitating optimum oral bolus preparation, pharyngeal and oesophageal and bolus motility, and for comfort. When postural stability and control are problematic during eating, care should be taken to provide seats that are an appropriate size. Seat depth, height of chair back and seat height should be appropriate to allow for surfaces to stabilize trunk, hips and feet. Height of the eating surface, whether table or wheelchair lap tray, should be optimum for resting arms on the surface and for self-feeding. The plan includes any special instructions for seating and for assisting in maintaining correct upper body and head-neck alignment and stability during eating (Sheppard, 1995). The physical or occupational therapist may provide consultation for appropriate seating (Woods, 1995).

Diet

Diet recommendations for this population, as for other adult populations, are specific to the signs and symptoms of the disorder. In order to compensate for impairment and deficiencies in swallowing or facilitate improved swallow function stipulations may be provided for food temperature, tastes, viscosity, and texture. In addition, recommendations may be made for liquid replacements, increasing calorie density in foods and high calorie, full nutrient supplements to compensate for swallowing and feeding deficiencies. The dietitian provides management for dietary needs.

Utensils and equipment

Adaptive utensils and equipment may be recommended to facilitate self-feeding and oral preparation and to regulate bolus size. These may include specially shaped, sized or coated spoons, forks, cups and straws as well as pads that stabilize plates, cup holders and specially designed plates. The occupational therapist may provide consultation for managing adaptive equipment and self-feeding strategies.

Communication strategies

Effective communication during the meal is essential for maintaining health, safety, and skills and expressing lifestyle choices. Consideration is given to the preferred modality for expression and the special needs for reception, as well as the skills of the carer as a communication partner. To achieve the goal of optimum communication it may be necessary to use augmentative communication systems and personal communication dictionaries to facilitate effective interactions during the meal (Bloomberg and Johnson, 1991; Bloomberg, 1996; McLean et al., 1999).

The appropriate focus of communications during an eating activity depends on the feeding and swallowing capabilities of the individuals concerned as well as their level of communication competency. Communications may be limited to supporting calm, alert, focused attention to the eating task, or to supporting cooperative interactions between individuals regarding the eating activity – activities such as passing foods. When communication, attending, and swallowing and feeding skills permit, the content of the interactions may include social exchanges that are not directly related to the current activity. Special training for carers and patients may be needed to generate sensitivity to the effects of communication on the eating task. The SLP manages the communication issues.

Feeding techniques

Feeding techniques are selected to address specific needs of the individual. Techniques used in this context are cueing strategies that assist the individual or facilitate optimum performance of the eating behaviour. A strategy is typically selected to improve one or more task components of the swallowing and feeding behaviour. Optimally, strategies should improve performance in the short term. They should provide a compensatory advantage, and improve overall competency in the long term – i.e. have a therapeutic effect.

The task components that are addressed most frequently are:

- body postural control and alignment;
- movements that culminate in reception of the bolus;
- containment of the bolus in the mouth;
- bolus preparation including mixing with saliva and chewing;
- oral transport;
- initiation of swallowing;

- airway protection;
- pharyngeal clearance; and
- independence.

The strategies may include assisting, touch, visual or verbal cueing, and supervising for compliance. Special techniques for dependent feeding include adaptive spooning and cup strategies that are selected to facilitate more competent oral preparation and containment of the bolus. The SLP may collaborate with the occupational therapist in developing a routine that will best support oral pharyngeal function and optimum independence.

After-eating care

After-eating care may be prescribed to facilitate an increased frequency of saliva swallowing immediately following the end of the meal (Sheppard et al., 2003). Sliding an empty, room temperature or chilled spoon in the mouth facilitates swallowing and is used for individuals who tend to cough on saliva following eating. Positioning restrictions following eating may be prescribed to alleviate signs or symptoms of GERD or oesophageal dysmotility.

MANAGING THE ORAL HYGIENE BOLUS

The oral hygiene plan is part of comprehensive dysphagia care in this population. Maintaining optimum oral hygiene is important for minimizing the risk for pulmonary infection in individuals who are known to aspirate (Langmore et al., 2002; Langmore et al., 1998)). Adaptive brushing strategies may be needed in individuals with neuromuscular or sensory impairments in the mouth and pharynx in order to avoid aspiration of the oral hygiene bolus and to achieve good oral hygiene (Altabet et al., 2003).

The oral hygiene plan may include stipulations for body position during brushing – standing, seated or side lying, and head-neck alignment. The brushing device and the dentifrice may be specified. Brushing techniques may be selected to facilitate access to the mouth, to allow the accumulating oral hygiene bolus to drain from the lips, and to assure tolerance of the procedure.

ADMINISTERING ORAL MEDICATIONS

Taking oral medications is often a daily, routine activity for the adult with developmental disability. If the individual has dysphagia, the procedure for administering oral medications will typically follow the same procedures as those specified in the IMP with respect to independence of the individual in taking the medication, postural alignment and stabilization, utensil, texture and viscosity of the medications preparation, bolus size, and choice of liquid or solid used to clear the medication from the oesophagus. The generally accepted guidelines for upright posture during swallowing and minimum of 60 ml of wash down following the medication are appropriate (Barks and Sheppard, 2005).

INCIDENTAL TRAINING AND IMPLICIT LEARNING

It is a challenging task for the clinician to change the behaviours of adults with developmental disability in activities that involve swallowing. Impairments in cognition, attention, communication, and regulation of emotional states are common in this population. Resulting deficiencies are apparent in their ability to learn, retain and comply with compensatory strategies and therapeutic routines. Implicit learning – learning that is the consequence of repeated daily experience – has been found to be more effective for facilitating learning in individuals with ID/DD than explicit learning (Krinsky-McHale et al., 2003; Vinter and Detable, 2003). Frequently used behavioural strategies are those that involve training during the target activity, and using cueing, feedback on performance adequacy, and reinforcement to train and maintain desired patterns of behaviour. This incidental training model has been observed to be promising for changing maladaptive eating and other swallowing behaviours.

THERAPY

There has been little attention in the literature to the efficacy of therapeutic strategies in treating dysphagia in adults with DD. However, there is some evidence from the paediatric literature and from the literature on adult onset, chronically disabled populations that may be considered relevant to the discussion of management of people with DD.

INDIRECT STRATEGIES

Indirect strategies – those that do not involve eating – include exercises that increase frequency of saliva swallow and those that have been found to be effective for improving underlying competency for swallowing. Strategies are selected that are tolerated by the individual and have some empirical or logical support for their use. Thermal stimulation has been shown to reduce aspiration in adolescents with developmental disability. Enhanced sensory input using flavoured powders and oral stimulation routines has been used to increase frequency of saliva swallow. Exercise strategies, such as the Shaker exercise, which are selected to increase strength and stability in the suprahyoid muscles have been found to improve swallowing in ageing individuals (Langmore and Miller, 1994). Similar exercise routines have been used in this population but their efficacy has not been tested. Oral motor exercises for improving lips, tongue, mandible, velum, and vocal folds are used, but efficacy remains to be tested. These strategies are implemented most frequently in individuals who are designated to be given 'nil by mouth', or tube fed and on reduced oral feeding. The goals are to maintain or improve swallowing capabilities for saliva and to introduce or increase oral feeding.

DIRECT STRATEGIES

Direct therapy strategies – those that involve food – may be used in this population for maintaining or improving independence and skills for oral preparation, and for improving oral initiation and pharyngeal phases of swallowing. Modified head-neck alignments may be used (Logemann, 1998) and are generally tolerated. However, it may be difficult to train this population to use swallowing manoeuvres such as the supraglottic swallow.

SURGICAL INTERVENTION

In cases of intractable aspiration and or nutritional failure that is associated with dysphagia, surgical interventions may be considered. A range of surgical options are appropriate including reconstructions of structures involved in swallowing to improve swallowing for oral feeding, surgical placement of a feeding tube – gastrostomy or jejunostomy to substitute for, or supplement, oral feeding and as a strategy of last resort, surgical closure of the larynx. In tube-fed individuals, as in those who are fed orally, aspiration may result during ingestion of food, during swallowing of oral secretions and during reswallowing of emesis. The role of the SLP in managing the tube fed individual is to maintain the adequacy of swallowing for saliva and, whenever possible, to develop a programme for therapeutic tastes, or return to partial or complete oral feeding.

SUMMARY

Adults with developmental disability and dysphagia have a challenging array of co-occurring medical problems and disabilities that complicate assessment and treatment. The combination of chronic paediatric and adult onset swallowing problems are identified and diagnosed by screening, clinical and instrumental assessments. Co-occurring problems that complicate management of dysphagia are identified. Special plans may be needed for managing daily needs for eating, saliva control, oral hygiene and swallowing oral medications. In addition, dysphagia therapy programmes are appropriate for preventing regression and optimizing skills for swallowing and feeding, maintaining swallowing adequacy for saliva in the tube fed individual, and for rehabilitating problems resulting from adult onset swallowing disorders.

CASE STUDIES

CASE STUDY 1

DA is a 42 year old with severe intellectual disability and developmental disability. He is ambulatory. He uses his limited speech for communication. He has an active seizure disorder controlled incompletely with medications. He becomes lethargic following seizure, unable to walk safely and with increased difficulty eating. He feeds himself. He will confiscate foods whenever they are available from the plates of his eating companions, the kitchen and canteen. He has a history of choking episodes that have required assistance (Heimlich manoeuvre, etc.) to resolve. Nutrition is within normal limits. Gastrointestinal and pulmonary systems are not remarkable. No adaptive eating equipment had been recommended. He prefers to eat his meals with a 7 ml-sized teaspoon and fingers.

CDA revealed oral preparatory deficiencies characterized by excessive size spoonfuls and bite size, excessive rate of placement of food in mouth, excessive drinking rate, chewing skills limited to bite sized, soft to chew, finger foods. Other chewable foods were swallowed without mastication. There was intermittent, brief coughing during eating and drinking. Modified Barium Swallow was performed following a choking episode to rule out physiological characteristics that may be contributing to choking. It confirmed reduced mastication and revealed mildly delayed initiation of swallowing on liquids and solid foods. Pharyngeal clearance was normal. Screening for oesophageal dysmotility during the MBS by oesophageal 'follow through' of a solid bolus ruled out oesophageal issues as contributing.

The conclusion was that DA had a moderate dysphagia (Dysphagia Management Staging Scale Level 3) (Sheppard, 1995), in that he needed diet modifications and adaptive feeding strategies to manage his disorder. Recommendations by the SLP dysphagia specialist were to prepare an individualized mealtime plan that would include incidental training strategies for reducing choking risk and reducing food confiscation behaviours during meals, and to refer to a behaviour modification specialist for evaluation and additional training recommendations.

The individualized mealtime plan for DA included:

- 'Mechanical soft' (soft to chew and mashed textures) diet with bread cut into bite size pieces, and nectar thick liquids. Condiments and seasonings were used to enhance flavours of food.
- Junior sized (4 ml) spoon with adult-sized handle.
- Cut-out ('Nosey') cup.
- One-on-one level of assistance/training.
- Feeding techniques to regulate behaviours were worded in 'person-centred' language. 'Help me to not overfill my spoon by using a spoon to wipe off the excess.' 'Help me to take only one piece of bread at a time.' 'Encourage me to take drinks throughout the meal.' 'Touch my arm to encourage me to stop drinking after three to four sips and swallows.' 'Place your hand on my shoulder and instruct me to eat

my own food if I reach for someone else's food.' 'Feed me if I am too tired to feed myself following a seizure.'

- Incidental training consisted of frequent praise for incidents of appropriately sized spoonfuls, reduced rate of eating, and refraining from food confiscation during a meal.

Initially, verbal, visual and tactile cues, assistance and reduction of environmental triggers were used to shape desired behaviours. Cueing and environmental controls were simplified as behaviours improved and stabilized. Level of supervision and training could be reduced and DA advanced to eating with a carer and two to three peers sitting at a table.

CASE STUDY 2

NK is a 20 year old with diagnoses of cerebral palsy quadriplegia, seizure disorder and dysphagia. She is non-ambulatory and non-verbal. Her respiratory health has been good. She is alert, enjoys eating, has normal food preferences and communicates with facial gestures and vocalizations at meals. Her diet consists of mashed table foods, cookies and regular liquids. She is a dependent eater. It takes approximately one hour for her to complete a meal. There was a recent weight loss of more than 10% of her body weight following two hospitalizations for seizures. There was a recent increase in coughing on solid and liquid foods. These events raised concerns about ongoing oral feeding and resulted in referral for comprehensive team evaluation. The family expressed their belief that continuing oral feeding was important for maintaining a good quality of life for NK. They were not willing to consider gastrostomy at this time. They were eager to participate in a nutritional management programme that might improve her chances for ongoing, successful, oral feeding.

The hospital-based, evaluating team consisted of SLP dysphagia specialist, medical doctor with specialty in developmental disability, radiologist, dietitian, and physical therapist. The assessments included an MBS and CDA. Significant findings were malnutrition with weight at 52% of ideal body weight, and marked oral neuromuscular involvement with associated difficulties swallowing saliva and solid and liquid food. Mastication was weak and incomplete. NK was unable to bite off pieces of food. She tended to laugh and vocalize while eating. Inflammation of the gingival mucosa was noted on oral examination. There was instability in head-neck and trunk interfering with sitting. A lap-tray was available for her wheelchair; however, it was not used consistently during eating.

The MBS revealed marked abnormalities in oral preparation, oral initiation and pharyngeal stages of swallowing with multiple swallows required to clear a single bolus. The cookie, a part of her typical diet, was swallowed whole. There was laryngeal penetration of solid and liquid boluses but no aspiration on the 12 swallows that were observed on fluoroscopy. These deficits were associated with a weak and delayed swallow, overall. However, liquids were managed somewhat better than solid foods.

The team conveyed the results of the evaluation to the family and counselled them that NK would do best if she had a feeding gastrostomy to supplement her oral feeding. In consideration of the family's wishes, however, a comprehensive NMP was proposed. It was presented to the family as an interim plan. The family was urged to reconsider placement of a feeding gastrostomy if, within three months, NK did not gain weight, experienced dehydration or experienced deterioration in her respiratory health.

- Nutritional management goals were to improve nutrition, reduce meal duration and increase effectiveness of swallowing. The nutritional management plan included consultation with dentist or periodontist.
- The diet recommendation of finely mashed, moist solid foods (reduced viscosity) and nectar-thick liquids. Liquid, full nutrient supplement was used to increase daily calorie intake. Cookies were prepared in a slurry by mixing them with milk and spooning.
- Use of a Hensinger collar and assistance during eating to maintain optimal, head-neck postural alignment and stability.
- Use of lap-tray consistently during eating to help stabilize the upper body.
- Shorter, more frequent meals and snacks.
- Adaptive strategies for spoon and cup placement in mouth and for clearing residual foods and saliva at end of meal.
- Verbal cueing to reduce laughing and vocalization during eating.
- Exercise programme to improve ability to stabilize the mandible in a closed-mouth posture, to increase frequency of saliva swallowing, and to improve ability to stabilize head-neck with a balance of flexion against extension.
- Individualized oral hygiene and oral medication administration plans.
- Training for family members and day placement staff.

NK gained weight and remained healthy. Oral feeding continued and placement of gastrostomy tube were deferred.

REFERENCES

Altabet S, Rogers K, Imes E, et al. (2003) Comprehensive approach toward improving oral hygiene at a state residential facility for people with mental retardation. Mental Retardation 41(6): 440–5.

Arvedson JC, Brodsky L (2002) Pediatric Swallowing and Feeding, Assessment and Management. Albany: Singular Thompson Learning.

Barks L, Sheppard JJ (2005). Eating and swallowing disorders (dysphagia) in adults and children. In Nehring WM (ed.) Core Curriculum for Nurses and Health Care Professionals Specializing in Intellectual and Developmental Disabilities. Boston: Jones & Bartlett.

Bloomberg K (1996) Practically Speaking. Videotape. Melbourne: Yooralla Society of Victoria.

Bloomberg K, Johnson HM (1991) Communication Without Speech: A Guide for Teachers and Parents. Hawthorne, Australia: ACER.

Bryan DW, Pressman H (1995) Comprehensive team evaluation. In Rosenthal SR, Sheppard JJ, Lotze M (eds) Dysphagia and the Child with Developmental Disabilities: Medical, Clinical, and Family Interventions. San Diego: Singular Publishing Group.

Burklow KA, Phelps AN, Schultz JR, et al. (1998) Classifying complex pediatric feeding disorders. Journal of Gastrointestinal Nutrition 27: 143–7.

Crocker AC (1989) The spectrum of medical care for developmental disabilities. In Rubin IL, Crocker AC (eds) Developmental Disabilities: Delivery of Medical Care for Children and Adults. Philadelphia: Lea & Febiger, pp. 10–22.

Enderby P (1997) Therapy Outcome Measures (TOM), Speech-Language Pathology, Technical Manual. San Diego: Singular Publishing Group.

Krinsky-McHale SJ, Devenny DA, Kittler P, et al. (2003) Implicit memory in aging adults with mental retardation with and without Down syndrome. American Journal on Mental Retardation 108(4): 219–33.

Kuhn DE, Matson JL (2002) A validity study of the screening tool of feeding problems (STEP). Journal of Intellectual Disability 27(3): 161–7.

Kurtz MB, Paraguya M, Fischer LS (1998) Dysphagia in the adult with developmental disability, enteral tube placement: criteria and outcomes. Paper presented at the Dysphagia Research Society Seventh Annual International Meeting, New Orleans.

Langmore SE, Miller RM (1994) Behavioural treatment for adults with oropharyngeal dysphagia. Archives of Physical Medicine and Rehabilitation 75: 1154–60.

Langmore SE, Skarupski KA, Park PS, et al. (2002) Predictors of aspiration pneumonia in nursing home residents. Dysphagia 17(4): 298–307.

Langmore SE, Terpenning MS, Schork A, et al. (1998) Predictors of aspiration pneumonia: How important is dysphagia? Dysphagia 13: 69–81.

Logemann JA (1998) Evaluation and Treatment of Swallowing Disorders (2nd edn). Austin: Pro-ed.

Love RJ, Hagerman EL, Taimi EG (1980) Speech performance, dysphagia and oral reflexes in cerebral palsy. Journal of Speech and Hearing Disorders 45: 59–75.

MacFarland SZC (2003) Current trends and issues in understanding adults with developmental disabilities. Seminars in Hearing 24(3): 171–8.

Marquis J, Pressman H (1995) Radiologic assessment of pediatric swallowing. In Rosenthal SR, Sheppard JJ, Lotze M (eds) Dysphagia in the Child with Developmental Disabilities: Medical, Clinical, and Family Interventions. San Diego: Singular Publishing Group.

McLean LK, Brady NC, McLean JE, et al. (1999) Communication forms and functions of children and adults with severe mental retardation in community and institutional settings. Journal of Speech and Hearing Research 42: 231–40.

Migliore LE, Scoopo FJ, Robey KL (1999) Fiberoptic examination of swallowing in children and young adults with severe developmental disability. American Journal of Speech-Language Pathology 8: 303–8.

Poon C (1995) Pharmacology. In Rosenthal SR, Sheppard JJ, Lotze M (eds) Dysphagia and the Child with Developmental Disabilities: Medical, Clinical, and Family Interventions. San Diego: Singular Publishing Group, pp. 337–402.

Pronsky ZM (2002). Food Medication Interactions (12th edn). Birchrunville: Food-Medication Interactions.

Reilly S, Skuse D, Poblete X (1996) Prevalence of feeding problems and oral motor dysfunction in children with cerebral palsy: a community survey. Journal of Pediatrics 129: 877–82.

Roberts IM (1989) Gastrointestinal problems. In Rubin IL, Crocker AC (eds) Developmental Disabilities: Delivery of Medical Care for Children and Adults. Philadelphia: Lea & Febiger.

Rogers B, Stratton P, Msall M, et al. (1994) Long-term morbidity and management strategies of tracheal aspiration in adults with severe developmental disabilities. American Journal on Mental Retardation 98(4): 490–8.

Rogoff M-L (1989) Psychotropic medication. In Rubin IL, Crocker AC (eds) Developmental Disabilities: Delivery of Medical Care for Children and Adults. Philadelphia: Lea & Febiger, pp. 348–53.

Rosenthal SR, Sheppard JJ, Lotze M (eds) (1995) Dysphagia and the Child with Developmental Disabilities: Medical, Clinical, and Family Interventions. San Diego: Singular Publishing Group.

Rubin IL, Crocker AC (1989) Developmental Disabilities: Delivery of Medical Care for Children and Adults. Philadelphia: Lea & Febiger.

Sheppard JJ (1987) Assessment of oral motor behaviours in cerebral palsy. Seminars in Speech and Language 8(1): 57–70.

Sheppard JJ (1991) Managing dysphagia in mentally retarded adults. Dysphagia 6: 83–7.

Sheppard JJ (1994) Clinical evaluation and treatment. In Rosenthal SR, Sheppard JJ, Lotze M (eds) Dysphagia and the Child with Developmental Disabilities: Medical, Clinical and Family Interventions. San Diego: Singular Publishing Group, pp. 37–76.

Sheppard JJ (2002) Swallowing and feeding in older people with lifelong disability. Advances in Speech-Language Pathology 4(2): 119–21.

Sheppard JJ, Guglielmo A, Burke LC, et al. (2003) Frequency of saliva swallowing in children before and after eating. Paper presented at the American Speech-Language-Hearing Annual Convention, Chicago.

Sheppard JJ, Hochman R (1989) Clinical symptoms of dysphagia in mentally retarded individuals. American Speech-Language-Hearing Association Annual Convention, St Louis MO, November.

Sheppard JJ, Liou J, Hochman R, et al. (1988) Nutritional correlates of dysphagia in individuals institutionalized with mental retardation. Dysphagia 3: 85–9.

Stewart JT (2003) Dysphagia associated with Risperidone therapy. Dysphagia 18(4): 274–5.

Vinter A, Detable C (2003) Implicit learning in children and adolescents with mental retardation. American Journal on Mental Retardation 108(2): 94–107.

Waterman ET, Koltai PJ, Downey JC, et al. (1992) Swallowing disorders in a population of children with cerebral palsy. International Journal of Pediatric Otorhinolaryngology 24: 63–71.

Westerinen H, Kaski M, Virta L, et al. (2004). Register based prevalence of intellectual disability (Abstract). Journal of Intellectual Disability Research 48: 488.

Woods EK (1995) The influence of posture and positioning on oral motor development and dysphagia. In Rosenthal SR, Sheppard JJ, Lotze M (eds) Dysphagia in the Child with Developmental Disabilities: Medical, Clinical, and Family Interventions. San Diego: Singular Publishing Group, pp. 153–88.

Zarate N, Mearin F, Hidalgo A, et al. (2001) Prospective evaluation of oesophageal motor dysfunction in Down's syndrome. American Journal of Gastroenterology 96(6): 1718–24.

11 Improving Swallowing Function: Compensation

JULIE CICHERO

INTRODUCTION

Swallowing, once damaged, can hopefully be improved either by *compensation* or *rehabilitation*. There is an important difference in these two terms and the strategies they employ to make the difference to the swallowing mechanism. It might assist if we take a brief look at the analogy of a broken leg. We can compensate for the broken leg by using a wheelchair or a set of crutches to mobilize. We still achieve the purpose of mobilizing but through different routes. It provides an immediate answer to the problem, but only a transient solution. We bypass the problem of the broken limb, we *compensate* for it. On the other hand, we may wish to mobilize again by using and repairing the broken leg – we want to effect permanent physiological change. In this case rehabilitation is employed. There is a period of time for the bone to mend but after that time the muscles of the legs must be strengthened and a range of motion exercises employed to ensure that the limb will function as normally as possible. This is the process of rehabilitation and the end product is a resumption of function as near as possible to the situation before the injury. Often, individuals who go on to rehabilitation begin with a period of compensation (using crutches). Even during the initial phases of rehabilitation they may still require their crutches. Gradually the ratio changes so that the compensatory mechanisms become fewer and the reliance on the limb becomes greater as function is restored. The eventual aim is that the compensatory strategies can be dispensed with when function is restored. Whether the function is the exactly the same as it was premorbidly is not the issue, although quality of life measures may show the patient to have different views on this matter. Hopefully this demonstrates that both compensation and rehabilitation are important aspects of the recovery of function.

This chapter will examine compensation in the improvement of swallowing. As with the broken limb analogy, compensatory techniques are often used during the acute and/or severe phases of recovery. It would be hoped that individuals would then progress to rehabilitation in order to improve the function of the swallowing mechanism – rehabilitation of swallowing is discussed in detail in Chapter 12. However, some individuals continue to rely on compensatory techniques for the long-term. Compensation can occur in the adaptation of:

Dysphagia: Foundation, Theory and Practice.   Edited by J. Cichero and B. Murdoch
© 2006 John Wiley & Sons, Ltd.

- posture;
- swallowing techniques;
- diet, temperature and taste;
- rate and route of intake;
- prosthetic devices and surgery.

These will now be expanded upon below.

POSTURE

Changing the posture of the individual with swallowing disorders can affect efforts to redirect the flow of food (body posture), alter postural stability associated with feeding (body posture) or change pharyngeal dimensions (head posture).

USING BODY POSTURE TO REDIRECT THE FLOW OF FOOD

One of the first rules the speech pathologist learns is that, for safe feeding, individuals should be sitting upright or the head of the bed should be at approximately 90°. Certainly this makes a great deal of sense. Gravity may assist in progressing the bolus through the pharynx more quickly. When lying down, the bolus travels more slowly through the pharynx and is more likely to adhere to the posterior pharyngeal walls. In the upright posture the bolus is projected in more of an anterolateral direction. Note that laryngeal protective responses do not appear to be affected when swallowing occurs in either the sitting or lying postures in healthy individuals when swallowing a small volume bolus (Barkmeier et al., 2002). The thyroaytenoid muscles are activated at the same time as or within milliseconds of activation of the submental complex that marks the initiation of the swallow. As yet there are no data to determine whether dysphagic individuals similarly have stable and consistent timing of laryngeal muscle onset regardless of body posture.

The upright position recommended to dysphagic individuals during feeding is also important to reduce the likelihood of reflux in susceptible individuals, because gravity again assists in keeping gastric contents in the stomach where they belong. When an individual lies down, the position of the abdominal contents shifts and pushes the diaphragm upwards. If there is material in the stomach it may push up against the lower oesophgeal sphincter (the junction between the oesophagus and the stomach) and creep back into the oesophagus. Once in the oesophagus, the bolus may exert pressure on the upper oesophageal sphincter (UES) and re-enter the pharynx. Intrabolus pressure in the supine position is significantly higher compared with an upright position (Shaker and Lang, 1994). This is most unsuitable as the refluxed bolus could dwell in the pharynx and be drawn into the open airway during tidal breathing. This would result in aspiration.

Postural stability and its association with safe feeding

The basic principles of eating and drinking in the upright position should not be viewed as absolute. It is important to remember that infants begin feeding in a position that is more horizontal than upright. Infants progress from feeding in a semi-lying and flexed position, progressing to an upright sitting position (~6 months to 8 months) and eventually to unassisted stable chair sitting. They require sitting balance and an ability to support the head and trunk in the upright position. If the trunk is unstable, this has a flow-through effect to the head. If individuals' attention is consumed with ensuring that they won't 'fall over', there is little room left to concentrate on swallowing. So how does this relate to posture during feeding? Basically the body must be supported and stable and the head should also be supported and stable. This provides the best base for the individual to be able to concentrate on swallowing.

Individuals with low muscle tone (i.e. hypotonus) are most likely to show poor ability to maintain head and trunk postural stability. Tamura et al. (1999) discuss the concepts of 'gravitational' and 'antigravitational' postures. An antigravitational posture is one where the body must support and maintain a substantial portion of its own weight. This necessitates prolonged muscle activity.

Sitting and standing are examples of antigravitational postures. When an individual lies down in a recumbent or supine position, the body does not have to support its own weight. The chair or bed bears the weight of the body. In individuals with severe disability, great effort is required to support their body weight to accomplish what healthy individuals consider as the simple act of sitting. An unstable trunk can in turn cause an unstable head. The platform for eating is unstable and this places the individual at risk of aspiration/penetration. There are measurable physiological signs that can alert the clinician that the mere act of trying to remain upright during feeding is 'hard work' for the individual.

Tamura et al. (1999) reported that, in individuals with severe disability, feeding in the upright position resulted in reduced oxygen saturation, and increased pulse rate. The increased pulse rate and also reports of increased respiratory rates are indicators that the body is trying to recover the reduction in available oxygen saturation levels. Again, the link between respiration and swallowing is quite pronounced.

The physiological changes reported by Tamura et al. (1999) only occurred during feeding. They did not occur when the individuals were simply sitting upright, showing that the act of eating and swallowing places additional demands on the cardiorespiratory system. What this should tell us, then, is that even though individuals should be sitting in as upright a position as possible to encourage safe swallowing, there is a delicate balance with the need to ensure that the very act of sitting does not put too much strain on the cardiopulmonary system. It is very likely that a supported reclined posture may in fact be more beneficial to individuals with impaired trunk and/or head control. The exact degree of recumbence has not, at this point, been determined. Dorsey (2002) presented information on this very issue. Dorsey (2002) found that upright positioning (70°–90°) in individuals with severe developmental disabilities was associated with aspiration. However, individuals who were supported and reclined (60°–35°) showed a reduction in aspiration. The change in posture was reported to shift the centre of balance from the pelvis up towards the trunk and shoulders. The effect was to increase stabilization of the jaw. Consequently the muscles of the lips, tongue and buccal region (cheeks) were able to work more effectively due to less effort, greater strength and coordination. These results have implications that stretch further than the cerebral palsy and developmental disability populations. Individuals who lose their ability to volitionally control head and trunk support through stroke, TBI or other acquired neurological or physical injury should also be afforded postural support during feeding. The act of sitting places muscular demands on the body. These demands must be kept to a minimum if the individual is to feed safely.

The clinical bottom line is that it is important that individuals be maintained in as upright a position as possible during feeding to (a) take advantage of the effects of gravity in propelling the bolus into the oesophagus, and (b) to make it harder for refluxed material to re-enter the pharynx after swallowing. However, where individuals are unable to support their head and/or trunk comfortably, measures must be taken to allow head and/or trunk support to occur. This may involve progressively reclining the chair/bed to an angle that best allows the body to be supported and reduce the 'physiological load' during eating. The exact degree of safe recumbency is yet to be determined.

HEAD POSTURES

Once the best 'body posture' for the individual has been determined, the clinician can then look at manipulating head position. Changes to head position can affect the direction of flow of the bolus and also the physical dimensions of the pharynx (make portions larger or smaller). These head postures are compensatory because, if effective, they should be employed for each and every swallow. The clinician must bear in mind the individual's (a) cognitive skills and ability to learn and remember to use head postures, and (b) the individual's physical reserve – whether fatigue will occur after a few swallows when using the compensatory pattern. These variables are important considerations when contemplating teaching an individual any compensatory technique. Can it be taught, can it be remembered faithfully and can it be maintained?

The following discussion outlines a selection of head postures that can be employed with individuals with dysphagia who have the requisite cognitive skills and physical reserve to use them. Note that the vast majority of these techniques were developed by Professor Jeri Logemann. These strategies have been developed with an understanding that a change to swallowing physiology is possible when there is a change to the anatomical alignment of the structures used during swallowing. She has been instrumental in the development of compensatory manoeuvres for dysphagic individuals.

CHIN TUCK

The chin tuck technique is probably one of the best-known head postures and is as its name suggests. Individuals are taught to *position their chin towards their chest and look down towards their knees.* Note, the head should maintain a midline posture; only the head moves. In using this manoeuvre, the larynx is brought further under the base of the tongue so as to physically bring it further away from the bolus. Remember that during resuscitation individuals are taught to bring the head backwards and extend it to open the airway. The chin tuck works on the principle that the airway is maximally protected if the head is flexed over the airway. When the head is in the chin tuck position, the oral part of the tongue is drawn forward (due to gravity) and the valleculae become bigger. Remember that valleculae are the spaces between the base of the tongue and the uppermost surface of the epiglottis (there are two valleculae – right and left). In this posture the tongue base, however, is afforded a closer position to the pharyngeal walls (Logemann, 1997).

Bulow et al. (1999) have also reported that when the chin tuck is employed there is a reduction in the distance between the larynx and the hyoid and between the hyoid and the mandible. During flexion, the entire distance of the pharynx is shortened. Note also that this shortening loosens the pharyngeal constrictor muscles. These muscles are responsible for advancing the bolus through the pharynx.

The chin tuck has been used when there is

- a delay in triggering the pharyngeal swallow; or
- if there is reduced posterior movement of the tongue base (Lazarus, 2000).

There are some contraindications. Note that extreme flexion (head forward) can make the airway prone to collapse. The mass of tissue behind the jaw and the hyoid may push into the airway causing this to happen (Wolf and Glass, 1992). Individuals who have a compromised respiratory system may find this posture somewhat suffocating and may be unable to sustain it or use it effectively. As noted above, Bulow (1999) points out that the act of flexion loosens the pharyngeal constrictors, making them potentially less effective in progressing the bolus through the pharynx. Individuals with weak pharyngeal constrictor muscles could be at risk for post-swallow residue and hence aspiration after the swallow if they employ the chin tuck technique. Note that individuals with impaired laryngeal excursion may also be at a disadvantage when using the chin tuck technique. The elevation and forward movement of the larynx is a key mechanical movement in effecting epiglottic closure. The effect of laryngeal excursion is to 'knock the feet' out from under the epiglottis. In the chin tuck position, an individual with poor laryngeal excursion will not effectively move the epiglottis to its horizontal position. The epiglottis will remain upright and, as the bolus is pushed towards the pharynx by the tongue, the bolus may follow the curves of the epiglottis up to the tip and then down the other side. The 'other side', however, is a route directly into the laryngeal vestibule and the airway below. An upright epiglottis provides an easy route for the bolus (particularly the liquid bolus) to reach the airway. Consequently, a reduction in laryngeal excursion should similarly contraindicate the use of the chin tuck.

HEAD ROTATION

The head rotation posture is also quite transparent. The posture involves the individual turning his or her head to the weaker side to the full extent of comfort. Note, only the head moves, the trunk should remain in the neutral position. The head movement effectively close off the weaker side and to physically encourage the bolus down the stronger side. This technique also has the effect of pulling the cricoid cartilage further away from the posterior pharyngeal wall. This reduces the resting pressure in the UES and may assist individuals who have UES dysfunction (Logemann, 1997).

Individuals with a unilateral weakness or who have undergone reconstruction of the pharynx may benefit from this technique. Individuals with difficulty opening the UES, such as those with the symptom of pyriform sinus residue post swallow may also benefit from this technique.

HEAD TILT

The head tilt posture uses the effect of gravity to move the bolus in the desired direction. The patient is instructed to tilt the head towards the stronger side during swallowing.

Individuals with unilateral oral weakness, or those with unilateral pharyngeal weakness may benefit from this technique. Note, the oral and pharyngeal weakness should be on the same side if the head tilt technique is to be employed. Individuals who have undergone head and neck surgery may also find this technique enables them to compensate for structures that may have been removed during surgery.

SIDE LYING

In the side-lying technique individuals are instructed to lie down on their side. This has the effect of reducing gravitational force, as discussed above. The bolus is more inclined to adhere to the posterior pharyngeal wall and stay away from the valleculae. Logemann (1997) reports that it is effective for individuals with reduced pharyngeal contractions, where one would see the symptom of diffuse pharyngeal residue post swallow.

This technique may benefit individuals with diffuse post-swallow pharyngeal residue as a result of pharyngeal weakness (unilateral or bilateral) and also individuals who have undergone head/neck surgery where the effectiveness of the pharyngeal muscles has been compromised.

However, this technique gives rise to issues concerning patient compliance. It cannot be adapted for social situations. It is also difficult to self-feed in this position, with the bolus spilling from the spoon before there is an opportunity to get it to the mouth.

NECK EXTENSION

In the neck extension posture, the individual is instructed to sit or stand in the upright position and when they are ready to transfer the bolus from the oral cavity to the pharynx to extend the neck backwards and lift the chin upwards. This technique uses gravity to clear the oral cavity (Logemann, 1997).

This technique is useful for individuals who have impairments in the oral transfer phase. They may show symptoms of post-swallow oral residue and bolus transfer problems.

The individual *must* have excellent airway protection abilities to safely use this technique. As noted above, the extended head position is effective in opening the airway. The individual must be able to protect the airway to use this technique. For this reason, it is suggested that only individuals with excellent cognitive skills and auditory comprehension be considered for this technique. It is often used in individuals who have undergone head/neck surgery. For these individuals, oropharyngeal structural impairment is the issue, not cognitive abilities. Note also that, in extending the neck, this action inhibits laryngeal excursion. This has the flow-on effect of inhibiting UES opening. The individual may need to be taught to adopt the neck extension technique only for the transfer phase from the oral to pharyngeal cavities and then quickly resume an upright head posture so as to reduce the impact on laryngeal elevation and UES opening.

The manoeuvres listed above are suitable for some but not all dysphagic individuals. Clinicians should be wary of 'always employing the chin tuck manoeuvre', for example. The manoeuvres should be applied on a case-by-case basis with careful thought given to the indications and also the contraindications of the techniques. A more conservative approach is warranted if the risks outweigh the benefits or indeed could make the situation worse.

AIRWAY PROTECTION STRATEGIES

The section above has focused on ways to improve swallowing function by changing the posture of the head or the body. A recurrent theme in this text is the interrelationship between respiration and swallowing. The following techniques focus specifically on protection of the airway during and/or after swallowing. There are three general airway protection strategies that can be employed in individuals with dysphagia. These are: the supraglottic swallow, the super-supraglottic swallow and pharyngeal expectoration. As with the head posture techniques described above, the clinician should give due consideration to the patient's ability to learn the techniques, be competent in using the techniques for each and every swallow and that the techniques are not likely to cause the patient to fatigue and decompensate their swallowing function. As with the postural techniques, the airway techniques will now be described below.

THE SUPRAGLOTTIC SWALLOW TECHNIQUE

During the supraglottic swallow the patients are instructed to take a breath gently and hold it, transfer the bolus into the oral cavity (the breath is still held) and swallow while holding their breath. Immediately after the swallow they are instructed to breathe out, cough or clear the throat. It is important that they understand that they should expel air immediately after the swallow before they take a breath in. If they take a breath in, residue in the pharynx is likely to be drawn into the laryngeal vestibule and the airway.

The effect of the supraglottic swallow is to bring the vocal folds together before and during the swallow, hence providing a mechanical barrier to penetrated/aspirated material. It provides conscious, volitional airway protection. It brings to conscious and volitional control the airway protection technique healthy individuals usually employ. Bulow et al. (1999) reported that the larynx starts to elevate as the individual inhales at the beginning of the supraglottic swallow technique and the prolonged laryngeal excursion assists also in prolonging relaxation and opening of the UES. Consequently this technique offers a dual role in mechanically protecting the airway via cord closure, but also better clearance of the pharynx with a longer period of UES opening and relaxation. It may be useful to teach this technique in stages. First of all, ask patients simply to hold their breath (no bolus, no swallow). Encourage them to hold their breath for particular periods of time (2 s, 5 s, 7 s). Then progress to hold the breath and then exhale forcefully (again no bolus is used). Once clinicians are satisfied that patients have sufficient respiratory reserve to support this technique and to understand the steps involved, they can introduce the swallow and the bolus. Finally the patient will progress to hold the breath, take the bolus in, swallow while holding the breath, then breathe out forcefully.

Individuals with reduced or delayed vocal fold closure and those with a delayed pharyngeal swallow might benefit from this technique (Logemann, 1997). Individuals with diagnosed 'silent aspiration' may be candidates for this technique. Individuals who have difficulty coordinating swallowing and respiration may find this technique successful as it provides a conscious structure to the patterning of swallowing and respiration.

Individuals with an already compromised respiratory status (e.g. chronic obstructive pulmonary disease) may find that they can only employ this technique for short periods of time. Fatigue may reduce the effectiveness of the technique. Note also that both the supraglottic swallow and the super-supraglottic swallow are contraindicated in individuals with a history of stroke or coronary artery disease, and those with acute congestive heart failure or uncontrolled hypertension. This is because of the stress that the breath-holding manoeuvres place on heart function (Chaudhuri et al., 2002).

THE SUPER-SUPRAGLOTTIC SWALLOW TECHNIQUE

The super-supraglottic swallow builds from the supraglottic swallow. This technique uses effortful breath holding and forceful exhalation or cough after the swallow prior to taking a breath in. The differences between the super-supraglottic swallow and the supraglottic swallow are in the effort of breath holding and the force used to expel the breath after the swallow. When effortful breath holding as opposed to voluntary breath holding is employed the arytenoids are tilted further forward, the vocal folds (true and false) come together and the laryngeal ventricles are obliterated. This provides a tight mechanical valve. In order to achieve effortful breath holding, the individual may be instructed to take a deep breath *and hold it*, rather than just holding his or her breath. As with the supraglottic swallow, breath holding (in this case effortful) is employed prior to and throughout the swallow. The effortful breathing out, or throat clearing or post-swallow coughing aims to use the subglottic pressure generated by that tight laryngeal valve to blow out any pharyngeal residue up towards the oral cavity. From here it can be swallowed again or expectorated. Bulow et al. (1999) make a good point regarding instructions for this expulsion of air out after the swallow. It is important that the individual be aware that the air should be *expelled*. In coughing we take a breath in to generate the subglottal pressures required to cough effectively. It may be safer to simply advise the individual to *blow the air out* after the swallow.

The indications for use of this technique is reduced closure of the airway entrance (Logemann, 1997). As with the supraglottic swallow above, individuals with a compromised respiratory system, may find that this technique causes fatigue and may decompensate while using it. In addition, those patients who have a history of stroke or coronary artery disease are not advised to use this technique due to potentially harmful cardiac consequences (Chaudhuri et al., 2002).

PHARYNGEAL EXPECTORATION

Pharyngeal expectoration (spitting out) is useful for clearing post-swallow pharyngeal residue. The instructions may be along the lines of bringing secretions up from the back of the throat or a 'truck driver's spit' (Huckabee, 2003). It relies on the individual having sufficient pharyngeal muscle strength to bring post-swallow residue from the pharyngeal region back up into the oral cavity. It aims to physically remove accumulated pharyngeal contents. If it can't go down, bring it back out of the mouth.

Individuals with reduced laryngeal excursion and therefore likely poor UES opening may benefit from this technique. People with poor laryngeal excursion are more prone to pyriform sinus residue. Those with poor base of tongue function who present with valleculae residue may also benefit from this technique.

Individuals with poor pharyngeal contractions may have trouble with the pharyngeal expectoration technique as it requires them to use the pharyngeal muscles to bring the bolus out of the pharynx and back into the mouth. It is socially rather an unpleasant sound, and the individual must also discreetly dispose of the material. For this reason it is likely that this technique is more of a short-term solution to pharyngeal residue.

OTHER COMPENSATORY MANOEUVRES

The manoeuvres discussed above fall neatly into postural change strategies or airway protection strategies. There are, however, two other manoeuvres that are not covered under these headings. These are the Mendelsohn manoeuvre and the effortful swallow. These are described below.

MENDELSOHN MANOEUVRE

The Mendelsohn manoeuvre is designed to address the problem of reduced laryngeal elevation during swallowing. The individual is instructed to hold the swallow at the height of vertical movement of the larynx. Translated to the patient it is like holding the swallow at the point where the base of the tongue is at its highest and stopping the swallow midway. The effect of catching the swallow 'midway' is that this is the height of laryngeal excursion. We know that, through hyolaryngeal excursion, the UES is able to open due to the pulling motion on the UES via the cricoid cartilage. With a prolonged period of hyolaryngeal elevation, the UES also remains open for longer. There is therefore a better possibility of the bolus passing fully into the oesophagus.

This manoeuvre is designed to be used with individuals who display reduced laryngeal elevation during swallowing.

This manoeuvre requires the individual to have exceptional cognitive abilities. In the author's personal experience I have found only one or two patients capable of understanding and then achieving the Mendelsohn manoeuvre.

THE EFFORTFUL SWALLOW

The effortful swallow involves instructing the patient to swallow very hard. I have often asked patients to think of it as 'trying to swallow the phone book'. The effort in employing the technique increases posterior tongue base movement (Logemann, 1997). It is suggested that it is appropriate for reduced pharyngeal strength as it uses the forceful movement of the tongue to increase external pressure on the bolus. This then moves the bolus through the pharynx more effectively and reduces the likelihood of residue. Bulow et al. (1999) noted that the muscle tension employed to use this technique causes muscle shortening, which subsequently causes early elevation, but decreased movement of the larynx and hyoid. The effortful swallow technique does effectively shorten the route for laryngeal elevation (Bulow et al., 1999).

It is suggested that the effortful swallow be used with individuals with reduced pharyngeal contractions or weakness of the pharynx.

COMBINATIONS: HEAD POSTURES PLUS COMPENSATORY MANOEUVRES

The clinician should be aware that the postures and manoeuvres outlined above need not occur in isolation. It is possible to combine manoeuvres where appropriate. The appropriateness of combining manoeuvres should be determined on a case-by-case basis taking into account the underlying physiology of the dysphagia. For example, it would be appropriate to combine a chin tuck with head rotation to the damaged side. It may also be suitable to combine the supraglottic swallow with the neck extension technique to be certain to protect the airway.

DIET

Physically changing the patient's posture or employing certain airway protection or head postures may assist the individual with dysphagia. However, there will be circumstances where it is not possible to teach individuals the postures or be sure that they will use the postures faithfully for every swallow. One of the first compensatory acts is to change the type or texture of food and/or fluid the dysphagic individual receives. Clinicians are aware, for example, that a thickened fluid is more cohesive than a thin liquid bolus and travels more slowly than a thin liquid bolus. Cohesiveness and slower transit hopefully equate to better oropharyngeal control of the bolus. The physiological changes that occur when swallowing a thickened fluid bolus have been described in detail in Chapter 3. For solids, the clinician should return to the process of transitional feeding in infants. Recall that infants begin their foray into solids by taking smooth, lump-free pureed foods. They then progress to minced food, finely chopped foods, soft foods and finally 'table foods' that healthy adults enjoy.

The transitional feeding progression in the child relates to maturation of the teeth and coordination of biting, chewing and mastication in the formation of a swallow-safe bolus. The brain is being taught and laying foundations for patterned responses in later life. When an individual presents with an acquired dysphagia, it is generally the case that, once again, we revert to the safe pureed foods and progress through the continuum back up to regular table foods.

The following section will briefly describe the types of foods and fluids that are recommended by speech pathologists for individuals with dysphagia. It is important to be aware that there is vast diversity in terminology for the gradations of foods and fluids used in dietary recommendations. The variations in terminology are not country specific – they are not even state specific, but may vary from hospital to hospital and nursing home to nursing home. The diversity in terminology makes it difficult to communicate the dysphagic individual's needs. The clinician should be diligent in ensuring that any terminology used is as transparent as possible – preferably giving descriptors to assist interpretation. Speech Pathology and Dietetic groups are moving towards standardization of terminology in the US (Clayton, 2002), Britain and Australia. It is likely that this process is also occurring in other countries.

The following is a *generic classification* of solids and liquids into broad terms, with examples provided to assist clarification. The classification progresses from the most modified textures to standard textures.

SOLIDS

Vitamized food

Food in this category is smooth and lump free. It does not require chewing and should hold together on the spoon (i.e. it is cohesive). Dysphagic individuals are likely to have trouble forming a bolus by themselves. Vitamized food could also be described as like mousse or pudding.

Examples of suitable foods are vitamized meat and vegetables (extra gravy may be required to make the food moist and less sticky), pureed pasta, pureed fruit, custard; smooth cooked cereals, yoghurt, pureed scrambled eggs. Examples of foods to avoid are bread, rolls, biscuits/crackers, muffins, dry cereals, cakes, pies, pastries, whole fruit, nuts, soups that have chunks (e.g. minestrone), lettuce, stringy vegetables, corn, baked beans, lollipops/candies that require chewing.

'Minced' food

Food in this category is soft and requires minimal chewing. The food is still moist and should be easy to form into a bolus. Foods in this category should be able to be deformed by using the tongue to squeeze the bolus against the palate.

Examples of suitable foods are those listed for the vitamized diet plus the following: minced or finely chopped meats and vegetables (extra gravy may still be required to add moisture to the food), puddings and custards, soft moist cakes, fork-mashed soft fruits, poached, scrambled or soft-cooked eggs, and well cooked soft and moist pastas.

Avoid dry or coarse cereals, dry or coarse cakes or biscuits/cookies, dried fruits, tough meats (e.g. bacon, sausages), sandwiches, potentially mixed textures (e.g. cereal with milk), hot or cold potato chips, corn, peas, beans, lettuce, nuts, lollipops/candies that require chewing.

'Soft' food

Food in this category is close to approaching regular table food. Due to the process of ageing or disease, some individuals may find firm or hard solid food difficult to bite and chew. Moreover, individuals with dentures often have difficulty biting and masticating hard foods, such as raw apples. Foods in this category are, therefore, modified to exclude items that are particularly hard, firm, brittle, sticky or crunchy. Adequate dentition and chewing ability are required. The elderly may naturally gravitate to this mild form of diet texture modification due to difficulties with dentition and mastication that are associated with normal ageing.

Examples of suitable foods are well-moistened cereals, soft-filled sandwiches (e.g. spread filling, not meat and salad filling for example), casseroles, rice dishes, canned and cooked fruits, eggs.

Examples of foods to avoid are tough and crusty breads, biscuits/cookies, dry cakes, dried fruit, hard fruit (e.g. apple, pear), stringy fruit; dry meat, fish or chicken dishes, raw vegetables, nuts, candies/lollipops that require chewing.

Regular or 'table' foods

There are no limitations to textures or types of foods in this category. Individuals would probably have fully functioning dentition (either their own teeth or well fitting dentures) and have no weakness of the oral musculature required for mastication.

Special categories

Liquid puree includes soups and foods that have been turned into a liquid format. *High energy fluids* are a category 'designed' by dietitians to meet the nutritional needs of individuals who are unable to cope with traditional purees. Foods in these categories may be used for oncology patients, jaw-wired patients or patients who have undergone maxillo-facial surgery.

FLUIDS

Thickened fluids can be purchased fully prepared from commercial distributors in tetra packs and larger containers. Thickened fluids can also be made up to the desired level of thickness using varying levels of commercially available powdered thickeners to reach the desired consistency. Depending on the thickening agent used, most varieties of fluids can be thickened, including hot and cold fluids. Carbonated fluids can be thickened, however, they tend to lose their carbonation in the thickening process and can taste quite syrupy. Although water can be thickened, it tends to acquire the taste of thickener (however mild) and tends no longer to taste like water. A weak flavouring (e.g. cordial) can mask the mild flavour of the thickener and also allow ingestion of more pleasant tasting thickened water. The clinician should be aware that the 'base substance' (i.e. juice, water, milk or dairy product) has an effect on how much thickener should be added to achieve the desired consistency. For example, less thickener is added to a juice-based drink than a milk-based drink for both drinks to achieve the same degree of 'thickness'. The clinician should also be aware that thick fluids have a 'standing time'. The standing time is the time taken for the thickened fluid to reach its stable level of 'thickness' after the powdered thickener is added to the fluid. For some fluids this time is 5 minutes, for others closer to 15 minutes. Some fluids then remain stable, whereas others continue to thicken on standing. This is when the fluid continues to thicken with time, even though no more thickener powder has been added. It can turn a nectar-like fluid into a semi-thickened fluid over the course of a day. Thickened fluids vary in their degree of thickness depending upon temperature. There are some everyday examples that illustrate this point nicely. Think of honey and also toothpaste. During summer the honey is very runny and it is very easy to squeeze the toothpaste from the tube. During colder months, however, the honey becomes thicker and the toothpaste becomes more viscous, hence a greater degree of pressure is required to squeeze it out of the tube. Thickened fluids behave in a similar fashion – they vary with temperature, often becoming thinner when heated. Some thickeners are designed to maintain the degree of thickness regardless of whether they are added to a hot liquid, or if the liquid is frozen. Individual thickeners should be scrutinized, however, for what they are able to achieve. Each of the variables detailed above should be considered by the clinician when teaching patients or their carers how to make up thickened fluids for home or community use. Further details about thickened fluids and the study of rheology and material characterization can be found in Chapter 3. In an ideal world individuals would receive a fluid that is thickened to precisely the amount they require to make it safe for them to swallow, but no more than that. Due to the mass production of thickened fluids that by necessity occurs in hospitals and aged-care facilities, it is common practice to use only two to three different levels of thickened fluids. Unfortunately, the economics allows little chance of individualization. Three levels of thickened fluids are described below.

- *'Full thick'* or *'pudding-like'* *thickened fluids.* These fluids are cohesive and hold a shape on a spoon. It is not possible to pour these fluids from a cup into the mouth. It is not possible to ingest this thickness of fluid using a straw. Spoon is the optimal method of ingesting this type of thickened fluid.
- *'Half thick'* or *'smooth drinking yoghurt consistency'* *thickened fluids.* These fluids are sometimes known as 'honey-thick consistency'. They are also cohesive, and pour slowly. It is possible to ingest these fluids directly from the cup; however, they do pour quite slowly. These fluids would pour in a slow, steady stream from a spoon. It would be very difficult to ingest this thickness of fluid using a straw, although it may be possible using a wide-bore straw.
- *'Quarter thick'* or *'nectar-like'* *thickened fluids.* Fluids in this category pour reasonably rapidly from a cup. They generally leave a residue in the cup after being poured out and may leave a 'coating feeling' in the mouth. It is possible to ingest this level of fluid thickness from a cup or using a straw.
- *'Regular'* or *'thin fluids'.* These are the fluids healthy individuals ingest on a daily basis. They are free flowing and fall rapidly when poured. They can be ingested easily by cup or straw.

Note, thick fluids are not an 'all-or-none' phenomenon. An individual may be eligible to test sips of thin fluids under strict supervision, while consuming thickened fluids at other time independently. Decisions such as these should be determined on a case-by-case basis.

DIET – OTHER CONSIDERATIONS

Administration of medications

The clinician should also give consideration to patient safety in swallowing oral medications. It is inappropriate for individuals who require full thick fluids and a vitamized diet to be expected to swallow 3–4 capsules or tablets per day. After consultation with the patient's medical doctor and pharmacist the following alternatives could be considered if appropriate:

- crushing the tablets and dispensing them in a spoonful of thickened fluid;
- liquid as opposed to tablet form;
- alternative methods of administration (e.g. suppository).

Note that some medications are unsuitable for crushing. For example, some medications have an enteric coating that prevents them from being 'broken down' and dispersed until they reach the stomach – it is inappropriate to crush such medications.

The patient's physician and pharmacist should be consulted with regards to administration of medications in the individual with dysphagia.

Oral hygiene

It is particularly important for individuals with dysphagia to have good oral hygiene. Langmore et al. (1998) found that dependency for oral hygiene and number of decayed teeth ranked as second and third on the list of 'best predictors' for a dysphagic individual to develop aspiration pneumonia. If there are concerns about patients swallowing their toothpaste, then a toothpaste with a smaller percentage of fluoride can be used – e.g. a toothpaste intended for paediatric use. Alternatively water can be used to moisten the toothbrush and dispense with the toothpaste altogether. Much like scrubbing the grime from a dirty floor, it is more the circular, abrasive action of the brush against the teeth that removes plaque than the toothpaste per se. Alternatively, the ability to hold a small amount of rinsing water in the mouth and then expectorating it could form quite a good therapeutic task for voluntary oral control of a volatile bolus (i.e. water). Rehabilitation strategies are discussed extensively in Chapter 12. Oral hygiene should be remembered, particularly with individuals who have a unilateral sensory loss and are prone to pocketing food in the buccal cavity.

RATE OF ORAL INTAKE AND ROUTE OF INTAKE

Swallowing compensation can also be achieved by altering the rate at which food or fluid is provided to the oral cavity and also the route of intake. Clinicians will generally want dysphagic individuals to slow down the rate at which they put food or fluid into their mouth. This is particularly the case with individuals following TBI or individuals who have a right hemisphere deficit – both groups are prone to impulsivity and poor self monitoring. Ways of reducing the speed of oral intake include:

- using a teaspoon rather than a standard-sized spoon (this also reduces volume);
- using a small cup (i.e. 100 ml capacity) rather than a standard-sized cup (250 ml capacity);
- using a cup with a lid and sipper moulding – with or without a one-way valve;
- use of wrist weights to encourage the individual to put the fork or spoon down between mouthfuls.

In addition to modifications by way of smaller versions of cups and spoons to adjust the amount of oral intake an individual receives, there are other devices that can assist the individual with dysphagia. For example, a 'dysphagia cup' has been designed. It is oval shaped so that the individual has sufficient room for his or her nose while tipping the cup up. It has a large handle on the side to assist individuals with less than optimal fine motor function. It is also weighted so that its base is heavy, encouraging the individual to put the cup down between mouthfuls. The heavy base also provides the cup stability, with it being less prone to being accidentally tipped over. Other methods of altering the way in which individuals receive their solids or fluids may have to be individually tailored. I had some success modifying a sauce bottle by attaching a piece of flexible straw-like tubing to its end so that individuals could use their hand to squeeze the fluid up the tubing and deliver it to the posterior of the oral cavity. The person for whom this adaptation was made had had a large proportion of the soft palate removed due to cancer. He was finding it difficult to manipulate the fluid so that it flowed down his stronger side. The task of drinking was much less taxing for this patient because he was able to deliver the bolus to the posterior of the oral cavity and direct it to his stronger side.

Despite our best efforts, it is not always possible for individuals to keep taking food and fluids orally. It is necessary for some individuals to be fed by non-oral methods. Aspiration is one reason why individuals may be fed for the short or longer term non-orally. Fatigue may also play a part in determining a role for non-oral feeding. Individuals who take 10 s or more to prepare every mouthful will be too fatigued to meet all of their nutritional needs orally. Some of these non-oral feeding methods include:

• nasogastric feeding (NGT);
• gastrostomy feeding (also known as PEG – for percutaneous endoscopic gastrostomy);
• total parenteral nutrition (TPN); and
• an intravenous line (IV).

A nasogastric tube allows for nutrition to be delivered to the individual without the added pressure of eating while the individual is recovering. The nasogastric tube is placed into the nose, passes down the pharynx, through the UES, and into the oesophagus. The NGT is generally considered a short-term solution. Agitated patients are prone to pulling their NG tubes out due to irritation. Patients with NG tubes are also prone to reflux. Percutaneous endoscopic gastrostomy are generally considered a long-term solution to the issue of non-oral feeding. Here a surgical incision places an entry point permanently into the stomach for direct placement of the nutritional bolus. Percutaneous endoscopic gastrostomies can be removed if patients improve to the point where they no longer need them. Complications with this procedure include, the risk of infection around the stoma site, soreness of the site and leakage out of the stoma. Total parenteral nutrition is reserved for patients who are unable to take nutrition via enteral means, i.e. via the stomach and digestive system. With TPN, a nutritionally complete solution is infused directly into the bloodstream. It is often administered via the subclavian vein. IV lines are used to provide the patient with hydration. It does not provide nutrition per se. Acutely ill individuals can tolerate a short period of time (~48 hours) with IV fluids only before a means of providing nutrition (oral or non-oral) must be achieved.

Note that oral and non-oral feeding are not 'all-or-nothing' phenomena. It is possible for an individual to receive non-oral feeding and, when safe, commence small amounts of oral intake. This is often done in the middle of the day when the individual is most alert and least likely to be fatigued. Non-oral feeds can be gradually reduced so that the individual experiences the sensation of hunger and is thus more likely to want to eat food orally.

PROSTHETIC DEVICES AND SURGERY

The use of surgery or prosthetic devices is another more radical form of compensation for dysphagia. In one case, an individual seen clinically who presented with surgical removal of the right portion of the soft palate, a surgical device provided both improved communication and improved swallowing. The speech pathologist accompanied the patient to a prosthedontist who designed and fitted an obturator for the patient. The obturator was a plate-like device that attached to the patient's existing upper teeth. It had a large bulbous portion at the posterior region that acted to fill the void left by surgical removal of the portion of soft palate tissue. The prosthesis required a tongue impression and it was reshaped so that it was individualized for the patient. Although speech therapy was still required to enhance communication after fitting the obturator, the patient's communication and swallowing skills were significantly improved when the obturator was used.

The obturator is also known as a *palatal augmentation prosthesis.* This device has most commonly been used for individuals who have sections of the oropharynx removed due to cancer, especially after glossectomy. It is also useful for individuals with impaired tongue mobility due to trauma or neurological disorders (Marunick and Tselios, 2004). The prosthesis allows for an augmented palate to be created. It is possible, for example, to 'build up' the prosthetic palate so that the vault of the hard palate is lowered. Hence the patient with limited tongue movement is more likely to be able to achieve tongue-to-palate contacts, which are required for both speech and swallowing. This type of prosthesis may particularly assist the oral stage of swallowing, assisting with more efficient food preparation and reducing the likelihood of oral residue (Light et al., 2001).

A *palatal lift* is another prosthetic device that may be considered when there is minimal or no elevation of the soft palate. In addition to extremely poor soft palate function, the potential candidate should also have a reduced gag reflex. This is to ensure that when the prosthesis is in place the device does not trigger a gag reflex. When the device is in place the incompetent soft palate is brought level with the hard palate. The uvula, however, is not covered. The width of the lift section varies from patient to patient (Light et al., 2001). This device is particularly useful for reducing nasal air emissions by providing a mechanical barrier for air leakage into the nasal cavity. In addition, intraoral air pressure is improved for speech. It is also possible to use the palatal lift prosthesis in combination with the palatal augmentation device. Together these devices may be useful for the treatment of speech and swallowing disorders where the deficit lies with the soft palate region (Light et al., 2001).

These prostheses have some disadvantages. They include:

• discomfort;
• poor mouth odour as a result of accumulated food residue on the prosthesis;
• continuing velopharyngeal insufficiency;

- elimination of sensory feedback from the intact mucosa of the hard palate, as the prosthesis now covers this portion;
- difficulty in social situations due to the large size of the prothesis (Sinha et al., 2004).

In order to address these issues, Sinha et al. (2004) have reported on the use of a *folded radial forearm free flap* to reconstruct the palate. This type of surgery is obviously only suitable for individuals who have had portions of the velopharynx surgically removed. This type of surgery would not be suitable for individuals with velopharyngeal insufficiency as a result of neurological deficit. The radial foream free flaps have the benefit of being able to restore sensation as one of the antebrachial cutaneous nerves is attached to the glossopharyngeal or greater palatine nerve. These flaps do not, however, restore dynamic function to the region. They work in the same way as the prosthesis, although they have the advantage of being permanent and re-establishing sensation where possible.

Selley (1985) has reported on the use of an intra-oral device called a *palatal training appliance*. The palatal training device is designed and fitted by a dental surgeon. The appliance consists of a 1 mm stainless steel piece of wire that is bent into a U shape. The device is bent to conform to the shape of the patient's resting soft palate, with the bottom of the U shape lightly touching the soft palate near the base of the uvula. The aim of the device, which is worn throughout the day, is to stimulate a reflexive swallow. The mere presence of the device in the mouth causes some initial increased salivation. It is possible that the increased sensory stimulus offered by additional saliva in the oral cavity may in fact be more of a catalyst for improving swallowing function, simply by increased practice!

CLINICAL CONSIDERATIONS

When considering a prosthesis or surgery for velopharyngeal deficits following surgery, trauma or neurological deficit, Marunick and Tselios (2004) suggest evaluation of the following:
(a) mobility and sensory status of the remaining structures (mandible, floor of mouth, tongue, lips, cheeks, velopharyngeal complex), (b) interach space, (c) maxillomandibular relations, (d) dentition, (e) alveolar ridges, (f) salivary function and (g) radiotherapy on soft tissue. In addition these should be evaluated in conjunction with swallowing studies, patient expectations, and patient motivation. These factors in combination will allow the determination of realistic treatment goals (Marunick and Tselios, 2004: 68).

SURGERY

Surgery and temporary surgical implants have been a consideration for individuals with poor airway closure due to paralysis of one of the vocal folds. *Medialization thyroplasty* has most often been associated with surgical restoration of voice; however, it may also be used for individuals with poor airway closure. An inability to protect the airway during swallowing places the individual at risk of aspiration. The concept behind medialization is that an additional bulk is added to the damaged vocal fold. This is done by either surgically inserting an implant (Type I thyroplasty), or injecting the damaged cord with Teflon or Gelfoam. For Type I thyroplasty the implant is placed between the thyroid cartilage and the vocalis muscle (Woo, 2000). Both the surgical and injection procedures are carried out by a qualified surgeon (e.g. an ENT surgeon). Some patients are not suitable candidates for medialization thyroplasty. These include those with bleeding disorders or compromised immune status, those undergoing chemotherapy and those with poor wound healing.

After vocal fold paralysis both biomechanical and histological changes occur. Apart from immobility of the damaged cord, there is also an absence of vocal fold tension and muscle atrophy begins. These factors work to change the position of the vocal fold. The medialization thyroplasty and injection procedures aim to reshape the position of the cord and also the stiffness of the damaged cord (Woo, 2000). With the damaged cord bulked up and in a more midline position, the functional cord has a better chance of contacting with it to provide adequate airway closure. *Arytenoid adduction* may also be performed in conjunction with medialization thyroplasty.

Even with successful medialization thyroplasty there may still exist a 'posterior chink' or opening. This posterior opening would mean that a portion of the cords was not entirely closed and could allow material to be aspirated through the opening. In order to address this problem, the surgical approach of arytenoid adduction may be used. Again, a qualified surgeon is best placed to recommend the type of surgery most suitable for individual situations.

As noted above, the medialization thyroplasty and injection procedures have been used predominantly for improvement in vocal quality; however, few objective data are available for swallowing outcomes (Bhattacharyya et al., 2002). Unilateral vocal fold immobility most commonly results from thoracic or cardiac surgery, followed by malignancy, with a small percentage associated with idiopathic origin, high vagal or intracranial causes or neck mass (Nayak et al., 2002). It is also more commonly left-sided (Bhattacharyya et al., 2002). Caution is warranted given that surgery may result in inadvertent trauma to the strap muscles, the superior laryngeal nerve or the ansa cervicalis. These could, in turn, lead to postoperative swallowing disorders associated with reduced laryngeal elevation or even reduced laryngopharyngeal sensation (Bhattacharyya et al., 2002). So it is possible for patients to present with adequate swallowing but poor voice quality before the procedure, and then after the procedure have better vocal quality but poorer swallowing performance (Bhattacharyya et al., 2002). It should also be fully ascertained via thorough assessment (see Chapter 8) that the swallowing problem does indeed arise from poor glottic closure. Deficits such as reduced laryngeal excursion or poor pharyngeal propulsion will not be improved by the surgical or injection techniques. Note also that the injection techniques may also pose problems if the substance injected strays from its intended location resulting in potential airway compromise

(Kelly, 2000). The clinician and the medical team should be very clear as to the cause of the problem before embarking upon treatment, with the treatment designed to address the specific problem. Further research is required to determine those who are most likely to benefit from the medialization thyroplasty or injection.

CRICOPHARYNGEAL MYOTOMY

Cricopharyngeal myotomy is probably the best-known surgical intervention for dysphagia. It is a surgical procedure whereby the fibres of the cricopharyngeal muscle are cut to permanently open the sphincter. It was first used in 1951 as a treatment for post-polio dysphagia and is designed to relieve pharyngeal obstruction (Kelly, 2000). Logemann (1998: 147) more completely describes the procedure as: 'an external incision through the side of the neck into the cricopharyngeal muscle, slitting the fibres from top to bottom, usually at the posterior midline'. Shin et al. (1999) explain that there are in fact two surgical approaches for myotomy – posterior section (as described above), and lateral section. Bilateral lateral section has been shown to be more useful than posterior section (Shin et al., 1999). The myotomy incision usually extends upwards to include part of the muscle and downwards into part of the oesophageal muscle. Extreme caution must be exercised due to the close proximity of the recurrent laryngeal nerve. Cricopharyngeal myotomy is most suited to individuals with disorders specific to the cricopharyngeal region. Kelly (2000) advocates use of the procedure when there is defective opening of the UES but with adequate hyolaryngeal excursion and adequate tongue and pharyngeal propulsion forces. Individuals selected for the procedure should also be medically and neurologically stable. The most common contraindication for the procedure is medical instability.

Cricopharyngeal myotomy is best used in individuals who present with cricopharyngeal spasm and also Zenker's diverticulum (Veenker et al., 2003). Cricopharyngeal spasm is where the cricopharyngeal muscle fails to relax adequately or completely, causing an anchoring effect on the larynx, preventing its normal movement of lifting upward and forward (Logemann, 1998). Zenker's diverticulum is an outpouching of the oesophageal mucosa through Killian's triangle anatomically located between the transverse fibres of the cricopharyngeus and the oblique fibres of the inferior pharyngeal constrictor (Veenker et al., 2003). The studies that advocate use of myotomy for these conditions have small subject numbers (Kelly, 2000; Veenker et al., 2003).

Cricopharyngeal myotomy has been used in the paediatric (newborn) population for primary cricopharyngeal achalasia. The achalasia results from the cricopharyngeal muscle failing to relax at the appropriate time in the swallowing process, despite an absence of motor abnormalities (Korakaki et al., 2004). The authors in the study report, however, that dysphagia persisted for up to 5 months after surgery and was likely linked to concurrent oesophageal abnormalities. The disorder is relatively rare and difficult to diagnose. Symptoms appearing in the weeks after birth may include coughing, choking, regurgitation of saliva and milk, nasal reflux, recurrent aspiration, pneumonia and failure to thrive (Korakaki et al., 2004). Korakaki et al. (2004) report that feeding can commence on the first day after surgery although it may take some time for the infant to sustain adequate nutrition purely by oral means. Supplementary feeding by way of nasogastric tube or gastrostomy may be required to ensure that the infant continues to thrive.

Cricopharyngeal myotomy has also been used in the motor neurone disease population (MND), also known as amyotrophic lateral sclerosis (ALS). It is a surgical intervention that is aimed at promoting oral intake for as long as possible in this population. The success rate, however, is 30% to 50%, with improvement often only being temporary (Shin, et al., 1999; Ryuzaburo et al., 2002). The authors of this study strongly advocate that the oral and pharyngeal phases of swallowing should be evaluated using both videofluoroscopy and manometry. Each technique (described further in Chapters 7 and 8) provides complementary information. In practice, videofluoroscopy is the most common method of diagnosis together with a thorough patient history. Radiographically the clinician may see an obstruction to thick fluids or solids or a hypopharyngeal bar that obstructs greater than 50% of the lumen. Manometry, an advantageous adjunct, is often not available (Kelly, 2000). Ryuzaburo et al. (2002) suggest that cricopharyngeal myotomy is not recommended for motor neurone disease/ALS patients who present with poor tongue function or, those with weak pharyngeal strength but a normally relaxing UES. Cricopharyngeal myotomy is not a cure-all. It must be tailored to specific cricopharyngeal dysfunction to be effective. Note that UES tone is not abolished during the procedure but is reduced by about 50%. Moreover, myotomy does *not* increase the prevalence of regurgitation in patients who undergo the procedure for pharyngeal dysphagia (Williams et al., 1999).

LARYNGEAL SUSPENSION

Laryngeal suspension is another type of surgical procedure that may be suitable when there is severely inadequate or even absent elevation of the larynx during swallowing. The complications of this may be insufficient opening of the cricopharyngeus or UES, and also aspiration. The aim of surgery in this case is the permanent positioning of the larynx in an elevated and anterior position to physically move it out of the way of the incoming bolus. During surgery, the larynx may be fixed to the hyoid bone or suspended from the mandible by wire or thread. By elevating the larynx in this manner, the UES is opened. The larynx in its new position is also resting up high under the base of the tongue. The close location of the base of tongue to the opening of the larynx may cause the patient respiratory difficulties (e.g. dyspnea) so, again, the surgeon will exercise extreme caution in the final positioning of the structures.

Note that surgery and injection should be considered *only after natural recovery has ceased and all therapy techniques have been exhausted*. The prosthetic, surgical and injection treatments are included in this chapter as they are a way of compensating for physiologic insufficiency. In performing the procedure they effect permanent change. Some may see this more as a rehabilitative procedure; however, it is included here for the sake of completeness.

REFERENCES

Barkmeier J, Bielamowicz S, Tekeda N, et al. (2002) Laryngeal activity during upright vs.supine swallowing. Journal of Applied Physiology 93(2): 740–5.

Bhattacharyya N, Kotz T, Shapiro J (2002) Dysphagia and aspiration with unilateral vocal cord immobility: Incidence, characterization, and response to surgical treatment. The Annals of Otology, Rhinology and Laryngology 111(8): 672–9.

Bulow M, Olsson R, Ekberg O (1999) Videomanometric analysis of supraglottic swallow, effortful swallow, and chin tuck in healthy volunteers. Dysphagia 14: 67–72.

Chaudhuri G, Hildner CD, Brady S, et al. (2002) Cardiovascular effects of the supraglottic and super-supraglottic swallowing maneuvers in stroke patients with dysphagia. Dysphagia 17: 19–23.

Clayton J (ed.) (2002) National Dysphagia Diet Task Force. National Dysphagia Diet: Standardization for Optimal Care. Chicago IL: American Dietetic Association.

Dorsey LD (2002) Effects of reclined supported postures on management of dysphagic adults with severe developmental disabilities. Dysphagia 17(2): 180.

Huckabee M-L (2003) Topics in Dysphagia Management. Course Presentation: Speech Pathology Australia, Brisbane, 20–21 June.

Kelly JH (2000) Management of upper esophageal sphincter disorders: Indications and complications of mytomy. American Journal of Medicine 108(4a): 43S–46S.

Korakaki E, Hatzidaki E, Manoura A, Velegrakis G, Charissis G, Gourgiotis D, Giannakopoulou C (2004) Feeding difficulties in a neonate with primary cricopharyngeal achalasia treated by cricopharyngeal myotomy. International Journal of Pediatric Otorhinolaryngology 68: 249–53.

Langmore SE, Terpenning MS, Schork A, et al. (1998) Predictors of aspiration pneumonia: how important is dysphagia? Dysphagia 13(2): 69–81.

Lazarus CL (2000) Management of swallowing disorders in head and neck cancer patients: Optimal patterns of care. Seminars in Speech and Language 21(4): 293–309.

Light J, Edelman S, Alba A (2001) The dental prosthesis used for intraoral muscle therapy in the rehabilitation of the stroke patient: a preliminary research study. New York State Dental Journal 67 (5): 22–8.

Logemann J (1997) Role of the modified barium swallow in management of patients with dysphagia. Otolaryngology, Head and Neck Surgery 116(3): 335–8.

Logemann J (1998) Evaluation and Treatment of Swallowing Disorders (2nd edn). Austin TX: Pro-Ed.

Marunick M, Tselios N (2004) The efficacy of palatal augmentation prostheses for speech and swallowing in patients undergoing glossectomy: a review of the literature. Journal of Prosthetic Dentistry 91 (1): 67–74.

Nayak V, Bhattacharyya N, Kotz T, et al. (2002) Patterns of swallowing failure following medialisation in unilateral vocal fold immobility. Laryngoscope 112(10): 1840–4.

Ryuzaburo H, Niro T, Takeshi W, et al. (2002) Videomanoflurometric study in Amyotrophic Lateral Sclerosis. Laryngoscope 112(5): 911–17.

Selley WG (1985) Swallowing difficulties in stroke patients: a new treatment. Age and Ageing 14: 361–5.

Shin T, Tsuda K, Takagi S (1999) Surgical treatment for dysphagia or neuromuscular origin. Folia Phoniatrica et Logopaedica 51(4/5): 213–19.

Sinha UK, Young P, Hurvitz K, et al. (2004) Functional outcomes following palatal reconstruction with folded radial forearm free flap. Ear, Nose and Throat Journal 83(1): 45–8.

Tamura F, Shishikura J, Mukai Y, et al. (1999) Arterial oxygen saturation in severely disabled people: effect of feeding in the sitting position. Dysphagia 14: 204–11.

Veenker EA, Anderson PE, Cohen JI (2003) Cricopharyngeal spasm and Zenker's diverticulum. Head and Neck 25(8): 681–94.

Williams RBH, Ali GN, Hunt DR, et al. (1999) Cricopharyngeal myotomy does not increase the risk of esophageal acid regurgitation. American Journal of Gastroenterology 94(12): 3448–54.

Wolf LS, Glass RP (1992) Feeding and Swallowing Disorders of Infancy. Tuscon: Therapy Skill Builders.

Woo P (2000) Voice disorders and phonosurgery I: aryteniod adduction and medialisation laryngoplasty. Otolaryngologic Clinics of North America 33(4): 817–40.

12 Swallowing Rehabilitation

JULIE CICHERO

It is unquestionable that eating and drinking are activities required to sustain life. However, the vast majority of our *social activities* revolve around eating and drinking too. Celebrations and meetings are often set around meal times. For older individuals who no longer work, time of day is determined by meal time. Even from our own experiences, when on holidays for example, decisions regarding food take a pleasant priority. The aim then of any swallowing treatment is to maximize participation in these life events. The previous chapter provided discussion about swallowing *compensation*. It was likened to using a crutch to allow the individual to eat or drink with an aid. Note, however, that the aid must always be present, and without it they would not be able to eat or drink successfully. Rehabilitation on the other hand aims to improve substantially – or, preferably, permanently fix – the underlying disorder. In this way the individual resumes eating and drinking in as normal a manner as possible. The task may be achieved slightly differently, for example, by using different muscles or muscle sets to assume the function of damaged muscles, but the outcome is independence in safe eating and drinking. Behavioural treatment for swallowing disorders has been described in the literature since the mid 1970s, with a dramatic increase in literature pertaining to dysphagia treatment since the early 1990s (Langmore and Miller, 1994). There has also been a change to the administrator of swallowing rehabilitation in this time frame. Earliest swallowing therapists tended to have a background in occupational therapy and nursing. It is only since the early 1980s that speech pathologists have had a stronger presence in the field (Langmore and Miller, 1994).

Logemann (1999) states that the best treatment for swallowing is swallowing! Individuals must practise the task that they are wishing to improve in order to be successful. Consequently, this chapter commences with a summary of information from the field of human movement studies, and the principles of rehabilitation of function. Exercises specific to swallowing function are also discussed. The use of technology with swallowing rehabilitation is discussed, with particular reference to surface electromyography (sEMG) and electrical or neuromuscular stimulation. It is also important to remember the role of our instrumental assessment techniques in this chapter and to determine how these assessments can be used therapeutically. In conclusion, the chapter provides special mention of the non-oral patient and why treatment of this population is critical.

In our quest for new treatments for individuals with dysphagia, speech pathologists need to look at the evidence base for what it is we do. This evidence is required to

Dysphagia: Foundation, Theory and Practice.   Edited by J. Cichero and B. Murdoch
© 2006 John Wiley & Sons, Ltd.

allow us to reach a decision about optimal care for our patients. Dysphagia treatment is relatively new (Reilly, 2004), and as such we are in the process of developing the evidence base for what we do. Evidence is required to demonstrate efficacy. It is acknowledged, however, that there may not always be evidence for what we do. Often times clinicians begin a course of treatment that 'seems to work'. This does not constitute an evidence base. It can, however, be used to generate clinically relevant research questions and hypotheses that should be tested. These are powerful questions because they have been driven by 'real world' experiences (Barbui, 2005). However, research rigour is required in order to 'prove' their efficacy. Where no evidence base exists for a particular type of swallowing therapy, for example, it is appropriate to look at other disciplines where evidence does exist and use these as a starting point to generate our own discipline-specific evidence. It cannot be implemented without modification, but can allow the researcher and clinician a framework to commence the development of evidence. In addition, where no evidence exists, the clinician and researcher should also ask the question 'Should this treatment be beneficial?' In order to answer this question, the researcher and clinician needs a sound understanding of the principles that underpin the proposed therapy and the nature of the impairment that is targeted (Clark, 2003). Principles of evidence-based practice and bridges and barriers to their implementation are discussed now to set a framework for the remainder of the chapter.

EVIDENCE-BASED PRACTICE IN SWALLOWING REHABILITATION

Evidence-based practice is defined as a 'conscious, explicit and judicious use of current best evidence in making decisions about the care of individual patients' (Knottnerus and Dinant, 1997, p. 1109). Simply stated, clinicians should use techniques for treatment that have a proven track record. This track record should be based on large numbers of individuals, where studies have been well designed, well controlled, and scientifically analysed. It is tempting to continue along a particular path for historical reasons, using the 'that's the way it has always been done' philosophy. This approach, however, does not constitute evidence, and adherence to its philosophy presents as a barrier to proven techniques. For example, the chin tuck technique has been used as a generalized treatment for all individuals with dysphagia. It is broadly based on the premise that tucking the chin is a mechanical method for protection of the larynx because it narrows the airway entrance and reduces the distance between the tongue base and pharyngeal wall (Poertner and Coleman, 1998). Logemann has been reported as saying that the chin tuck is often a first line of management for oropharyngeal dysphagia, with effective elimination of aspiration more than 50 per cent of the time (Bulow et al., 1999). If we extend the neck backwards during resuscitation to open the airway, then logically in flexing the head forward, we offer mechanical protection to the airway. However, research conducted in 1999 has shown that the chin tuck technique is contraindicated in certain populations; specifically individuals with weak pharyngeal constrictor muscles

(Bulow et al., 1999; Bulow et al., 2001). Chin tuck with this population increases the likelihood of aspiration rather than preventing it. The effect of loosening the pharyngeal constrictors was noted with both healthy and dysphagic individuals. Yet there are many clinicians, nurses and carers who routinely use a chin tuck technique with *all* individuals with swallowing disorders, believing they are acting in their best interests. It is noted that the data base for the Bulow et al (1999; 2001) studies is very small with only eight participants in each of the control and dysphagia groups. However, the research methodology was thorough and sound.

It is acknowledged that research may be difficult to design so that it meets the dual purpose of clinical validity and research rigour. Often studies are undertaken on homogenous populations in an attempt to rule out confounding variables presented by different aetiologies. However, in the real world, patients may present with several problems, or co-morbidities. As a result these individuals are often underrepresented in the research literature, yet make up the larger portion of the clinician's clinical caseload (Knottnerus and Dinant, 1997). Randomized clinical controlled trials have been in the process of development for 50 years, with clinical questions bent to fit their framework, rather than controlled clinical trials designed to fit the clinical situation (Knottnerus and Dinant, 1997). Knottnerus and Dinant (1997) suggest that quasi-experimental methods that respect the principles of the randomized clinical controlled trials may be of more benefit in the 'real world'.

THE PATH FROM GENERATION OF RESEARCH EVIDENCE TO CLINICAL APPLICATION

Haynes and Haines (1998) have put forward a pathway from generation of research evidence to the application of evidence in the clinical setting. They correctly state that much research and new innovations start in laboratories. Many remain there, either unsuitable for clinical implementation due to cost or technology, or are simply discarded. Those techniques that pass the initial laboratory type assessments should then undergo *trials* in the clinical arena to assess benefit and harm. Again it is at this stage where more techniques will either fail and be discarded or be deemed to provide benefit and progress to larger scale controlled trials with note of clinical outcomes. It is at this point that efforts should be made to disseminate the findings and promote application of the new technique. Introduction of techniques before they have been properly evaluated runs the risk of implementation, which is then very difficult to withdraw from practice even when the utility of the technique has been disproved (Haynes and Haines, 1998).

Clinicians are now better educated about looking for research evidence to strengthen their decision-making. They do not always have the specific skills to determine good from poor research design. Publication in a journal does not always guarantee high-level research rigour. Clinicians need to be mindful of properly evaluating the literature before implementation of new techniques. In saying this it is acknowledged that this is a time-consuming task which is difficult to incorporate in conjunction with the important task of assessing and treating clients. Haynes and

Haines (1998) reported that new 'abstracting services' are evolving in which studies with direct clinical impact are critically appraised. These short appraisals are then summarized in a journal. The international peer-reviewed journal *Dysphagia* includes a section titled 'Comments on selected recent dysphagia literature'. This is the beginning of such a service. To the best of my knowledge a dedicated abstracting service has not yet been developed for dysphagia or speech pathology treatment. As a profession, however, we should prioritize such a service. The Cochrane Collaboration summarizes all randomized controlled trials of healthcare interventions; however, it does not cover the quasi-experimental studies discussed above. There are also many excellent texts that have recognized the importance of this task (Reilly et al., 2004); however, access to an online up-to-date database of critically appraised studies with clinical impact critiqued by professional clinical researchers would be most beneficial.

MAKING 'BEST PRACTICE' CLINICAL DECISIONS

There are a number of elements that are critical to making 'best practice' clinical decisions. These include: (a) remembering the evidence correctly at the right place and time, (b) defining each patient's unique circumstances, (c) asking the patient's preferences, and understanding the patient's values and rights (Haynes and Haines, 1998). Exploring these in more detail, clinicians need to commit to continuing professional development to ensure that they are aware of reputable 'best practice'. They need to be responsible for understanding the circumstances where treatments should and should not be applied. Each individual patient is unique. Thorough assessment is required to determine what specifically is wrong with the patient and assess how this affects the individual. Clinicians also need to determine whether there are any other problems that might influence choice of treatment, and the treatment that will be the safest and most effective. For example, the supraglottic swallow is used as an airway protection technique (see Chapter 11). For individuals without sufficient cognition or new learning abilities, as in the case of multiple strokes, severe head injury or dementia, the use of this technique is not recommended. Apart from cognition, the clinician also needs to consider complicating factors such as expressive or more importantly receptive language disturbances (dysphasia). These deficits may affect the individual's ability to understand the clinician's instructions. The patient's insight into their problem is also critical. If they don't perceive that they have a problem their motivation and compliance with treatment will be significantly reduced to non-existent. Complicating factors such as depression can also reduce motivation to complete therapy. These aspects of rehabilitation are discussed further below. Evaluation of these factors requires clinical experience and expertise. All of this needs to be tempered with the client's preferences and rights to accept or refuse treatment. Given all of this, it should be obvious that to design a meaningful treatment plan for an individual is a unique, patient-specific task. No cookbook will ever produce a meaningful treatment plan. The following information provides basic principles in rehabilitation; however, the clinician *must* tailor the information to the client in front of them. Evidence from the literature will be critically analysed in this chapter to assist the clinician in interpreting the evidence base for swallowing rehabilitation.

EXERCISE PHYSIOLOGY AND THERAPY FOR INDIVIDUALS WITH DYSPHAGIA: BASIC PRINCIPLES

Human swallowing is a complex task requiring the coordination of numerous muscles and cranial nerves. While it is tempting to look at the rehabilitation of individual muscles, the clinician must understand that it is the coordinated action of sets of muscles that allows the act of swallowing to be successfully achieved. As noted above, therapy should be patient-specific. It should come as little surprise then that evidence relating to swallowing therapy is population specific, with the largest populations reported being cerebral palsy, stroke and Parkinson's disease (Reilly, 2004). Unlike many drug trials, the numbers of participants in the swallowing therapy studies are often comparatively small. Therapy reported revolves around a small number of quite specific exercises that either address one aspect of the swallowing process (e.g. oral motor exercises) or combined compensatory and rehabilitation approaches (see Table 12.1). Often the clinician may need to apply a combination of compensatory strategies (as discussed in Chapter 11) in addition to rehabilitation exercises. The balance between the two may shift as the patient improves in function. So for example, a higher proportion of compensation may be required initially when dysphagia is most severe and gradually reduced as swallowing function improves. However, to produce the improvement, rehabilitation strategies need to be employed. With a relatively short history in dysphagia therapy, we are still learning about the rehabilitation process (Huckabee and Pelletier, 1999). As newcomers to the field of rehabilitation, it is logical that we can learn much from discipline fields devoted to human movement. These are variously termed: human movement studies or science, kinesiology or sport and exercise science. These fields encompass an understanding of how people move, why they move and factors that limit or enhance our ability to move (Abernethy et al., 2005). It requires an understanding of functional anatomy, biomechanics, exercise physiology, motor control and exercise psychology.

Table 12.1 Different types of therapy reported in the literature

Muscle or muscle group exercises/therapy	Combined therapies (includes 'therapy' + compensatory strategies)
• Oral motor exercises	• *Diet modification* and 'exercises'
• Masako manoeuvre	• *Thermal stimulation + supraglottic*
• Shaker or 'head lift' exercises	*swallow* + bolus propulsion exercises
• Mendelsohn manoeuvre	• *Diet modification* + 'exercises' + *counselling*
• Effortful swallow manoeuvre	• *Diet modification* + oral motor
	exercises + *swallowing techniques* + *positioning*

Source: adapted in part from Reilly (2004).

It is outside of the scope of this chapter to apply each of these aspects to swallowing. However, it is strongly advocated that the direction swallowing rehabilitation should take is one where speech pathologists work collaboratively with exercise physiologists or human movement scientists to provide the best outcomes for our patients. Table 12.1 provides a taste of how our two disciplines can work for the betterment of individuals with dysphagia.

ACQUIRING MOTOR SKILLS FOR THE FIRST TIME

The field of human movement studies tells us that to become experienced in a motor skill takes many years (i.e. 10 years) or 10,000 hours or millions of trials of practice (Abernethy et al., 2005). When watching children learn to walk, we notice their resilience as they learn the new task. They fall down, they struggle to get back up, and then repeat this process endlessly until they eventually master the skill. There are of course a number of factors underpinning the success of the process; sufficient strength and stability of the body's structure and frame and the basic ability to programme the movement in the first place. But with those things as a given, the child learns through many repetitions to achieve the task, and learns to apply the skills to different terrains (grass, concrete, dirt, sand) and to move at different speeds (e.g. walk vs. run). If we apply this observation regarding walking to how children eat or drink, it makes sense then that, as the child moves from one texture to another, there will be a period of 'lesser performance'. Moving from a smooth, lump-free texture to a lumpy texture challenges the patterns that the child has acquired. They effectively start again with this new texture, but with the expertise gained from the previous texture, and adapt their skills to accommodate the new texture. The child needs to adjust the way the mandible moves to allow the tongue maximum range of motion to manipulate the bolus to become a smoother consistency. The 'feeling' that the bolus is sufficiently smooth (i.e. a form that their sensory system recognizes) is evidence of success and they can then apply the motor pattern for swallowing to it. The same pattern of new learning starts again with soft solids and then hard textures. Note always that the child is learning to bring the new texture back to a form that their sensori-motor system recognizes. With this 'expert' skill level comes the ability to 'cope' with subtle variations. As an adult the experience of swallowing an inadequately masticated hard texture such as a corn crisp results in pharyngeal pain as we apply the normal motor swallowing pattern for a smooth bolus. The pain reminds us that this type of bolus needs to be prepared better for swallowing in order to have a pain-free swallowing experience.

With the ability to master the act of swallowing and become 'experts' at it, we also gain the ability to 'multi-task'. That is we can carry on a conversation while having a meal. We can manipulate the food using a knife and fork while chewing a bolus and then swallowing it. We become so good at the 'task' of swallowing that we can mix textures – take a mouthful of solids and then add liquids and mix the textures orally. Even more difficult still we can coordinate the process of taking a mixed texture into the mouth, segment the textures and swallow them separately.

For example when swallowing a fruit punch with fruit pieces, as 'experts' we can take the fruit and liquid consistency into the mouth, hold the fruit orally and swallow the liquid, then move on to masticating and swallowing the fruit. It is 'expert' levels of swallowing skill (perhaps in varying gradations) that are lost in individuals that have had a stroke, neurological injury or surgery to the swallowing system. For some, the entire process must be relearned, i.e. they become novices again. This is particularly difficult though because they have previously been 'experts' at their task. We as clinicians have to work very hard to change the ingrained pattern of learned behaviour. That pattern of behaviour required a 'normal' structural, muscular and neural response system; some, or all of those factors may be affected, which means that the patterns previously used may not result in the desired response. The outcome of attempting to apply the learned motor pattern when the foundations of the system are faulty may result in aspiration, or the inability to take sufficient food/fluid in because of the effort required to achieve the task. Our role is huge, difficult, challenging, exciting and frustrating. Individuals must first understand that just as they once learned to walk, they also learned to swallow – it's just that we do this so early in life that we have no adult memory of the process. It is so fundamental to survival that it is required from the moment we enter the world. Patients have often commented that they can't believe they have 'forgotten' how to swallow.

PRINCIPLES OF LEARNING A NEW TASK: A HUMAN MOVEMENT PERSPECTIVE

So if we were to conceptualize learning a new task, what would it look like? Literature shows us that learners go through at least three distinguishable phases in progressing from being a novice at the 'new task' to being an expert. These are: (a) the 'verbal-cognitive' phase, (b) the associative phase, and (c) the autonomous phase (Prosiegel et al., 2000; Abernethy et al., 2005).

Stage 1 – the 'verbal-cognitive' phase or, shaping the behaviour

Traditionally in the 'verbal-cognitive' phase, the movement task to be learned is completely new. In the adult dysphagia populations, however, this is only partially true because they have had many years of experience in swallowing. Where it is applicable, however, is that dysphagic individuals need to alter their learned programme of response in order to accommodate the changes in sensation, or motor strength or coordination. Learning a new swallowing manoeuvre, for example the Mendelsohn manoeuvre, involves learning a new task (the Mendelsohn manoeuvre is discussed in detail below). Abernethy et al. (2005) suggest that at this stage the learner is preoccupied with understanding the requirements of the task – what is it that needs to be done to successfully perform the skill? The learner needs to put all of their concentration into issues such as the position of their body and limbs, what position do they need to be in to get repetitive or ongoing feedback about how they are managing the task and most importantly how does the correct movement feel? They are learning to plan the task.

The role of the speech pathologist in re-educating the 'expert swallower' is first of all an ability to explain to the individual that they are now relearning this task. Individuals with dysphagia and their carers need to understand that they need to be in the best overall trunk, shoulder girdle, neck, jaw and head position to be maximally stable and optimized proprioceptively to manage the task. As noted in Chapter 11, if body position is so poor that the trunk is unstable, the individual will focus more on the feeling that they are going to fall than the act of swallowing, hence significantly limiting their ability to concentrate on the new task to be learned. At this stage the goals are positioning, thinking and planning movement.

What can we do to help? The individual needs excellent verbal instruction in addition to demonstration and prompt feedback on what is 'right', so that they know when they have achieved the goal of safe swallowing. They need to experience success in the task so that they can attempt to replicate the successful actions and postures over and over again, and once again become experts at the task of swallowing. We begin now to understand the extreme challenge of this phase for individuals with brain injury or neurological deficits that undermine their ability to understand verbal or gestural instruction. There are also issues surrounding insight. Does the person understand and acknowledge that they are no longer expert at swallowing and need to relearn this task? Do they have sufficient motivation? Do they have the stamina to do the 'practice' required to make them experts again? What are their arousal and anxiety levels like?

Abernethy et al. (2005) explain that the initial attempts at the new task are based on movement patterns extracted from existing skills. So 'old habits' become reshaped and reworked to become new patterns. Unlike congenital swallowing disorders where babies have not had the 'experience' of normal swallowing patterns, adults with acquired injuries have 'old swallowing patterns' that they can use as a foundation for modification. The astute clinician must highlight the similarities and also the differences between the 'old swallowing pattern' and the 'new swallowing pattern'. Let's look at an example. Assuming that cognition is adequate, and that insight, motivation and stamina are profound, the clinician decides to teach an individual the supra-glottic swallow technique. This technique is described in detail in Chapter 11 and also further below. The supraglottic swallow is in fact a bringing to consciousness the unconscious swallow-respiratory cycle discussed in Chapter 4. We take food or fluid into the mouth, halt breathing, swallow, then exhale and recommence tidal breathing. We do this without thinking – we have become experts at this task. The supraglottic swallow reteaches the individual the task using verbal instruction and perhaps biofeedback. Re-education of the swallow-respiratory cycle by way of the supraglottic swallow is discussed in detail later in this chapter. Notice that this rehabilitation task does not focus on one specific muscle; it focuses on the whole process of airway protection during swallowing. The task can be broken down into smaller units and practised in portions before being put together as a whole task.

Stage 2 – fine tuning the movement task (swallowing behaviour)

Abernethy et al. (2005) explain that in the next phase of learning the task the performance of the new task is more consistent because the learner has settled on a particular strategy or approach. The individual eventually settles on the body and oral posture that through trial and error they have determined to be the 'one' to fine tune, rather than switching from one movement pattern to another. For the clinician the skill is in identifying when the individual has hit upon that 'successful swallow pattern'; the one that just needs fine tuning. So now that the individual has found the correct pattern, they now need to practise it over and over and over again. And then they need to adapt it to different conditions where the movement will be performed. So again with swallowing, the individual may first learn their movement patterns in the clinician's office where it is quiet and without distractions. Once they have some mastery in this environment, it must be generalized to eating in a quiet room with others, then eating in a noisy room with others etc. There is an endless range of permutations that we could work on (see Table 12.2 for some suggestions).

Table 12.2 Incremental adjustment of factors affecting feeding and swallowing: suggestions

---

Environment

- Quiet single room (patient + therapist)
- Quiet single with low-volume radio or television background noise
- Quiet single room with low-level background noise (patient + therapist + another person – patient to concentrate on tasks while therapist and other person have intermittent conversation)
- Quiet dining room (2–3 individuals share the table with the dysphagic individual)
- Normal dining room situation
- Family gathering
- Café, restaurant, shopping centre
- Party

Bolus type

- Saliva
- Thin liquid (most difficult if delayed pharyngeal swallow or reduced airway closure)[a]
  - Alter flavour, temperature, other – eg. carbonation
  - Cup size – small cup size (30 ml medicine cup) promotes small sip, gradually increasing cup size (50 ml, 100 ml, 150 ml, 200 ml, 250 ml) allows gradual incremental increase in sip size
  - Straw (length of straw, diameter of straw, type of liquid ingested using the straw)
- Thick liquid (most difficult if reduced tongue strength, range or coordination of movement or reduced pharyngeal wall contraction)[a]
  - Degree of thickness (nectar → half or honey thick → full or pudding thick)
  - Alter flavour, temperature, other – eg. carbonation
- Texture modified foods
  - Vitamised or puree food (most difficult if reduced tongue strength, range or coordination of movement or reduced tongue base movement or reduced pharyngeal wall contraction)[a]
  - Degree of texture modification (vitamised or puree → minced → soft → normal food)

Table 12.2 *(Continued)*

- ° Alter flavour, temperature
- ° Mixed textures (fluids plus solids) [more challenging]
- Quantity
  - ° Specific number of teaspoonfuls, dessertspoonfuls or sips
  - ° Where supplemented non-orally (e.g. nasogastric tube or gastrostomy) aim for increasing increments
  - ° Commence with meals where patient is most alert (e.g. breakfast or morning tea)
  - ° Small meals frequently (6 × per day)
- Medication
  - ° Viscous liquid, small tablet, capsule, large tablet
  - ° Multiple medications
  - ° Carrier fluid for the medications (thick liquids or thin liquids)

Positioning

- Full support for thorax, shoulder girdle, neck and head to provide stability (external)
- Liaise with physiotherapist for external supports
- Seating situation
  - ° Bed, armchair, dining room chair, wheelchair

Dependence for feeding

- Full dependence
  - ° Full supervision and assistance → close supervision → moderate supervision → far supervision → intermittent supervision → no supervision
- Self-feeding
  - ° Maximally assisted self-feeding (liaise with occupational therapist) +/− adaptive utensils (rocker knife, plate guard, thick handled cutlery, dysphagia cup) → gradually reducing level of assistance
- Feedback (verbal, visual, acoustic)-gradually reducing

ª Logemann (1995)

By increasing task complexity we continually fine tune the task and allow the person to develop the skills to cope in a range of situations. Now it may be that ideally they should sit in a quite room by themselves to eat the majority of the meal, but perhaps the aim should also be that they can participate, even for a small time, in the more 'complex/difficult' situation of a family meal situation. This brings to the fore the holistic nature of eating and issues surrounding social isolation. The inability to participate in mealtimes, which are social events, affects an individual's mental, physical, social, emotional and financial well-being (Huckabee and Cannito, 1999; Nguyen et al., 2005). Huckabee and Cannito (1999) directly quote a dysphagic patient as saying 'Since I equated eating with living, I thought I was just marking time until I died' (p. 104). Social isolation may also contribute to depression which will have a negative impact on the ability to participate in a rehabilitation programme. Poor performance in home swallowing therapy activities has been linked to depression in one case study (Huckabee and Cannito, 1999). This is the time to employ the techniques and strategies that are specific to the difficulties the person is experiencing, whether they be in the oral phase, pharyngeal phase, both phases and/or protection of the airway during swallowing.

Stage 3 – automatism (of swallowing)

Some individuals may regain this 'instinctive' level of skill, where the ability to swallow appears largely automatic again. In this phase the movement appears to be able to be controlled without the person paying attention to it. Abernethy et al. (2005) explain that at this level the task is performed so consistently and so precisely that the need to monitor the action constantly to ensure that it is correctly performed is significantly reduced. The very rapid sequences of coordinated movements necessary for safe swallowing require efferent commands to be constructed in advance. Abernethy et al. (2005) call this 'open-loop' control. It is different to 'closed-loop' control whereby control of movement is based on feedback. Our difficulty then is initially trying to turn an 'open-loop' system, which is what successful swallowing requires, into a temporarily closed loop system so that we can provide feedback to improve the speed accuracy and control. This is an extremely difficult task. Add to this that, for rapid open-loop systems, the time taken to initiate the movement is directly proportional to the amount of preplanning that needs to take place. While we can borrow concepts from the field of physiotherapy with re-education of limb control, this is quite a different task to the rapid responses of the larynx and pharynx required during swallowing. Clinically, individuals with dysphagia that have a slow oral phase and perhaps even a slow pharyngeal phase but where control and concentration is high are likely to be safer swallowers than dysphagic individuals who are impulsive. Impulsive individuals attempt to use the open-loop system without the control they previously had, and consequently are likely to be more at risk of aspiration. Our goal then may be to teach the individual to slow down, to regain control and once they have mastered this, then speed it back up again.

Once we have an effective open-loop system, where the motor programme operates on a pre-structured set of commands, it allows us to build bigger and better motor programmes. In this way more elements are under the control of a single programme. Once might postulate that this is in effect what happens very early in life with swallowing and respiration. The motor patterns for breathing are clearly laid down very early. When a baby is born its first task is to inflate the lungs and begin the process of breathing. Not too long after it also requires sustenance in order to thrive. Breathing and swallowing use the biological time-share structure of the pharynx for successful feeding; that is an ability to cease respiration during the swallow and then resume it afterwards (see Chapter 4 for further details). It could be argued that this is a very well-developed open-loop system. When insult or injury occurs, the motor programmes that had previously worked in synchrony have become disjointed. They may never work again as a high-powered open-loop system, but rather as a number of smaller open-loop systems. The result, then, is that the ability to multi-task (e.g. have a conversation while eating) is lost and for some the ability to multi-task may never be recovered.

Abernethy et al. (2005) explain that once we reach this autonomous stage of learning it is extremely difficult, if not impossible, to change a movement pattern where an error in technique has become ingrained. The movement control operates below the level of consciousness and consequently it is very difficult to verbalize how they are performing the skilled movement. Perhaps this is why the rehabilitation of dysphagia is so difficult. To take something that this so subconscious and make it a conscious task, and provide the verbal and kinaesthetic feedback to make it a conscious task – at least for long enough for the individual to relearn correct movement patterns – is a sizeable challenge.

IMPROVING MOTOR LEARNING

There are a number of factors that should be remembered when considering rehabilitation. These include the specific skill that you want the patient to acquire; the role of perception and decision-making; the amount and type of practice and the type of feedback provided.

Specificity of motor skills

Skill acquisition is highly specific and it is acknowledged that 'there is usually little or no transfer of training from one motor skill to another' (Abernethy et al. 2005, p. 261). Applying this principle, the function of the tongue in speech does not give the clinician an accurate idea of tongue function for bolus control or swallowing initiation. Therefore, while it is necessary to break a task down, the very best rehabilitation for swallowing has to be swallowing. Skills need to be practised under the condition that is the closest to the demands of the situation in which the skill will eventually be performed. This brings into question the efficacy of oral motor exercises and all exercises that focus purely on one muscle group. Indeed the evidence base for oral motor therapy is decidedly lacking and with good reason (Clark, 2003; Reilly, 2004).

Muscles are of course critical to the movements required for successful swallowing and it may be tempting to look at the rehabilitation of individual muscles. However, we know that the process of swallowing requires the coordination of many movements and the dynamic function of many muscles. The discussion above relating to open-loop systems reminds us that the act of swallowing is very fast and for non-dysphagic individuals it occurs at an automatic or subconscious level. It makes sense then to think about rehabilitation of *movement patterns* rather than individual muscles per se. Basmajian (1982) provides a wonderful visual example of the role of muscles in movement. He describes muscles as actors on a stage. The actors all work together to provide a performance. 'They have their entrances, play their part and then exit' (p. 117). *But*, when one of the muscles becomes paralysed, it upsets the sequence and affects the ability of the other muscles to perform their roles. He says that unlike an actor, for the muscles, there are no 'understudies', thus the ability to perform the whole action may be significantly compromised. In swallowing rehabilitation, if we choose just to focus on one of the 'actors', we must also be sure that we are focusing on the specific part that it plays during the swallowing process. Remember that many of the muscles we use for swallowing are also used for speech; however, the roles they play are vastly different.

Perception and decision-making

It may be tempting to think that poor performance is a result of poor movement execution. If this were the only fault then 'practise, practise, practise' might be the answer.

However, poor perception or poor decision-making can equally cause errors in performance. A *perceptual error* such as incorrect judgement of speed of movement of the thin liquid in the oral cavity my cause the individual to be unable to control the liquid; provide insufficient time for the respiratory system to be protected and result in penetration or aspiration of the bolus. Perception requires an ability to recognize patterns and anticipate outcomes. In swallowing, we are aware that chewing a steak bolus for three seconds will not significantly deform its structure and will likely result in the bolus being too large to swallow safely. We recognize the *pattern* of insufficient mastication and the *outcome* being a potential choking hazard. Some individuals with dysphagia, perhaps due to altered sensation, lose this ability to recognize the pattern and anticipate the outcome. In this situation the challenge is to reteach the individual to interpret how the bolus feels in the oral cavity and use this information to decide whether it is safe to swallow and the best way to swallow the bolus. The clinician should be particularly alert for perceptual difficulties in individuals who have frontal lobe damage, traumatic brain injury, right hemisphere stroke or dementia.

Apart from poor perception, a *decision-making error* may also result in aspiration. For example, over-filling the oral cavity with more food before the previous bolus has been swallowed may also result in a choking hazard. In swallowing we have a small margin for error and so decisions need to be made accurately. The same population types that may have difficulty with perception may similarly have difficulty with decision-making. So we need to be aware that the ability to execute the swallow pattern may well be normal, and in fact it may be the perceptual or decision-making skills that require rehabilitation. Particularly for swallowing, decision-making needs to occur very rapidly, almost unconsciously. Add to this scenario conditions that slow movement, such as ageing, injury or disease. Here more than ever, the decision-making and perceptual skills must be at their peak in order to compensate for a delay in movement initiation.

Practice

We have all been taught that the best way to improve our skills is to practise them, and this is certainly true; but what is the best way to practise? Research shows us that there are different types of practice: constant, random and blocked. These are best explained using a concrete example: imagine yourself at the golf driving range; you can repeat the same task over and over (constant), for example, hitting a bucket of balls using only the driver. In blocked practice you might hit 15 balls using the driver, then 15 balls using the sand wedge, then 15 balls using the seven iron and so on. In random practice you might start with the sand wedge, then use the driver, then the seven iron and so forth, with no particular pattern being used. The literature shows that if you want to be very good at the practice task (e.g. hitting golf balls), then constant practice is the way to go. Certainly there is a higher degree of success and consistency at the task gained from constant practice than the blocked or random techniques. However, if you want to be able to transfer those skills to the golf course, the research shows that random practice provides poor to average skills during *practice* but superior retention and transfer ability (Dick et al., 2003; Holladay and Quinones, 2003). Empirically this makes sense. In a game of golf you use a number of different clubs depending on where the ball has landed rather than using the same club over and over for the same distance shot (Abernethy et al., 2005).

Let's relate the literature now to normal mealtimes. Healthy individuals will alternate different textures of food, and intersperse eating with drinking. So, if we want our patients to be able to participate in a normal meal, the practice tasks should focus not just on the fluids but also on the food and any combinations of these that might be employed. Practising swallowing saliva will help the individual improve saliva swallowing but is unlikely to transfer to bolus swallows. Practising swallowing of thickened liquids will help improve swallowing of thickened liquids. For individuals with a severe dysphagia, the clinician could vary the presentation by using different textures, flavours and temperature of the bolus (see Table 12.3). Note also though that the only way to improve swallowing a thin liquid will be to practise swallowing a thin liquid. It may be that the task can be broken down into smaller steps before embarking on the total act; however, it will be necessary to use thin fluid trials if this is the desired outcome.

Interestingly, the argument for random practice schedules does not hold for individuals with Alzheimer's disease. Random practice places a higher cognitive demand on the participant than blocked or constant practice. This is not to say, however, that individuals with Alzheimer's disease do not benefit from therapy. Dick

Table 12.3 Block vs random practice tasks in golf and swallowing

Block practice tasks (drills)		Random practice tasks	
Golf	Swallowing	Golf	Swallowing
Use the same club (e.g. driver) to hit a bucket of balls at a driving range	Trial teaspoons (5ml increments) of one cup (250ml) of full thick fluids (i.e. 50 trials)	Hit a bucket of golf balls at a driving range in the following order: a driver, a 7 iron, a sand wedge and a putter	Trial in the following order: one spoonful of full thick fluids, one saliva swallow, one spoonful of vitamized meat, one spoonful of vitamized vegetables, two teaspoons of full thick fluids, one sip of water

Source: adapted from Abernethy et al. (2005).

et al. (2003) reported that motor learning is relatively preserved throughout the course of Alzheimer's disease. Specifically they found though that these individuals improve using constant practice, and did not benefit the way other individuals did from variable practice. They recommended that daily activities such as eating should be practised in a repetitious and invariable manner, and included individuals of moderate-severe stages of dementia in this recommendation. Given this information, it would appear that practice schedules that are random may be better for individuals with dysphagia who do not have a cognitive overlay (e.g. head and neck patients). Certainly for individuals with dementia, the constant practice paradigm would seem to be recommended.

Block or constant practice may be required when a new task is being learned initially. Research has shown that deliberate attention and conscious step-by-step monitoring of performance can impede function rather than improve it for individuals who have developed a high level of skill. The reverse is true of the novice. These individuals initially require deliberate attention and conscious effort to succeed (Beilock et al., 2002). The skill for the clinician is knowing when to ease off on overt feedback and allow the individual to move towards greater autonomy.

Feedback

There are many errors in the first stage (verbal-cognitive) of new skill acquisition. Many new movement strategies may be tried to gain an idea or a feeling of what success 'feels like'. It is imperative that the individual receives some success though, or motivation will rapidly decline. Without motivation the individual will not even attempt the task. The single most important role here may be the instructions and feedback to establish a correct pattern. Note, however, that while specific instruction is useful initially and may benefit practice tasks, specific instructions impair performance of skills that have become more automatic (Beilock et al., 2002). The provision of specific instructions means that the learner has to 'think less' to process the task, because the 'coach' is doing that for them. In the long run, however, the goal is for independence (stage 3 – automatism, described above). Goodman and Wood (2004) reported that individuals who receive more specific feedback have more opportunities to learn what to do when things are going well, but fewer opportunities on what to do when things are going poorly. People who received less specific feedback spent more time responding to errors during practice. Unfortunately, more errors during practice are viewed negatively and seen as failure which then interrupts effective problem solving strategies. Certainly the suggestion is that both aspects need to be experienced in order to cope with problems that might occur during the task. The authors give the example of machine operators. If the machine operators can only operate with well-functioning equipment, they may not have the skills to cope when the equipment malfunctions. Swallowing is somewhat similar and the stakes are high.

It may be that individuals need to experience some degree of failure (i.e. pharyngeal residue, penetration or aspiration) in order to learn how to cope (i.e. coughing to clear the airway). However, our margin for acceptable 'failure', i.e. amount of 'acceptable' aspiration, is quite small because of the consequences. Nevertheless, individuals should be given feedback to promote the behaviours that we want to see, but also be given 'controlled' or safe opportunities to experience small failure so that we can help them to develop strategies for coping if 'failure' occurs. As another analogy, it is no good teaching someone how to walk, if they are also not taught how to get up if they fall over. An inability to cope with failure has the potential to lead to high levels of anxiety which then paralyses future attempts. Goodman and Wood (2004) also found that the rules for learning how to respond to poor performance were different to the processes of learning how to respond to good performance. Clearly further research in this area, and particularly how it might apply to rehabilitation of swallowing, is required. One further comment on the topic of feedback is that both explicit instruction and guided discovery, where learners are given opportunities to explore different solutions to the problem, have been found to improve performance on real-world motor tasks (Williams et al., 2002).

Psychological variables affecting rehabilitation

In addition to the variables listed above, the clinician also needs to bear in mind psychological variables that can either make or break rehabilitation. These variables may in fact be at the core of whether an individual is even a candidate for rehabilitation. As noted above, an individual's insight into their difficulty is important. For example, research has shown that in the stroke population, individuals with dysphagia rarely perceive that they have a swallowing problem (Parker et al., 2004). If the individual doesn't perceive that he or she has a problem, they will not be motivated to fix the problem. The clinician's first task may be to demonstrate to the patient that they do indeed have a problem swallowing! Instrumental assessments such as videofluoroscopy and fiberoptic endoscopic evaluation of swallowing (FEES) may be critical in assisting the clinician to demonstrate the presence of a swallowing disorder.

Motivation

Motivation is critical to complete any task and a lack of motivation is demonstrated by low compliance. Motivation is driven by direction, intensity and persistence (Abernethy et al., 2005). An example will be used to explain these concepts more clearly. Mr Jones presents to the speech pathologist with a complete dense right hemiplegia. There is right facial weakness and a moderate dysarthria. Swallowing function is moderately impaired. Mr Jones is very motivated towards learning to walk again. Although his speech is dysarthric, he is able to make himself understood. He is tolerating a modified diet and half or honey thick fluids safely and efficiently. Mr Jones is motivated by learning to walk again. His focus, or direction is on his physiotherapy sessions. He invests a lot of energy on his physiotherapy sessions and is quite persistent in his efforts to relearn to walk. Although Mr Jones may be motivated to improve his speech and swallowing, he demonstrates a greater motivation and persistence towards learning to walk again. Abernethy et al. (2005) explain that it is possible to enhance motivation. Direction or the desire to participate can be improved by making the experience enjoyable. Choosing a particular food or fluid type that Mr Jones particularly enjoys may make him more motivated towards swallowing therapy. Intensity of practice can increase by explaining *why* he is doing a particular activity. Finally, Mr Jones is more likely to persevere with the therapy tasks if he can see a long-term benefit, for example being able to resume a normal diet and fluids.

Anxiety

Anxiety is something that we tend not to hear about in dysphagia rehabilitation, and yet it may be more prevalent than we might expect. Anxiety is a subjective feeling of apprehension, and it is usually accompanied by increased arousal levels (tense muscles, higher blood pressure, heart rate or respiratory rate). It usually occurs when people perceive a situation as threatening. In the case of dysphagia a perceived inability to swallow a particular food or fluid texture may cause fear and anxiety. Anxiety is quite subjective, so that faced with the same situation, one individual may find the situation a little bit challenging while another may find it extremely threatening (Abernethy et al., 2005). Increased anxiety is detrimental to performance. A fear of swallowing or choking will most likely paralyse the person with fear and make them incapable of the task, even if they are physically able to achieve it. Sheppard advocates teaching individuals how to remove an unwanted bolus from their mouth (Sheppard, 2005). This skill provides them with some degree of oral control over the bolus and may also decrease anxiety levels.

Goal setting

Once the psychological issues have been addressed, the clinician should set about the task of goal-setting. Setting a goal gives you something to aim for. The goal needs to be the patient's goal – not the therapist's goal. We are more likely to be motivated to achieve the goal if we have a stake in it. Achievement of goals also gives the feeling of success which is important for perseverance. Goals need to be attainable or realistic, but also challenging. The clinician will also need to determine strategies to achieve the goal (practice, feedback, breaking the task into smaller or easier components). You also need to know when you have achieved your goal. (See also Chapter 16 regarding outcome measures in dysphagia.) It may be that a number of short-term goals are required to reach the final long-term goal. Aim to set a goal that is specific to the behaviour you want to promote. In a study that looked at patient dissatisfaction with rehabilitation, Liu et al. (2004) found that individuals were more likely to be dissatisfied if they had a higher proportion of non-achieved goals. In addition, they found that conflicting aims between the therapist and the patient was another major source of patient dissatisfaction with the rehabilitation process. Expectations on admission were also a factor in determining subsequent levels of satisfaction. Pain, anxiety and fatigue did not, however, affect patient satisfaction with rehabilitation. Given this information, clinicians need to appreciate the importance of patient-driven goal setting. Skill must also be used to ensure that these patient-orientated goals are realistic to provide appropriate expectations. For example, for an individual with severe oral and pharyngeal dysphagia where primary nutritional intake is via non-oral means (e.g. a PEG), the goal may be for tastes of favourite foods that have been pureed and small amounts of thickened liquids at meal times to enhance socialization. The clinician may also employ some lateral thinking to make the experience more pleasurable by thickening a cup of tea or another favourite drink to promote satisfaction and enhance motivation.

FOCUS AT THE MUSCULAR LEVEL FOR REHABILITATION OF SWALLOWING

It may be tempting to focus on strengthening particular muscles to improve swallowing function. It is the premise of oral motor exercises to improve the strength, speed and range of movement of the lips, tongue and jaw through repetitive movements of these structures in a drill-like fashion. As noted above in the discussion regarding specificity of motor skills, muscle groups work in synchrony. Some muscles may be postural supports during speech, yet prime 'actors' for swallowing. While there may be some place for muscle strengthening, it is more important that the muscle complex be strengthened by doing the desired task than attempting to strengthen individual muscles. In addition, it is important to understand that muscle strength is but one of a triad of properties required for muscle 'fitness'.

Muscle fitness

In addition to strength, muscle power and endurance are all required for 'muscle fitness' (Abernethy et al., 2005). Strength refers to the maximum force that can be produced by a muscle or muscle group in a single movement while muscle power refers to the interplay between force and speed of movement. Muscle endurance is particularly important for the dysphagia population; it refers to the ability of the muscle to generate force repeatedly, or continuously over time. The three key areas of strength, power and endurance are interrelated. It is important to understand that improvement in one area does not imply that improvements to the other areas will follow. For example, oral motor exercises aimed at improving muscle strength will not necessarily enhance power or indeed endurance. For individuals with dysphagia, the problem of sustained endurance may be one of the most challenging that the clinician has to deal with. Exercises repeated with low levels of resistance may increase endurance.

Muscle tone

Muscle tone should be addressed by the dysphagia clinician. Tone refers to the tendency of the muscle to resist passive stretch. It is possible to assess tone in the limbs by determining the amount of resistance when the examiner passively extends or flexes the limb. The same, however, is not true of the musculature for speech and swallowing because the muscles are (a) often small and inaccessible, (b) situated in overlapping muscle groups and (c) not straightforward by way of agonist/antagonist relationships. Note also that there will be different exercises to increase tone(flaccidity) than those where there is too much tone (spasticity). For example, massage has been reported to be effective in reducing increased tone (Clark, 2003).

Muscle strength

Muscle strength has been described above and is important for basic functions such as posture, balance and coordination. Strength can be defined as the capacity of a muscle or group of muscles to produce the force necessary for initiating, maintaining and controlling movement (Ng and Shepherd, 2000). Muscle strength will increase when there are complex interactions between neural, structural and metabolic activities in skeletal muscle. It is closely related to the size of the muscle and also muscle fibre type (fast or slow twitch fibres). In order to improve strength, reasonably forceful contractions are required. This can be achieved by 'resistance' training (Clark, 2003). However, exercise needs to occur to the point of fatigue or 'overload' to cause a change to the muscular system. Once the muscles have fatigued, they also need time to recover. There is no data available on recovery time of the swallowing muscles after strength training to the point of fatigue. Using the principles of motor learning described above, the task is to overload impaired muscle groups during functional tasks and then allow them time to recover to achieve best outcomes. In skeletal muscle, muscle bulking (hypertrophy) occurs approximately 6–8 weeks after strength training (Abernethy et al., 2005). When looking at general exercise principles suitable for an ageing population Abernethy et al. (2005) noted that where there is impaired coordination or slower action times, simple movements and supported exercise should be considered. Due to the effects of ageing, clinicians should expect slower progress and improvement in exercise capacity. Note also that strength training is contraindicated for certain populations; namely motor-neuron disease and multiple sclerosis. In these conditions strength training is not beneficial and may even be harmful (Clark, 2003).

Muscle weakness

Weakness on the other hand is a reduction in force and the concept of fatigue is closely associated with it (Clark, 2003). Weakness is often seen in individuals with swallowing disorders. However it is very difficult to predict the degree of functional limitation from the severity of weakness observed. Measurement of this weakness is also very difficult in objective terms. Note that immobility and disuse of muscles has been implicated as a cause of muscle weakness in the stroke population, with the researcher pointing out that patients can have learned non-use and 'helplessness' in a non-stimulating rehabilitative environment (Ng and Shepherd, 2000). Disuse atrophy specifically of the superior constrictors has been postulated by Perlman et al. (1989) following disruption to the sensory side of the sensori-motor pattern. Perlman et al. (1989) claim that this disuse atrophy exacerbated by insufficient sensory stimulation could limit or delay recovery of swallowing function.

Muscle actions

Most voluntary muscles are attached to bone (Basmajian, 1982). Muscles cross joints so that when they contract, they cause movement. When a muscle contracts it pulls two bony attachments closer together. For example, anterior and superior movement of the larynx during swallowing occurs as a result of contraction of the anterior belly of the digastric, posterior belly of the digastric, geniohyoid, omohyoid, stylohyoid and mylohyoid muscles (Moore and Dalley, 1999). The action of muscle contraction is termed 'concentric' movement. 'Eccentric' actions on the other hand occur when a muscle is activated but is lengthening. It is lengthening because other forces prevent the muscle from shortening. Abernethy et al. (2005) explain that this situation occurs in order to control movement, to stabilize or to decelerate the body. The final action is 'isometric' activity. This is where the muscle is activated but the overall length of the muscle-tendon complex does not change. Thus isometric contractions are important for stabilization and maintenance of posture. Importantly, Abernethy et al. (2005) point out that the descriptions of muscle movement found in anatomy textbooks are based on the assumption that movement is produced by concentric muscle action. This is indeed the case with the Curtis et al. (1988) study where fresh cadaver speci-mens were used to simulate the actions of paired muscles to define their roles during swallowing. While the study is very detailed, it does not take into account the chang-ing roles of the *muscle complexes* required for swallowing. It also cannot simulate the actions required for swallowing any bolus, let alone boluses of different textures and viscosities. The study treats the muscles required for swallowing as one might view a set of musical scales for the piano. Each note is included in the scale, but it is the organization of those notes in a particular order at a particular time that forms a so-nata. Similarly it is the organization of a particular set of muscles in a particular order at a particular time that determines the act of swallowing rather than a record of indi-vidual muscle actions engaged in one activity (concentric movement) in isolation.

IS THERE A CASE FOR ORAL MOTOR EXERCISES FOR SWALLOWING REHABILITATION?

Many clinicians continue to use oral motor exercises under the misguided belief that these movements will improve general muscle strength and thence improve mus-cle function during speech and swallowing. Oral motor exercises typically include tongue protrusion, lateralization, and elevation; and pursing and spreading of the lips in a drill-like fashion. First and foremost, there is insufficient evidence to sup-port the use of oral motor exercises to improve swallowing function (Langmore and Miller, 1994; Clark, 2003; Reilly, 2004). Literature that is reported for oral motor exercises often (a) lacks control groups, (b) provides results from single case studies or small numbers of subjects and (c) often combines the approach with other thera-pies, negating a case for its use in isolation. The aforementioned notes on specificity of motor task should also indicate that drill exercises of the oral musculature are of dubious value. If the task is to improve tongue protrusion, then one would practise protruding the tongue. In swallowing there is no function for such an act. As noted above, therapy and practice should be contextual. Based on the lack of evidence for oral motor exercises and the lack of theoretical underpinnings for their use in dysphagia rehabilitation, oral motor exercises are *not* recommended for rehabilitation of swallowing. However, active range of movement exercises may be beneficial in preventing the formation of restrictive scar tissue (Clark, 2003). This is particularly relevant in the head and neck population where the formation of scar tissue following surgery or chemo and/or radiotherapy is an issue.

REHABILITATION OF SWALLOWING: A FUNCTIONAL APPROACH

The previous discussion should indicate that in order to rehabilitate swallowing the clinician should identify specific aspects of swallowing for improvement. For example, based on assessment results the clinician may work on (a) aspects of the oral phase, (b) aspects of the pharyngeal phase, (c) both aspects of swallowing function, (d) swallow-respiratory coordination, or (e) removing the bolus from the oral cavity or pharynx. The non-oral patient presents as a special case in point, and this will be discussed separately. Traditionally therapeutic tasks such as oral motor exercises (discussed above) or swallowing manoeuvres are discussed under separate headings. In the following discussions, they will be included where they are applicable under the general headings below.

REHABILITATION OF THE ORAL PHASE

After a thorough examination of the oral phase of swallowing, there are many different aspects of the sensori-motor programme that may be targeted. These include:

- opening the mouth to accept a bolus;
- taking the bolus from a cup or spoon (or fork);
- lip closure to contain the bolus within the oral cavity;
- manipulation of the solid bolus for effective deformation or preparation (including mastication);

  ○ control of the solid bolus for positioning between the molars during preparation;

- control of the liquid bolus to ensure that it remains in the oral cavity until it is ready for swallowing;
- effective swallow reflex initiation and propulsion;
- velopharyngeal competency for intra-oral pressure (sucking);
- clearance of the oral cavity of residue after the primary bolus swallow;

Opening the mouth to accept a bolus

Opening the mouth to accept a bolus will be facilitated by a pleasant stimulus! Motivation will be enhanced if the individual would truly like to take the bolus into the mouth. This is where goal-setting and understanding the patient's likes and dislikes are important. The clinician may find that placing the bolus close to the patient's nose so that they can experience the aroma may entice mouth-opening behaviour. Gentle repetitive pressure of the cup or spoon on the lower lip may also enhance lip and then jaw opening. Wherever possible, if the individual can self-feed, this may also be a positive motivating factor in getting the bolus into the oral cavity. Collaborative work with an occupational therapist is recommended where self-feeding is one of the goals of treatment. Where there is spasticity in the muscles of the face it may be appropriate to use massage to reduce the tone to allow the jaw to open (Clark, 2003). Verbal instruction to open the mouth should also accompany any assistive actions by the therapist.

Taking the bolus from a cup, spoon or fork

Taking the bolus from a cup, spoon or fork requires lip closure around the device. The task can be graded such that the clinician may move from large spoons to smaller spoons to allow the individual to increase amount of lip closure. Similarly progression from a medicine style cup (30ml capacity) to increasingly larger capacity cups may assist with the process of lip closure around a cup. Physical assistance to bring the cup or spoon to the mouth could be offered and then phased out as the individual becomes more independent with the task. Note that there will be considerably more closure required to use a spout cup or a straw. With straws the bore size (i.e. diameter) of the straw can also be manipulated from larger to smaller.

Lip closure to contain the bolus

Lip closure to contain the bolus within the oral cavity requires that the lips come together with sufficient strength and tone. Where there is severely limited volitional movement, the clinician could manually assist the patient by closing the lips for them. Where there is volitional movement and sufficient cognitive capacity, the clinician could also use a lollipop placed within the oral cavity and ask the individual to close their lips around it to encourage lip closure. Alternatively the clinician could use tethered shapes made out of acrylic or Teflon as these will not deform within the oral cavity. Round shapes are more comfortable during oral manipulation (Jacobs et al., 1998). The clinician could also try and remove the lollipop from the oral cavity while the patient resists this movement using lip closure to include resistance exercise into the task. Lifesavers (candy) anchored using string (Huckabee and Pelletier, 1999) or dental floss have also been suggested for this manoeuvre; however, the clinician needs to be mindful of melting the Lifesaver with exposure to saliva and likely sucking actions and thinning of the material allowing it to break, and lose the tether. Sugar-free lollies are advocated to reduce the likelihood of exacerbating dental caries or the proliferation of 'bad' oral pathogens. Aspiration of bacterial pathogens in saliva is associated with an increased risk of developing aspiration pneumonia where dysphagia is also present (Langmore et al., 1998). Clinicians therefore must be diligent in ensuring that the oral cavity is well cleaned at the completion of any food or fluid trials, but particularly with those that are likely to increase dental caries (e.g. increased sugar content).

Other methods of promoting lip closure include holding a straw or tongue depressor with the lips and gradually increasing the length of time the individual holds the item between their lips to improve endurance (Sheppard, 2005). To increase strength then resistance needs to be employed. The clinician could attempt to remove the straw or tongue depressor while the patient grips it with their lips. The clinician could also ask the patient to press down firmly on the tongue depressor using their lips, repeating the motion until fatigued. The clinician could also ask the patient to use their lips (protrusion and retraction activities) to pull a strip of moistened gauze into the mouth (Huckabee and Pelletier, 1999). Note that these tasks aim at keeping the bolus within the oral cavity and attempt to minimize drooling the material (liquid, solid or saliva) from the oral cavity. They do not address control of the bolus within the oral cavity.

Manipulation of a solid bolus for deformation

Manipulation of the solid bolus for effective deformation requires tongue agility, buccinator tone and lip and jaw closure. Once again adherence to functional tasks is recommended. Individuals could be given large items to manipulate such as large pieces of gauze or lengths of liquorice (Logemann, 1998). The individual could be asked to use the tongue to 'grip or hold' the item to start with. Following this they could be asked to move the bolus to either side of the mouth and position it between the teeth or place it into the buccal cavities and then retrieve it from these positions. Use of the tip of the tongue in particular should be encouraged, as this is one of the most densely innervated areas of the body (Jacobs et al., 1998). The aim of these tasks would be to improve endurance and accuracy of controlled movement. Once successful with large items, the clinician could progress to smaller tethered items. For example, a piece of chewing gum could be wrapped in gauze and tethered using dental floss or string for manipulation. This has the added effect of using taste as a stimulant. Paste substances could be placed by the clinician on the palatal, buccal or dental surfaces with instruction to use the tongue to wipe the surfaces clean. When it is time to progress to an untethered bolus, the clinician could initially use small portions of items that will dissolve in the oral cavity (e.g. buttery biscuits such as shortbread etc.). Mechanoreceptors in the periodontal ligament are primarily responsible for the tactile function of teeth (Jacobs et al., 1998). These receptors are important for coordinating jaw muscles during biting and chewing. In order to activate receptors in the jaw musculature items with a thickness of 5mm or more are required. For this reason, a bulky but secured item such as the gauze-covered chewing gum may be advantageous in providing tactile input. The clinician can also use a heavy bolus to stimulate the occlusal surface. Better stereognostic abilities are indicated in individuals who are able to detect small differences in weight interdentally (between the teeth). Untethered boluses will eventually be required for successful reintroduction of chewing. Note also that chewing typically occurs on one favoured side, thus treatment to improve chewing can be taught on that one side (Yamada et al., 2005).

From the point of view of safety and to reduce anxiety, it may also be beneficial to teach the patient specifically how to remove an unwanted bolus from the oral cavity (Sheppard, 2005). This could be combined with a bolus control activity. For example, the clinician could place a straw into the patient's oral cavity and ask the patient to use their tongue and lips to expectorate the straw. Small portions of the straw could initially be placed into the mouth, moving towards progressively longer lengths of straw. The clinician could also position paste or puree into the buccal cavities and ask the patient to use their tongue to retrieve and then expectorate the bolus. Failing the use of the tongue for this manoeuvre, the clinician could teach the patient to use their finger to remove the residue. This technique is also called 'lingual sweep' (Huckabee and Pelletier, 1999).

Control of a liquid bolus within the oral cavity

Control of a liquid bolus within the oral cavity is a natural progression. Once a cohesive bolus can be safely controlled then a more volatile and less cohesive bolus such as liquid can be attempted. In this regard moving from very viscous fluids to progressively less viscous fluids to reach the consistency of water is suggested. Patients may be instructed to take a spoonful of fluid into the mouth and hold it in the mouth before expectorating it. The clinician can increase the amount of time the individual holds the liquid bolus in the mouth before expectorating it. With good control the patient may be asked to move the bolus around the mouth without swallowing it (Logemann, 1998). Note that a slightly larger bolus (e.g. at least 5ml or larger) may be required for individuals where there is reduced intra-oral sensation. Small volumes (e.g. 1–2ml) may otherwise not be sufficient to alert the patient that there is anything in their mouth, which is a potentially hazardous situation. In individuals with reduced intra-oral sensation, therapy may progress from larger and heavier boluses to smaller and lighter boluses that mimic saliva (e.g. 1–2ml).

Swallow initiation and bolus propulsion

Swallow initiation and bolus propulsion require the bolus to be maintained in the oral cavity until the bolus is sufficiently prepared for swallowing. Movements relating to tongue control, stabilization and posture are critical at this point following successful oral containment. Exercises in the previous paragraphs will assist in preparing the oral musculature for containment so that the bolus is well controlled prior to the swallow. At this point, however, the best activity for swallow initiation and bolus propulsion is using these actions with a bolus. A heavy cohesive bolus may be suggested as a starting point progressing to more challenging materials such as less cohesive boluses (liquids). Optimal use of compensatory strategies (e.g. taste, texture and temperature) is also advocated at this stage (see Chapter 11).

Intra-oral pressure

Effective function of the soft palate is required to generate the intra-oral pressure needed for sucking (e.g. straw drinking). There is limited information on specific exercises to improve palatal function and there is no information regarding functional carry-over for tasks such as straw drinking. The act of straw-sucking, with graded difficulty levels may promote velopharyngeal closure to assist in generating the required intra-oral pressure to succeed at the task. Where trials with a fluid bolus are not feasible, the clinician may start with asking the patient to suck through a narrow bore straw to lift up a piece of tissue paper. The task can be made more difficult by drawing up a heavier object, such as a cotton wool ball. Note that this task also requires good lip seal, buccal tone and tongue movement (see notes above). When progressing to fluids, the clinician can make the task harder by asking the patient to suck up a very viscous fluid because this requires more effort to draw it up the straw. A wide bore (i.e. diameter) straw will be needed with viscous fluids. The diameter and length of the straw can also be manipulated to make the task easier or more difficult. Length of the straw allows the clinician to manipulate the duration that the individual is sucking through the straw. The clinician can then progress to sips that are brought up the straw and then released back into the cup. Then small sips, large sips and multiple sips, can be introduced again varying viscosity as required. Note also, that this task requires very good swallow-respiratory coordination. See notes below in improving respiratory capacity and swallow-respiratory coordination.

Continuous positive airway pressure (CPAP)

CPAP or continuous positive airway pressure is an instrumental technique that may be assistive in improving velopharyngeal function. CPAP delivers a calibrated amount of continuous air into the nasal cavity. The air pressure provides a resistance which the muscles of the soft palate must overcome to elevate the soft palate and draw the pharyngeal walls in to achieve velopharyngeal closure. The idea is that the muscles must overcome the resistance to function and that this practice using resistance will build up muscle strength. Kuehn (1997) explains that to build biceps strength an individual will lift weights; but rather than attaching a weight to the soft palate, a column of air is injected that the muscles need to work against. A water manometer attached to the CPAP machine allows the clinician to determine the strength of the air pressure. CPAP has predominantly been used to treat sleep apnoea by preventing collapse of the upper airway, but has also been used to treat hypernasality of speech. It has not been specifically used to treat swallowing disorders. Initial results of the technique indicate some speech improvement but variable function in a well-designed study investigating the use of CPAP to reduce hypernasality in a cleft palate population (Kuehn et al., 2002). In addition, the use of CPAP as a treatment for hypernasality following traumatic brain injury has been reported (Cahill et al., 2004). In these three case studies, the authors found that CPAP could be effective in treating moderate-severe hypernasality following traumatic brain injury (Cahill et al., 2004). Of note was the finding that one of the three individuals studied reported an improvement in swallowing function both during and after the CPAP treatment. The authors postulated that the effort from increased velopharyngeal effort had a flow on effect to the swallowing system. As noted above, the CPAP technique requires the soft palate and the pharyngeal muscles to respond to the air pressure. The subject indicated that following CPAP treatment he found that swallowing was less effortful.

Both the Cahill et al. (2004) and Kuehn et al. (2002) studies are true to the principles of exercise physiology for focus on improvement of strength noted above. Both studies varied the air pressure (e.g. started with pressure of 4cm H_2O and progressed gradually to 7.5 cm H_2O over a four week period) to increase resistance gradually. They also graduated the time the individual spent using the CPAP therapy (e.g. initially 10 minutes, leading up to 22 minutes). Finally, the CPAP treatment was applied during a representative task, i.e. during speech. Based on the very limited information available regarding the use of CPAP with dysphagia, it would appear that the technique may be of some benefit where the aim is to improve velopharyngeal function, movement of the superior pharyngeal constrictors and intra-oral pressure. Note that the principles of varying the difficulty of the task (water pressure), the time required (fatigue factor) and use during a functional task (e.g. straw sucking or swallowing) are indicated by the exercise physiology literature.

Clearance of residue from the oral cavity

Clearance of residue from the oral cavity after the primary swallow occurs commonly and subconsciously throughout mealtimes. Therapy activities described above relating to using the tongue to clean palatal, buccal and dental surfaces are suggested. The clinician could place paste, thickened liquids, cold ice chips or small amounts of lemon sorbet into the buccal cavity for retrieval and expectoration. Once successful at expectoration, the individual could retrieve and then swallow the items. Interestingly a technique used to improve respiratory support and vocal intensity in individuals with Parkinson's disease has also been demonstrated to have a positive effect on swallowing. Pre and post treatment analysis of a group of individuals with Parkinson's disease using videofluoroscopy showed improved oral transit time and a reduction in post swallow oral residue after participating in the Lee Silverman Voice Treatment (LSVT®) programme (Sharkawi et al., 2002). Clinicians are required to attend a course to be accredited in using the LSVT®. It is a prescribed programme of 16 sessions run over a four-week period. Treatment occurs four times per week with sessions of 50–60 minutes duration. Three daily exercises include: maximum duration of sustained phonation, maximum fundamental frequency range and maximum functional speech loudness drills. Individuals are encouraged to use a louder voice while speaking and are encouraged to 'feel and think loud' (Sharkawi et al., 2002). To date, the research has been conducted with individuals with Parkinson's disease; however, the technique may be applicable to other populations who present with post swallow oral residue. It was also noted that there was improved oral tongue and tongue base activity during the oral and pharyngeal phases of swallowing in addition to increased vocal intensity. Further research is required to document the efficacy of the LSVT programme in the rehabilitation of dysphagia in other populations.

PHARYNGEAL PHASE

Targeted areas for rehabilitation of the pharyngeal phase of the swallow may include:

- closure of the soft palate to prevent nasal regurgitation during or after the swallow
- effective hyolaryngeal excursion

  ○ Mendelsohn manoeuvre
  ○ head lift exercise
  ○ falsetto exercise

- effective pharyngeal shortening and contraction to strip the bolus from the pharynx

  ○ Masako exercise
  ○ effortful swallow manoeuvre

- effective opening of the upper oesophageal sphincter

  ○ Mendelsohn manoeuvre

- closure of the laryngeal vestibule (including arytenoid movement, vocal fold closure and epiglottic deflection)
- respiratory capacity to cope with swallowing
- swallow-respiratory coordination

  ○ supraglottic swallow
  ○ super-supraglottic swallow

Closure of the soft palate during swallowing

Closure of the soft palate during swallowing is required to reduce the likelihood of nasal regurgitation. Nasal regurgitation is only occasionally seen in individuals with dysphagia, with the difficulty being attributed more to deficits of the pharyngeal constrictors than the soft palate per se (Huckabee and Pelletier, 1999). Treatment strategies for improvement of soft palate function and enhancing movement of the superior pharyngeal constrictors has been discussed above. The proposed treatment strategies relate to straw drinking and CPAP therapy.

Effective hyolaryngeal excursion

Effective hyolaryngeal excursion is required to manually protect the airway during swallowing. The mechanism for this process has been described earlier in this text (see Chapters 1 and 4). Exercises that have been proposed to improve hyolaryngeal excursion in the dysphagia literature include: the Mendelsohn manoeuvre; head lift manoeuvre and falsetto exercises. Note that the Mendelsohn manoeuvre and the head lift manoeuvre may also be implicated in improved opening of the upper oesophageal sphincter (UES) due to the biomechanical arrangement of the hyolaryngeal complex with the UES. Specifically pulley-like traction from the hyoid and its connections with the larynx triggers opening of the UES due to attachment of the inferior portion of the larynx with the UES.

The Mendelsohn manoeuvre is reportedly designed to increase the extent and duration of laryngeal elevation, thereby increasing the duration and width of UES opening (Kahrilas et al., 1991). This function allows the bolus to travel into the oesophagus and minimize residue in the pyriform sinuses post swallow. The evidence base for the technique is derived from a small number of studies, some of which have measured the effectiveness of the technique with healthy individuals (Kahrilas et al., 1991) and some have applied the technique to individuals with dysphagia (Huckabee and Cannito, 1999; Prosiegel et al., 2000). The technique is true to the principles of exercise physiology where the target is improvement in range of movement, not force, however. The technique where the individual is required to hold the larynx up at the height of the swallow (described previously in Chapter 11) requires some strength because the larynx is held by the muscles against the resistance of gravity. Prosiegel et al. (2000) performed a very rigorous study based on kinematic analysis of laryngeal movements in in-patients with neurogenic dysphagia. The authors demonstrated that measurable changes in laryngeal excursion were associated with functional improvement in feeding status. In addition, some of the patients who participated in the study revealed that they had learned the skilled movement so well (indeed had become expert in it), they that were no longer aware that they were using the technique.

The Mendelsohn manoeuvre does, however, require excellent cognitive skills and considerable muscular control. It will provide the clinician with a challenge in teaching the execution of the technique to suitable candidates. Note also that Huckabee and Pelletier (1999) suggested that the Mendelsohn manoeuvre should be used only as an exercise technique rather than employed during mealtimes. Given that the technique upsets the temporal duration of the normal swallow, they suggest that individuals may be more prone to aspiration. However one can also view that the manoeuvre is a 'new' way of swallowing. As such the individual may indeed aspirate as they learn, much as the child falls over many times before they stand and walk. The research by Prosiegel et al. (2000) does not state whether the therapy programme required the subjects to perform the Mendelsohn manoeuvre with saliva bolus swallows, only that assessment of the technique occurred using saliva swallows. To err on the side of caution, the clinician could teach the mechanics of the technique then employ it with saliva swallows. Chewing gum or paraffin wax will increase saliva flow to allow the individual more opportunities to practise with a saliva bolus.

The *head lift manoeuvre* was developed by Shaker et al. (1997). The technique is proposed to strengthen the suprahyoid muscle complex (specifically the mylohyoid, geniohyoid, and digastric muscles). It requires the individual to lie flat on a bed or the floor and perform three sustained head raisings for one minute each from the supine position. The exercises have a one-minute rest interval between each head lift. The sustained head lifts are then followed by 30 consecutive head lifts from the supine position also. For both the sustained and repeated head lifts subjects are instructed to raise the head high and forward enough to see their toes without raising their shoulders from the bed or floor (as applicable). As reported by Shaker et al. (1997; 2002) the exercise is performed three times each day.

The technique is based on sound exercise physiology biomechanics. It focuses on a muscle complex that is required functionally for swallowing. It uses an isometric-isokinetic exercise design. As described above, however, it does not follow a pattern of gradually increasing level of difficulty by varying either the number of repetitions or the number of times performed per day over a treatment period. The subjects in the Shaker et al. (2002) study performed the exact exercise three times a day for six weeks and in doing so both biomechanical and functional swallowing improvement was noted. Efficacy of the technique was further demonstrated when the sham exercise group, who showed no improvement in hyolaryngeal excursion, were crossed over to the real exercise programme, where improvement was demonstrated (Shaker et al., 2002). To be true to the principles of exercise physiology, future efforts should be aimed at determining a step-wise programme (fewer repetitions initially, increasing to more repetitions and more practice cycles). The concept of fatigue should be incorporated into the task by progressively making the task harder in order to cause muscle hypertrophy. Unlike learning mediated by performing the task during an environment similar to the task, the head lift manoeuvre should not be performed while attempting to swallow. It is then, an exercise technique purely designed to strengthen the suprahyoids, with the hope that the strengthened muscles will perform better during the target task of swallowing. Note also that the evidence base for the technique is quite small with numbers of 31 healthy elderly and 27 dysphagic individuals studied (Shaker et al., 1997; Shaker et al., 2002).

The *falsetto exercise* has been advocated by Logemann (1998) to improve laryngeal elevation. The exercise rests on the premise that during the production of falsetto the larynx elevates almost as much as it does during swallowing. Consequently the clinician asks the patient to slide up the pitch scale as high as possible and then hold the high note for several seconds with as much effort as possible (Logemann, 1998). This exercise does not have an evidence base to support its use for swallowing rehabilitation. Technically does it make sense? It is questionable whether practising this task will result in improved laryngeal excursion during *swallowing*, given that it uses muscle complexes that are pattern generated for *speech*. As previous discussions have highlighted, while the same muscles may be used for phonatory and deglutitory functions, they play different parts and enter and exit at different times to perform these complementary but quite different roles. The falsetto exercise requires good respiratory support and vocal fold closure and both of these are also necessary for swallowing. However, during swallowing we do not phonate. Further examination of the biomechanical and exercise physiology principles of this technique is required before its efficacious use in swallowing therapy can be demonstrated. In addition, well-designed research studies need to occur to demonstrate its validity.

Effective pharyngeal shortening and contraction

Effective pharyngeal shortening and contraction is required to move the bolus efficiently through the pharynx. Once the swallow reflex has been initiated, the pharyngeal stage of the swallow is not under voluntary control, which makes rehabilitation of this phase of the swallow very challenging. Perlman et al. (1989) demonstrated, using hooked wire electrodes inserted into the superior pharyngeal constrictor muscle, that swallowing itself produced the greatest amount of activity. The next greatest level of superior constrictor activity as recorded using electromyography was the production of the sound /k/ held for several seconds (Perlman et al., 1989). There are two techniques that have been advocated for use specifically with the aim of improving the efficiency of the pharyngeal phase of the swallow. These are the Masako exercise and the effortful swallow manoeuvre.

The *Masako exercise* is designed to exercise a portion of the superior constrictor (glossopharyngeus muscle) which is believed to be responsible for tongue base retraction and medialization of the pharyngeal constrictors at the level of the tongue base (Logemann, 1998). To improve muscle or muscle complex strength requires resistance, which is achieved using this technique. It requires the individual to hold approximately 1.5cm of the tongue tip between the teeth and swallow with the tongue held in this anchored position. In doing so the base of tongue movement is inhibited while increased pharyngeal wall movement is required to compensate for the lack of tongue base movement. The patient should feel a pulling at the back of the throat when performing the exercise. It is suggested that this exercise only be used with saliva swallows rather than a food or fluid bolus (Huckabee and Pelletier, 1999). The evidence base for this technique is scant and relies on the results of only 10 healthy subjects (Huckabee and Pelletier, 1999). Its rationale is based on biomechanical evidence of changes in swallowing function following base of tongue resection, whereby the pharyngeal walls medialize more towards the tongue base to compensate for the lack of tongue base movement towards them. The biomechanical rationale behind the technique appears to be sound and the exercise itself uses resistance to generate strength. Exercise programmes using the technique should adhere to principles described above using graduated programmes of (a) repetitions, (b) number of sets of repetitions per day, (c) overall length of programme and (d) building fatigue and recovery from fatigue into the programme.

The *effortful swallow manoeuvre* is a technique designed to increase posterior movement of the tongue base during swallow reflex initiation. In doing so it should improve bolus clearance from the valleculae. It requires the individual to 'squeeze hard with all of your muscles' (Logemann, 1998) or swallow as if you are swallowing a telephone book (i.e. a large object). The aim then is to encourage the active and conscious use of force to help propel the bolus. There is very limited evidence for the efficacy of the use of this technique. Biomechanically the exercise is sound, and can be employed during the target activity (i.e. swallowing food or fluid). Bulow et al. (2001) found that the technique seemed effective in reducing the degree of penetration in a group of individuals with moderate to severe pharyngeal stage dysphagia. The technique did not, however, reduce residue in the pharynx post swallow which was one of the original postulations of the technique. Bulow et al. (2001) also found that four of their eight participants experienced difficulty in performing the technique. Bulow et al. (2001) noted that there was reduced hyoid elevation during the swallow because of early hyoid elevation pre-swallow while performing the manoeuvre. As a result there was a reduction in laryngeal excursion during the swallow. This is not optimal for airway protection and neither is it good for UES opening. Here we can see that a change to improve one aspect of the swallowing complex significantly affects the normal function of another part of the swallowing complex. Further studies are required in the implementation of these techniques using videofluoroscopy and where possible concurrent manometry to detail how the techniques affect the biomechanics of swallowing. Given that the current evidence rests on only eight healthy and eight dysphagic individuals, further studies using much larger numbers are required. At a minimum it is recommended that the effects of the postures be demonstrated on videofluoroscopy to ensure that the patient is truly benefiting from the technique.

Opening of the upper oesophageal sphincter

Opening of the upper oesophageal sphincter is mediated via the biomechanics of hyolaryngeal excursion. Techniques listed above to improve the range of movement for laryngeal excursion should also have a knock-on effect with improved duration or diameter of UES opening. These techniques include the head lift exercise and the Mendelsohn manoeuvre. Bulow et al. (1999) also found preliminary indications that the use of the supraglottic swallow (described below) appeared to improve laryngeal excursion and UES opening; however, further studies with larger numbers are required.

Closure of the larynx and laryngeal vestibule

In order to protect the airway during swallowing there is mechanical closure of the arytenoids, vocal cords and epiglottic deflection over the laryngeal vestibule (see also Chapter 4). Effort closure of the larynx while compressing the thoracic and abdominal contents causes (a) the arytenoids to be brought to the midline, (b) the false vocal folds to be brought together, (c) obliteration of the laryngeal ventricle because the false vocal folds are drawn down tightly against the true vocal folds, and (d) the thyroid cartilage is elevated and approximates the hyoid bone as sub-glottic pressure increases (Aronson, 1985). This type of effort closure occurs during coughing, throat clearing, vomiting, urination, defecation and parturition, in addition to lifting and pushing. Teaching individuals to cough or clear their throat effectively should also be a suitable rehabilitation exercise because it is protective and may assist in removing a misdirected bolus. The individual will require sufficient respiratory support, and glottic closure in order to achieve these tasks. Note that vocal fold adduction is not as important for safe swallowing as arytenoid closure and epiglottic deflection and a functional pharyngeal stripping activity (Huckabee and Pelletier, 1999). It was demonstrated in Chapter 3 that there are varying patterns of vocal fold adduction in healthy individuals, all of which are considered normal.

Note also that aggressive treatment using cough or throat clearing activities is not recommended for individuals with a history of stroke or coronary artery disease due to effects on cardiac status (Chaudhuri et al., 2002). Liaison with a physiotherapist is advisable given their expertise in pulmonary rehabilitation. Epiglottic deflection occurs as a combination of tongue base retraction and hyolaryngeal excursion (discussed further in Chapter 4). Thus suitable biomechanical exercises that improve these functions may also assist in promoting more effective epiglottic deflection. Given that the arytenoids, vocal folds and epiglottis function in a very specific way during the act of swallowing, it is likely that the best rehabilitation for these structures will be in practice swallowing, as previously described.

RESPIRATORY SUPPORT FOR SWALLOWING

Respiratory support for swallowing is critical. When we breathe we don't swallow and when we swallow we don't breathe. The body will always choose to breathe over eating and drinking. This is highlighted in conditions such as Chronic Obstructive Pulmonary Disease (COPD) where there is a 30–50 per cent incidence of pneumonia (Langmore et al., 1998; see also Chapter 9). Halting of respiration is required for a minimum of 0.3–0.6 seconds for thin liquids and 3–5 seconds or more during continuous cup drinking (Logemann, 1998). Liaison with a physiotherapist is suggested in the rehabilitation of respiratory support for swallowing due to their expertise in pulmonary rehabilitation. As a starting point, the clinician may gather baseline data of respiratory support for swallowing, such as the duration that an individual can comfortably hold their breath. Treatment may include holding the breath for progressively longer periods of time although no longer than 5 seconds is suggested in de-conditioned individuals. The clinician may also use some of the straw exercises described above, the goal being to blow a piece of tissue paper or cotton ball successively larger distances. Then the patient could be taught to use the straw to lift the tissue paper and then cotton ball up for one second, progressively increasing the duration (2 secs, 3 secs etc.). This is a resistance exercise that will become more challenging with successively 'heavier' items to be lifted via the straw. Components of the LSVT programme for improving vocal intensity in individuals with Parkinson's disease may also prove useful in generally increasing respiratory resilience and capacity in other individuals.

Coordination of respiration and swallowing

Not only is sufficient respiratory reserve and support necessary for safe swallowing, but coordination between the swallowing and respiratory systems is essential. The swallow-respiratory cycle has been described earlier in Chapter 4. The *supraglottic swallow* and the *super-supraglottic swallow* techniques bring to the conscious level slight variations on what normally happens when the swallow-respiratory system works harmoniously. These techniques have been described as airway protection strategies in Chapter 11. They are compensatory strategies used for rehabilitation until they have been internalized (achievement of stage 3 – automatism). The purpose of the *supraglottic swallow* is to effect closure of the vocal folds before and during swallowing in order to protect the airway (Logemann, 1998). It is a technique which is true to the principles of exercise physiology because it makes conscious what was once an unconscious task. It relies on the coordination of many patterns, the largest patterns being the overall synchrony between swallowing and respiration. For safety and in the context of the swallow-respiratory cycle, the individual should be instructed to take a breath and hold it, place the bolus in the oral cavity while continuing to hold the breath, keep holding the breath while swallowing and then immediately after the swallow, breathe out or cough.

For some patients the instruction to 'hold your breath' does not result in vocal fold closure, with the individual instead ceasing chest wall movement, but leaving the airway open. Logemann (1998) suggests that if this is suspected, the clinician can ask the patient to take a breath, then say 'ahhh', stop voicing and hold the breath, and continue with the remainder of the task. Individuals with significant muscle weakness or poor endurance may find this exercise quite difficult (Bulow et al., 1999).

The task of swallow-respiratory coordination can be broken down into smaller tasks. The individual can be taught to hold their breath for increasing increments of time. Following this, they can then be taught to hold the breath, then forcibly breathe out. Then the individual may progress to utilizing the task with a saliva bolus, and finally with food and fluid boluses. Given that this task reasonably neatly mimics the usually subconscious swallow-respiratory pattern, it should prove relatively easy for an individual to acquire. In fact, Zuydam et al. (2000) reported on a case where an individual post surgery to the posterior third of the tongue used a supraglottic swallow technique without being instructed to do so. Given that it is so much like the normal swallow-respiratory pattern, the clinician will need to bear in mind the fading out of feedback when it is no longer required, as feedback once the task has been accomplished serves to impair ('analysis paralysis') rather than enhance performance (Goodman and Wood, 2004).

The *super-supraglottic swallow* is a variation on the supraglottic swallow. The patient is instructed to inhale and hold their breath very tightly while bearing down. They are encouraged to continue to bear down while swallowing and then exhale forcefully or cough after the swallow (Logemann, 1998). The concept of bearing down is used for the benefit of vocal closure described above; that is, more forward arytenoid movement and closure of the false vocal folds in addition to true vocal fold closure. Cardiac arrhythmia has been reported during swallowing sessions, utilizing the supraglottic and super-supraglottic swallow manoeuvres in individuals with stroke or coronary artery disease and dysphagia (Chaudhuri et al., 2002). Based on a small study, the authors advocated that the effects of the supraglottic and super-supraglottic swallow techniques were dangerous for individuals with a medical history of stroke (including cardiac arrhythmia or coronary artery disease), acute congestive heart failure and uncontrolled hypertension. On investigation of the effect of the technique in healthy individuals, Bulow et al. (1999) and Ohmae et al. (1996) found that laryngeal elevation was prolonged and there was a subsequent prolongation of UES opening. In the dysphagic population also, laryngeal elevation was increased (Bulow et al., 2001). As noted above, the evidence base for the use of both the supraglottic swallow and the super-supraglottic swallow is scant and based on exceedingly small numbers. Generalization is therefore cautioned, particularly in the populations noted above.

IS THERE A CASE FOR ELECTRICAL STIMULATION THERAPY IN DYSPHAGIA REHABILITATION?

Electrical stimulation has in some places been embraced as a new and exciting method of rehabilitating swallowing function. The most familiar use of electrical stimulation has been with upper and lower limb movement where muscles are considerably larger and more easily isolated than those found in the head and neck (Grill et al., 2001). Electrical stimulation is the application of low voltage electrical currents to muscle tissue, thereby causing contraction of the muscle fibres (Clark, 2003). The neuromuscular response is influenced by (a) the characteristics of the electrical current, (b) whether stimulation is continuous or intermittent, (c) placement of the electrodes, (d) the length of the treatment session (i.e. dose), (e) use in isolation or during a functional task and (f) the regularity of the treatment. Many of these parameters are yet to be rigorously investigated. Clark (2003) reported that high frequency stimulation produces the most forceful contractions; however, these can cause rapid fatigue. On the other hand, lower frequency stimulation produces lower forces and thus reduces the likelihood of fatigue. There is limited information available about the use of electrical stimulation parameters suitable to provide high or low force contractions for the various muscle groups necessary for swallowing. It has been suggested that electrical stimulation (also known as functional neuromotor stimulation- FNS) is most suitable for an intact neuromuscular system with impaired central nervous system control (Ludlow et al. 2000).

Pattern of motor recruitment is different in electrical stimulation to the usual pattern in functional tasks

One of the biggest problems with electrical stimulation is that the pattern of motor unit recruitment is different to what occurs during volitional movement of the muscles. During volitional movement smaller Type I fibres (slow twitch) are activated first, followed by Type II (fast twitch) fibres as additional force is required (Clark, 2003). There are different subtypes of the Type II fast twitch fibres. Type IIA fibres are noted to be fast resistant fibres, whereas Type IIB are fast fatigue fibres (Kimura, 2001). As an example, the thyroarytenoid muscle is a rapidly contracting fast Type II muscle. These characteristics allow the thyroarytenoid to close the vocal folds rapidly for airway protection during swallowing (Ludlow et al., 2000). During electrical stimulation, a larger proportion of Type II fibres are recruited, altering the normal pattern of recruitment that would occur with volitional use. Thus active exercise in functional tasks would appear to be better than electrical stimulation of muscles as this allows the normal recruitment pattern of the different muscle fibres. Note also that because the muscles in the head and neck are small and overlapping, there can be little certainty of correct placement of the electrodes where palpation is used to determine placement. Clark (2003) suggests that electrical stimulation should perhaps be reserved for individuals unable to participate in an active exercise programme. Further, it may be better if the stimulation is paired with a functional task. However, considerably more research is required to provide exact levels of electrical current suitable for use, dose and duration of sessions.

There is another major problem underpinning the application of electrical stimulation in the rehabilitation of swallowing. The muscles of the oral cavity, pharynx and larynx are unique due to their many very different functions such as speech, breathing, swallowing, and coughing (Ludlow, 2005). These muscles have multiple roles and at present there is limited information to determine which muscles are stabilizers and which are agonists and antagonists during these very different roles. Table 12.4 shows the very different effects that bilateral afferent block of the internal branch of the superior laryngeal nerve using anaesthesia has on swallowing, Valsalva manoeuvre, cough and voice (Ludlow, 2005). The results suggest that the afferents that supply the internal branch of the superior laryngeal nerve are essential for swallowing, but not voice production. As another example, note that the cricoarytenoid muscle is associated only with vocal fold opening during a sniff, whereas during speech the cricoarytenoid and the thyroarytenoid are correlated with both opening and closing actions. For coughing, the thyroarytenoid and lateral cricoarytenoid were only correlated with vocal fold closing. Put simply, the cricoarytenoid muscle works in different patterns and with different muscles to achieve different roles. It is also worth bearing in mind that Burnett et al. (2003) found that stimulation to some areas of a muscle produce movement in one direction, while stimulation to the same muscle but in a different area could produce a movement in a different direction. Previous discussions relating to motor learning indicate that muscle contractions in one activity cannot be expected to translate reliably to improvement in another activity. The discussion regarding the cricoarytenoid serves to highlight the intrinsic difficulties in designing an electrical stimulation programme. It provides further support for the use of electrical stimulation in enhancing function in *the functional context of swallowing*.

There are also difficulties associated with intra-individual variation of anatomical configuration in the application of electrical stimulation. Considerable training is required to ensure correct placement of the electrodes. Burnett et al. (2003) used

Table 12.4 Effect of bilateral afferent block using anaesthetic of the internal branch of the superior laryngeal nerve on swallowing, Valsalva, cough and voicing function

Swallowing	Cough	Valsalva	Voice
• Swallowing = effortful	• No effect	• No effect	• Minimal effects
• Increased frequency of laryngeal penetration			
• Increased frequency aspiration			
• Incomplete laryngeal closure			

Source: Ludlow (2005).

hooked wire electrodes to determine whether single, bilateral or combined muscle stimulation provided the best results for laryngeal elevation. They found that while all three methods improved laryngeal elevation that paired muscle stimulation provided the best results, although no one muscle or muscle pair achieved the greatest laryngeal elevation in all participants. Note also that the study was conducted on a small number of healthy individuals. The researchers recommended that optimal stimulation sites should be determined on a patient-by-patient basis.

Potential for nerve damage

Damage to the nerve is another area of concern when contemplating electrical stimulation. Mann et al. (2002) reported two case studies where electrodes implanted into laryngeal nerves resulted in scar tissue around the nerve in one case and recurrent laryngeal nerve paralysis in another. The authors were therefore wary of direct electrical stimulation of peripheral nerves, however, application of electrical current into a muscle was seen as a safer alternative. Mann et al. (2002) looked at the use of electrical stimulation of the genioglossus muscle to increase the dimensions of the hypopharyngeal airway for individuals with obstructive sleep apnoea. While the technique proved successful and it was suggested that intra-muscular stimulation of the muscle provided equivalent results to direct stimulation of the hypoglossal nerve, it was found that if the electrodes slipped into the geniohyoid, for example, posterior tilting of the epiglottis was noted. The accurate placement of the electrodes is therefore very important, particularly with hooked wire electrodes. Note also though that while some types of stimulation can enhance swallowing, too much stimulation can produce inhibitory changes which are associated with detrimental changes to healthy swallowing patterns (Power et al., 2004). The results of the study, looking at only three different parameters of frequency (5 Hz, 1 Hz or 0.2 Hz with 0.2ms pulse width, 280V) of electrical stimulation of the faucial pillars for 10 minutes, suggested that the pattern of stimulation is very important in promoting 'plastic' changes in the brain. Note also that the authors had postulated that 5Hz frequency would induce optimal changes, where in fact the 5Hz frequency produced inhibitory responses. As further support of the need to define therapeutic parameters clearly, Fraser et al. (2002) further found that excitability can be increased or decreased depending upon the frequency, duration and intensity of electrical sensory stimulation. The Fraser et al. (2002) study cautiously promoted positive effects of sensory electrical stimulation with the effect of stimulation being linked to improved swallowing function lasting from one hour after the initial 10 minute application.

There is also literature to support the fact that if denervated muscle is stimulated at levels greater than 6V that this stimulation results in tissue damage and/or electrode corrosion in implanted electrodes (Ludlow et al., 2000). Chronic muscle stimulation can change fast muscle fibres into slow muscle fibres, affecting their physiological function, and histological and neurochemical characteristics (Ludlow et al., 2000). For this reason, intermittent stimulation designs may assist by providing a period of rapid stimulation, followed by a period of rest to allow the muscle to recover. Ludlow et al. (2000) conducted an extremely thorough investigation of chronic electrical stimulation of the thyroarytenoid muscle in a dog model. An animal model was required prior to use on humans. The size and proportion of the laryngeal structures of canines is the closest to those of humans and it was for this reason that dogs were used in the study. Ludlow et al. (2000) specifically sought to provide information pertaining to effects of chronic muscle stimulation and the extent of tissue damage. Ludlow et al. (2000) found that in their sample of six canines that had been chronically intermittently stimulated with implanted electrodes for 8 hours a day, 5 days a week for up to 8 months, there were small differences between stimulated and non-stimulated muscles. However, the authors note that the sample sizes were small and that the 16 hours that the stimulation was withheld daily would have contributed to muscle recovery. Failure of relaxation of the muscle results in persistent shortening of the muscle causing contractures. This is clearly not something that would assist swallowing recovery. Considerably more research into the long-term effect of electrical stimulation is required with larger sample sizes.

Electrical stimulation for swallowing rehabilitation using surface electrodes

Electrical stimulation to improve swallowing function has also been employed using surface electrodes. Leelamanit et al. (2002) reported surface electrode placement over the submandibular gland in order to stimulate the thyrohyoid muscle in order to improve laryngeal elevation. The justification for choice of site of placement and target muscle group was not well demonstrated. Patients in this study were stimulated for four hours a day until they fulfilled the criteria for improved swallowing or until it was demonstrated that other interventions were required. There was no justification provided for the length of time that stimulation occurred. There was also no justification of the pulse type, pulse frequency or size of the stimulating electrodes despite the fact that the authors recognized and reported that these parameters were critical to 'successful neuromuscular electrical stimulation rehabilitation'.

Freed et al. (2001) applied electrodes to the skin surface in an attempt to justify use of the technique for rehabilitation of swallowing. The authors compared the electrical stimulation protocol with a thermal-tactile stimulation protocol. There was no control group. The authors included both inclusion and exclusion criteria. There were different numbers of patients assigned to the electrical stimulation and thermal stimulation groups, making it difficult to compare the two techniques for efficacy. The patient characteristics in the two groups was also quite different. For the electrical stimulation group two different electrode placement patterns were used. One had placement of the electrodes on either the right or left side with 'the upper electrode placed above the lesser horns of the hyoid bone on the digastric muscle, and the lower electrode placed on the thyrohyoid muscle at the level of the top of the cricothyroid cartilage' (Freed et al., 2001, p. 469). This position was used for the majority of patients. For patients with tracheostomies or whose anatomy prevented use of the previous configuration, the following placement parameters were used: 'on either side of the midline, above the lesser horns of the hyoid bone on the digastric muscle'

(Freed et al., 2001, p. 469). These are obviously quite different placement and comparability of results gained from the two placements is questionable. For both placements a physical therapist and a speech pathologist applied the electrodes. The authors note that the electrodes were repositioned until muscle fasciculations occurred or the 'strongest contraction was observed during the swallowing response'. There appears to be little scientific basis for this criteria for electrode placement.

Note also that current intensity was 'set at the patient's tolerance and comfort level'. However, it is also noted that some individuals who participated in the study had aphasia. The authors do not demonstrate how they determined whether aphasia affected the individual's ability to indicate comfort level reliably. Intensity of the electrical signal was increased in increments of 2.5mA up to a maximum of 25mA to the individual's comfort and tolerance level. Of concern the authors state that 'when ES was successful in obtaining a voluntary swallow response, the patient was asked to attempt to swallow...' a specific fluid consistency (p. 469). The concern is that the intensity of the stimulation appears to have been ramped up until a response was gained with little checks in place to ensure that skin damage or indeed muscle damage did not also occur. The stimulation was reported to have been delivered for 60 minutes, in a continuous mode with a one second pause between each minute. There is insufficient detail to be sure (a) how often the individual was required to swallow during the electrical stimulation (i.e. participate in a functional task) or (b) if the stimulation occurred continuously, regardless of whether the person was swallowing or not. Research from the exercise physiology literature would question the utility of the latter. This study did not vary the amount of stimulation offered (dose) per patient nor did it gradually increase the duration of the stimulation on a daily basis. In this context it is very difficult to agree with the author's interpretations of the results. Further well-designed research is required in this field.

Contraindications for use of electrical stimulation

The literature supports the statements that electrical stimulation is contraindicated in patients with (a) carotid sensitivity, (b) evidence of heart block, (c) patients using pacemakers, (d) patients who are pregnant, (e) those with hypersensitive skin, and (f) those recovering from surgery at or very close to the site of intended electrode placement (Huckabee and Pelletier, 1999; Leelamanit et al., 2002). The head and neck are densely vascularized and innervated, consequently skill and expertise is required for accurate placement of the electrodes in addition to consideration of populations to avoid (e.g. cancer, radiotherapy, chemotherapy).

Electrical stimulation can also cause (i) chemical burns if applied to injured skin or for a prolonged duration, (ii) heat burn due to the intensity of the current, (iii) potential for electrical shock, (iv) spreading of infection due to the muscle excitation effect, and (v) muscle soreness with prolonged and intensive use (Leelamanit et al., 2002). The use of electrical stimulation in patients following radiotherapy should also be cautioned if the intended site of placement of the electrodes is within the radiotherapy field.

Many of the electrical stimulation studies provide insufficient data to determine the voltage and amperage used in their studies. Moreover where some of these values are recorded, there is little consistency in them! Both of the studies using surface electrical stimulation techniques are poorly designed, with thin hypotheses, insufficient information about inclusion and exclusion criteria, no use of randomization or control groups and results confounded by natural recovery. There is insufficient information to state whether surface stimulation has a primary effect on the muscle beneath it, peripheral nerves attached to the muscle or near to the muscle or some combination of both. In addition, both studies applied the stimulation in block fashion for either one hour or four hours, without pairing the stimulation with functional swallowing tasks (Freed et al., 2001; Leelamanit et al., 2002). Both studies serve nothing more than to show there may be potential for the use of electrical stimulation in the rehabilitation of swallowing, but there are a significant number of questions to be answered before it is routinely applied in the clinical setting. Issues of training accreditation also need to be addressed.

BIOFEEDBACK IN THE REHABILITATION OF SWALLOWING

Biofeedback is an external means of providing feedback to a patient and is intended to increase the rate of motor learning, thus improving the efficiency of treatment (Crary et al., 2004). That feedback may be provided in the form of (a) specific comments from the therapist, (b) a visual image while performing a task (e.g. endoscopy, videofluoroscopy, visual display attached to electromyography device), or (c) auditory feedback (e.g. cervical auscultation). Biofeedback has been shown to enhance new learning. It is a method of providing additional input to internal sensorimotor feedback and allows an individual to shape their behaviour based on what they see, hear or feel. Biofeedback is encouraged as a useful adjunct for rehabilitation of function and is designed to be used in combination with the therapeutic exercises and compensatory strategies described elsewhere in this text. It is a temporary adjunct that gives the patient information about 'the right way' for them to swallow or prepare the bolus safely. Surface electromyography is often cited as a useful biofeedback device for swallowing rehabilitation. The evidence base for its use is small, however, the principles underlying why it should be useful are sound. Videofluoroscopy and endoscopy of swallowing and cervical auscultation can also be used in varying degrees to provide biofeedback.

SURFACE ELECTROMYOGRAPHY – sEMG

Surface electromyography (sEMG) is a means of measuring the myoelectric impulses generated by the muscle just before it contracts (Abernethy et al., 2005). The signal generated is fed into a device that produces a visual signal of a raw waveform that is then smoothed to provide a more 'user-friendly' visual display for the patient. Typically the amplitude or strength of the movement is depicted along the vertical axis and the timing of the contraction is displayed along the horizontal axis. In the surface format EMG is applied using electrodes onto the skin surface. However

EMG can also be applied invasively, using hooked wire electrodes into the body of the muscle (Sonies 1991; Sonies and Baum, 1988). Intramuscular placement is required to use EMG in a diagnostic format. It requires considerable skill, training and knowledge of head and neck anatomy. Given its invasive nature, intramuscular EMG is not widely used in clinical practice. sEMG on the other hand is non-invasive and provides the clinician with an accurate indication of the functional activity of the muscles it overlies (Huckabee and Pelletier, 1999). With the electrodes placed on the surface and due to the high degree of overlapping muscles in the face and neck, it is very difficult to isolate a single muscle. In fact it is more often a group of muscles that are being recorded. For this reason, sEMG should not be used for diagnostic purposes, but should be reserved for rehabilitation via biofeedback. In addition, due to vast intra-individual variability, patients should serve as their own controls. sEMG has been advocated to (a) promote a reduction in tone where spasticity appears likely, (b) improve coordination and motor patterning, and (c) assist development of muscle recruitment where the muscle/s appear to be weak or paralysed (Huckabee and Pelletier, 1999). The reader is referred to Huckabee and Pelletier (1999) for a detailed account of the use of sEMG for rehabilitation of swallowing. Some brief points are presented below.

Huckabee and Pelletier (1999) explain that the biofeedback afforded by sEMG facilitates a patient's awareness of muscular contractions associated with swallowing. In clinical practice electrodes are most often placed on the submental muscles to facilitate feedback on swallow initiation and the suprahyoids to facilitate feedback on laryngeal excursion (Huckabee and Cannito, 1999). Electrode placement is critical. Electrodes need to be placed on the belly of the muscle rather than the points of insertion. While this is obviously easier with large muscles in the limbs, the task becomes much more difficult with the small and overlapping muscles of the face, floor of mouth and throat. The distance that the electrodes are placed apart is also important, because the electrodes will measure as deep as the active and referent electrodes are spaced apart. Thus the closer together the electrodes are placed the smaller the amount of information gleaned, while further distance apart may enhance the signal (Huckabee and Pelletier, 1999). Finally it also matters whether the electrode is large or small. Smaller electrodes tend to provide a more specific measurement than larger ones. With larger electrodes a greater surface area is recorded and the specificity of the measurement is therefore reduced (Huckabee and Pelletier, 1999). Huckabee and Cannito (1999) reported some of the characteristics of the oscilloscope display one might expect when different swallowing manoeuvres are employed. For example, they state that during employment of the Masako exercise, the visual display shows a high peak amplitude for a short duration, deemed representative of rapid contraction, and relaxation of the suprahyoids during swallowing. In contrast, during the Mendelsohn manoeuvre a typical oscilloscope display may show a rapid onset rise in amplitude followed by a sustained high amplitude trace (while the larynx is elevated against gravity) for a few seconds before an abrupt drop in amplitude signalling the end of the manoeuvre (larynx returns to rest) and return to rest.

sEMG has been reported in two recent clinical studies aimed at rehabilitation of swallowing in individuals with chronic dysphagia (symptoms >6 months)

(Huckabee and Cannito, 1999; Crary et al., 2004). Huckabee and Cannito (1999) used a small sample of individuals with chronic dysphagia secondary to brain stem injury. Information regarding placement of the electrodes was inconclusive, stating only that submental and suprahyoid muscles were targeted. Treatment was intensive, utilizing one hour of direct therapy each morning and mid-afternoon with a rest period of 3–4 hours between sessions. Treatment continued for five consecutive days. In addition, patients were given a home programme to be carried out three times during the week which relied on independent sessions using the sEMG of 15 minutes' duration. It could be argued that the benefit of the home programme may well have been negligible given the short and inconsistent duration of the home treatment. Treatment was patient specific and utilized sEMG in conjunction with swallowing manoeuvres such as the Mendelsohn manoeuvre, Masako exercise, the head-lift manoeuvre and effortful swallow as required. Direct oral intake was also incorporated as early as was safely possible into the treatment programme. This type of programme is quite well designed; it makes use of biofeedback, physiologically sound manoeuvres and a contextual setting (trials of food). The results of the small study showed that there were improvements in swallowing physiology, pulmonary status and type of foods and fluids the patient was able to safely eat. Interestingly the patients that improved reported that they were no longer using compensatory techniques to swallow safely. This does not appear to have been formally investigated, and much like the Prosiegel et al. (2000) study, the patients may in fact have been using the techniques without conscious awareness. That is, they may have achieved stage 3 – the automatism phase of learning.

Crary et al. (2004) investigated a mixed population of stroke and head/neck surgical individuals with dysphagia symptoms in evidence for more than six months. In this study, individuals participated in daily 50-minute clinical sessions. In addition, the patients were asked to complete two home therapy sessions per day; however, there was no indication of the suggested time frame for these home therapy sessions. Number of therapy sessions ranged from four to 28. Therapy was discontinued when both the patient and the clinician agreed that further improvement was unlikely. Electrodes were placed on the anterior neck between the hyoid bones and the superior border of the thyroid cartilage. The ground electrode was placed over the thyroid notch area, with each active electrode placed to the right and left of the ground electrode. A very functional approach was employed where sEMG was used to facilitate techniques to improve bolus control and airway protection. True to the principles of exercise physiology, an ascending threshold approach was employed whereby the patient had to progressively increase swallow effort to obtain an auditory signal indicating success. Bolus volume and viscosity were also systematically manipulated. The results of the study indicated that the structural behavioural programme was most beneficial for the stroke population. Crary et al. (2004) suggest that the swallowing pattern is more amenable to rehabilitation when the dysphagia is physiologically based rather than mechanically based, as in the case of head/neck surgery. The authors suggested that 'head/neck patients may be less likely to have the physiologic capability to change swallowing patterns' (p. 164), however, I would argue that with cognition preserved, these individuals are better candidates for swallowing re-education. The challenge for the therapist is in assisting the patient to find new patterns, or strategies to help them achieve functional swallowing.

PHARYNGEAL EMG

EMG activity of the pharyngeal phase of swallowing is rarely undertaken due to the difficulties in placement of the electrodes. Previous investigators have reported recording EMG activity from the superior pharyngeal constrictors using hooked wire electrode placement directly into the muscle (Perlman et al., 1989). A more novel and less invasive approach has been described by Palmer et al. (1989) where bipolar suction electrodes were adhered to the mucosa of the posterior pharyngeal wall and provided information from the stable underlying constrictor muscles. The researchers indicated that choice of electrode type (hooked wire electrode, needle electrode or bipolar suction electrode) was dependent on the purpose of the study and the muscles selected for study. Indeed some of the electrode types were better for certain muscles than others. The ability to reliably record from cricopharyngeus remains technically challenging, however. Further research is required to develop normative data for recruitment patterns using these EMG devices. Certainly reliable and minimally invasive pharyngeal EMG may be very helpful in providing feedback to individuals with pharyngeal stage dysphagia.

Other biofeedback mechanisms for swallowing rehabilitation

As noted above, videofluoroscopy and endoscopy of swallowing may provide useful biofeedback. It is more difficult to use videofluoroscopy in a biofeedback modality due to the ethical issues of keeping radiation exposure to a minimum. However, if the patient is taught a rehabilitative manoeuvre or exercise (e.g. Mendelsohn manoeuvre etc.) the clinician can use the images to show the individual the result of applying the manoeuvre, perhaps allowing the individual to better visualize what it is they are trying to achieve. Endoscopy of swallowing affords more real-time use of biofeedback. For example, the monitor can be positioned so that the patient can clearly see copious secretions in the pharynx, be instructed to swallow and then see and feel the result of a successful swallow in clearing the secretions. Techniques such as the supraglottic swallow can be taught in segments using endoscopy. For example, the patient can be taught the breath hold and release component of the task and can watch as the cords close. They can also see and experience the difference between the supraglottic swallow and the more forceful super-supraglottic swallow. Even for individuals without the cognitive skills to perform these manoeuvres, the ability to see food or fluid residue in the pharynx prior to or after the swallow and then see the result of a clearing swallow in removing the residue may allow them to better learn a prophylactic clearing swallow.

Cervical auscultation can also be used for biofeedback. Attachment of a small throat microphone to a portable amplifier will allow both clinician and patient to determine the synchrony of swallowing and respiration. It allows them to hear a primary swallow and any clearing swallows; with clearing swallows encouraged if this is required. It also allows them to hear for changes in respiration quality (wet) and speed (fast) post swallow. Changes to swallowing sounds and post swallow respiratory sounds can also be monitored during the employment of swallowing manoeuvres or exercises to determine whether they assist, hinder or make no difference to the swallow-respiratory cycle.

A POPULATION OF SPECIAL NOTE – TREATMENT OF THE PATIENT WHO IS NIL BY MOUTH (NBM)

Individuals with severe dysphagia, reduced or fluctuating levels of alertness or frail medical condition are often placed nil by mouth (NBM). Often times these individuals have an IV line placed and a nasogastric tube (NGT) to meet their nutritional needs, with the NGT aimed at being a temporary measure. For the dysphagia clinician, it is imperative that individuals who are placed nil orally are placed as high priority for dysphagia rehabilitation and prophylactic measures to reduce the likelihood of the development of aspiration pneumonia. Akner and Decerholm (2001) reported that greater than 80 per cent of patients hospitalized for more than 21 days had difficulty eating and that half of all patients referred to stroke rehabilitation were malnourished.

Tube feeding is considered a predictor for the development of aspiration pneumonia (Langmore et al, 1998). The reasons for this are as follows. Salivary flow rate is reduced in the NBM patient due to the fact that food and fluids no longer stimulate saliva production. This reduction in saliva flow allows the colonization of pathogenic organisms in the oral cavity. If these pathogenic organisms are aspirated, a chest infection is the likely outcome unless the patient's immune response can deal with the organisms. However, if the immune function is compromised by malnutrition, then the risk of infection is higher (Perry and McLaren, 2003). In addition to this, note the previous discussions relating to disuse atrophy of muscles. Without a reason to swallow (i.e. food and fluid intake), the individual has fewer opportunities to use these muscles in a functional context. The elderly population may already be de-conditioned and thus at higher risk for malnutrition prior to hospitalization. Further, dehydration and malnutrition cause reduced muscle strength, high levels of fatigue, and reduced immunological function (Olde Rikkert and Rigaud, 2003) and therefore, a cycle of systematic decline. Consequently if the patient is sufficiently alert, the clinician should aim at providing activities to induce at least saliva swallows (e.g. tastes of lemon ice or sucking on a lollipop – see previous discussion). The 'move it or lose it' concept needs to be uppermost for the dysphagia clinician. Note also the importance of good oral hygiene to reduce the likelihood of colonization of pathogenic oral bacteria. In a recent cost analysis study it was reported that a single hospitalization for aspiration pneumonia presents an average cost of US$6,000 (Waters et al., 2004). The dysphagia clinician should make every effort to advocate for early nutrition and hydration, good oral hygiene, and short bursts of rehabilitation treatment as soon as the patient is able to tolerate it. These strategies may help reduce the likelihood of the development of aspiration pneumonia specifically due to nil oral status, which benefits the individual by improving quality of life and potentially decreases morbidity and mortality (Waters et al., 2004). Thus rather than waiting for the patient to improve, the clinician should actively treat the NBM patient as early as possible to maximize recovery.

SUMMARY

This chapter discusses the importance of evidence-based practice for dysphagia rehabilitation. It shows that the 'evidence' for dysphagia rehabilitation is based on a small number of studies that often have small sample sizes. Where evidence does not exist, the clinician should ask whether the proposed treatment technique has solid foundations that support a view that it 'should' work. This chapter provided a treatment style that is based on the principles underpinning exercise physiology and motor learning in a functional context. It also highlighted the psychological issues surrounding rehabilitation such as patient insight, motivation and active participation in goal-setting. Using a different approach to most texts, this chapter aimed to provide clinicians with a starting point for functional rehabilitation of swallowing function. It also described the role of feedback and biofeedback in rehabilitation. Finally it concluded with discussions regarding the NBM patient. It is particularly important that NBM patients receive every opportunity to participate in a rehabilitation programme or modified rehabilitation programme to ensure that muscles used in swallowing are not further depleted by disuse atrophy. Clinicians should read this chapter together with Chapter 11 regarding compensation, as the majority of patients, and particularly those with dysphagia of neurological origin will require judicious use of both principles in achieving oral intake. Oral intake should be the clinician's goal to maximize an individual's ability to participate in social activities that are imperative for healthy physical, social, mental and psychological well-being. Research into the field of rehabilitation of dysphagia is in its infancy and individuals and researchers are strongly encouraged to add to the evidence for its efficacy. It will be prudent to liaise with experts in human movement studies to obtain the best outcomes for our patients.

REFERENCES

Abernethy B, Hanrahan SJ, Kippers V, Mckinnon LT, Pandy MG (2005) The Biophysical Foundations of Human Movement (2nd edn). Lower Mitchum SA: Human Kinetics.
Akner C, Decerholm T (2001) Treatment of protein-energy malnutrition in chronic non-malignant disorders. American Journal of Clinical Nutrition 74: 6–24.
Aronson AE (1985) Clinical Voice Disorders: An Interdisciplinary Approach (2nd edn). New York: Thieme.
Barbui C (2005) Evidence-based medicine and medicine-based evidence. Neurological Science 26: 145–6.

Basmajian JV (1982) Primary Anatomy (8th edn). Baltimore: Williams & Wilkins.

Beilock SL, Carr TH, MacMahon C, Starkes JL (2002) When paying attention becomes counterproductive: Impact of divided versus skill-focused attention on novice and experienced performance of sensorimotor skills. Journal of Experimental Psychology Applied 8(1): 6–16.

Bulow M, Olsson R, Ekberg O (1999) Videomanometric analysis of supraglottic swallow, effortful swallow, and chin tuck in healthy volunteers. Dysphagia 14: 67–72.

Bulow M, Olsson R, Ekberg O (2001) Videomanometric analysis of supraglottic swallow, effortful swallow and chin tuck in patients with pharyngeal dysfunction. Dysphagia 16(3): 190–5.

Burnett TA, Mann EA, Cornell SA, Ludlow CL (2003) Laryngeal elevation achieved by neuromuscular stimulation at rest. Journal of Applied Physiology 94: 128–34.

Cahill LM, Turner AB, Stabler PA, Addis PE, Theodoros DG, Murdoch BE (2004) An evaluation of continuous positive airway pressure (CPAP) therapy in the treatment of hypernasality following traumatic brain injury. Journal of Head Trauma Rehabilitation 19(3): 241–53.

Chaudhuri G, Hildner CD, Brady S, Hutchins B, Algia N, Abadilla E (2002) Cardiovascular effects of the supraglottic and super-supraglottic swallowing manoeuvers in stroke patients with dysphagia. Dysphagia 17: 19–23.

Clark HM (2003) Neuromuscular treatments for speech and swallowing: A tutorial. American Journal of Speech-Language Pathology 12(4): 400–15.

Crary MA, Carnaby GD, Groher ME, Helseth E (2004) Functional benefits of dysphagia therapy using adjunctive sEMG biofeedback. Dysphagia 19: 160–4.

Curtis DJ, Braham SL, Karr S, Holborow GS, Worman D (1988) Identification of unopposed intact muscle pair actions affecting swallowing: Potential for rehabilitation. Dysphagia 3: 57–64.

Dick MB, Hsieh S, Bricker J, Dick-Muehlke C (2003) Facilitating acquisition and transfer of a continuous motor task in healthy older adults and patients with Alzheimer's disease. Neuropsychology 17(2): 202–12.

Fraser C, Power M, Hamdy S, Rothwell J, Hobday D, Hollander I et al. (2002) Driving plasticity in human adult motor cortex is associated with improved motor function after brain injury. Neuron 34: 831–40.

Freed ML, Freed L, Chatburn RL, Christian M (2001) Electrical stimulation for swallowing disorders caused by stroke. Respiratory Care 46(5): 466–74.

Goodman JS, Wood RE (2004) Feedback specificity, learning opportunities, and learning. Journal of Applied Psychology 89(5): 809–21.

Grill WM, Craggs MD, Foreman RD, Ludlow CL (2001) Emerging clinical applications of electrical stimulation: Opportunities for restoration of function. Journal of Rehabilitation Research and Development 38(6): 641–53.

Haynes B, Haines A (1998) Getting research findings into practice: Barrier and bridges to evidence based clinical practice. British Medical Journal 317 (7153): 273–6.

Holladay CL, Quinones MA (2003) Practice variability and transfer of training: the role of self-efficacy generality. Journal of Applied Psychology 88(6): 1094–1103.

Huckabee ML, Cannito MP (1999) Outcomes of swallowing rehabilitation in chronic brainstem, dysphagia: A retrospective evaluation. Dysphagia 14: 93–109.

Huckabee ML, Pelletier CA (1999) Management of adult neurogenic dysphagia. San Diego: Singular.

Jacobs R, Serhal CB, van Steenberghe D (1998) Oral stereognosis: A review of the literature. Clin Oral Invest 2: 3–10.

Kahrilas PJ, Logemann JA, Krugler C, Flanagan E (1991) Volitional augmentation of upper esophageal sphincter opening during swallowing. American Journal of Physiology 260: G450–G456.

Kimura J (2001) Electrodiagnosis in diseases of nerve and muscle: Principles and Practice. 3 edn. Oxford: Oxford University Press.

Kuehn DP (1997) The development of a new technique for treating hypernasality: CPAP, American Journal of Speech-Language Pathology 6: 5–8.

Kuehn DP, Imrey PB, Tomes L, Jones DL, O'Gara MM, Seaver EJ et al. (2002) Efficacy of continuous positive airway pressure for treatment of hypernasality. Cleft Palate-Craniofacial Journal 39(3): 267–76.

Knottnerus JA, Dinant GJ (1997) Medicine based evidence, a prerequisite for evidence based medicine. British Medical Journal 315 (7116): 1109–10.

Langmore DE, Miller RM (1994) Behavioural treatment for adults with oropharyngeal dysphagia. Archives of Physical Medicine and Rehabilitation 75: 1154–60.

Langmore SE, Terpenning MS, Schork M, Chen Y, Murray JT, Lopatin D et al. (1998) Predictors of aspiration pneumonia: How important is dysphagia? Dysphagia 13: 69–81.

Leelamanit V, Limsakul C, Geater A (2002) Synchronised electrical stimulation in treating pharyngeal dysphagia. The Laryngoscope 112: 2204–10.

Liu C, Thompson AJ, Playford ED (2004) Patient dissatisfaction: Insights into the rehabilitation process. Journal of Neurology 251: 1094–7.

Logemann JA (1995) Dysphagia: Evaluation and treatment. Folia Phoniatrica et Logopopaedica 47: 140–64.

Logemann JA (1998) Evaluation and Treatment of Swallowing Disorder (2nd edn). Austin, Texas: Pro-Ed.

Logemann JA (1999) Behavioural management for oropharyngeal dysphagia. Folia Phoniatrica et Logopaedica 51(4/5): 199–213.

Ludlow CL (2005) Central nervous system control of the laryngeal muscles in humans. Respiratory Physiology and Neurobiology 147: 205–22.

Ludlow CL, Bielamowics S, Rosenbuerg MD, Ambalavanar R, Rossini K, Gillespie M et al. (2000) Chronic intermittent stimulation of the thyroarytenoid muscle maintains dynamic control of glottal adduction. Muscle and Nerve 23: 44–57.

Mann EA, Burnett T, Cornell S, Ludlow CL (2002) The effect of neuromuscular stimulation of the genioglossus on the hypopharyngeal airway. The Laryngoscope 112: 351–6.

Moore KL, Dalley AF (1999) Clinically Oriented Anatomy (4th edn). Philadelphia: Lippincott Williams & Wilkins.

Ng SSM, Shepherd RB (2002) Weakness in patients with stroke: Implications for strength training in neurorehabilitation. Physical Therapy Reviews 5: 227–38.

Nguyen NP, Frnak C, Molitz CC, Voc P, Smith HJ, Karlsson U et al. (2005) Impact of dysphagia on quality of life after treatment of head-and-neck cancer. International Journal of Radiation Oncology Biology Physics 61(3): 772–8.

Ohmae Y, Logemann JA, Kaiser P, Hanson DG, Kahrilas PJ (1996) Effects of two breath-holding manoeuvres on oropharyngeal swallowing. Annals of Otology Rhinology and Laryngology 105: 123–31.

Olde Rikkert MGM, Rigaud A-S (2003) Malnutrition research: High time to change the menu. Age and Ageing 32: 241–3.

Palmer JB, Tanaka E, Siebens AA (1989) Electromyography of the pharyngeal musculature: Technical considerations. Archives of Physical Medicine and Rehabilitation 70: 283–7.

Parker C, Power M, Hamdy S, Bowen A, Tyrrell P, Thompson DG (2004) Awareness of dysphagia by patients following stroke predicts swallowing performance. Dysphagia 19: 28–35.

Perlman AL, Luschei ES, Du Mond CE (1989) Electrical activity from the superior pharyngeal constrictor during reflexive and nonreflexive tasks. Journal of Speech and Hearing Research 32: 749–54.

Perry L, McLaren S (2003) Nutritional support in acute stroke: the impact of evidence-based guidelines. Clinical Nutrition 22(3): 283–93.

Poertner LC, Coleman RF (1998) Swallowing therapy in adults. Otolaryngologic Clinics of North America 31(3): 561–79.

Power M, Fraser C, Hobson A, Rothwell JC, Mistry S, Micholson DA et al. (2004) Changes in pharyngeal corticobulbar excitability and swallowing behaviour after oral stimulation. American Journal of Physiology Gastrointestinal and Liver Physiology 286: G45–G50.

Prosiegel M, Heintze M, Wagner-Sonntag E, Schenk T, Yassouridis A (2000) Kinematic analysis of laryngeal movements in patients with neurogenic dysphagia before and after swallowing rehabilitation. Dysphagia 15: 173–9.

Reilly S (2004) The evidence base for the management of dysphagia. In S Reilly, J Douglas, J Oates (eds) Evidence Based Practice in Speech Pathology. London: Whurr (pp. 140–84).

Shaker R, Kern M, Bardan E, Taylor A, Stewart ET, Hoffman RG et al. (1997) Augmentation of deglutitive upper esophageal sphincter opening in the elderly by exercise. American Journal of Gastrointestinal Liver Physiology 272: G1518–G1522.

Shaker R, Easterling C, Kern M, Nitschke T, Massey B, Daniels S et al. (2002) Rehabilitation of swallowing by exercise in tube-fed patients with pharyngeal dysphagia secondary to abnormal UES opening. Gastroenterology 122: 1314–21.

Sharkawi A, Ramig L, Logemann J, Pauloski B, Rademaker A, Smith C et al. (2002) Swallowing and voice effects of Lee Silverman Voice Treatment (LSVT$REG;): A pilot study. Journal of Neurology, Neurosurgery and Psychiatry 72(1): 31–6.

Sheppard JJ (2005) Treating neuromotor feeding and swallowing disorders: Children and adults with developmental disability. Workshop, AGOSCI National Conference, Brisbane, Australia: 31 August–3 September.

Sonnies BC (1991) Instrumental procedures for dysphagia diagnosis. Seminars in Speech and Language 12(3): 185–97.

Sonies BC, Baum BJ (1988) Evaluation of swallowing pathophysiology. Otolaryngologic Clinics of North America 21(4): 637–48.

Waters TM, Logemann JA, Roa Pauloski B, Rademaker AW, Lazarus CL, Newman LA et al. (2004) Beyond efficacy and effectiveness: Conducting economic analyses during clinical trials. Dysphagia 19: 109–19.

Williams AM, Ward P, Knowles JM, Smeeton NJ (2002) Anticipation skill in a real-world task: Measurement, timing and transfer in tennis. Journal of Experimental Psychology Applied 8(4): 259–70.

Yamada Y, Yamamura K, Inoue M (2005) Coordination of cranial motorneurons during mastication. Respiratory Physiology and Neurobiology 14: 177–89.

Zuydam AC, Rogers SN, Brown JS, Vaughan ED, Magennis P (2000) Swallowing rehabilitation after oro-pharyngeal resection for squamous cell carcinoma. British Journal of Oral and Maxillofacial Surgery 38: 513–18.

Part IV Aetiologies, Assessment and Treatment of Children with Swallowing Disorders

13 Clinical Signs, Aetiologies and Characteristics of Paediatric Dysphagia

ANGELA MORGAN and SHEENA REILLY

Increasingly, since the mid-1990s, feeding and swallowing disorders in children have been recognized independently from dysphagia in the adult population. This change is long overdue. Aetiologies associated with paediatric dysphagia are widespread, and many causes are extremely rare (Munro, 2003; Desuter et al., 2004). Further to the child's primary medical diagnosis there are a range of other factors that may be causing or complicating the dysphagia, as paediatric feeding and swallowing are typically compounded by a variety of developmental stressors. Dysphagia during childhood occurs in a context of neurological maturation, increasing nutritional needs, rapid physical growth, and cognitive and psychosocial development. The situation may be further complicated by the fact that many children are unable to communicate their own clinical symptoms (Kramer and Monahan-Eicher, 1993). In part this might be related to developmental age (e.g. young infants) but many children with dysphagia have coexisting communication disorders. Such infants and young children are therefore heavily reliant on parents and therapists observing and inferring the presence and extent of the child's dysphagia.

A multidisciplinary focus on dysphagia is therefore of paramount importance in the paediatric population to ensure that discipline-specific professionals are observing and reporting features from their specialist areas. The evaluation of dysphagia must not only focus on the child's primary medical diagnosis and presenting pathology but must also be related to the age of the patient and the typical development of feeding and swallowing for that age (Dusick, 2003). Early detection is crucial for achieving optimal outcomes (Schurr et al., 1999), and in order to ensure efficient diagnosis and treatment, each member of the multidisciplinary team must be cognizant of potential clinical signs or symptoms of dysphagia that typically present in infants and children. In addition, the team must be aware of the potential aetiologies for dysphagia, and the characteristics of dysphagia noted in various diagnostic groups. Through the collaboration of expert opinions within a developmental framework, the team is able to produce a more complete picture of the presenting swallowing issues for a particular child. Given these considerations, it is the aim of the present chapter to detail:

- patterns of referral for dysphagia;
- the aetiological basis for paediatric dysphagia;

Dysphagia: Foundation, Theory and Practice.   Edited by J. Cichero and B. Murdoch
© 2006 John Wiley & Sons, Ltd.

- the characteristics of children who present with dysphagia; and
- to review, where possible, the clinical signs and symptoms suggestive of dysphagia in various conditions.

REFERRAL PATTERNS FOR PAEDIATRIC DYSPHAGIA

Children are referred for assessment of dysphagia for a variety of reasons, all of which are driven by a problem with either:

- safety for oral feeding;
- adequacy of nutritional intake;
- efficiency and coordination of oral feeding.

When the safety of oral feeding is compromised children may demonstrate coughing/ choking, recurrent chest infection or pneumonia, apnea, or recurrent bronchospasm, all indicating that the child is at high risk for airway compromise or aspiration (Kramer, 1985; Loughlin, 1989; Tuchman, 1989; Kramer and Monahan-Eicher, 1993). Children who are referred for a lack of oral intake typically exhibit signs or food refusal, gagging or vomiting during or after feeds, failure to thrive, or weight loss (Kramer and Monahan-Eicher, 1993; Jolley et al., 1995; Dusick, 2003). Issues of feeding efficiency or coordination typically result from oral-motor dysfunction. Oral-motor dysfunction is characterized by lack of coordination of the jaw, lips, teeth, cheeks, tongue or palate resulting in an inability to perform the movements of biting, chewing, drinking and swallowing (Gisel et al., 1998). It is described in greater detail below. Finally, children may be referred because of reduced efficiency for feeding as a result of underlying respiratory or cardiovascular issues. Children presenting with acute pulmonary or cardiac issues may not have enough energy to eat (Gisel et al., 1998), and fatigue readily during feeding, resulting in increased length of feeds and often reduced oral intake. It must be remembered that whilst dysphagia may present in isolation, it is more conventionally seen as one component of difficulty in a child with a multitude of impairments (Kramer, 1985).

CLINICAL SIGNS AND SYMPTOMS OF PAEDIATRIC DYSPHAGIA

Clinicians typically begin their evaluation of dysphagia by investigating the presence of clinical indicators to help define the location and severity of the problem, or perhaps even to determine whether the disorder exists. However caution must be exercised when using feeding history and clinical observations for early identification of dysphagia (Arvedson et al., 1994). A seminal study by Arvedson et al. (1994) investigated the relationship between aspiration, feeding concerns and developmental diagnoses in a group of 186 children with severe developmental disability. A total of 48 children in the study were found to aspirate. Arvedson et al. (1994) found poor values (33% to 38%) for predicting aspiration based on the clinical signs and symptoms of: cough, choke or respiratory problems; concern for aspiration; and dependence on others for feeding.

Based on their finding of 94% silent aspiration in this group, the authors also surmised that silent aspiration can be overlooked if the clinician is intent on finding overt clinical signs such as coughing, choking or respiratory distress during the oral feeding trial (Arvedson et al., 1994). Perlman (1999) also warns against overinterpretation of the signs and symptoms, highlighting that not having any or all clinical signs does not always suggest that a patient is safe for oral intake.

Clinical signs and symptoms vary from person to person (Rosenbek et al., 1996), and are dependent upon a range of factors including age and the type of underlying disease or disorder (Loughlin, 1989). In relation to age, the response to episodes of aspiration is age dependent (Mercado-Deane et al., 2001). Just as the coordination of the swallowing mechanism improves with age, protective reflexes of this system also develop over time. The cough reflex becomes the primary mechanism for protecting the airway as an infant grows (Loughlin and Lefton-Greif, 1994). However, neonates have not yet developed a cough reflex and they typically respond to aspiration by ceasing breathing (apnea) and closing the airway until the aspirated material has cleared (Mercado-Deane et al., 2001). Apnea is very uncommon in older children (Loughlin and Lefton-Greif, 1994) who rely on the cough reflex to protect their airway. Independent of age, a cough reflex may also be absent due to desensitization resulting from frequent aspiration (Mercado-Deane et al., 2001), or as a result of neurological impairment (Arvedson et al., 1994). Thus it may be difficult to determine whether a child has an absent cough reflex due to immaturity, neurological impairment or as a result of frequent aspiration, complicating the dysphagia diagnosis. As noted previously, it may be difficult to determine the basis of the actual signs and symptoms themselves, making it possible to misinterpret clinical signs as being indicative of dysphagia when they may be signalling some other type of response to a medical disorder. It is imperative that children have a full medical assessment prior to a feeding evaluation, in order to determine the presence of any underlying medical diagnosis that may be contributing to the clinical symptoms (Perlman, 1999).

Knowledge of any underlying diagnosis is important but the clinician must also be alert to the presence of other symptoms that may be unrelated to the primary medical aetiology. Reilly and Carr (2001) reported a case study of a child with dysphagia and severe developmental disability. The child had built up a behavioural pattern of food refusal over time that was assumed by the health professionals working with the child to be due to the child's developmental disability. However, further investigation of the swallowing mechanism via videofluoroscopic swallowing assessment revealed that the child had ingested a foreign body. It was the discomfort of the foreign body misplaced in the child's swallowing mechanism that was causing the child's aversive response to feeding. This case study provides a perfect example of additional signs/symptoms contributing to a feeding disorder independent of the known primary medical diagnosis.

Despite having highlighted that caution is required when interpreting the significance of clinical signs and symptoms, the clinician still relies heavily on these factors for determining the presence of dysphagia (Perlman, 1999). The clinician forms a hypothesis regarding the location and severity of dysphagia, dependent on the clinical history of symptom onset and based on when signs and symptoms occur in relation to the mealtime (Arvedson and Lefton-Greif, 1998). For example, if the child demonstrated marked post-swallow oral residue and required multiple swallows to clear the material, it would be reasonable to suspect a problem with the oral phase of the swallow, whereas marked pulmonary congestion and altered post-feed vocal quality might indicate potential pharyngeal phase difficulties, or aspiration. Clinical signs and symptoms can therefore help guide the clinician in determining areas for further investigation in their initial evaluation. Common clinical signs and symptoms of dysphagia associated with various aetiologies are reported throughout the body of this chapter. The reader is referred to the following papers for commonly reported clinical signs and symptoms of paediatric dysphagia associated with various aetiologies: Loughlin, 1989; Rogers et al., 1993; Arvedson et al., 1994; Kohda et al., 1994; Loughlin and Lefton-Greif, 1994; McColley and Carroll, 1994; Jolley et al., 1995; Brodsky, 1997; Arvedson and Lefton-Greif, 1998; Darrow and Harley, 1998; Gisel et al., 1998; Mercado-Deane et al., 2001; Reilly and Cass, 2001; Dusick, 2003.

ORAL STRUCTURE AND FUNCTION

Oral-motor impairment is a frequent cause of disruption to the feeding mechanism, and typically presents in all children with dysphagia regardless of diagnosis. Common clinical signs noted in children with oral-motor impairment are:

- lack of energy or endurance for oral feeding;
- significant amount of oral residue remaining in mouth post-swallow;
- excessive drooling/sialorrhea;
- drooling in addition to speech/language delays;
- prolonged mealtimes (>30 minutes on average);
- excessive gagging on oral secretions during feeds;
- lip retraction/limited upper lip movement;
- poor labial seal for sucking/removing food from spoon/preventing anterior spillage;
- jaw thrust/jaw clenching/jaw retraction/jaw instability/tonic or phasic bite reflex;
- tongue thrust, retraction, hypotonia, deviation, limited movement;
- reduced buccal tone/reduced buccal sensory awareness;
- reduced bolus formation and transport;
- delayed or difficult initiation of swallow;
- multiple swallows required to clear oral cavity.

In order to assess oral-motor function adequately, the clinician must understand normal oral-motor development. Oral-motor function develops with age, with distinct skills being acquired at different times. These changes are intricately linked to neurological maturation, changes to oral structure, and postural development in the young infant. As one might expect, different skills are acquired in parallel with the introduction of new types of foods/fluids in conjunction with new methods of presentation (e.g. spoon or cup versus breast/bottle). For example, young infants are heavily dependent upon the breast or bottle delivering fluids, and they must have adequate sucking skills to allow efficient stripping of fluid into the oropharynx for swallowing in order to achieve adequate oral intake for growth. As solid foods are introduced via a spoon, alongside fluids delivered via a cup, the child must develop more mature patterns of lip, tongue and jaw movement in order to again achieve efficient and successful oral intake for nutrition and survival. The present review details three primary stages of oral-motor development: sucking skills in infants less than six months of age, the transitional feeding period from six months up to three years, and the continued maturation of juvenile oral-motor skills to approximate adult oral-motor patterns.

ORAL-MOTOR ABILITY IN INFANTS LESS THAN 6 MONTHS OF AGE

Optimal oral-motor function in the infant is crucial for facilitating sucking and ensuring efficient and adequate oral intake. Initially, the infant's movement patterns are bound largely by reflexes, which gradually develop from automatic into more refined voluntary feeding patterns (Stevenson and Allaire, 1991). Adequate structure and movement of the tongue, lips, cheek, jaw and palate is required in order for an infant to attain an optimal suck, and therefore to achieve efficient feeding and adequate oral intake. Any disruption in the structure or movement of these areas may result in disruption to the sucking mechanism, and typically in inefficient and reduced oral intake, see Tables 13.1a and 13.1b.

Suckle feeding

Suckling involves the rhythmical compression of the lower jaw and tongue against the upper jaw and palate, and the lips forming an anterior seal with the nipple, resulting in the generation of negative intraoral pressure and thus suction (Herbst, 1983; Morris, 1989; Tuchman, 1989; Gisel et al., 1998). During suckling the tongue moves in a primitive extension-retraction pattern. Tongue movement is partly limited due to the decreased size of the oral cavity, where it is bound laterally by the fatty buccal pads, posteriorly by the high position of the larynx, and anteriorly by the relatively small mandible (Stevenson and Allaire, 1991). A true suck is achieved later as greater lip pressure is developed to seal off the oral cavity, and the tongue moves up and down synchronously with the jaw achieving greater intraoral pressure and a more efficient sucking pattern (Morris, 1989; Stevenson and Allaire, 1991). Gewolb, Vice et al. (2001) have demonstrated that the basic rhythmical nature of pharyngeal swallowing stabilizes prior to sucking rhythmicity, with swallowing patterns stabilizing at around 32 weeks postmenstrual age. The sucking rhythm, however,

Table 13.1a Normal and abnormal infantile oral-motor structures at rest

Oral structure at rest	Normal	Abnormal	Contributing factors/ impact of abnormal oral-motor function
Tongue	• Soft, flat, relatively thin, rounded tip • Slight central groove in anterior-posterior direction • Tongue sitting in bottom of mouth behind lower gum ridge (newborn tongue may cover gums and tongue inside of lower lip)	• Tongue-tip elevated to upper gum ridge or behind alveolar ridge • Tongue humped in anterior-posterior direction • Tongue bunched in lateral direction • Tongue tip and body retracted posteriorly in mouth • Tongue protrusion with limited shaping/resistance when touched (tongue likely to be excessively soft and wide) • Asymmetry of tongue with deviation to dominant side	• Elevated tongue-tip may block nipple placement, and prevent feeding. • Elevated tongue-tip may be due to high tone, or low postural tone whereby the infant fixes the tongue to gain head and neck stability. • Humped, bunched, or retracted tongue often due to high tone. • Prevents central grooving, may result in poor control of bolus, and premature spillage of fluid over tongue base. • Retracted tongue position inhibits contact between the tongue and the nipple and results in inadequate sucking pressure. • Tongue protrusion at rest indicates general hypotonia. Child may have problems with anterior containment of bolus, problems with stabilizing the nipple during sucking, or in forming a central groove (see above). • Asymmetry may cause problems with central grooving, impacting upon intra-oral pressure generation for sucking.
Jaw	• Neutral jaw position with upper and lower jaw loosely opposed so lips touch	• Recessed jaw: lower gum ridge is posterior to upper gum ridge • Asymmetry/deviation of resting position to one side • Open mouth posture	• May cause tongue retraction also, and may result in tongue falling back into pharyngeal airway leading to respiratory distress. • May cause problems with compression of teat/nipple as jaw may not have direct opposition to gum ridges. • May be due to muscle tone increase on one side, or may be due to structural deficits, or from poor in utero positioning. • Open mouth position at rest may be due to low tone, where the mouth will be loosely open. • Open mouth posture with increased extensor tone, signals high tone. • Open mouth posture results in poor lip seal, inadequate compression of the teat/nipple, inadequate negative intraoral pressure, and potentially anterior spillage of the bolus if any liquid is expressed.

Table 13.1a (*Continued*)

Oral structure at rest	Normal	Abnormal	Contributing factors/ impact of abnormal oral-motor function
Lips and cheeks (circumoral structures)	• Lips and cheeks should be soft at rest. • Lips should loosely shape to nipple with slight pressure at the corners of the mouth. • Fat pads present in cheeks to provide stability up until 6–8 months of age.	• Retracted lips: lips pulled back tightly • Pursed lips: lips pursed tightly • General hypotonia of lips • General hypotonia of cheeks	• Lip retraction occurs more commonly in the older child with neurological impairment and is rarely seen in the infant with hypertonia. • Pursed lips most common in infants with high tone. • Pursed/tight lips may make nipple insertion difficult. • Hypotonia of the lips results in poor lip seal, reduced ability to generate intra-oral pressure for sucking, and therefore reduced feeding efficiency. • May see breaks in suction due to poor lip seal, characterised by smacking sounds. • Anterior spillage of liquid from the lips is also common. • Poor buccal/cheek tone results in reduced ability to generate negative intra-oral pressure, again compromising sucking and reducing feeding efficiency. • Poor buccal tone impairs lip seal, also impacting on the generation of intra-oral pressure, and possibly resulting in anterior spillage of fluid.
Palate	• Intact and smoothly contoured. • Shape of palate should approximate shape of tongue.	• Cleft • Bifid uvula • Narrow • High-arched • Flat • Anomalies/asymmetry of grooves of alveolar ridge	• Cleft of the palate leads to an inability to create intra-oral pressure, and therefore interferes with the generation of sucking. • A bifid uvula may result in incomplete velopharyngeal valving, and thus nasopharyngeal reflux. • Narrow, high-arched palates typically result from prolonged oral intubation of the newborn. • Most children can over-come palatal anomalies of narrow/high-arched or flat palate in order to feed successfully in the absence of other factors contributing to feeding dysfunction. • However, palatal anomalies may interfere with in-utero tactile exploration of the tongue and palate, potentially impacting on oral-motor development of such skills as flattening, cupping, flaring and elevation of the tongue.

Source: Alper and Manno (1996); Marshalla (1985); Morris (1982); Morris (1985); Morris (1989); Wolf and Glass (1992).

Table 13.1b Normal and abnormal infantile oral-motor structures during movement

Oral structure during movement	Normal	Abnormal	Contributing factors/impact of abnormal oral-motor function
Tongue	• Touch to middle of tongue from tip to back: should cause tongue to cup around finger, or a flattening and flaring of the tongue with elevation of the tip and lateral margins and simultaneous depression of the midline. This response is present in 2/3 of infants at birth; common 5–12 months. • Tongue lateralisation response: touch to side of tongue between 0–9 months should cause elevation of mid-section of tongue, and a gross-rolling action of the tongue toward the stimulus. • Tongue movements should be 'in' and 'out' or 'up' and 'down'. • The 'in' excursion should be of greater force than the 'out'. • All tongue movements should be of small excursion with a rhythmical quality.	• Flat tongue unresponsive to touch • Any deviations from the expected pattern of movement. • Tongue thrust: 'in' and 'out' pattern with a strong 'out' excursion. • Clonus noted before sucking or during sucking pauses. • Fasciculations observed	• The hypotonic flat tongue may not create a central groove, thus inhibiting the ability to channel fluid to the oropharynx, placing child at risk for premature spillage of fluid over the base of tongue. • Impaired tongue function and movement in general may inhibit oral preparation and transit of the bolus, resulting in inefficient sucking and feeding. • Tongue thrust normally due to increased tone, particularly increased extensor tone, and possible CNS abnormalities. • Tongue thrust inhibits teat/nipple compression, adequate lip seal and the ability to achieve negative intra-oral pressure. • Tongue thrusting may also inhibit appropriate posterior movement of the bolus into the oropharynx, with attempts at oral transit typically resulting in anterior spillage of the bolus.
Jaw	• Normal jaw movement is smooth, occurs in small excursion, with a rhythmical quality.	• Large excursions • Abnormal jaw thrust • Lack of range of jaw movement • Tonic biting: jaw clenching with no/extremely delayed release • Phasic biting: intermittent jaw clenching with delayed release • Clonus/tremors	• Large jaw excursions signal poor jaw stability and poorly graded jaw movement • Forceful downward movement of the jaw where the jaw appears to jut forward is typically a result of increased tone. This jaw thrusting motion may also appear as large jaw excursions, but they have far more force and far less rhythm than the pattern of poorly graded large jaw

Table 13.1b (*Continued*)

Oral structure during movement	Normal	Abnormal	Contributing factors/impact of abnormal oral-motor function
		• Lack of range of jaw movement	excursion. These infants often present with abnormal jaw opening also. • If the child has a passive range of movement, but limited active range of movement, initiation of feeding may be difficult.
		• Tonic biting	• Tonic biting is a problem of active movement that limits mouth opening, whereby the infant appears to get stuck in a pattern of mouth closure for extended periods of time.
		• Phasic biting	• The infant demonstrating phasic biting appears to get stuck in a pattern of mouth closure, however, for a reduced period of time compared to a tonic bite. • Biting may be secondary to increased tone, but may also reflect infants attempt to hold nipple in place when tongue movement is not functional.
		• Clonus	• Clonus or tremor of the jaw may be noted during jaw movement.
Rooting reflex	• Adaptive reflex. Touch to baby's lips or cheeks causes child to turn head to source of stimulus and open mouth.	• Poor rooting reflex.	• Orally intubated child or child whose NG tube is taped to side of face may not exhibit strong rooting reflex which is likely due to decreased sensory response from repeated tapings.
Sucking reflex	• Adaptive reflex. Elicitation can vary depending upon stimulus (e.g. nutritive vs non-nutritive). A light touch from nipple/finger to baby's lips/tongue should initiate sucking response. Non-nutritive suck should have brisk onset in response to stimulation and should occur at rate of two sucks per second.	• Disorganisation and arrhythmicity. • Weak suck.	• Common in neurologically impaired infants receiving tube feedings, the tongue is often thick and bunched with a lack of central grooving for bolus passage, or the tongue may be retracted and fixed against the palate for stability.

Table 13.1b (*Continued*)

Oral structure during movement	Normal	Abnormal	Contributing factors/impact of abnormal oral-motor function
	• Nutritive suck should have brisk onset in response to stimulation and should occur at rate of two sucks per second.		
Gag reflex	• Protective reflex. Elicited by touch to anterior 1/3 of tongue. Present at birth, reduces in strength around 7 months of age, persists into adulthood.	• Nil reflex may be denoted as abnormal in the young infant.	• Not proven to be a requirement for safe feeding in adults, but thought to help prevent large foreign objects from entering the trachea. Gag reflex may be heightened due to prolonged intubation or a nasogastric feeding. Enhanced gag reflex may prevent oral intake.
Cough reflex	• Protective reflex. Elicited by foreign objects. Reflex begins with stimulation of the cough receptors by viruses, aeroallergens and chemicals. Not expected in neonate who uses apnea to avoid aspiration of foreign material.	• Reduced or absent cough reflex.	• Poor or absent cough reflex may increase the risk of aspiration of food or fluid. May see silent aspiration in the presence of absent cough reflex. May see reduced cough reflex due to prolonged orotracheal intubation or nasogastric feeding tube placement, from neurological impairment, or frequent aspiration.

Source: adapted from Alper and Manno (1996); Chow (2000); Lifschitz (2001); Marshalla (1985); Mercado-Deane et al. (2001); Morris (1982); Morris (1985); Morris (1989); Wolf and Glass (1992).

stabilizes during the period from 32 to 40 weeks, and maturation of sucking should result in increased aggregation into suckle runs, increased length of suckle runs, and increased rate of sucking (Gewolb et al., 2001). Sucking should be rhythmical and there should be good coordination of sucking, swallowing and breathing, with approximately one cycle per second (Wolff, 1968).

Problems with sucking

The relative contribution and integration of the tongue, lips, jaw, buccal cavity and palate as documented in this review highlights how a disruption in either the anatomical structure, or the physiological movement may result in oral-motor dysfunction. Oral-motor impairment is likely to lead to inefficient sucking, and potentially poor oral intake, weight loss or an inability to gain weight, and failure to thrive. A list of potential problems occurring with sucking is documented below. Premature infants and infants with congenital heart disease are particularly at risk for developing sucking difficulties, and these are also discussed.

Organization/arrhythmicity

One common problem noted with sucking is disorganization or arrhythmicity of the sucking pattern. This difficulty may occur due to general neurological disorganization, mild respiratory problems, or a nipple flow rate that is incompatible with the infant's sucking characteristic (Wolf and Glass, 1992). Morris (1989) noted that disorganization and arrhythmicity were characteristic of the majority of neurologically impaired infants. This is not surprising given that very premature infants who do not yet have the neurological maturity for sucking tend to demonstrate disorganized sucking patterns, which take longer to mature into the coordinated sucking patterns typically seen at around 35 weeks postmenstrual age (Gewolb, Bosma et al., 2001). Ineffective tongue movement or protrusion may interfere with the child's sucking or compression mechanism. Whilst impairment of any oral structure may affect the coordination of sucking, swallowing and breathing, poorly graded or poorly controlled jaw movement significantly disrupts the rhythmical movements of the lips, cheeks and tongue due to the close anatomical attachment of these structures (Morris, 1989). Children with respiratory problems may also demonstrate lack of coordination of the sucking mechanism due to disruption to the rhythm and timing of breathing. Disorganized or arrhythmic sucking may be characterized by irregular bursts of sucking, random pauses, and possibly coughing or choking depending on the level of disorganization.

Weak suck or reduced endurance

A weak suck is characterized by limited generation of intraoral pressure and hence poor suction, and also by poor compression, leading to reduced liquid flow. Poor liquid flow results in poor efficiency of oral feeding with infants needing to take a longer time to consume adequate oral intake, and typically expending as much energy as they are consuming. A weak suck of muscular origin typically occurs due to generalized muscle weakness or immature muscle development (e.g. in premature infants) and specific conditions that result in muscular weakness (e.g. myasthenia gravis or neonatal myotonic dystrophy). Other medical conditions may result in a weak suck, where the child may be too ill or fatigued to generate adequate sucking pressure and compression, e.g. respiratory disorders, congenital heart disease. Children may begin with a strong suck initially which becomes weak over the duration of the feed (Wolf and Glass, 1992).

Poor initiation of sucking

Some children may not initiate feeding easily, being sleepy and hard to arouse, or showing limited appetite. The child with congenital heart problems or respiratory problems may commonly display this pattern of feeding behaviour. Other children may have excessive rooting to the stimulus of the nipple and be unable to inhibit the reflex in order to attach and begin sucking (Wolf and Glass, 1992). Neurologically impaired infants may be unable to attach properly due to extreme problems of oral and postural tone and aversive oral reflexes preventing mouth closure over the nipple.

Other factors influencing sucking

Postural stability, mobility, and sensorimotor development all influence oral-motor development. Sensorimotor development in particular is closely related to oral-motor development in the child from birth to approximately 8 months of age (Macie and Arvedson, 1993). Stability of the head, neck and shoulder girdle is required for adequate oral-motor function (Gisel et al., 1998). The sucking pads, small intraoral space, and larynx high in the neck provide adequate stability for oral movement in newborns who have not yet developed postural stability. Postural stability begins around the temperomandibular joint, and facilitates improved jaw control, which is required for further refinement of oral mobility and precision (Morris, 1982). Dysfunction or instability of the temperomandibular join has been documented to result in oral-motor problems in children (Bonjardim et al., 2003).

Children with impairment of muscle tone affecting the body present with specific deficits in oral movement that reflect their dominant tonal patterns (Sheckman-Alper and Manno, 1996). Either flexion or extension can lead to poor oral-motor movement and thus compromise oral intake. For example, hyperextension of the neck reduces jaw stability clinically associated with wider movements of the jaw, and jaw thrusting, whereas flexion of shoulder girdle is associated with jaw clenching (Morris, 1989).

THE TRANSITIONAL PHASE IN CHILDREN AGED FROM 6 MONTHS TO 3 YEARS

The weaning or transitional period of feeding is typically characterized by the change from suckle feeding and the sole intake of liquids, to the introduction of solids, starting from around 6 months of age and continuing into the child's second or third year (Bosma, 1985). The transitional stage encompasses the development of chewing skills, and the initiation of spoonfeeding and cup drinking.

Development of chewing skills

Tongue and jaw movement begin with movements in straight planes of extension and flexion in the infant, in and out and up and down (Morris and Klein, 1987). At around 5 to 6 months, tongue movements increase in range to include lateral excursion and the tongue begins to move independently of the jaw (Bosma, 1985; Stolovitz and Gisel, 1991). In parallel with this oral-motor development, children are able to eat food with tiny lumps from approximately 7 to 10 months of age (Carruth and Skinner, 2002). Rotary jaw movement begins at around 10 to 12 months and will continue to develop into the child's second year (Alexander et al., 1993; Pinder and Faherty, 1999). At approximately the same time, the tongue will begin to move laterally and diagonally to bring the food to the cutting edge of the teeth if further chewing is required, and to assist in oral preparation of the bolus (Stevenson and Allaire, 1991; Alexander et al., 1993; Green et al., 1997). In conjunction with this development, children are able to begin chewing and swallowing firmer foods without choking from approximately 10 to 14 months of age (Carruth and Skinner, 2002). Controlled rotary jaw movements and tongue lateralization should be noted by approximately 2 years of age (Stevenson and Allaire, 1991). Thus, the increase in tongue lateralization typically occurs when jaw stability has developed. Movement of the lips, jaw and tongue become more differentiated so that in place of the rhythmical up-and-down movement of these structures noted during sucking, the jaw is now able to perform the finer graded movements required for chewing, being slightly more independent of the lips and tongue, and the lips and tongue in turn can also move independently of the jaw. A mature pattern of swallowing with tongue tip elevation is also noted at 12 months of age, and lip control develops so that the corners of the lips are actively drawn in to help in bolus transit (Stevenson and Allaire, 1991). Not surprisingly, chewing has been shown to become more efficient during this period of increased tongue mobility and jaw stability from 6 months to 2 years (Stolovitz and Gisel, 1991). In fact, feeding times have been found to decrease on all food textures with increasing age and greater maturation of oral-motor function (Gisel, 1990).

Spoonfeeding

Spoonfeeding has been reported to begin at around 5 months of age and is characterized in the initial stages by infants suckling the pureed food from the spoon. Active spoonfeeding develops at approximately 6 months, with the child actively using the upper lip to clear the spoon. Much work has focused on the development of tongue movement and chewing skill, little focus has been given to the development of lip closure or lip pressure. Lip closure is important for efficient oral feeding at all stages of feeding development. In the transitional phase of feeding, lip closure or pressure is needed for maintaining an anterior seal and for removing food from the spoon. Chigira et al. (1994) evaluated lip pressure using a strain-gauge transducer in 104 normally developing children ranging from 5 months to 5 years. Chigira et al. (1994) reported that lip pressure developed steadily from 5 months to 3 years of age and continued to increase, but more slowly, from 3 to 5 years of age. Lip closure around the spoon develops relatively early, but patterns of lip closure during swallowing typically do not present until 12 months of age (Stevenson and Allaire, 1991).

Cup drinking

The same pattern of infant suckle feeding is seen during initial attempts at cup drinking. For most young children, cup drinking starts at 6 months of age. Choking and coughing may occur initially whilst the child starts to coordinate the suckle, swallow and breathing. Tongue protrusion under the cup may occur and biting down on the cup may be used to help compensate for the lack of jaw stability not seen until 2 years of age (Stevenson and Allaire, 1991).

The critical period of oral-motor development

Stolovitz and Gisel (1991) found that younger children show more mature feeding skills for solid foods, which require that the tongue work independently of the jaw to enable adequate chewing and oral preparation of the bolus. In contrast, they reported that younger children would typically revert back to sucking behaviours with puree or softer consistencies, which did not require such differentiated movement of the lips, jaw and tongue for preparation (Stolovitz and Gisel, 1991). This finding has implications for the development of oral-motor skills. It is clear that children should be offered foods of a texture that require chewing during this optimal period of 6 months to 2 years in order to develop the required oral-motor skills. Many authors have agreed with the argument, initially proposed by Illingworth and Lister (1964), that there is a 'critical period' for oral-motor development. Illingworth and Lister (1964) suggested that delayed introduction of spoonfeeding and cup drinking may lead to delayed oral-motor development, resistance to developing the necessary skills following introduction after the optimal period of 6 to 7 months of age, and potential behavioural feeding issues. Whilst this argument has not been proven empirically, many clinicians support the existence of a critical period based on anecdotal evidence and personal experience (Tuchman, 1988).

ORAL-MOTOR DEVELOPMENT IN CHILDREN FROM 2 YEARS OF AGE AND BEYOND

In regard to the development of oral-motor skills beyond the transitional period, research has focused more on the expected patterns of tongue movement during eating. Schwaab et al. (1986) reported that 2-to-4 year old children largely hold their tongue behind their teeth when mouth opening in anticipation of food. A more forward pattern of tongue movement during anticipation of food is typically noted in some 2- and 3-year-old children, with the tongue behind the teeth pattern being used more consistently by four years of age (Schwaab et al., 1986). Lip pursing or closed lips during swallowing has also been reported to begin in 2- and 3-year-old children (Schwaab et al., 1986). Further work in this area by Gisel (1988) found a consistent pattern of tongue positions and movements, with the tongue predominantly held in a resting position behind the teeth (68–82%), followed by tongue on top of teeth (8–18%), retracted 5 mm more (4–13%), and on or beyond the lower lip (3–8.5%). She also reported that swallowing changes during the 2- to 8-year-old period, from open mouth swallowing with circumoral musculature contraction to smooth swallowing without any noticeable circumoral activity. Papargyriou et al. (2000) evaluated the chewing development of 47 children over a 6-year period from age 9 years to 15 years. They reported that total chewing cycle duration, opening and closing time of the chewing cycle, and the three-dimensional closing distance increased during the growth period, whilst the closing time of the chewing cycle, the two-dimensional lateral and vertical distances, and both the opening and closing velocity decreased (Papargyriou et al., 2000). Therefore it can be noted that the chewing cycle continues to undergo change during growth, possibly due to anatomical changes, central nervous system maturation, and altered functional demands (Papargyriou et al., 2000). Recent and earlier kinematic studies of oral-motor development have suggested that children show greater variability in the production of oral-motor movements up until 12 years of age (Wohlert and Smith, 2002). Wohlert and Smith (2002) propose that this flexibility in oral-motor production in later childhood may be due to the continued neurophysiological and biomechanical changes occurring from adolescence up until adulthood.

PAEDIATRIC DYSPHAGIA: CLINICAL CHARACTERISTICS ASSOCIATED WITH MEDICAL DIAGNOSES

Dysphagia may arise in children due to a number of different medical diagnoses, including: prematurity; congenital neurological disorder/disease; aerodigestive/ respiratory problems, gastroesophageal reflux, traumatic brain injury, behavioural feeding problems, prematurity/failure to thrive, and congenital heart disease/disorder. Some children are referred with obvious signs and/or symptoms of oral intake difficulty, others may be referred with minimal or no current clinical signs and/or symptoms indicative of dysphagia. Such children are typically referred because the aetiology, or medical diagnosis may place the child at substantial risk of dysphagia. The potential impact of a range of diagnoses on the swallowing mechanism, and the presenting characteristics, clinical signs and symptoms of dysphagia, will be discussed.

PREMATURITY

Prematurity is the leading cause of perinatal mortality and morbidity (Romero et al., 2003). Infants born prematurely typically do not have the neurological maturation nor physiological development required for adequate feeding. Efficient oral feeding in infants requires coordination of rhythmic sucking, swallowing and respiration (Bosma, 1985; Gewolb et al., 2001; Lau and Hurst, 1999). The suck rhythm develops from 32 to 40 weeks in premature infants, and by 40 weeks they have reached a level of development that cannot be differentiated from term infants. During this 8-week maturational period, increasing aggregation into suckle and swallow runs, stabilization of suckle, rhythm and faster and longer suckle runs develop (Qureshi et al., 1999; Gewolb et al., 2001). Because the lungs of premature infants are immature and not be able to produce enough surfactant, the infants are at increased risk of respiratory distress. Hyaline membrane disease and infant respiratory distress syndrome may result. Aside from neurological immaturity and respiratory issues, premature infants are typically tube fed initially until oral feeding skills mature. When oral feeding is introduced it is common to observe increased oral sensitivity in some infants (due to repeated insertion of feeding tubes and aversive oral experiences) and motor problems of oral function that appear to be related to lack of oral experience. Given all of these potential problems, it is not surprising that prematurity may give rise to a range of factors that can cause dysphagia in premature infants. Wolf and Glass (1992) report on potential problems that may result in the premature infant:

- Reduced coordination of sucking, swallowing and breathing, as a result of either poor respiratory control, or due to poor neurological and physiological maturation.
- Reduced endurance for feeding due to respiratory problems and subsequent lack of oxygen and energy for feeding.
- Reduced strength and control of oral structures, resulting in poor build up of intraoral pressure and compression for sucking, resulting in a weak inefficient suck, prolonged feeding times, and likely reduced oral intake.
- State modulation/alertness problems where infants do not spontaneously wake for feeding and, when they do feed, they show little interest and return quickly to sleep. This problem is distinguished from lack of endurance for feeding where the child may initially show interest, and then fatigue.
- Reduced oral-motor control or oral hypersensitivity, typically due to poor maturation or lack of oral experience, resulting in poor sucking.

Disorders affecting feeding associated with prematurity

The potential morbidity associated with infants born before 35 to 36 weeks include: intraventricular haemorrhage, necrotizing enterocolitis, and bronchopulmonary dysplasia (Sherer et al., 1998; Noerr, 2003; Stoelhurst et al., 2003; Ward and Beachy, 2003). All three disorders can have a significant impact on infant feeding, potentially leading to growth failure and failure to thrive, affecting neurological and physical development. Such potential morbidity arising from the premature infant is of great concern, as survival rates of even the most premature newborns have increased from 0% to 65% in some centres over the last 20 years (Ward and Beachy, 2003). Therefore the neonatal intensive care unit has been faced with increasingly complex management problems regarding these infants in recent times.

Intraventricular haemorrhage

Intraventricular haemorrhage (IVH) has been estimated to occur at a rate of 40% in infants born prior to 32 weeks of gestation (Volpe, 1997). Increased survival rates for more premature infants is of significance in relation to IVH in particular, as the incidence of IVH is directly related to gestational age, with very premature infants being at an increased risk of IVH. Intraventricular haemorrhage may lead to long-term neurological impairment and decreased survival, particularly if it is associated with posthaemorrhagic hydrocephalus (Ward and Beachy, 2003). As with any form of brain damage, bleeds may impact on oral and pharyngeal function dependent upon the site of the bleed and the resultant neuropathology.

Necrotizing enterocolitis

Necrotizing enterocolitis is a gastrointestinal disease, the exact pathogenesis of which is unknown. Typically the disease involves a pathogenic organism, enteral feedings and bowel compromise resulting in bowel injury in the neonate (Noerr, 2003). Clinical symptoms may range from mild feeding intolerance and abdominal distension to bowel perforation, peritonitis and cardiovascular collapse (Noerr, 2003). Necrotizing enterocolitis does not impact directly on the oral feeding mechanism but has complications of nutritional support and typically produces many long-term feeding problems (Ward and Beachy, 2003). Tolerance of enteral feedings may be poor, and experimental attempts at improving tolerance may take place over long periods of time. Typically children with necrotizing enterocolitis do not experience normal oral exploration and this may lead to reduced oral-motor development and oral-sensory issues.

Bronchopulmonary dysplasia

Bronchopulmonary dysplasia (BPD) is a chronic lung disease of premature infants typically arising from infant respiratory distress syndrome, barotrauma from positive pressure ventilation, oxygen toxicity and respiratory infections (Abman and Groothius, 1994; Hisplop, 1997; Hulsmann and van den Anker, 1997). Premature infants born from 23 to 31 weeks of gestation have been found to be at a 3.4-fold increased risk for developing bronchopulmonary dysplasia (Regev et al., 2003). Despite improved medical management including prenatal corticosteroid treatment and postnatal surfactant administration, large numbers of premature infants still develop BPD (Ward and Beachy, 2003). Lung function improves during childhood but residual abnormalities may be found in young adults (Hulsmann and Van den Anker, 1997). Long-term morbidity of pulmonary function is decreasing with improved ventilation equipment and management of ventilation (Ward and Beechy, 2003). Bronchopulmonary dysplasia can have a significant impact on growth; 30% to 67% of infants with BPD are reported to have growth failure in the first few months following discharge from hospital (Vohr et al., 1982; Kurzner et al., 1988). Due to the presence of BPD and the resultant increased respiratory effort, the child with BPD often presents with increased energy requirements at 10% to 20% above those of other infants (Putet, 1993). In addition, there is a further subgroup of infants with BPD who experience growth failure and present with even higher energy expenditure than infants with BPD without growth failure (Kurzner et al., 1988). Hypoxemia has also been reported to occur during oral feeding in infants with BPD, adding further to respiratory stressors and metabolic demands on the children (Singer et al., 1992; Shiao et al., 1996).

Physiologically based feeding problems and problems of mother–infant interaction are two main areas potentially contributing to impaired oral intake in children with BPD (Johnson et al., 1998). The types of physiologically based problems reported in infants and young children experiencing BPD include poor sucking patterns and aspiration with feeding (Lifschitz et al., 1987; Pridham et al., 1989; Martin and Pridham, 1992). Craig et al. (1999) reported poor stability of breathing in infants with BPD during feeding. As mentioned earlier, there is a maturational period for sucking seen from 32 to 40 weeks whereby a stable sucking rhythm develops including increasing aggregation into suckle and swallow runs, stabilization of suckle rhythm and faster and longer suckle runs (Qureshi et al., 1999; Gewolb et al., 2001). However, infants with BPD do not develop the anticipated maturation of suck and swallow rhythms compared with age-matched pre-term controls without BPD. Premature infants with BPD demonstrate reduced stability of suckle rhythm, decreased aggregation into suckle runs, and decreased length of suckle runs (Gewolb et al., 2001; Gewolb et al., 2003). Gewolb et al. (2001) proposed that this lack of development may be due to respiratory problems interfering with the establishment of suckle rhythms, or due to neurological issues which are common in premature infants.

Children with BPD have significant feeding problems due to their neurological and respiratory difficulties but, as with any chronically ill child, potentially negative psychosocial issues may exist between the mother and child, impacting upon feeding interactions. In particular, feeding interactions may be compromised for infants with BPD and other premature infants (Singer et al., 1996). A study of 55 very low birthweight infants, and 52 term infants evaluated feeding behaviour and maternal self-report of depression (Singer et al., 1996). Mothers of premature infants, regardless of the presence of BPD, reported more clinically significant symptoms of depression and anxiety than mothers of term infants (Singer et al., 1996). The infants with BPD also required more prompting to return to feeding, which may be problematic as mothers with depression and anxiety may be less likely to verbally prompt their children (Singer et al., 1996). It is clear that maternal psychosocial symptoms should be considered when assessing feeding issues in premature infants.

For further reading on mother–child interactions during feeding for infants with chronic illness, or failure to thrive, refer to: Ammaniti et al., 2004; Feldman et al., 2004; Parkinson, Wright and Drewett, 2004; Stewart and Meyer, 2004.

CONGENITAL HEART DISEASE

Children with congenital heart disease (CHD) are at a higher risk of failure to thrive, or growth failure compared to other infants largely because of their poor oral intake and higher-than-average resting metabolic rate (Jackson and Poskitt, 1991; Thommessen et al., 1992; Barton et al., 1994; Hofner et al., 2000). There are three main categories of heart disease including acyanotic, cyanotic and obstructive heart defects. However limited data are available to indicate whether feeding differs according to the type of congenital heart disease. Varan et al. (1999) investigated the effects of cardiac diagnosis on growth and nutrition. They compared four varying groups: acyanotic patients with pulmonary hypertension (n = 26), acyanotic patients without pulmonary hypertension (n = 5), cyanotic patients with pulmonary hypertension (n = 16) and cyanotic patients without pulmonary hypertention (n = 42). They found that cyanotic patients with pulmonary hypertension were more likely to present with moderate to severe malnutrition and failure to thrive than the other three groups. The acyanotic patients with pulmonary hypertension were the second most affected group, displaying mild or borderline malnutrition (Varan et al., 1999). It would appear that the presence of hypoxia and pulmonary hypertension may be factors for predicting which groups of children with heart disease may be more susceptible to experiencing feeding problems. Regardless of specific diagnosis, infants with congenital heart disease have been reported to be at risk of feeding difficulties arising from both physiological problems and from problems with infant–mother feeding interaction as discussed below.

Physiological feeding issues

Wolf and Glass (1992) have reported two main feeding issues that may present in children with congenital heart disease: poor endurance and early satiety.

Poor endurance

Infants with heart disease may present with poor feeding endurance due to disruptions in blood flow, an inability to increase blood flow during feeding, or mixing of oxygenated and unoxygenated blood, all resulting in insufficient oxygen levels and thus little energy for feeding (Wolf and Glass, 1992). Infants will typically fatigue easily and may stop feeding before consuming efficient oral intake. Clemente et al. (2001) reported that children with congenital heart disease have significantly more breathing problems during feeding and also tend to vomit more frequently during feeds than other infants. These are factors that would also increase the energy expended during mealtimes leading to fatigue. Some infants may initially appear interested in feeding, however infants with severe cardiac lesions and markedly reduced energy levels may not even rouse spontaneously for feeding.

Early satiety

Children with congenital heart disease have been reported to have poor appetite. Thus, not only do they have suboptimal intake but they also appear to lack the drive to eat (Thommessen et al., 1992). Gastrointestinal issues may also coincide with congenital heart disease, including delayed gastric emptying and gastrointestinal hypomotility that may provide infants with a feeling of early satiety and thus decrease their appetite prior to adequate energy being consumed (Wolf and Glass, 1992).

Psychosocial factors

Mothers of infants with congenital heart disease experience maternal fatigue and anxiety (Lambert and Watters, 1998). Parents have also reported that feeding infants with CHD is difficult, taking more time than feeding other infants, and causing anxiety (Thommessen, Heiberg and Kase, 1992). Lobo and Michel (1995) studied 20 mother–infant pairs, 10 with CHD and 10 controls, and found that subtle disengagement cues were more common for infants with CHD. Lobo (1990) also found that mothers of infants with CHD scored lower on a rating of social emotional growth and infants with CHD scored lower on a measure of responsiveness to caregiver and clarity of cues. Clemente et al. (2001), however, studied the feeding issues of 64 children with CHD and 64 healthy controls and concluded that the feeding problems were related to the organic heart condition and not specifically to the mother-infant interaction. Indeed the issues of mother-infant interaction reported in the literature are significant, and psychosocial issues must be considered in assessing feeding in a child with CHD. Interestingly, the problems do appear similar to those that occur during the feeding interactions of mother and infant in many infants with chronic illness.

CONGENITAL NEUROLOGICAL DISORDERS

Dysphagia is prevalent in children with congenital neurological disorders, and developmental disability. Because both groups have a predisposition to oral-motor dysfunction and gastroesophageal reflux (Reilly et al., 1996; Schwarz et al., 2001; Gisel et al., 2003; Munro, 2003; Werlin, 2004) they are the most common populations to present with dysphagia. A wide range of feeding issues is reported in children with developmental disability. Field et al. (2003) studied 91 children with developmental disability, including autism (n = 26), Down syndrome (n = 21) and cerebral palsy (n = 44). Children in all three groups demonstrated food refusal, food selectivity by type or texture, oral-motor delay and dysphagia (defined as problems with swallowing). The characteristics of dysphagia in a range of congenital neurological disorders/developmental disabilities will be explored.

Cerebral palsy

Children with cerebral palsy are at risk of reduced oral intake for a number of reasons, including: oral-motor dysfunction, pharyngeal phase problems associated with aspiration, and communication difficulties that reduce their ability to request food and drink (Reilly et al., 1996). Early feeding problems are significant in this population; mothers sometimes report that feeding problems, including difficulty with positioning for feeding, are the first sign that something is wrong with their child (Reilly and Skuse, 1992; Reilly et al., 1996; Motion et al., 2002). Motion et al. (2002) set out specifically to define the type of early feeding difficulties characteristic of children later diagnosed with cerebral palsy. They found that whereas many parents report problems feeding their infants in the first four weeks, the reports from parents of children with cerebral palsy were qualitatively different. Specifically, such children demonstrated exhaustion with feeding and their feeding problems persisted up to and beyond 6 months of age, with greater neurological and growth impairment at school age (Motion et al., 2002).

Types of cerebral palsy and dysphagia

Although dysphagia may coexist in all types of cerebral palsy, the children most at risk are those with more severe neurological and four-limb involvement (quadriplegia or tetraplegia). Children with diplegia and hemiplegia are less likely to have significant dysphagia (Motion et al., 2002). Reilly et al. (1996) found that tetraplegia was associated with moderate and severe oral-motor dysfunction, and diplegia was more commonly associated with mild oral-motor difficulties. In addition, those children with diplegia were more likely to demonstrate texture-specific problems, whereas children with tetraplegia typically had some level of difficulty with all textures (Reilly et al., 1996). Potential reasons for the child with spastic quadriplegia to be at an increased risk for dysphagia include the fact that they are dependent feeders and are often unable to communicate (Casas et al., 1994; Reilly et al., 1996), as well as having more severe neurological involvement and associated problems such as epilepsy and other postural problems likely to interfere with good feeding (e.g. scoliosis). Dependent feeders and those with limited communication skill are not in control of the selection of consistency, rate or volume of their oral intake (Casas, McPherson and Kenny, 1994; Reilly, Skuse and Poblete, 1996). Assessment of the mealtime routine and interactions between the caregiver and child with cerebral palsy are an extremely important component of ensuring that the nutritional needs and appropriate requirements of the child are being met (e.g. positioning, alterations of diet consistency).

Importance of mealtime observation

Reilly et al. (1992, 1996) demonstrated the importance of observing mealtime interactions between the child with cerebral palsy and the caregiver in their home. Reilly and Skuse (1992) found that children with cerebral palsy (n = 12) had mealtimes of equal duration to their matched controls despite parents of children with cerebral palsy reporting excessively long feeding duration. They suggested that feeding difficulties often place extreme stress on the parent responsible for feeding, with mealtimes becoming a tense and unpleasant experience (Reilly and Skuse, 1992; Reilly et al., 1996). The discrepancy in reported mealtime duration was suggested to be due to the mental health status of the mothers, with 10 out of 12 mothers of children with cerebral palsy, and only two out of 12 mothers of matched controls, scoring below average on a mental health scale (Reilly and Skuse, 1992). In addition to differences in reported mealtime length, differences were also noted between the two groups in regard to oral intake. Children with cerebral palsy were offered less food and consumed less over a 24-hour period (Reilly and Skuse, 1992). Reduced intake may have been a result of brief mealtimes, poor positioning, severe oral-motor dysfunction, and parents offering food of poor caloric density (Reilly and Skuse, 1992). In a later study on children with cerebral palsy, Reilly et al. (1996) reinforced that children with severe oral-motor dysfunction typically had briefer meals than those with mild or no oral-motor dysfunction. Mealtime duration was so short in some instances that children would not have been able to consume sufficient calories in that time (Reilly et al., 1996). Futhermore, they supported their previous assumption that many parents offered food of poor caloric density, finding that many parents used powdered foods, which helped them to achieve an appropriate diet consistency but were low in calories.

Pre-oral, oral and pharyngeal phase involvement

There is debate in the literature regarding the extent of involvement of the pharyngeal phase in children with cerebral palsy. It is largely agreed that the most significant impairments are seen in the pre-oral and oral phases of deglutition (Casas et al., 1995). Impairments in these phases are seen predominantly in those children with damage to the corticospinal/corticobulbar tracts, which modulate these voluntary stages of deglutition (Casas et al., 1995). A study by Casas et al. (1995) investigated 20 children with spastic cerebral palsy, and 20 neurologically normal children. They found statistically significant differences between the preoral and oral phases between the two groups and no difference in the pharyngeal phase between groups. However, an earlier study by McPherson et al. (1992) found differences in the pharyngeal phase of children with cerebral palsy involving the respiration-deglutition cycle. These differences were significant as they lead to an increased risk for aspiration. For example, many children in their cerebral palsy group (n = 22) were found to inspire at any time during the cycle, including at the end of the swallow. Children with cerebral palsy are also noted to have pharyngeal residue (Helfrich-Miller et al., 1986). Thus, given that pharyngeal residue is commonly noted, and the potential for children to inspire after swallowing, these children may be at risk of aspiration after swallowing. Hypoxemia has also been found during oral feeding in those children with cerebral palsy who have an abnormal respiratory rate, or in those who experience excessive fatigue with meals (Rogers et al., 1993).

Texture selectivity

Children with cerebral palsy have been reported to have more problems with liquid than with solid food consistencies (Casas et al., 1994; Rogers et al., 1994; Casas et al., 1995). Children with CP appear to have more problems controlling the liquid bolus due to their oral-motor difficulties, whereby the bolus typically flows directly to the pharynx via gravity to trigger a swallow (Kenny et al., 1989). Obviously, larger liquid bolus amounts are handled worse than smaller amounts, and children with CP have also been reported to require more time during eating or drinking in order to help them organize the bolus (Casas et al., 1994). A recent study by Furkim et al. (2003) reported aspiration occurred more commonly with liquids before and after swallowing.

Summary

An early assessment of swallowing function in children with cerebral palsy is of paramount importance in order to detect problems so that prevention and intervention programmes can be instigated. Clinicians particularly aim to prevent growth retardation and respiratory complications subsequent to aspiration. Whilst many children are reported to have difficulty with liquids, some children may have problems with other textures, so that a full feeding assessment evaluating all textures is required. Children with cerebral palsy often require gastrostomy feeding due to any of the afore-mentioned potential areas of feeding difficulty, including: malnutrition, aspiration and associated respiratory disease, insufficient food or fluid intake due, or excessive effort and stress during oral feedings due to dysphagia (Rogers, 2004). Gastroesophageal reflux is also commonly noted in children with cerebral palsy (Rogers, 2004), and this complication comes with further potential risk of aspiration. Continued monitoring is vital for this population, as some children with cerebral palsy present with normal feeding skills for a number of years before developing feeding problems. Thus, the child with CP may be at risk for dysphagia later in life, and not simply from birth, or during the more susceptible transitional stages where they have also been noted to experience feeding difficulty. Commonly reported oral and pharyngeal phase impairments in children with cerebral palsy are listed in Table 13.2.

Moebius sequence

The main diagnostic feature of children with Moebius sequence is congenital palsy of the facial (VII) and abducens (VI) nerves (Sjogreen et al., 2001). Other commonly associated features of the disorder include involvement of the glossopharyngeus (IX) and hypoglossus (XII), craniofacial and orofacial anomalies, and limb malformations (Sjogreen et al., 2001). The aetiology remains unknown, but the use of the term 'sequence' describes multiple anomalies resulting from one structural or mechanical factor, usually subsequent to many aetiologies (Stromland et al., 2002).

Table 13.2 Commonly reported oral and pharyngeal phase impairment in children with cerebral palsy

Oral/pharyngeal phase	Commonly reported difficulties
Oral phase	Limitation of lateral movement of tongue for solid food
	Excessive tongue thrusting and pumping
	Poor expulsion of liquid from nipple during bottle feeding
	Delays in oral phase (>3 seconds for posterior propulsion from base of tongue to tonsillar pillars)
	Oral hypersensitivity
	Prolonged exaggerated bite reflexes
	Poor functioning of cheek and lip musculature
	Poor lip seal
	Excessive drooling
	Temperomandibular joint contracture
Pharyngeal phase	Nasal aspiration
	Slow swallow initiation/swallow trigger delay
	Multiple swallows to clear pharyngeal residue
	Piecemeal deglutition
	Hyperactive and hypoactive gag reflexes
	Aspiration before during or after the swallow
	Most commonly aspirate on liquid
	Absent or reduced cough reflex
	Cricopharyngeal dysmotility

Dysphagia and aspiration are the most life-threatening problems of individuals with Moebius sequence (Cohen and Thompson, 1987).

Feeding problems are commonly associated with the Moebius sequence as a result of cranial nerve involvement and orofacial malformations (Meyerson and Foushee, 1978; Cohen and Thompson, 1987; Amaya et al., 1990; Rizos et al., 1998; Sjogreen et al; Stromland et al., 2002). More specifically, cleft palate, tongue weakness/palsy, pharyngeal dysfunction, macroglossia, micrognathia and generally poor health of the neonate have been reported as the likely causes for feeding problems (Sjogreen et al., 2001).

Oral and pharyngeal phase involvement

Sjogreen et al. (2001) evaluated the feeding and swallowing function of a group of 25 patients with Moebius sequence aged from 2 months to 54 years. All 25 patients presented with oral phase problems, and only three patients demonstrated pharyngeal phase difficulties. The oral phase was characterized by reduced lip function resulting in poor removal of food from the spoon; anterior spillage of the bolus from the corners of the mouth; neglecting to chew large pieces of food, swallowing them whole; and markedly reduced oral transit time (Sjogreen et al., 2001). Impairments of lip and tongue function are the two main deficits of the oral phase in this population. In regard to lip function, the inability to seal the lips due to facial weakness/

palsy causes the most difficulties. Tongue movement and strength may also be markedly reduced due to asymmetry, structural deficits causing atrophy, and hypoplasia (Sjogreen et al., 2001; Stromland et al., 2002).

Pharyngeal phase problems, most likely due to the bulbar paralysis, included clinical signs of aspiration such as coughing with liquids and choking on food consistencies. The bulbar paralysis in this population has been linked to aspiration and subsequent pneumonia and respiratory complications (Haslam, 1979). Despite this profile of impairment, Sjogreen et al. (2001) reported that the majority of patients were maintaining a functional solid diet. This finding implies that despite persistent feeding impairment, individuals with Moebius sequence are able to compensate for their feeding problems to allow them to achieve a normal oral diet.

Relationship between age and feeding impairment

Feeding problems may begin from birth in infants with Moebius sequence, and the nature of the impairment typically changes with age. Infants with a facial palsy alone may breast feed successfully and may experience only minor sucking difficulties. The caregiver may simply be required to provide facilitation using their fingers to help the infant achieve adequate lip seal around the nipple (Sjogreen et al., 2001; Stromland et al., 2002). However, children with orofacial anomalies in association with facial palsy often demonstrate more significant sucking problems (Sjogreen et al., 2001; Stromland et al., 2002). Overall, impaired tongue function (if glossopharyngeal and hypoglossal nerves are involved) is typically the greatest debilitating factor contributing to sucking problems (Sjogreen et al., 2001).

Feeding difficulties have been reported to improve with age in individuals with Moebius sequence (Sjorgreen et al., 2001), however changes in the manifestation of the feeding problem may also occur between young children and adults. Whilst impaired lingual function is most debilitating for infants and young children, poor lip closure is the greater problem for older children and adults. Not only does poor lip seal impact on the efficiency of eating, making it difficult to prevent anterior spillage of food and fluid – this impairment also has social implications. Excessive drooling, thought to be linked in part to poor lip seal, is very socially limiting for adults and older children. Furthermore, Sjogreen et al. (2001) found that older children would prevent anterior spillage by using a hand to keep the food in the oral cavity. Adults, however, were reported to use a napkin for the same purpose. Whilst such strategies provided good functional outcomes for the individuals with Moebius sequence, management of the underlying impairment may help to reduce the need for such socially limiting compensatory strategies.

Prader-Willi syndrome

The clinician involved in the dysphagia management of a child with Prader-Willi syndrome from birth to childhood will witness an extraordinary change in the feeding behaviour of the child. Prader-Willi syndrome is a neurogenetic disorder characterized by hypotonia and feeding problems in early infancy, followed by hyperphagia and obesity from early childhood. Children with Prader-Willi syndrome present with dysmorphic facial features, hypogenitalism, short stature, behavioural problems, and mental retardation (Bray et al., 1983; Airede, 1991; Gillessen-Kaesback et al., 1995; Lindgren et al., 2000). The clinical presentation of hypotonia, feeding difficulty and dysmorphic appearance is often strong enough to suggest the presence of the disorder in infancy (Dubowitz, 1969).

The dysphagia specialist may be heavily involved with the management of children with Prader-Willi syndrome from birth and throughout the first month when feeding problems are most debilitating, and to a lesser degree throughout the remainder of infancy when the feeding problems reduce in severity (Airede, 1991). The feeding problems in early infancy are described as poor appetite and an inability to suckle, resulting in the need for supplemental tube feeding (Airede, 1991; Haig and Wharton, 2003). However, around the age of 2 years, tone begins to normalize and the child with Prader-Willi syndrome develops an insatiable appetite and typically becomes obese (Airede, 1991; Cassidy, 1992; Haig and Wharton, 2003). No data are reported on the specific type of feeding difficulties experienced in infancy, nor on the feeding abilities of the children following the development of hyperphagia in early childhood. At this time however, behavioural feeding management is required, along with emotional support for the family, to deal with the child's voracious appetite and obsession with food (Haig and Wharton, 2003). The intense preoccupation with food is thought to be due to a lack of satiation. The Prader-Willi syndrome phenotype also includes symptoms similar to obsessive compulsive disorder, which may also interact to result in food obsession (Dimitropoulos et al., 2000; Lindgren et al., 2000).

Brachmann de Lange syndrome/Cornelia de Lange syndrome

Brachmann de Lange syndrome, or Cornelia de Lange syndrome, is most commonly recognized by forehead hirsuitism, fish-mouth facial appearance, and synophrys (bushy-eyebrows in continuance). In addition, hypoplastic mandible, microcephaly, long curly eyelashes, small nose with anteverted nostrils, delayed dentition, high arched palate, and variable limb reduction deficits are typically present (Hart et al., 1965; Kumar et al., 1985; Braddock et al., 1993). Children with Brachmann de Lange present with feeding problems related to oral-motor dysfunction, lack of swallowing coordination, recurrent vomiting, gastroesophageal reflux and poor oesophageal motility, which may result in failure to thrive and life-threatening aspiration pneumonia (Hawley et al., 1985; Cates et al., 1989; Bull et al., 1993). Improved methods of diagnosis and management have improved the outcome of children affected with this condition (Bull et al., 1993). Aggressive medical and surgical intervention has been advocated for those with gastrointestinal problems or failure to thrive, to prevent complications of dysphagia, oesophagitis, or malnutrition and to ensure an optimal outcome for these children (Bull et al., 1993). A number of authors have recognized the relationship between recurrent chest infections or pneumonia and the presence of feeding problems and gastroesophageal reflux/vomiting (Lachman et al., 1981; Filippi, 1989). Medical and surgical treatment includes the use of nasogastric and gastrostomy tubes to supplement feeding, and Nissen fundoplication to prevent reflux and vomiting.

Coffin–Siris syndrome

Coffin–Siris is a genetic syndrome characterized by mental deficiency, intrauterine growth retardation, hypoplastic fifth fingers and nails, hirsuitism, and initial feeding and respiratory problems (Coffin and Siris, 1970; Carey and Hall, 1978; Schinzel, 1979; Lucaya et al., 1981; Qazi et al., 1990). Very few data are available detailing the specific nature of the feeding difficulties for children with Coffin–Siris syndrome. However, feeding difficulty is reported to begin at birth with the presence of poor sucking and swallowing (Schinzel, 1979; Qazi et al., 1990; McGhee et al., 2000). Nasogastic and gavage tube feeding are commonly reported in the first few months (Carey and Hall, 1978; Schinzel, 1979; Qazi et al., 1990), with one case of gastrostomy being reported in the literature (Tunnessen et al., 1978). Little mention is made in any study regarding the resolution of the feeding and swallowing problems, nor of the type of outcome for oral intake achieved. However data seem to indicate that feeding issues largely resolve after infancy (Carey and Hall, 1978; Schinzel, 1979; Lucaya et al., 1981). The majority of studies document the first few years of life for children with Coffin–Siris syndrome, however the study by McGhee et al. (2000) documented the features noted in a child of age 11, and interestingly found the child to be obese. No mention was made as to the type of oral intake the child was receiving. Severe feeding problems had been reported over her first month of life only, and were reported to improve gradually. McGhee et al. (2000) proposed that the development of obesity in late childhood may be part of the natural history of the disorder, but called for further long-term evaluation of weight issues in this population.

Further potential complications for feeding disorder in this population may include: cardiac anomalies, marked respiratory problems, and gastrointestinal disorders (Coffin and Siris, 1970; Carey and Hall, 1978; Lucaya et al., 1981; Tunnessen et al., 1978). The impact of heart disease and respiratory issues on feeding skills in the infant is noted elsewhere in this chapter. Recurrent upper and lower respiratory tract infections are also frequent in the first few years of life in children with Coffin-Siris syndrome (Qazi et al., 1990).

CHARGE

'CHARGE' (Coloboma of the eye, Heart defect, Atresia of the choanae, Retarded growth, development and/or CNS anomalies, Genital hypoplasia, and Ear anomalies and/or deafness) is an acronym that describes an association of multi-system abnormalities of which choanal atresia is a component (Davenport et al., 1986). Since the association was first described, many other abnormalities have been found to occur, with the main features including facial palsy, cleft lip and palate, velopharyngeal incompetence, tracheoesophageal atresia, thymic and parathyroid hypoplasia, and renal abnormalities (Davenport et al., 1986; Oley et al., 1988). Despite seminal papers stating that aspiration of secretions due to pharyngolaryngeal impairment may represent the major incremental risk factor for mortality, there remain few data specific to feeding or swallowing problems in this population that are not of a purely structural or anatomical nature (Blake et al., 1990; Morgan et al., 1992).

Aetiologies for feeding issues associated with CHARGE

The two main issues potentially leading to swallowing impairment, aside from a cleft palate, include airway complications and gastrointestinal issues (Tellier et al., 1998). The presence of heart disease and airway difficulties may also impact on feeding skills in children with CHARGE.

Airway difficulties

Nasopharyngeal, hypopharyngeal and laryngopharyngeal abnormalities may all lead to airway instability in children with CHARGE (Coniglio et al., 1988; Asher et al., 1990; Morgan et al., 1992). Nasopharyngeal deformities may include bilateral choanal atresia, an abnormally contracted nasopharynx in the lateral and/or vertical dimension, and an abnormally prominent medial pterygoid lamina and thickened posterior nasal septum (Oley et al., 1988). Children with CHARGE have been reported to have a range of laryngotracheal anomalies including laryngomalacia, tracheomalacia, tracheoesophageal fistula, subglottic stenosis, laryngeal clefts, and vocal cord palsy (Blake et al., 1990; Morgan et al., 1992; Tellier et al., 1998). Laryngomalacia is reported to be the most frequent congenital laryngeal anomaly noted in children with CHARGE, manifesting in stridor and feeding difficulties that typically resolve by 18 months of age (Morgan et al., 1992). Subglottic stenosis may be congenital, or in some cases where children have had a number of minor surgical operations and prolonged periods of intubation, granulation tissue, mucosal ulceration and fibrosis may occur from intubation trauma causing acquired subglottic stenosis (Hollinger, 1982).

Gastrointestinal problems

Commonly reported signs of gastrointestinal difficulty noted in children with CHARGE include vomiting and choking. Underlying problems found to induce these signs include pharyngo-oesophageal dysmotility and gastroesophageal reflux (Blake et al., 1990; Morgan et al., 1992; Tellier et al., 1998). Asher et al. (1990) reported that all patients with CHARGE in their study (n = 16) demonstrated swallowing difficulties, with patients reporting pooled secretions, vomiting and choking. Whilst they did not report the cause of these symptoms, they proposed that the combination of anatomical defects and physiological impairment was likely to lead to a deleterious airway event, or aspiration. Morgan et al. (1992) recommend the use of tracheostomy where required to avoid aspiration, a common cause of death in these children.

Smith-Lemli Opitz syndrome

Smith-Lemli Opitz is an autosomal recessive disorder of cholesterol biosynthesis that manifests in multiple congenital anomalies (Cunniff et al., 1997; Nowaczyk and Waye, 2001; Tierney et al., 2001; Prasad et al., 2002). The main characteristics first proposed by Smith et al. (1964) included a distinct craniofacial appearance, cleft palate, ptosis, cataracts, postaxial polydactyly and hypoplasia. Language, cognitive and motor development are also typically delayed along with attentional issues, and behavioural problems including tantrums, aggressive outbursts and self-injuring behaviours (Tierney et al., 2001). Cormier-Daire and colleagues (1996) noted that, although the clinical manifestations of Smith-Lemli Opitz are extremely variable, several features are typically present in children with classical presentations of the disorder, including: micrognathia, severe microcephaly, major ante and postnatal growth retardation, and feeding problems. They also reported that the major ante and postnatal growth retardation seen in children with Smith-Lemli Opitz was due to feeding difficulties (Cormier-Daire et al., 1996).

Feeding difficulties associated with Smith-Lemli Opitz

Often a dysphagia specialist may be one of the first health professionals involved in the management of a child with Smith-Lemli Opitz. Prasad et al. (2002) reported on a child referred to a medical team at six-and-a-half months due to hypotonia, poor feeding and poor weight gain. The nature of the feeding difficulties for children with Smith-Lemli Opitz may be diverse and varied, potentially arising from craniofacial anomalies, tonal issues, gastrointestinal problems, respiratory issues, congenital heart defects, and/or metabolic issues.

Impact of craniofacial anomalies on feeding

Children with Smith-Lemli Opitz presenting with craniofacial anomalies such as micrognathia or cleft palate will present with feeding issues. Further craniofacial anomalies specific to this group of children with Smith-Lemli Opitz include: a high arched palate and narrow hard palate, broad and ridged alveolar ridges, and redundancy of sublingual tissues (Donnai et al., 1986; Curry et al., 1987). Whilst such anomalies might not impact markedly on feeding ability, the SLP might expect to note these features during an oromotor examination.

Further issues affecting feeding

The hypotonia present in infancy has been reported to resolve with age but it often develops into hypertonia, contractures and orthopaedic problems for children who are non-ambulatory (Nowaczyk and Waye, 2001). Such physical issues impact markedly on oral-motor function, and as a result may reduce oral intake. Gastrointestinal abnormalities complicate feeding issues further, whereby pyloric stenosis, vomiting, gastroesophageal reflux, gastrointestinal irritability, feeding intolerance, and allergies are common (Kelley and Hennekam, 2000). Laryngomalacia and tracheomalacia may be present (Nwokoro and Mulvihill, 1997). Congenital heart defects may also be present in approximately 50% of children with Smith-Lemli Opitz (Lin et al., 1997), having potentially deleterious effects on feeding – see above. Further compounding issues of oral-motor dysfunction, gastrointestinal issues, efficiency and fatigue for feeding are metabolic/caloric intake considerations, given that a hypermetabolic state has been noted in many patients with Smith-Lemli Opitz (Kelley and Hennekam, 2000). Hypersensitivity and tactile defensiveness has also been reported for the hands, feet, extremities, and the oral region (Tierney et al., 2000). Not surprisingly, given the many factors that may cause feeding difficulty in children with Smith-Lemli Opitz, recurrent episodes of pneumonia are common (Cunniff et al., 1997; Ryan et al., 1998). Enteral feeding is commonly used to offset malnutrition in children with Smith-Lemli Opitz, with gavage feeding needed in newborns, followed by short-term nasogastric feeding, and then longer-term gastrostomy feeding in many children (Cormier-Daire, 1996; Nowaczyk and Waye, 2001; Prasad et al., 2001).

Down syndrome

The presence of feeding difficulties in children with Down syndrome is of significant concern, given that a lack of mobility or feeding skills have been more accurate predictors of early death than the medical problems associated with congenital heart disease in the syndrome (Eyman and Call, 1991). Historically the feeding difficulties noted in children with Down syndrome were reported to occur as a result of delayed development. Palmer et al. (1978) proposed that the following features were subsequent to the delayed development of oral reflexes and self-feeding: poor sucking and swallowing in infancy, drooling, open-mouth posture during feeding, delayed transition to solid food, and the persistence of the protrusion reflex past the first or second year. In more recent times however, the pattern of oral-motor dysfunction in children with Down syndrome has been suggested to occur largely as part of an aberrant developmental path, rather than due to developmental delay (Spender et al., 1996).

Specific feeding difficulties associated with Down syndrome

Oral-motor and feeding dysfunction is reported to be most marked in children with Down syndrome from the ages of 9 months to three years (Spender et al. 1996). The main feeding issues occur as a result of dysfunction, specifically hypertonicity, of the jaw, lips, and tongue (Howard and Herbold, 1982; Limbrock et al., 1991; Spender et al., 1995). In particular, a pattern of persistent tongue protrusion is the overriding feature, causing anterior spillage or, in more severe presentations, preventing any food from entering the oral cavity (Gisel et al., 1984a; Spender et al.,

1995). Hypoplasia of the mandible and maxilla has been reported to be the main factor contributing to the tongue protrusion noted in these children (Fischer-Brandies, 1989). Tongue protrusion may occur on all textures, but some parents report food refusal and behavioural issues relating to specific food textures (Spender et al., 1995). Gisel et al. (1984a) found that tongue protrusion was most marked with puree and least marked with cracker consistency. Adding further to issues of oral containment, children with Down syndrome are frequently mouth breathers due to heavy nasal congestion, and thus typically present with a persistently open-mouth posture during eating (Howard and Herbold, 1982). Texture selectivity has also been noted, with children avoiding solid foods and refusing to chew (Field et al., 2003). The aversion to chewable foods has been suggested to be largely due to oral-motor delays whereby children avoid foods due to difficulty chewing, but also due to potential episodes of gagging or choking when foods are not chewed properly (Field et al., 2003).

Oral-motor delays resulting in chewing difficulty

Poor rhythmicity of the jaw, lips and tongue affect mastication for children with Down syndrome. Gisel et al. (1984b) found that children with Down syndrome spent longer in each chewing cycle for raisins and cracker consistencies and had a greater number of chewing cycles for the puree consistency. Spender et al. (1995; 1996) found an immature pattern of anterior-posterior suckling persisting in place of the mature up-down vertical sucking pattern that should be present from around 8 months. Such problems have implications for the efficiency of oral intake for children with Down syndrome, with children potentially taking longer to consume adequate amounts of energy. Poor feeding skills occur in children with Down syndrome, but good developmental feeding outcomes have been reported for some in this population depending upon the factors contributing to the feeding impairment. Cullen et al. (1981) reported that, of 89 children with Down syndrome whom they evaluated for mastery of feeding skills, younger children attained most feeding milestones much earlier if they had no, or only mild congenital heart disease, if their parents followed through with guidance, and if they had 'good' muscle tone.

Rett syndrome

Rett syndrome occurs in 1:10,000 women, arising from a mutation on the X chromosome (Hagberg, 1985; Sugarman-Isaacs et al., 2003). Rett syndrome is not usually evident in the neonate or young infant. Instead the majority of females with Rett syndrome are reported to have normal development during infancy. However a regression is noted in development around 2 to 3 years, and delays become noticeable, including problems with feeding (Hagberg, 1985; Morton et al., 1997; Willard and Hendrich, 1999). Specifically, there appears to be regression in oral-motor ability, particularly with decreased lateralization of the anterior tongue and an open-mouth posture, which results in poor chewing skills, and often also results in anterior spillage of food. Morton et al. (1997) also found that the time taken to swallow a mouthful of liquid or solids gradually increases with age, reflecting the inefficiency of bolus preparation and the oral stage of feeding.

It is extremely difficult to determine a reason for dysphagia in Rett syndrome, with the likely aetiologies being complex and multifactorial (Reilly and Cass, 2001). Reilly and Cass (2001) propose that the decreases in growth and oral-motor function with increasing age may be related to declining postural stability, a pattern noted in children with cerebral palsy.

Issues of poor growth and texture tolerance

Cass et al. (2003) reported on the oromotor and feeding abilities in a group of 87 females with Rett syndrome aged between 2 years 1 month and 44 years 10 months. Interestingly, Cass et al. (2003) reported that despite 83.9% of the parents of the females with Rett syndrome reporting that their children had good appetites, weight loss was reported to be a problem in approximately 20% of the participants. This weight loss may be associated with the poor chewing skills and restricted range of oral intake demonstrated by children with RS. Sugarman et al. (2003) studied 22 girls with RS and suggested that the texture of foods eaten may be important in predicting future nutritional status. When texture tolerance for chewing, crunchy, viscous foods and beverages is high, a larger variety of foods is more likely to be consumed, resulting in higher nutrient intakes. Limited texture tolerance is a potential predictor of poor oral ability in managing food and thus the child may demonstrate self-restricted eating patterns and a subsequent low nutrient intake (Sugarman et al., 2003). Budden et al. (1990) reported on 20 girls with Rett syndrome, aged 3 years 11 months to 19 years 4 months, and found that, apart from one subject who required a gastrostomy, all the girls were eating pureed or soft foods and had difficulty chewing food and using their tongues effectively.

Oral and pharyngeal feeding problems

Aside from the marked chewing problems identified in children with Rett syndrome, other oral-phase difficulties have been reported to include poor tongue lateralization, involuntary dyskinetic tongue writhing, mouth breathing at rest and during feeding, anterior spillage of fluids, intermittent drooling, poor bolus formation, poor mid and posterior tongue movement resulting in inefficient oral transit and piecemeal deglutition, poor glossopharyngeal seal with the palate resulting in premature spillage into the pharynx, oral residue, and a delayed swallow trigger (Budden et al., 1990; Morton et al., 1997; Motil et al., 1999).

Whilst feeding problems of the oral phase, including chewing, are most frequently reported, dysphagia in Rett syndrome has also been reported to occur at the pharyngeal level as well. Budden (1995) reported that 49 of the 60 females they studied with RS had dysphagia; 25 (41%) had oral stage problems, and 12 (20%) had oral and pharyngeal problems. In regard to the pharyngeal phase, Morton et al. (1997) reported three episodes of aspiration out of 20 subjects (15%). The aspiration was noted to occur largely prior to a swallow with premature spillage of the liquid bolus over the base of the tongue, or aspiration of solids due to a delayed pharyngeal phase swallow. Two subjects aspirated a small amount after the swallow due to significant and persistent pharyngeal residue. All three subjects had a history of more than three chest infections in the past year, compared with an average of only 0.5 infections per year among the subjects in whom aspiration was not detected. By contrast, none of the subjects in the study by Motil et al. (1999) displayed aspiration, or had a history of recurrent lower respiratory tract infections. However, reduced oropharyngeal clearance was noted by Motil et al. (1999), with pooling of liquids and solids in the valleculae and pyriform sinuses before swallowing, and the persistence of residue in these sinuses after swallowing, both of which increase aspiration risk. Laryngeal penetration was also noted during swallowing, particularly in subjects who were hypertonic or hypotonic (Motil et al., 1999).

Breathing patterns of children with Rett syndrome

Breathing difficulties are commonly reported in children with Rett syndrome, in particular apnea or 'breath-holding', not just in sleeping hours, and hyperventilation. Cass et al. (2003) reported apnea and hyperventilation to be the most common breathing difficulties in their study. They found that fewer breathing problems were noted in the younger (<5-year) and older (>20-year) age groups, and the greatest range and frequency of problems were noted for those aged 5–9 years and 10–19 years. For more information on respiration patterns during feeding, the reader is referred to Chapter 4.

Pierre Robin sequence

Pierre Robin sequence is characterized by micrognathia and glossoptosis, which leads to respiratory distress due to the large tongue being limited in anterior placement by the small jaw, causing it to fall back into the pharynx (Marques et al., 2001; Li et al., 2002; Wagener et al., 2003). Pierre Robin sequence can occur in isolation, or in association with other congenital anomalies or syndromes (Shprintzen, 1992). Pierre Robin sequence typically occurs with a cleft palate, and is most frequently associated with Stickler syndrome (also called hereditary arthro-ophthalmopathy), and velocardiofacial syndrome (Shreiner et al., 1973; Van den Elzen et al., 2002). Airway obstruction and feeding difficulties are the two main problems associated with Pierre Robin sequence (Wagener et al., 2003). Children with Pierre Robin sequence typically present with noisy breathing, snoring, stridor, cyanosis, feeding problems and aspiration pneumonia (Li et al., 2002).

Feeding difficulties associated with structural anomalies

The feeding problems noted in children with Pierre Robin sequence are usually secondary to the airway obstruction (Marques et al., 2001). Airway obstruction is thought to occur largely due to the tongue falling backward into the oropharynx (Robin, 1923; Shprintzen, 1992). In order to try and prevent the tongue falling back into the pharynx, one suggested treatment method has been the use of prone position. Takagi and Bosma (1960) found an improved suck and improved co-ordination of tongue and mandible movement in the prone position. Early treatment and intervention is important as the degree of feeding problem is usually related to the extent of the airway problem, thus solving the airway problem can lead to a rapid resolution of the feeding problems (Marques et al., 2001; Li et al., 2002). The reader is referred to Schaefer et al. (2004) for a recent algorithm for the most appropriate management technique for specific patients.

The prognosis regarding feeding difficulties is positive, with most neonates outgrowing such problems by 6 months of age (Benjamin and Walker, 1991). The improvement in oropharyngeal function has been linked to neurological maturation and subsequent increases in the neuromuscular control of the tongue and growth of the mandible (Takagi and Bosma, 1960; Sher, 1992). The feeding problems are thought to be due not only to the airway obstruction but also to the retroposition of the tongue itself and the size of the tongue (Marques et al., 2001). Prognosis is positive for return to oral intake and the development of feeding skills, but respiratory effort and feeding problems caused by respiratory distress, lingual retroposition and potential cleft palate may lead to failure to thrive (Shprintzen, 1992). The feeding problems tend to include vomiting and aspiration with consequent protein-energy malformation (Marques et al., 2001).

Feeding difficulties associated with physiological problems

The above discussion has focused mainly on feeding issues due to airway problems, but a number of studies have proposed that the feeding problems associated with Pierre Robin sequence are actually not subsequent to the airway obstruction but are actually due to the presence of underlying poor sucking skills and poor tongue movement (Cruz et al., 1999; Baudon et al., 2002). Many infants with Pierre Robin sequence have been reported to experience lack of coordination of the oral and pharyngeal phases of swallowing (Renault et al., 2000). Caouette-Laberge et al. (1996) reported that the feeding problems with Pierre Robin sequence appeared to be due to decreased tongue movement or impaired muscular co-ordination during swallowing. Baudon et al. (2002) reported that in a series of 28 patients with Pierre Robin sequence (aged 15 days to 45 days), 24 infants had feeding problems. A severe feeding problem was noted in 12 infants, characterized by an absence of sucking and inactive or tonic pharyngeal phase. A further six infants had moderate sucking and swallowing problems, and the remaining six had mild feeding issues.

NEUROMUSCULAR JUNCTION DISORDERS

A number of neuromuscular junction diseases are associated with dysphagia in children, including myasthenia gravis and botulism (Kosko et al., 1998).

MYASTHENIA GRAVIS

Myasthenia gravis is a progressive immune-mediated disorder affecting acetylcholine receptors located on muscle membranes at the neuromuscular junction (Kosko et al., 1998). In the neonate, myasthenia gravis can present as transient neonatal myasthenia gravis or as a congenital syndrome (Koenigsberger and Pascual, 2002; Gurnett, Bodnar, Neil and Connolly, 2004). There is also a juvenile form of myasthenia gravis in children characterized by specific clinical features differing from those seen in the adult (Garofalo-Gomez et al., 2002). Myasthenia gravis in the infant is characterized by constipation, poor feeding, weak crying, hyporeflexia, respiratory distress and sucking problems (Faroux et al., 1992; Verspyck et al., 1993; Papazian, 1992; McCreery et al., 2002). The respiratory involvement and dysphagia are significant causes of morbidity and mortality in myasthenia gravis (Thomas et al., 1997). Bulbar muscle weakness is common in myasthenia gravis resulting in dysphagia and thus weakness and fatigue of the lips, tongue and jaw may result in poor sucking and chewing skills for infants and young children.

BOTULISM

Infantile botulism occurs infrequently and is caused by the ingestion of Clostridium botulinum spores that occur in honey or soil products (McMaster et al., 2000; Krishna and Puri, 2001; Cox and Hinkle, 2002). The toxin is absorbed and it binds to acetylcholine receptors on motor nerve terminals at the neuromuscular junction, damaging neuromuscular junction function (Cox and Hinkle, 2002). The infant becomes progressively weak, hypotonic and hyporeflexic with bulbar and spinal nerve abnormalities (Cox and Hinkle, 2002). Symptoms include: constipation, lethargy, weak cry, poor feeding, dehydration, and respiratory difficulty (Wilson et al., 1982; Cox and Hinkle, 2002; McMaster et al., 2000; Ravid et al., 2000; Krishna and Puri, 2001).

AERODIGESTIVE TRACT

Whilst it has been established that any aetiology causing disruption to the swallowing mechanism may potentially lead to respiratory complications, structural or functional airway problems may have a more direct impact on both swallowing and respiratory function due to their shared anatomy. The following section will refer to structural or functional problems of the aerodigestive tract, or specifically the oropharynx, nasopharynx, larynx, trachea, pharynx and oesophagus. A brief discussion of a number of special problems such as tracheostomy, muscular disorder, neoplastic causes, and infectious disorders affecting the swallowing mechanism will be included. Many of these defects indirectly impact on swallowing by disrupting the co-ordination between respiration and swallowing, rather than directly impacting upon deglutition itself (Arvedson and Lefton-Greif, 1998; Dinwiddie, 2004).

Table 13.3 Aerogidestive tract anomalies that may impact upon feeding/dysphagia in the paediatric population

Area of aerodigestive tract	Disorder/disease/anomaly
Nasopharynx	Choanal atresia
	Nasal cysts (e.g. dermoids, gliomas, encephaloceles)
	Tumours
	Deviated septum
	Nasal aperture
	Midnasal stenosis (e.g. Crouzon craniostenosis)
	Midface hypoplasia (e.g. Crouzon and Apert)
Oropharynx	Cleft lip
	Mandibular hypoplasia (e.g. Robin sequence)
	Adenotonsillar hyperplasia
	Epiglottitis
	Penetrating trauma
	Tumour
	Cyst
Larynx	Laryngeal/subglottic stenosis
	Laryngomalacia
	Vocal cord paralysis
	Laryngeal cleft
	Laryngeal web
Pharynx	Pharyngeal paralysis
	Pharyngitis
	Peritonsillar abscess
	Retropharyngeal abscess
Trachea/Esophagus	Tracheosophageal fistula/oesophageal atresia
	Oesophageal masses
	Mechanical obstruction
	LES or UES sphincter dysfunction
	Oesophagitis
	Oesophageal compression
Miscellaneous	Neuromuscular junction diseases (e.g. myasthenia gravis, botulism)
	Muscular disorders
	Neoplastic causes (e.g. hemangioma, lymphangioma, papilloma, leiomyoma, neurofibroma)
	Traumatic injury
	Foreign body ingestion

Source: adapted from Arvedson and Lefton-Greif (1990); Brodsky (1997); Brodsky and Volk (1993); Dinwiddie (2004); Kosko et al. (1993); Keilly and Carr (2001).

See Table 13.3 for common aerodigestive tract diagnoses that may cause or further complicate dysphagia.

NASOPHARYNX

The majority of structural deficits of the nasopharynx obstruct the nasal cavity, thereby impacting on the infants, who are obligatory nose breathers up until six months of age, resulting in stridor and laboured respiration. Common structural anomalies of the nasopharynx include choanal atresia (see the section on CHARGE above), nasal cysts, deviated septum, mid-nasal stenosis, and cystic (e.g. meningoencephalocele, gliomas) and solid lesions (e.g. haemangioma, neurofibroma). Typically, this pattern of strained respiration increases during feeding, and thus may disrupt the co-ordination of respiration and swallowing (Brodsky and Volk, 1993; Brodsky, 1997; Arvedson and Lefton-Greif, 1998). Not only bilateral, but also partial obstruction and stenosis may affect feeding (Kosko et al., 1998).

Crouzon syndrome and Apert syndrome

Crouzon syndrome and Apert syndrome are two autosomally inherited craniofacial anomalies most commonly presenting with midface hypoplasia (Brodsky and Volk, 1993). Both syndromes have been associated with the fibroblast growth factor receptor 2 (FGFR2) gene (Abou-Sleiman et al., 2002; Van Ravenswaaij et al., 2002). Children presenting with Crouzon or Apert syndromes demonstrate altered nasopharyngeal anatomy, including: reduced pharyngeal height, width and depth, increased thickness and length of the soft palate, and decreased length of the hard palate (Peterson-Falzone et al., 1981). The combination of reduced nasopharyngeal space and poor patency of the posterior nasal choanae typically results in respiratory problems, particularly in the young child (Peterson-Falzone et al., 1981). The common clinical presentation involves marked respiratory distress, stridor and severe expiratory obstruction and wheezing (Beck et al., 2002). Breathing becomes more laboured and noisier during feeding in children with Apert or Crouzon syndrome due to the increased respiratory effort required (Brodsky and Volk, 1993). These children may also present with tracheal cartilaginous sleeve (TCS), a congenital anomaly involving fusion of a small number of tracheal arches, the entire trachea, or from beyond the carina into the bronchi (Cohen and Kreiborg, 1992; Scheid et al., 2002). Midface advancement conducted as early as three years of age can improve the airway of children with Apert or Crouzon syndrome, with tracheostomy insertion up until that time (Brodsky and Volk, 1993; Scheid et al., 2002). Not surprisingly, given the potential expanse of areas of obstruction in Apert and Crouzon syndrome, both upper and lower airway compromise may lead to early mortality in some cases (Cohen and Kreiberg, 1992; Beck et al., 2002).

Hemifacial microsomia

Hemifacial microsomias typically present without cleft palate but they tend to occur with obstruction of the oropharynx, causing prolonged noisy feeds and grunting (Brodsky, 1997). Hemifacial microsomia has been reported as the second most common congenital facial anomaly second to cleft palate (Salvado et al., 2003). Hemifacial microsomia is thought to arise from anomalous development of the first two branchial arches during development, and results in varying degrees of unilateral hypoplasia of the mandible, macrostomia and ear deformity. Neurological deficits and feeding issues are commonly seen in children with hemifacial microsomia.

OROPHARYNX

Cleft lip and palate

Cleft lip and/or palate are the most commonly occurring craniofacial anomalies with one in 700 newborns experiencing cleft lip and or palate (Kaufman, 1991), and one in 2000 newborns experiencing isolated cleft palate (Kosko et al., 1998). The main feeding issue for infants with cleft palate is the inability to generate adequate intra-oral pressure for sucking due to an inability to close off the nasopharynx (Brodsky and Volk, 1993; Kosko et al., 1998). Nasopharyngeal regurgitation may occur, how-ever this feature is not commonly reported in children with cleft palate (Kosko et al., 1998). Cleft lip may impact upon the development of intraoral pressure due to poor lip seal, resulting in reduced generation of sucking pressure. Often modifications in feeding practice can offset this feeding difficulty by altering the fluid delivery method so that less effort is required by the infant to increase the ingested calories and reduce energy output during feeding (Redford-Badwal et al., 2003). However in some cases where the infant is at risk of failure to thrive, supplemental feeding may be advocated. For a systematic review of feeding interventions in cleft palate, refer to Glenny et al. (2004)

Pandya and Boorman (2001) reported an increasing rate of failure to thrive de-pendent upon the diagnoses of cleft in children undergoing primary cleft procedures. They reported that children with unilateral cleft lip and palate had the lowest rate of failure to thrive at 32%, followed by 38% for bilateral cleft lip, and 49% for cleft palate. Following this investigation, Pandya and Boorman (2001) instated a special-ist feeding nurse and then recorded the number of children with cleft presenting with failure to thrive years later. They found a large decline in the number of children ex-periencing failure to thrive with 9% for cleft lip and palate, 20% for bilateral cleft lip and palate, and 26% for cleft palate. This demonstrated the importance of special-ized feeding management in offsetting the potential risk of failure to thrive in these infants, but also reinforced that failure to thrive was still relatively high in infants with isolated cleft palate. In agreement with this finding, Oliver and Jones (1997) reported that children with isolated cleft palate were more frequently associated with the need for nasogastric feeding than children with other cleft diagnoses. The Pierre Robin sequence (see above) is one of the more severe craniofacial anomalies, presenting with a U-shaped cleft palate.

Adenotonsillar hyperplasia

Those children with enlarged tonsils, or adenostonsillar hyperplasia, also exhibit oropharyngeal obstruction and typically exhibit a pattern of mouth breathing, snor-ing, and refusing to eat harder textures such as meat (Brodsky and Volk, 1993; Brod-sky, 1997). Children with hyperplasia of the tonsils/adenoids may present with failure to thrive as a result of the increased feeding and swallowing problems (Darrow and Siemens, 2002). Failure to thrive occurs due to the increased energy demands placed on these children during feeding due to the increased work of breathing to overcome the obstruction (Brodsky and Volk, 1993). Tonsillectomy and/or adenoidectomy will almost always relieve the obstruction (Potsic and Wetmore, 1990; Potsic and Wetmore, 1992; Darrow and Siemens, 2002).

LARYNX

Any lesion of the endolarynx such as laryngomalacia, laryngeal web or subglottic stenosis can obstruct or impair the airway, resulting in stridor and increased respiratory effort, longer feeding times and poor feeding skills, and thus failure to thrive due to increased energy expenditure and lack of oral intake (Brodsky and Volk, 1993; Brodsky, 1997). Choking and coughing is common early post-feed in children with dysphagia due to laryngeal anomalies (Brodsky and Volk, 1993).

Laryngomalacia

Laryngomalacia is the most common cause of airway obstruction, stridor and respiratory distress in infants (Ungkanont et al., 1998; Baljosevic et al., 2002). Laryngomalacia presents with a high-pitched inspiratory stridor when the infant feeds or cries, with the condition involving the collapse of the arytenoids, aryepiglottic folds and the epiglottis into the airway (Brodsky, 1997). Gastroesophageal reflux is also frequently seen with laryngomalacia, further complicating the dysphagia noted in these infants (Brodsky, 1997). Laryngomalacia typically resolves within the first year of life.

Vocal fold paralysis

Vocal fold paralysis and an inability for the vocal folds to adduct and adequately protect the airway could lead to aspiration. Vocal fold paralysis has been reported as the second most common congenital anomaly following laryngomalacia (Ungkanont et al., 1998; Friedman et al., 2001), and can be unilateral, bilateral, congenital or acquired (Dinwiddie, 2004). Children often demonstrate functional voicing, but have inspiratory stridor which may progress to complete respiratory obstruction (Takamatsu, 1996; Friedman et al., 2001). Aspiration is most frequently noted in unilateral paralysis, alongside hoarseness (Kosko et al., 1998). Bilateral vocal fold paralysis is typically associated with inspiratory or biphasic stridor that worsens with feeding (Kosko et al., 1998). Whilst some children recover completely following growth, others may require tracheostomy (Takamatsu, 1996).

Posterior laryngeal cleft

Posterior laryngeal clefts are rare congenital anomalies that account for a small percentage of laryngeal abnormalities (Ungkanont et al. 1998; Kennedy et al., 2000). They develop from an absence of fusion of the posterior cricoid lamina and possibly the tracheoesophageal septum (Fitzpatrick and Guarisco, 1999). There is a strong

Table 13.4 Benjamin and Inglis (1989) classification system of congenital laryngeal cleft in infants

Cleft type	Criterion
Type I	Supraglottic interarytenoid
Type II	Extending below the level of the glottis but only partially involving the cricoid itself
Type III	Extends into the cervical trachea
Type IV	Laryngotracheoesophageal cleft extending into the thoracic trachea

association between laryngeal cleft and tracheoesophageal fistula (Kosko et al., 1998). There are a number of classification systems for laryngeal cleft, including those by Armitage (1984), and Benjamin and Inglis (1989), with the latter being most commonly used – see Table 13.4. Evans et al. (1995) reported on 44 patients with laryngeal cleft and noted that the majority were type 1 (n = 26), followed by type 2 (n = 8), type 3 (n = 9), and type 4 (n − 1). Evans et al. (1995) also reported that children with type 1 cleft presented with recurrent chest infections, inspiratory stridor due to arytenoids or the mucosa overlying the arytenoids collapsing into the airway on inspiration, and/or cyanosis during feeding. Infants with cleft types 2, 3 and 4 were characterized by the same group of symptoms, however they also had degrees of aspiration proportional to the severity of the cleft (Evans et al., 1995).

Laryngeal web

Laryngeal webs occur infrequently and arise through poor embryological develop-ment of the larynx (Milczuk et al., 2000). The impact of the laryngeal web on the airway is highly variable, hence the resultant feeding difficulties and level of sur-gical management may vary between patients depending on the extent of airway obstruction (Hisa et al., 1989; Milczuk et al., 2000). Laryngeal web has recently been associated with a chromosome 22q11 deletion (McElhinney et al., 2002).

TRACHEA/OESOPHAGUS

Tracheosophageal fistula (TEF)/oesophageal atresia

Tracheosophageal fistula (TEF) and/or oesophageal atresia are the most common con-genital aerodigestive tract anomalies. Surgical repair is required in all cases (Kosko et al., 1998). Oesophageal atresia and tracheoesophageal fistula may exist separately but the majority of infants experience both (Kovesi and Rubin, 2004). Oesophageal atresia is an interruption to the oesophageal lumen, and a tracheoesophageal fistula is a connection between the airway and the oesophagus (Fine and Ma, 1985; Thilo and Rosenberg, 1999). A tracheoesophageal fistula may occur due to anomalous de-velopment of the tracheo-oesophageal septum (Lancaster et al., 1999). The difficul-ties that arise from this problem are obvious, with the communication between the trachea and oesophagus allowing for food/fluid to pass directly via the trachea and into the lungs. Tracheosophageal fistula may be congenital or acquired (Brodsky and Volk, 1993). The acquired form may occur following trauma, foreign body aspiration, or following surgery, e.g. tracheotomy (Brodsky and Volk, 1993). Dysphagia, coughing, choking, cyanosis and airway hyperreactivity is commonly associated with TEF, along with recurrent aspiration pneumonia (Kovesi and Rubin, 2004). Tracheomalacia may occur following TEF repair, resulting in continued distress of the airway and stridor (Brodsky and Volk, 1993).

Tracheostomy

Tracheostomy is a surgical opening running from the neck through to the trachea in order to bypass an upper airway obstruction, to help manage secretions, or to provide a means for ventilation for patients with life-threatening apnea (Brodksy, 1997). The typical placement of the tracheostomy tube (between the second and third tracheal rings) makes the pharyngeal phase more difficult because the larynx may not elevate properly, reducing protection against aspiration. Moreover, Shaker et al. (1995) have reported that the presence of a tracheostomy decreases vocal fold closure, again increasing aspiration risk (Brodsky, 1997). Young children typically have a cuffless tracheostomy tube because their small airways cannot accommodate a cuffed tube, whilst allowing enough lumen to breath adequately (Brodsky, 1997). Rosingh and Peek (1999) found that post-operatively following tracheostomy placement, 31/34 children had dysphagia and avoidance behaviours such as expelling food, gagging and vomiting, and only half of this group could have feeding problems explained by an underlying diagnosis. Granulation tissue needed treatment in 16/34 cases (47%) (Rosingh and Peek, 1999). Rozsai et al. (2003) also reported granulation tissue to be a common local problem following tracheostomy tube insertion. Tracheostomy may interfere with normal laryngeal function during swallowing and predispose the child to aspiration (Buckwalter and Sasaki, 1974). As in children without an artificial airway, chronic bronchitis, wheezing, congestion, and recurrent bacterial tracheitis should raise concern about chronic recurrent aspiration (Loughlin and Lefton-Greif, 1994). Taniguchi and Moyer (1994) state that the relationship between the presence of a tracheostomy and aspiration pneumonia is thought to be related to impaired swallowing caused by prolonged endotracheal intubation (Gilbert et al. 1987; Nash, 1988). Aspiration is a well recognized complication in patients with tracheostomy (Peruzzi et al. 2001; Gross, Mahlmann and Grayhack, 2003; Rozsai et al., 2003).

INFECTIONS CAUSING DYSPHAGIA

Persistent infections of the tonsils, retropharyngeal space or other head and neck spaces may cause abscesses and lead to dysphagia (Kosko et al., 1998). Ungkanont et al. (1995) reviewed 117 children undergoing management for head and neck space infections and found that peritonsillar and retropharyngeal infections were most common, followed by submandibular, buccal, parapharyngeal and canine abscesses.

Deep neck space abscesses in infants are often rapidly progressive, typically present with fever and neck mass, and often cause airway compromise (Cmerjrek et al., 2002; Dawes et al., 2002). Foreign body ingestion may lead to deep neck space abscess. Common medical management involves incision and drainage (Cmejrek et al., 2002). The common clinical signs are drooling, neck swelling and tenderness, fever, dysphagia and/or poor oral intake, refusal to swallow and torticollis (Ouoba et al., 1994; Lee et al., 2001; Cmejrek et al., 2002; Dawes et al., 2002; Kelly and Isaacman, 2002; Khan et al., 2004).

MUSCULAR DISORDERS

Myotonic dystrophy is an autosomal dominant inherited disease and is the most common muscular disease involving the skeletal and cardiac musculature, including the pharyngeal and gastrointestinal smooth and striated muscles (Sartoretti et al., 1996). Given the musculature involved in this disease, dysphagia is one of the most common sequelae (Odman and Kiliaridis, 1996; Marcon et al., 1998; Chiapetta et al., 2001). Major swallowing problems result from alteration in orofacial and pharyngeal musculature including impaired mastication, taking longer chewing time and more chewing cycles than normal; choking; aspiration; decreased pharyngeal contractions; impaired UES opening; delayed pharyngeal swallow trigger (Penarrocha et al., 1990; St Guily et al., 1994; Saito et al., 1995; Ertekin et al., 2001). Aspiration pneumonia is a common morbidity in individuals with myotonic dystrophy (Bodensteiner and Grunow, 1984; Saito et al., 1995; Sartoretti et al., 1996; Chiappetta et al., 2001). In neonates, poor sucking, choking, regurgitation, dysphagia and aspiration are common (Bodensteiner and Grunow, 1984). In the infant, myotonic dystrophy is usually characterized by facial diplegia, generalized muscular hypotonia and muscular respiratory failure (Bodensteiner and Grunow, 1984). There are many types of muscular dystrophy (Duchenne's, Steinert), and many other types of muscular disease including inflammatory myopathies (Polymyositis, Dermatomyositis) – the reader is referred to the following articles for further information on these issues, which occur infrequently in young children: Bruguier et al. (1984); Camelo et al. (1997); Chiappetta et al. (2001); Dalakas (1998); Marie et al. (1999); Metheny (1978); Tilton et al. (1998).

NEOPLASTIC CAUSES

Neoplastic or space occupying lesions of the aerodigestive tract can cause compression to both the airway and oesophagus and typically result in dysphagia (Brodsky, 1997; Kosko et al., 1998). Paediatric neoplasms include hemangioma, lymphangioma, leiomyoma, neurofibroma and papilloma (Mbakop et al., 1991; Osborne et al., 1991; Boas et al., 1996; Wang et al., 2002; Lee et al., 2003).

Hemangiomas

Hemangiomas are infrequently occurring benign tumours that may occur in infantile and adult forms (Berkes and Sente, 1998). Infantile hemangiomas typically occur in the subglottic region, and cause stridor, dyspnea, cough and dysphagia (Goldsmith et al., 1987; Lee et al., 2003). These tumours may occur in the glottis, supraglottic larynx and hypopharynx and are typically mixed or cavernous type hemangiomas that may experience dramatic growth during the proliferative phase (Yellin et al., 1996). Desuter et al. (2004) report two cases of postcricoid hemangioma and report symptoms such as: stridor, massive regurgitations, respiratory distress, feeding difficulties and a delayed growth curve. The impact of hemangiomas on feeding and swallowing is dependent on the location and volume of the mass, with those occurring in subglottic locations being the most life-threatening (Desuter et al., 2004). Treatment options include surgical excision, corticosteroids, interferon, laser therapy, or observation when symptoms are less severe; however, often treatment involves trying to control the tumour and relieve symptoms rather than being able to completely remove the lesion (Kosko et al., 1998; Lee et al., 2003).

Lymphangiomas

Lymphangiomas are the second most common neoplasm in children. Lymphangiomas are benign tumours, with the most common form being cystic hygroma (Charabi et al., 2000; Kardon et al., 2000). Cystic hygromas are large congenital malformations that typically occur in the posterior triangle of the neck and axilla in children less than 2 years of age (Osborne et al., 1991; Ricciardelli and Richardson, 1991; Charabi et al., 2000). Hygromas of the head and neck can be extremely difficult to manage given the serious potential complications of airway obstruction and feeding impairment (Ricciardelli and Richardson, 1991). Early treatment involving surgical excision and possibly debulking is advocated in children with these potentially rapid growing masses (Osborne et al., 1991; Ricciardelli and Richardson, 1991).

Leiomyoma

Leiomyoma is a cyst most commonly occurring in the oesophagus (Wang et al., 2002; Zahid et al., 2003). The primary symptom is dysphagia (Wang et al., 2002; Zahid et al., 2003). Leiomyoma of the oesophagus is a rare benign condition seen in children in which smooth muscle proliferation leads to a marked thickening of the distal wall of the oesophagus (Kosko et al., 1998). Patients with severe dysphagia are usually treated with oesophagectomy or oesophagogastrectomy (Kosko et al., 1998).

Other neoplasms

Two other infrequently occurring neoplasms include: laryngeal papilloma and neuofribroma. Laryngeal papilloma tends to occur in adult and juvenile forms. Clinically patients present with dysphonia, dyspnea, cough, foreign body sensation in throat and dysphagia (Mbakop et al., 1991). Neurofibroma of the larynx typically presents with stridor and dysphagia (Boas et al., 1996). Surgical excision and/or debulking is a treatment option in this rare condition (Boas et al., 1996).

Physical damage to swallowing structures

Complications may arise with dysphagia as a result of physical damage to the aero-digestive tract, including oral, pharyngeal, laryngeal and oesophageal structures. Common examples of structural trauma that may co-occur with traumatic brain injury include: fractures of the jaw, affecting jaw opening and movement; laryngeal trauma, which may lead to reduced laryngeal elevation or closure; ingestion of caustic substances potentially causing scar tissue on the tissues of the pharynx, leading to possible pooling or reduced pharyngeal wall movement; and wounds to the chest, which may cause oesophageal perforation or fistula formation (Logemann et al., 1994). Particularly in the initial stages of acute hospital management, the co-existence of such physical damage can significantly affect swallowing function and impede, or even delay, the initial stages of swallowing rehabilitation.

GASTROESOPHAGEAL REFLUX DISEASE

Gastroesophageal reflux is the regurgitation of gastric contents, which pass back through the lower oesophageal sphincter into the oesophagus (Ida, 2004). Refluxed material may be seen in the form of emesis, but in some cases, reflux is 'silent' with no obvious symptoms occurring during a reflux episode (Hyman, 1994). Reflux episodes occur in normal infants and they may display many of the symptoms of reflux disease (Orenstein et al., 1995; Putnam, 1997). Gastroesophageal reflux is diagnosed as a disease entity when the reflux noted is with consequence and at the far end of a continuum of normal infant physiology (Orenstein et al., 1995; Putnam, 1997).

WHAT CAUSES GASTROESOPHAGEAL REFLUX DISEASE?

Gastroeosphageal reflux disease is thought to occur due to two main reasons:

- failure of the normal means of preventing reflux; and
- failure of the means of clearing any reflux that occurs (Hyman, 1994; Kawahara et al., 1997; Putnam, 1997; Sullivan, 1997).

Young infants are more prone to developing gastroesophageal reflux disease (GORD) as the lower oesophageal sphincter, oesophageal peristalsis, and the general anatomy of the oesophagus matures with age (Hyman, 1994). Infants with appropriate development of the lower oesophageal sphincter (LES) are able to maintain adequate LES pressure to prevent reflux between swallows (Werlin et al., 1980). Alternatively, infants with GORD experience transient relaxation of the LES between swallows, lasting from seconds to minutes, and this has been reported to be the most significant aetiology for GORD in children (Kawahara et al., 1997; Putnam, 1997). A number of infants and children with GORD have also been found to have low or absent basal LES pressure which allows reflux to occur (Kawahara et al., 1997).

The stomach is lined with a specialized type of mucosa that is resistant to acid, but the mouth, pharynx and oesophagus are not protected against refluxed material (Putnam, 1997). Following an episode of reflux, adequate functioning of clearance mechanisms are crucial in actually moving the refluxed material and preventing prolonged contact with mucosal surfaces that have no acid resistance (Putnam, 1997). There are two main clearance mechanisms for moving reflux:

- oesophageal persitalsis; and
- stomach emptying.

Oesophageal peristalsis is important in returning reflux to the stomach (Putnam, 1997). Children with reduced oesophageal peristalsis will be at an increased risk of GORD. Delayed stomach emptying means that reflux may still occur, but when the stomach contents have passed into the small intestine, reflux cannot occur (Putnam, 1997).

CLINICAL SIGNS OF GORD

Two main types of clinical symptoms are noted with GORD:

- airway symptoms; and
- feeding symptoms (Carr et al., 2000) – see Table 13.5.

Respiratory complications associated with GORD include aspiration, reflux-induced laryngospasm, reflux bronchospasm and reflex central apnea (Sullivan, 1997; Ida, 2004). In particular, airway symptoms are thought to include stridor, cough, wheezing, nasal congestion, hoarseness, obstructive apnea and pneumonia

Table 13.5 Clinical signs and symptoms of dysphagia associated with gastroesophageal reflux disease (GORD)

Type of GORD symptom	Clinical signs/symptoms of dysphagia associated with GORD
Respiratory	Stridor
	Wheeze
	Cough
	Nasal congestion
	Hoarseness
	Aspiration
	Reflux central apnea
	Reflux-induced laryngospasm
	Reflux bronchospasm
Feeding related	Frequent vomiting during and post-feeds
	Choking/gagging
	Back arching
	Drooling
	Irritability with feeding
	Wet burps
	Failure to thrive

(Krishnamoorthy et al., 1994; Orenstein et al., 1995; Sullivan, 1997; Carr et al., 2000). Feeding related symptoms have been reported as: frequent vomiting, choking/gagging, food refusal, arching, drooling, irritability, wet burps and failure to thrive (Shepherd et al., 1987; Orenstein et al., 1992; Dellert et al., 1993; Orenstein et al., 1995; Carr and Brodsky, 1999; Carr et al., 2000; Ida, 2004).

Historically, feeding-related symptoms such as failure to thrive, frequent vomiting, and gagging have been the most commonly recognized symptoms of GORD; however, symptoms related to the aerodigestive tract have been recognized in more recent times (Carr and Brodsky, 1999; Carr et al., 2000). The GORD is thought to cause airway problems through a combination of microaspiration of refluxate and reflex bronchospasm, laryngospasm, central apnea and bradycardia (Orenstein and Orenstein, 1988).

All children with GORD may exhibit some of these symptoms, but Carr et al. (2000) distinguished the following as pathologically significant symptoms, in order of significance:

- frequent vomiting;
- failure to thrive;
- stertor;
- cyanotic spells; and
- choking/gagging.

HOW IS REFLUX TREATED?

Chronic GORD (e.g., frequent vomiting, apnea, choking, failure to thrive, dysphagia, feeding problems) is treated pharmacologically and/or surgically (Putnam, 1997). Pharmacological intervention involves medications that either neutralize acid or prevent acid production (Putnam, 1997). Nonpharmacologic practices have also been advocated. Orenstein (1983) advocated keeping the child in an upright or prone position as this was found to reduce reflux events compared to supine or seated positions. Historically, thickening feedings was also thought to increase caloric density and reduce regurgitation (Orenstein et al., 1987). However, others argue that there is a lack of efficacy in using thickened feeds as a treatment for GORD (Bailey et al., 1987). The Nissen fundoplication is the most commonly used surgical procedure for controlling GORD (Sullivan, 1997).

ASPIRATION AND GORD

Those children who present with aspiration due to oral-pharyngeal dysfunction in conjunction with reflux are difficult to manage (Putnam, 1997). There is an increased risk of aspirating refluxed contents in this population as they may aspirate when swallowing to clear the refluxed material (Putnam, 1997). Fundoplication is typically employed alongside gastrostomy in these children, however this anti-reflux surgery is commonly related to dysphagia (Munro, 2003).

HOW DO FEEDING PROBLEMS ARISE FROM GORD?

The relationship between swallowing and reflux is complex and probably poorly understood. As with many children who are unable to communicate their clinical symptoms, it is difficult to state definitively the reasons for the occurrence of dysphagia following reflux in the preverbal child. The prolonged presence of refluxed material in the oesophagus leads to inflamed oesophageal mucosa and often oesophageal bleeding. The pain associated with the oesophagus is thought to be the cause of food refusal in infants (DiScipio et al., 1978; Hyman, 1994; Sullivan, 1997; Williams et al., 1994). Following a series of painful reflux episodes, an infant learns to associate the pain with eating and thereby refuses to eat (Hyman, 1994; Mayer and Gebhart, 1994).

Subsequently, children will have reduced oral intake, and depending on the child's level of food refusal and weight loss, failure to thrive may result (Dellert et al., 1993). Other manifestations of this pain include irritability, arching, grimacing, head turning, physical refusal of bottle by pushing it away, and gagging (Shepherd et al., 1987; Orenstein et al., 1994; Putnam, 1997). Unfortunately, the behavioural response of food refusal has been conditioned, and the infant may persist with food refusal after the reflux and oesophagitis have been treated (Putnam, 1997).

The food refusal mechanisms present differently in the older child (Catto-Smith et al., 1991). Older children often report that they feel that food is stuck and feel that they need to drink fluids to help 'dislodge' the food (Catto-Smith et al., 1991). Typically, videofluoroscopy will reveal no stricture in the oesophagus, however it is thought to be due to non-specific disruptions to oesophageal peristalsis that prevent effective oesophageal emptying, impacting on the swallowing mechanism, and on the ability to clear refluxed material (Cucchiara et al., 1990). In some cases, however, chronic inflammation of the oesophageal wall may lead to thickening, and a fibrous oesophageal stricture may develop, resulting in either food impaction or regurgitation (Rode et al., 1992). Therefore, videofluoroscopic swallowing study (VFSS) may be advocated for an older child with a history of prolonged, uncontrollable GORD who reports such symptoms as discomfort after swallowing, and the inability to swallow certain consistencies of food (solids, meat).

FEEDING PROBLEMS IN INFANTS WITH GORD

Mathisen et al. (1999) investigated the specific feeding problems noted in 20 infants (mean age 6 months) with GORD, and 20 matched controls. Feeding problems were assessed by maternal interview, 24-hour diet analysis, a standardized test for oral-motor function (Feeding Assessment Schedule), and a rating scale of infant behaviour during feeding (Tester's and Maternal Rating Scale of Infant Behaviour during feeding-TRIB and MRIB). Eleven of the GORD infants were also assessed using VFSS. Mathisen et al. (1999) confirmed that children with GORD have significant feeding problems compared with controls. The feeding problems were characterized by oral-motor dysfunction, oral dysphagia, transitional phase problems, and negative feeding experiences for the mother and child.

Oral phase

A number of problems have been identified with the oral phase in children with GORD, via both clinical and radiological assessment. Oral phase problems have been found to include: food refusal, fewer self-feeding and readiness behaviours for solids, oral hypersensitivity, immature lip, tongue and jaw control, food loss, poor lip closure, poor bolus containment, few oral problems with liquids, but problems with puree and semisolid foods, prolonged holding of the bolus on the tongue, uncoordinated tongue movement, and delayed oral transit (Mathisen et al., 1999). Pharyngeal phase problems have been reported to include silent aspiration and delayed pharyngeal transit time (Mathisen et al., 1999).

Children with GORD have a greater number of choking episodes and panic reactions, and less smooth feeding sequences (Mathisen et al., 1999). During the transitional phase children begin to accept solid foods and increase the variety of textures consumed in parallel with the development of chewing and cup drinking, as discussed above. Mathisen et al. (1999) found that the 6-month-old infants with GORD had none of the readiness cues for transitioning. Of greater significance was that the transitional phase also relied on the caregiver (Morris, 1982; Carruth et al., 1993), and the caregivers of GORD infants were stressed and not enjoying feeding experiences with their children. Mathisen et al. (1999) also proposed that the transitional and oral phase problems may be due to the interaction of intrinsic oral-motor function, impoverished early oral experience and learned aversive behaviour. GORD infants are known to have resistance to feeding and oral hypersensitivity (Dellert et al., 1993), which decreases the infants' desire to use the mouth for exploratory play or the intake of food.

BEHAVIOURAL FEEDING PROBLEMS

The issue of behavioural feeding problems and the role of the speech pathologist in dealing with difficulties in this area is complex. Estimates of the proportion of preschool children presenting with behavioural feeding problems have ranged between 12% and 35% (Palmer et al., 1975; Minde and Minde, 1986; Blissett and Harris, 2002). Behavioural issues can arise with a number of other aetiologies. The feeding problems of 103 infants were categorized into specific aetiologies, with behavioural issues more often coded (85%) than neurological conditions (73%), structural abnormalities (57%), cardiorespiratory problems (7%), or metabolic dysfunction (5%) (Burklow et al., 1998). The high prevalence of behavioural feeding issues is of particular significance for two reasons. Firstly, a large number of children with behavioural feeding problems may demonstrate reduced oral intake, poor/reduced weight gain, or malnutrition, with subsequent failure to thrive and deleterious effects on neurological and physical development (Bithoney and Dubowitz, 1985; Skuse, 1993; Arvedson, 1997). Secondly, food and mealtimes are integral to family life and society, and disruptions in the feeding routine can impact upon the intellectual, social and emotional growth of the child, as well as overall family functioning (Chatoor et al., 1988; Archer and Szatmari, 1990; Mathisen et al., 1999).

Despite the prevalence of behavioural feeding problems, and the potential negative impact of this type of feeding disorder, very little is reported in the literature in this area. In particular, there is little agreement on the type of intervention programme to be implemented for children with food refusal or selectivity. Dahl and Sundelin (1986) state that the management of behavioural feeding problems is problematic, involving a wide variety of disciplines in the absence of a defined, agreed framework from which to view these issues. The reader is referred to Brown and Ogden (2004) and Reed et al. (2004) for recent investigations of the behavioural management of food refusal. Common clinical signs of behavioural feeding problems are:

- frowning or falling asleep during feeds to express resistance/fear of accepting foods or liquids;
- panic in facial expression of older children in response to feeding utensil approaching;
- head turning;
- hiding face;
- struggling to avoid being fed;
- selective food refusal/food resistance;
- reduced appetite/lack of oral intake;
- failure to accept age-appropriate foods (e.g. refusal to accept new foods, textures);
- excessive adaptations required to encourage feeding (e.g. thickening liquids, only offering smooth textures);
- sudden refusal to eat and drink;
- sudden loss of appetite;
- gradual change in eating habits or patterns;
- gradual or sudden onset of 'difficult' mealtime behaviour.

WHAT CAUSES CHRONIC FOOD REFUSAL/BEHAVIOURAL FEEDING PROBLEMS?

The causative factors for behavioural feeding disorders are complex and often multifactorial, rarely having a single cause (Werle et al., 1993). Many organic factors have been identified for feeding problems, including physiological abnormalities, neuromuscular conditions, allergies and acute infection, and various syndromes (Illingworth and Lister, 1964; Linscheid, 1992; Keng et al., 2002). A defining feature of food refusal is that medical or organic causes have been ruled out as being significant enough to explain the problems persistence (Chatoor et al., 1985; Williamson et al., 1987; Ginsberg, 1988). Instead, non-organic environmental factors such as behavioural mismanagement of children during feeding and aversive feeding experiences are presumed to play an integral role. The purpose of the present review is to focus on non-organic factors. It is acknowledged, however, that mixed

organic and non-organic factors can result in feeding refusal. In fact, many authors
have found that mixed organic and non-organic psychosocial feeding problems occur more frequently than straight non-organic feeding issues (Budd et al., 1992;
Burklow et al., 1998). It is acknowledged that children can develop behavioural feeding aversions through organic aetiologies (e.g. gastroesophageal reflux disease, as
discussed above), this section will focus on the behaviourally manifested feeding
problems that persist after medical treatment and not the feeding issues that exist
during organic involvement.

Aside from behavioural problems arising from medical illness or congenital
developmental delay, two other main aetiologies for chronic food refusal exist. The
first set of factors relates to delayed development, lack of oral experience, or failure
to move into the transitional period of feeding at the normal developmental time.
These problems result in children failing to successfully achieve the feeding skills
they require at certain stages in oral-motor progression. As a result children develop negative behavioural responses to their failure. The second factor relates to
psychosocial issues, including negative patterns of mother-child interaction, and/or
behavioural mismanagement.

Lack of oral experience/developmental delay

Skuse (1993) discussed the impact of sensitive periods for taste and texture. In relation to the sensitive period for taste, it appears that there is a period of opportunity
when the child is aged between 4 and 6 months when infants will typically accept
new tastes. It is hypothesized that if children experience a taste during this time,
they will carry a tolerance for these tastes into later childhood (Birch and Marlin,
1982; Skuse, 1993). Thus, to delay the introduction of tastes until after six months
may lead to food refusal, and particularly in children who are predisposed to behavioural problems by being 'temperamental' (Skuse, 1993). Similarly, a 'sensitive
period' has been proposed where children are typically exposed to solids around
6 to 7 months (Illingworth and Lister, 1964). If children do not experience foods of
increasing texture during this time, they may later develop food refusal for lumpy/
textured foods (Skuse, 1993).

Skuse (1993) proposed an additional factor related to this transitional phase of
feeding and later behavioural difficulties. He states that those children who have not
experienced more textured foods and have not developed more mature, fine movements of tongue and jaw for mastication may not chew food adequately for swallowing, resulting in aversive gagging or choking, and potentially leading to refusal
of solid foods (Skuse, 1993). Many authors have also highlighted populations at
increased risk for delayed exposure to oral exploration and the transitional phase of
feeding. That is, children who are fed for prolonged periods via a nasogastric tube,
where there may not be continued oral stimulation or oral sensory input, or where
aversive oral stimulation occurs such as nasotracheal suctioning or repeated passage
of the nasogastric and endotracheal tubes (Morris, 1989; Skuse, 1993; Willging,
2000). Furthermore, any children with severe medical illness where they may be

in the sterile hospital environment for long periods of time may also be at risk of delayed oral-motor development. Failure of a child to receive nutritive stimulation during the critical period whilst experiencing negative feeding experiences (e.g. choking) places the child at risk for developing feeding refusal, oral aversion or gagging/vomiting with attempts to feed orally (Budd et al., 1992; Willging, 2000). Willging (2000) noted that this combination of oral restrictions and aversive oral stimulation during early development is common in neonatal intensive care unit settings, promoting the dysfunctional feeding abilities of many of these children. Thus, even if foods are used with nasogastric feeds, children may not get positive input so that feeding is largely not a pleasurable experience, leading to food refusal.

Psychosocial factors

Successful feeding in the infant and young child is heavily reliant on both the child's own oral-motor skills, and also the skills of the parent in interpreting the child's needs. In relation to the child's skill level, if a child exhibits some pathological form of feeding difficulty, which the parent is unable to recognize, the parent may misinterpret the child's feeding behaviour as being based on temperament rather than pathology. This may lead the caregiver to feel negatively towards the child and the feeding experience (Arvedson, 1997). In regard to parental skills, the caregiver must be able to read and respond to subtle cues during the feeding process (Arvedson, 1997). For detailed descriptions of the types of expected caregiver responses during the stages of infancy (homeostasis, 2 to 3 months; attachment, 2 to 6 months; and separation/individuation, 6 to 36 months), the reader is referred to Chatoor et al. (1984) and Satter (1990). Failure of caregivers to understand their children's needs and their own role during the feeding process may lead to aversive feeding practices and behavioural feeding problems (Harris and Booth, 1992; Arvedson, 1997). Unsuccessful caregiver-infant feeding interactions have wider reaching implications than impacting on the child's physical growth, being linked to the child's cognitive and linguistic competence, securing attachment to major caregivers (Barnard et al. 1989; Arvedson, 1997).

Behavioural mismanagement for feeding is usually the result of parental anxiety about ensuring that their children maintain sufficient oral intake, or increase their oral intake (MacDonald et al., 1991; Harris and MacDonald, 1992; MacDonald et al., 1997; Blissett et al., 2000, 2001). Unfortunately, the strategies used by some parents to increase their children's intake exacerbate the feeding problems and make mealtimes more negative for all concerned (Harris and Booth, 1992; Skuse, 1993; Blissett et al., 2000). There is much debate over the correct way to handle food refusal but there is agreement regarding inappropriate ways to treat these problems, including reliance on bribery, force feeding, or playing excessive distracting games, as all of these behaviours could exacerbate the child's food refusal. For further principles and treatment protocols for remediation see the following: Archer and Szatmari, 1990; Greer et al., 1991; Werle et al., 1993; Ahearn et al., 1996; Arvedson, 1997; O'Reilly and Lancioni, 2001; Blissett and Harris, 2002.

TRAUMATIC BRAIN INJURY

Traumatic brain injury (TBI) is the most frequent cause of acquired disability in the paediatric population, leaving a large proportion of those who survive with multiple long-term impairment (Michaud et al., 1993). Dysphagia is one common consequence following brain injury in children and adults (McLean et al., 1995; Mackay et al., 1999). Morgan et al. (2003) reported a dysphagia incidence figure of 5.3% across all paediatric brain injury admissions over a 5-year period. When the population was broken down according to injury classification by Glasgow Comas Scale score, dysphagia incidence figures increased with increasing injury severity levels. Sixty-eight per cent of children with severe TBI presented with dysphagia, as opposed to dysphagia incidence figures of only 15% for children with moderate TBI, and 1% for children with mild TBI.

NEUROPATHOLOGY ASSOCIATED WITH DYSPHAGIA

Both primary and secondary neuropathophysiological effects of head injury may impact on the swallowing mechanism. Primary neuropathology including skull fracture, contusion, cerebral concussion and diffuse axonal injury may result in focal, multifocal or diffuse cortical and/or brain stem damage affecting the neurological control, and therefore functioning of the swallowing mechanism. Dysphagia may also occur through secondary neuropathology, depending on the area and degree of neurological damage. Significant metabolic/hypoxic changes can occur to produce functional disturbances such as rapid and inefficient respiration and possible circulatory failure. The association between respiratory/circulatory problems and fatigue has obvious implications for feeding in the child with brain injury, given the highly coordinated swallowing and respiratory processes. Pituitary disorders arising from damage to the hypothalamus and pituitary gland may cause electrolyte disturbances, problems with the satiety cycles of swallowing and/or hyperventilation. The presence of hyperventilation has implications for swallowing function, again due to the inter-relationship between swallowing and respiration. For a review of the neurological control of swallowing, and the functional impact of damage to any of these areas, refer to Chapter 1.

IMPACT OF TRAUMATIC BRAIN INJURY ON THE SWALLOWING MECHANISM

Oral intake can be markedly reduced by dysphagia following TBI, subsequently impacting upon the patient's nutritional status and compromising the recovery process (Mackay et al., 1999). The impact of dysphagia on recovery in children post-TBI is of particular concern, given that children already have additional energy requirements in order to ensure continued growth, and thus have added difficulties maintaining nutrition in the hypermetabolic state (Burd et al., 2001; Newman, 2001). Furthermore, secondary complications arising from dysphagia such as aspiration pneumonia are widely recognized as being major contributing factors to mortality and morbidity in TBI (Morgan, 1992; Morgan, 1994).

Oral and pharyngeal phase impairment

The dysphagia present post-TBI typically involves both oral and pharyngeal phases of swallowing (Rowe, 1999; Morgan et al., 2002). Specific impairments noted both clinically and via videofluoroscopic evaluation of swallowing in the paediatric population post-TBI include: reduced lingual control, hesitancy of tongue movement, inefficient repetitive tongue pumping in an attempt to propel the bolus posteriorly into the oropharynx, aspiration (including silent aspiration), delayed pharyngeal swallow reflex, reduced laryngeal elevation and closure, and reduced pharyngeal contractions.

Cognitive-behavioural deficits affecting feeding

A pattern of impaired cognition and altered behaviour related to feeding during the acute phase of rehabilitation has been noted in children with moderate-severe TBI (Morgan et al., 2004a). Field and Weiss (1989) proposed that the ability to follow directions and judgement of the rate and amount of intake are affected by cognitive status. These cognitive-behavioural deficits contribute to dysphagia in unpredictable ways, as swallowing has a voluntary as well as a reflexive component (Field and Weiss, 1989). Ylvisaker and Logemann (1985) have stated that severe dysphagia may occur in the presence of a mild physiological deficit due to cognitive-behavioural factors. Morgan et al. (2004a) indicated that the acute clinical assessment should investigate cognitive-behavioural issues in order to determine the effect of cognitive status on the feeding process. In this way cognitive-behavioural deficits can be identified and appropriate management strategies be determined to reduce the impact of such issues on dysphagia outcome.

Postural stability

Poor postural stability has been reported for children with TBI during the acute phase. A study by Morgan et al. (2004a) found that all 14 subjects (100%) had abnormal postural control and tone, and unstable head, neck, and postural control for trunk movement, ambulation or phonation. Subsequently, almost 80% of participants were unable even to orientate their head to the spoon upon presentation of food. Given the severity of tonal and postural impairment resulting in head and neck instability, it is not surprising that this population also had significant impairment in respiratory, laryngeal, lip, jaw and tongue function (Morgan et al., 2004a). The inability to achieve respiration adequate for phonation was noted in almost 90% of participants, and this, alongside issues of poor laryngeal closure on the clinical bedside evaluation, resulted in an inadequate cough reflex. Thus, the clinician is unable to rely on clinical signs of the presence of food or fluid on the vocal folds, or aspiration risk, such as cough during the clinical bedside evaluation. This is of major concern, as silent aspiration has been noted in the paediatric population post-TBI (Morgan et al., 2002), and again highlights the potential need for more objective radiological assessment to determine the presence of silent aspiration in this population.

Feeding efficiency

The severely compromised oral-motor integrity of the mandibular, facial, labial and lingual musculature demonstrated by children with moderate to severe TBI markedly affects feeding efficiency. Reduced facial tone may lead to food collecting in the cheeks, and large amounts of oral residue, placing the individual at an increased risk of passive food loss into the airway, or actively inhaling material. Problems with lip seal make removing the food from the spoon difficult, and these children also commonly display inactivity of the lips during sucking, munching or chewing, affecting intraoral pressure and bolus transit. Poor lip seal may also lead to anterior food loss. These oral-motor problems affect the efficiency or endurance aspects of mealtimes in children with dysphagia post-TBI, resulting in longer mealtime duration required to consume sufficient oral intake. Reductions in feeding efficiency are of particular concern in the TBI population where patients are already at risk of malnutrition subsequent to markedly increased nutritional demands to enable recovery.

Predictive factors for dysphagia and long-term dysphagia prognosis

Miller and Groher (1997) recognize that one of the most difficult aspects of working with neurogenic dysphagia is the diversity of the nature and extent of swallowing deficits that can arise even in patients with similar neuropathology. There are many factors in addition to neuropathology which may determine the presence and severity of dysphagia following TBI, including: extent of injury, presence or tracheostomy and/or duration of ventilation, and cognitive-behavioural impairment (Cherney and Halper, 1989; Halper et al., 1999; Mackay et al., 1999). Morgan et al. (2003) reported that significant factors for determining the presence of dysphagia in the paediatric population with TBI included a Glasgow Coma Scale score of 8 or less (indicative of severe TBI) and a ventilation period in excess of 1.5 days.

With regard to long-term prognosis of dysphagia, Morgan et al. (2004b) reported that across a patient group of 13 children with moderate/severe TBI (aged 4 years 1 month to 15 years, $M = 7$ years 4 months, $SD = 3$ years), oral-motor deficits and swallowing function resolved to normal status, and resolution to normal diet status was achieved by 12 weeks post-injury. Thus, based on these preliminary data, there would appear to be a positive prognosis for the return to a normal oral diet post-TBI for children who presented similarly to the rather homogenous group in the study by Morgan et al. (2004b). Seven children had haematoma, two presented with cerebral oedema and two with multifocal or diffuse injuries. The dysphagia outcome for children with brain stem impairment however appears less favourable than for those with neurological lesions confined to the cerebrum. Another study by Morgan et al. (2004c), however, reported on the swallowing outcome at 10 months post-injury for a 14-year-old female after a brain stem injury. The dysphagia presented by the child was found to resolve quickly for the initial two weeks post-injury, slowed to gradual progress for weeks 12 to 20, and then plateaued with mild clinical oral-motor and swallowing impairment up until 10 months post-injury where VFSS assessment revealed persistent aspiration on thin fluids. Fluid supplementation was still required by percutaneous endoscopic gastrostomy at 10 months after injury. Rowe (1999) has also reported on a paediatric case with brain stem injury that had longer term persistent swallowing deficits than children with other types of neuropathology. A prognosis of long-term rehabilitation prior to the return to oral feeding after brain stem injury is not surprising given the potential interruption of the complex relationship between the cranial nerve nuclei, nerve tracts and reticular interneurons found within the brain stem for the control of swallowing. Disruption of this relationship has been reported to potentially result in severe dysphagia that is resistant to spontaneous recovery in the adult population (Huckabee and Cannito, 1999). Thus it appears that the nature of the dysphagia after TBI is highly variable upon a range of factors including neuropathology and medical treatment.

A range of factors may result post-TBI in the paediatric population including cognitive-behavioural impairment, hypersensitivity, hyper or hypotonicity, oral-motor dysfunction, and oropharyngeal dysphagia, including silent aspiration. Until we understand more about the mechanisms of TBI and their potential impact upon the swallowing mechanism, children should be treated based on their individual symptomatology, as assessed using both VFSS and a clinical bedside evaluation, rather than their neuropathology or medical variables.

CONSEQUENCES OF DYSPHAGIA IN CHILDHOOD

The two major potential complications arising from dysphagia are malnutrition and aspiration with resultant respiratory complications. Whilst the complication of malnutrition can be successfully offset in the majority of cases by supplemental nutrition, the management of aspiration and subsequent respiratory compromise is more complex. Due to the shared anatomy of swallowing and respiration, problems related to swallowing can manifest in respiratory symptoms, and swallowing problems can exacerbate respiratory difficulties (Brodsky, 1997). Given the inter-relationship between respiration and swallowing, determining the cause of dysphagia in a child with breathing problems is complex. Airway problems may arise from dysphagia of any aetiology, so that assessment of this problem requires evaluation not only of the airway, but also of the child's cardiovascular function, neurodevelopmental status, and gastrointestinal function (Brodsky, 1997).

HOW DOES ASPIRATION AFFECT RESPIRATORY FUNCTION?

There are two main ways in which dysphagia and aspiration may lead to respiratory disease. The first is direct oropharyngeal aspiration of food or saliva into the trachea before, during or after swallowing (McColley and Carrol, 1994; Morton et al., 1999). The second is aspiration of gastric contents into the trachea following gastroesophageal reflux or an episode of vomiting (McColley and Carrol, 1994; Morton et al., 1999). Gastroesophageal reflux without aspiration has also been implicated in respiratory disease (McColley and Carrol, 1994), with clinical symptoms such as coughing, wheezing and recurrent pneumonia (Bauer et al., 1993). Taniguchi and Moyer (1994) suggest that if there are respiratory problems with gastroesophageal reflux, then oropharyngeal problems are likely to coexist. There is much debate regarding which mechanism of aspiration is most commonly associated with more serious consequences. Morton et al. (1999) reported that oral and pharyngeal motor dysfunction was the major cause of respiratory tract infection in children with severe neurodisability, and that oropharyngeal dysfunction led to an increased likelihood of direct aspiration. They also found that patients were at even higher risk of severe respiratory tract infections, and likely gastrostomy and fundoplication placement, if gastroesophageal reflux and aspiration of stomach contents were present in addition to oropharyngeal dysphagia (Morton et al., 1999). Taniguchi and Moyer (1994) also found that factors associated with an increased risk of pneumonia in a group of 142 patients with dysphagia of mixed aetiology were: presence of oropharyngeal aspiration, presence of gastroesophageal reflux, and the presence of a tracheostomy tube.

This fact is not surprising given that the development of respiratory problems is linked to the acidity of the material aspirated. A relatively small volume of aspirate can lead to significant respiratory issues if the pH is low, whereas larger volumes of neutral pH aspirate can be tolerated (Raidoo et al., 1990; Taniguchi and Moyer, 1994; Terry and Fuller, 1989). The texture of the food/fluid aspirated has also been linked to respiratory outcome in children. Taniguchi and Moyer (1994) found that children who aspirated pureed consistencies had nine times the risk of developing pneumonia compared to children who did not aspirate this consistency. Children who aspirated thickened liquids had the second greatest risk of developing pneumonia and children who only aspirated thin liquids did not have a statistically significant increase in pneumonia risk (Taniguchi and Moyer, 1994).

The clinical manifestations of dysphagia and/or aspiration differ between infants and children (Loughlin and Lefton-Greif, 1994). Apnea and bradycardia are the major symptoms noted in infants. They are rarely noted in older children who present more frequently with cough, congestion, wheezing, bronchitis, atelectasis and pneumonia (Loughlin and Lefton-Greif, 1994). The most serious clinical manifestation of aspiration is bacterial pneumonia; however, other chronic symptoms can be persistent and frustrating such as coughing and wheezing (McColley and Carrol, 1994). Some children presenting with chronic aspiration have been found to present with wheezing that cannot be remedied with bronchodilator therapy. Symptoms of aspiration with respiratory complication include: apnea, stridor or hoarseness, recurrent episodes of fever and dyspnea, atelectasis or infiltrates noted on chest x-ray, noisy congested breathing, coughing, and choking on feeds (Loughlin and Lefton-Greif, 1994; McColley and Carrol, 1994). Apnea is a protective response to prevent aspiration, but if it persists post-swallow, or if a delay in the clearance of the bolus occurs in a protracted apneic episode, hypoxemia or secondary bradycardia may occur (Loughlin and Lefton-Greif, 1994).

Some populations with already compromised respiratory function are at particular risk of further respiratory complications subsequent to dysphagia. Children with bronchopulmonary dysplasia (BPD), asthma and cystic fibrosis often have gastroesophageal reflux and appear to be at high risk for respiratory complications of dysphagia as a result (McColley and Carroll, 1994). The reader is also referred to Chapter 4 for further discussion of the interplay between respiration and swallowing.

CHAPTER SUMMARY

The current chapter highlights the vast range of primary diagnoses associated with paediatric dysphagia, and the multitude of secondary factors that may also cause or complicate feeding and swallowing disorders in this population. It is inappropriate, however, to assume that the underlying cause of dysphagia is a result of either the primary or secondary medical diagnoses alone. Reilly and Carr (2003) provided an example of this error in reporting a paediatric case whose food refusal was initially related to his primary diagnosis of developmental disability, but later correctly determined to be due to a lodged foreign body that was causing the child great irritation. It is also clear from the current chapter that many of the clinical characteristics, signs and symptoms of dysphagia are similar across medical populations. Thus although the clinician is reliant on observing and interpreting the presence and extent of dysphagia based on signs and symptoms during their initial clinical assessment of the child, these features may fail to provide an aetiology for the child's problems. Extra caution must also be used when interpreting from these signs in a paediatric population that is often unable to communicate its own difficulties, and whose underlying problems may be further compounded by a variety of developmental stressors. In conclusion, it is critical that the management of children with dysphagia involve multiple professionals working within a developmental framework. In this way, a comprehensive picture of the presenting feeding and swallowing issues can be documented for a particular child, enabling optimal assessment and treatment planning, and leading to optimal dysphagia outcomes for each individual.

REFERENCES

Abman SH, Groothius JR (1994) Pathophysiology and treatment of bronchopulmonary dysplasia: current issues. Pediatric Clinics of North America 41(2): 277–315.

Abou-Sleiman PM, Apessos A, Harper JC, et al. (2002) Pregnancy following preimplantation genetic diagnosis for Crouzon syndrome. Molecular Human Reproduction 8(3): 304–9.

Ahearn WH, Kerwin ML, Eicher PS, et al. (1996) An alternating treatments comparison of two intensive interventions for food refusal. Journal of Applied Behaviour Analysis 29(3): 321–32.

Airede KI (1991) Prader-Willi Syndrome: a case report. East African Medical Journal 68(10): 831–7.

Alexander R, Boehme R, Cupps BT (1993) Normal Development of Functional Motor Skills: The First Year of Life. Tucson AZ: Therapy Skill Builders.

Amaya LG, Walker J, Taylor D (1990) Mobius syndrome: a study and report of 18 cases. Binocular Vision 5: 119–32.

Ammaniti M, Ambruzzi AM, Lucarelli L, et al. (2004) Malnutrition and dysfunctional mother-child feeding interactions: Clinical assessment and research implications. Journal of the American College of Nutrition 23(3): 259–71.

Archer LA, Szatmari P (1990) Assessment and treatment of food aversion in a four year old boy: A multidimensional approach. Canadian Journal of Psychiatry 35(6): 501–5.

Armitage EN (1984) Laryngotracheo-oesophageal cleft: a report of three cases. Anaesthesia 39(7): 706–13.

Arvedson JC (1997) Behavioural issues and implications with pediatric feeding disorders. Seminars in Speech and Language 18(1): 51–69.

Arvedson JC, Lefton-Greif MA (1998) Pediatric Videofluoroscopic Swallow Studies. San Antonio TX: Communication Skill Builders.

Arvedson J, Rogers B, Buck G, et al. (1994) Silent aspiration prominent in children with dysphagia. International Journal of Pediatric Otorhinolaryngology 28(2–3): 173–81.

Asher BJ, McGill TJI, Kaplan L, et al. (1990) Airways complications in CHARGE association. Archives of Otolaryngology Head and Neck Surgery 116(5): 594–5.

Bailey DJ, Andres JM, Danek GD, et al. (1987) Lack of efficacy of thickened feeding as treatment for gastroesophageal reflux. Journal of Pediatrics 110(2): 187–9.

Baljosevic I, Subarevic J, Subarevic V, et al. (2002) Surgical tracheotomy in congenital anomalies of the larynx. Srpski Arhiv Za Celokupno Lekartsvo 130: S37–S39.

Barnard KE, Hammond MA, Booth CL, et al. (1989) Measurement and meaning of parent child interaction. In Morrisson F, Lord C, Keating D (eds). Applied Developmental Psychology. New York: Academic Press.

Barton JS, Hindmarsh PC, Scrimgeour CM, Rennie MJ, Preece MA (1994) Energy expenditure in congenital heart disease. Archives of Disease in Childhood 70(1): 5–9.

Baudon JJ, Renault F, Goutet JM, et al. (2002) Motor dysfunction of the upper digestive tract in Pierre Robin sequence as assessed by sucking-swallowing electromyography and esophageal manometry. Journal of Pediatrics 140(6): 719–23.

Bauer ML, Figueroa-Colon R, Georgeson K, et al. (1993) Chronic pulmonary aspiration in children. Southern Medical Journal 86(7): 789–95.

Beck R, Sertie AL, Brik R, et al. (2002) Crouzon syndrome: association with absent pulmonary valve syndrome and severe tracheobronchomalacia. Pediatric Pulmonology 34(6): 478–81.

Benjamin B, Inglis A (1989) Minor congenital laryngeal clefts: diagnosis and classification. Annals of Otology, Rhinology, and Laryngology 98(6): 417–20.

Benjamin B, Walker P (1991) Management of airway obstruction in Pierre Robin. International Journal of Pediatric Otorhinolaryngology 22(1): 29–37.

Berkes B, Sente M (1998) Adult Laryngeal Hemangiomas. Medicinski Pregled 51(11–12): 547–50.

Birch LL, Marlin DW (1982) I don't like it; I never tried it: effects of exposure on two-year-old children's food preferences. Appetite 3(4): 353–60.

Bithoney WG, Dubowitz H (1985) Organic concomitants of non-organic failure to thrive: implications for research. In Drotar D (ed.) New directions in failure to thrive: implications for research and practice. NewYork: Plenum, pp. 47–68.

Blake KD, Russell-Eggitt IM, Morgan DW, et al. (1990) Who's in CHARGE? Multidisciplinary management of patients with CHARGE association. Archives of Disease in Childhood 65(2): 217–23.

Blissett J, Harris G, Kirk J (2000) Growth hormone therapy and feeding problems in growth disorders. Acta Paediatrica 89(6): 644–9.

Blissett J, Harris G, Kirk J (2001) Feeding problems in Silver Russell Syndrome. Developmental Medicine and Child Neurology 43(1): 39–44.

Blissett J, Harris G (2002) A behavioural intervention in a child with feeding problems. Journal of Human Nutrition and Dietetics 15(4): 255–60.

Boas SR, Bloom MD, Bonilla JA (1996) Infantile laryngeal neurofibroma presenting as stridor and dysphagia. Clinical Pediatrics 35(3): 151–3.

Bodensteiner JB, Grunow JE (1984) Gastroparesis in neonatal myotonic dystrophy. Muscle and Nerve 7(6): 486–7.

Bonjardim LR. Gaviao MB, Carmagnani FG, et al. (2003) Signs and symptoms of temperomandibular joint dysfunction in children with primary dentition. Journal of Clinical Pediatric Dentistry 28(1): 53–8.

Bosma JF (1960) Glossopharyngeal respiration as a part of focal seizures of the pharyngeal area in an infant. Acta Paediatrica 49: S56–S61.

Bosma JF (1985) Postnatal ontogeny of performances of the pharynx, larynx, and mouth. American Review of Respiratory Disease 131: S10–S15.

Braddock SR, Lachman RS, Stoppenhagen CC, et al. (1993) Radiological features in Brachmann-de Lange syndrome. American Journal of Medical Genetics 47(7): 1006–13.

Bray GA, Dahms WT, Swerdloff RS, et al. (1983) The Prader-Willi Syndrome: a study of 40 patients and a review of the literature. Medicine 62(2): 59–80.

Brodsky L (1997) Dysphagia with respiratory/pulmonary presentation: assessment and management. Seminars in Speech and Language 18(1): 13–23.

Brodsky L, Volk M (1993) The Airway and Swallowing. In JC Arvedson, L Brodsky (eds) Pediatric Swallowing and Feeding: Assessment and Management. San Diego: Singular Publishing, pp. 93–122.

Brown R, Ogden J (2004) Children's eating attitudes and behaviour: a study of the modelling and control theories of parental influence. Health Education Research 19(3): 261–71.

Bruguier A, Texier P, Clement MC, et al. (1984) Pediatric dermatomyositis: Apropos of 28 cases. Archives Francaises de Pediatrie 41(1): 9–14.

Buckwalter JA, Sasaki CT (1974) Effect of tracheotomy on laryngeal function. Otolaryngologic Clinics of North America 17(1): 41–8.

Budd KS, McGraw TE, Farbisz R, et al. (1992) Psychosocial concomitants of children's feeding disorders. Journal of Pediatric Psychology 17(1): 81–94.

Budden S (1995) Management of Rett syndrome: a ten year experience. Neuropediatrics 26(2): 75–7.

Budden S, Meek F, Henighan C (1990) Communication and oral motor function in Rett syndrome. Developmental Medicine and Child Neurology 32(1): 51–5.

Bull MJ, Fitzgerald JF, Heifetz SA, et al. (1993) Gastrointestinal abnormalities: A significant cause of feeding difficulties and failure to thrive in Brachmann-de Lange Syndrome. American Journal of Medical Genetics 47(7): 1029–34.

Burd RS, Coats RD, Mitchell BS (2001) Nutritional support of the pediatric trauma patient: a practical approach. Respiratory Care Clinics of North America 7(1): 79–96.

Burklow KA, Phelps AN, Schultz JR, et al. (1998) Classifying complex pediatric feeding disorders. Journal of Pediatric Gastroenterology and Nutrition 27(2): 143–7.

Camelo AL, Awad RA, Madrazo A, et al. (1997) Esophageal motility disorders in Mexican patients with Duchenne's muscular dystrophy. Acta Gastroenterologica Latinoamericana 27(3): 119–22.

Caouette-Laberge L, Plamondon C, Larocque Y (1996) Subperiosteal release of the floor of the mouth in Pierre Robin sequence: experience with 12 cases. Cleft Palate Craniofacial Journal 33(6): 468–72.

Carey JC, Hall BD (1978) The Coffin-Siris syndrome. American Journal of Diseases in Children 132: 667–71.

Carr MM, Brodsky L (1999) Severe non-obstructive sleep disturbance as an initial presentation of gastroesophageal reflux disease. International Journal of Pediatric Otorhinolaryngology 51(2): 115–20.

Carr MM, Nguyen A, Nagy M, et al. (2000) Clinical presentation as a guide to the identification of GERD in children. International Journal of Pediatric Otorhinolaryngology 54(1): 27–32.

Carruth B, Skinner J, Nevling W (1993) Eating readiness: reading the cues. Pediatric Basics 63: 2–8.

Carruth B, Skinner J (2002) Feeding behaviors and other motor development in healthy children (2–24 months). Journal of the American College of Nutrition 21(2): 88–96.

Casas MJ, Kenny DJ, McPherson KA (1994) Swallowing/ventilation interactions during oral swallow in normal children and children with cerebral palsy. Dysphagia 9(1): 40–6.

Casas MJ, McPherson KA, Kenny DJ (1995) Durational aspects of oral swallow in neurologically normal children and children with cerebral palsy: an ultrasound investigation. Dysphagia 10(3): 155–9.

Cass H, Reilly S, Owen L, et al. (2003) Findings from a multidisciplinary clinical case series of females with Rett Syndrome. Developmental Medicine and Child Neurology 45(5): 325–37.

Cassidy SB (1992) Prader-Willi syndrome. Journal of Medical Genetics 34(11): 917–23.

Cates M, Billmire DF, Bull MJ, et al. (1989) Gastroesophageal dysfunction in Cornelia de Lange sundrome. Journal of Pediatric Surgery 24(3): 248–50.

Catto-Smith AG, Machida H, Butzner JD, et al. (1991) The role of gastroesophageal reflux in paediatric dysphagia. Journal of Pediatric Gastroenterology and Nutrition 12(2): 159–65.

Charabi B, Bretlau P, Bille M, et al. (2000) Cystic hygroma of the head and neck: a long term follow-up of 44 cases. Acta Oto Laryngologica 543: S248–S250.

Chatoor I, Conley C, Dickson L (1988) Food refusal after an incident of choking: a posttraumatic eating disorder. Journal of American Academy of Child and Adolescent Psychiatry 27(1): 105–10.

Chatoor I, Dickson L, Schaefer S, et al. (1985) A developmental classification of feeding disorders associated with failure to thrive: diagnosis and treatment. In Drotar D (ed.) New directions in failure to thrive: implications for research and practice. New York: Plenum Press, pp. 235–58.

Chatoor I, Egan J, Getson P, et al. (1988) Mother-infant interactions in infantile anorexia nervosa. Journal of the American Academy of Child and Adolescent Pscyhiatry 27(5): 535–40.

Chatoor I, Schaefer S, Dickson L, et al. (1984) Non-organic failure to thrive: a developmental perspective. Pediatric Annals 13(11): 829–43.

Cherney LR, Halper AS (1989) Recovery of oral nutrition after head injury in adults. Journal of Head Trauma Rehabilitation 4(4): 42–50.

Chiappetta AL, Oda AL, Zanoteli E, et al. (2001) Oropharyngeal dysphagia in the myotonic dystrophy: phonoaudiological evaluation and nasofibrolaryngoscopical analysis. Arquivos de Neuro Psiquiatria 59(2): 394–400.

Chigira A, Omoto K, Mukai Y, et al. (1994) Lip closing pressure in disabled children: a comparison with normal children. Dysphagia 9(3): 193–8.

Clemente C, Barnes J, Shinebourne E, et al. (2001) Are infant behavioural feeding difficulties associated with congenital heart disease? Child Care Health and Development 27(1): 47–59.

Cmejrek RC, Coticchia JM, Arnold JE (2002) Presentation, diagnosis and management of deep-neck abscesses in infants. Archives of Otolaryngology and Head and Neck Surgery 128(12): 1361–4.

Coffin GS, Siris E (1970) Mental retardation with absent fifth fingernails and terminal phalanx. American Journal of Diseases in Children 119(5): 433–9.

Cohen MM, Kreiborg S (1992) Upper and lower airway compromise in the Apert syndrome. American Journal of Medical Genetics 44(1): 90–3.

Cohen SR, Thompson JW (1987) Variants of Mobius syndrome and central neurologic impairment-Lindeman procedure in children. Annals of Otology, Rhinology and Laryngology 96(5): 93–100.

Coniglio JU, Manzione JV, Hengerer AS (1988) Anatomic findings and management of the choanal atresia and the CHARGE association. Annals of Otology, Rhinology and Laryngology 97(5): 448–53.

Cormier-Daire V, Wolf C, Munnich A, et al. (1996) Abnormal cholesterol biosynthesis in the Smith-Lemli-Opitz and the lethal acrodysgenital syndromes. European Journal of Pediatrics 155(8): 656–9.

Cox N, Hinkle R (2002) Infant botulism. American Family Physician 65(7): 1388–92.

Craig CM, Lee DN, Freer YN, et al. (1999) Modulations in breathing patterns during intermittent feeding in term infants and infants with bronchopulmonary dysplasia. Developmental Medicine and Child Neurology 41(9): 616–24.

Cruz MJ, Kerschner JE, Beste DJ, et al. (1999) Pierre-Robin sequence: secondary respiratory difficulties and intrinsic feeding abnormalities. Laryngoscope 109(10): 1632–6.

Cucchiara S, Staiano A, Boccieri A, et al. (1990) Effects of cisapride on parameters of oesophageal motility and on the prolonged intraoesophageal pH test in infants with gastro-oesophageal reflux disease. Gut 31(1): 21–5.

Cullen SM, Cronk SE, Pueschel SM, et al. (1981) Social development and feeding milestones of young Down syndrome children. American Journal of Mental Deficiency 85(4): 410–15.

Cunniff C, Kratz LE, Moser A, et al. (1997) The clinical and biochemical spectrum of patients with Smith-Lemli-Opitz syndrome and abnormal cholesterol metabolism. American Journal of Medical Genetics 68(3): 263–9.

Curry CJ, Carey JC, Holland JS, et al. (1987) Smith-Lemli-Opitz syndrome-type II: multiple congenital anomalies with male pseudohermaphroditism and frequent early lethality. American Journal of Medical Genetics 26(1): 45–57.

Dahl M, Sundelin C (1986) Early feeding problems in an affluent society: categories and clinical signs. Acta Paediatrica Scandinavica 75(3): 370–9.

Dalakas MC (1998) Controlled studies with high-dose intravenous immunoglobulin in the treatment of dermatomyositis, inclusion body myositis, and polymyositis. Neurology 51(6): S37–S45.

Darrow DH, Harley CM (1998) Evaluation of swallowing disorders in children. Otolaryngologic Clinics of North America 31(3): 405–18.

Darrow DH, Siemens C (2002) Indications for tonsillectomy and adenoidectomy. Laryngoscope 112(8): 6–10.

Dawes LC, Bova R, Carter P (2002) Retropharyngeal abscess in children. ANZ Journal of Surgery 72(6): 417–20.

Davenport SLH, Hefner MA, Mitchell JA (1986) The spectrum of clinical features in CHARGE syndrome. Clinical Genetics 29(12): 298–310.

Dellert S, Hyams J, Treem W, et al. (1993) Feeding resistance and gastroesophageal reflux in infancy. Journal of Pediatric Gastroenterology and Nutrition 17(1): 66–71.

Desuter GRR, Makhlouf KE, Francois GJ, et al. (2004) Postcricoid hemangioma: an overlooked cause of dysphagia in infants? A case report. Dysphagia 19(1): 48–51.

Dimitropoulos A, Feurer ID, Roof E, et al. (2000) Appetitive behaviour, compulsivity, and neurochemistry in Prader-Willi Syndrome. Mental Retardation and Developmental Disabilities Research Reviews 6(2): 125–30.

Dinwiddie R (2004) Congenital upper airway obstruction. Paediatric Respiratory Reviews 5(1): 17–24.

DiScipio W, Kaslon K, Ruben R (1978) Traumatically acquired conditioned dysphagia in children. Annals of Otology, Rhinology and Laryngology 87(4): 509–14.

Donnai D, Young ID, Owen WG, et al. (1986) The lethal multiple congenital anomaly syndrome of polydactyly, sex reversal, renal hypoplasia, and unilobar lungs. Journal of Medical Genetics 23(1): 64–71.

Dubowitz V (1969) The floppy infant. Clinical Developmental Medicine 31: 65.

Dusick A (2003) Investigation and management of dysphagia. Seminars in Pediatric Neurology 10(4): 255–64.

Ertekin C, Yuceyar N, Aydogdu I, et al. (2001) Electrophysiological evaluation of oropharyngeal swallowing in myotonic dystrophy. Journal of Neurology Neurosurgery and Psychiatry 70(3): 363–71.

Evans KL, Courteney-Harris R, Bailey CM, et al. (1995) Management of posterior laryngeal and laryngotracheoesophageal clefts. Archives of Otolaryngology Head and Neck Surgery 121(12): 1380–5.

Eyman RK, Call TL (1991) Life expectancy of persons with Down syndrome. American Journal of Mental Retardation 95(6): 603–12.

Faroux B, Trang H, Renolleau S, et al. (1992) Respiratory form of myasthenia gravis. Archives Françaises de Pédiatrie 49(7): 633–5.

Feldman R, Keren M, Gross-Rozval O, et al. (2004) Mother-child touch patterns in infant feeding disorders: Relation to maternal, child and environmental factors. Journal of the American Academy of Child, Adolescent Psychiatry 43(9): 1089–97.

Field D, Garland M, Williams K (2003) Correlates of specific childhood feeding problems. Journal of Paediatrics and Child Health 39(4): 299–304.

Field LH, Weiss CJ (1989) Dysphagia with head injury. Brain Injury 3(1): 19–26.

Filippi G (1989) The de Lange syndrome. Report of 15 cases. Clinical Genetics 35(5): 343–63.

Fine G, Ma CK (1985) Alimentary tract. In Kissane JM, Anderson WAD (eds) Anderson's Pathology. St Louis MO: Mosby.

Fischer-Brandies H (1989) Vertical development of the jaw in cases of trisomy 21: Interactions of form and function. Orthodontie Française 60(2): 521–6.

Fitzpatrick PC, Guarisco JL (1999) Posterior laryngeal cleft. Journal of the Louisiana State Medical Society 151(6): 300–3.

Friedman EM, DeJong AL, Sulek M (2001) Pediatric bilateral vocal fold immobility: the role of carbon dioxide laser posterior transverse partial cordectomy. Annals of Otology, Rhinology and Laryngology 110(8): 723–8.

Furkim AM, Behlav MS, Weckx LL (2003) Clinical and videofluoroscopic evaluation of deglutition in children with tetraplegic spastic cerebral palsy. Arq Neuropsiquiatr 61(3): 611–16.

Garofalo-Gomez N, Sardinas-Hernandez NL, Vargas-Diaz J, et al. (2002) Myasthenia gravis in infancy: a report of 12 cases. Revista de Neurologica 34(10): 908–11.

Gewolb IH, Bosma JF, Taciak VL, et al. (2001) Abnormal developmental patterns of suck and swallow rhythms during feeding in preterm infants with bronchopulmonary dysplasia. Developmental Medicine and Child Neurology 43(7): 454–9.

Gewolb IH, Vice FL, Schweitzer-Kenney EL, et al. (2001) Developmental patterns of rhythmic suckle and swallow in preterm infants. Developmental Medicine and Child Neurology 43(1): 22–7.

Gilbert RW, Bryce DP, McIlwain JC, et al. (1987) Management of patients with long-term tracheostomies and aspiration. Annals of Otology, Rhinology and Laryngology 96(5): 561–4.

Gillessen-Kaesbach G, Gross S, Kaya-Westerloh S, et al. (1995) DNA methylation based testing of 450 patients suspected of having Prader-Willi syndrome. Journal of Medical Genetics 32(2): 88–92.

Ginsberg AJ (1988) Feeding disorders in the developmentally disabled population. In Russo DE, Kedesdy JH (eds) Behavioural Medicine with the Developmentally Disabled. New York: Plenum, pp. 21–41.

Gisel EG (1988) Tongue movements in normal 2- to 8-year-old children: Extended profile of an eating assessment. American Journal of Occupational Therapy 42(6): 384–9.

Gisel EG (1990) Effect of food texture on the development of chewing in children 6 months to 2 years of age. Developmental Medicine and Child Neurology 33(1): 69–79.

Gisel EG, Birnbaum R, Schwartz S (1998) Feeding impairments in children: Diagnosis and effective intervention. International Journal of Orofacial Myology 24: 27–33.

Gisel EG, Lange LJ, Niman CW (1984a) Tongue movements in 4- and 5-year-old Down's syndrome children during eating: a comparison with normal children. American Journal of Occupational Therapy 38(10): 660–5.

Gisel EG, Lange LJ, Niman CW (1984b) Chewing cycles in 4- and 5-year-old Down's syndrome children: a comparison of eating efficacy with normals. American Journal of Occupational Therapy 38(10): 666–70.

Gisel EG, Tessier MJ, Lapierre G, et al. (2003) Feeding management of children with severe cerebral palsy and eating impairment: an exploratory study. Physical Occupational Therapy Pediatrics 23(2): 19–44.

Glenny A, Hooper L, Shaw W, et al. (2004) Feeding interventions for growth and development in infants with cleft lip, cleft palate or cleft lip and palate. Cochrane Database of Systematic Reviews (Issue 3), Art. no. CD003315.DOI:10.1002/14651858.CD00315.pub2.

Goldsmith MM, Strope GL, Postma DS (1987) Presentation and management of postcricoid hemangiomata in infancy. Laryngoscope 97(7): 851–3.

Green JR, Moore CA, Ruark JL, et al. (1997) Development of Chewing in Children from 12 to 48 Months: Longitudinal Study of EMG Patterns. Journal of Neurophysiology 77(5): 2704–16.

Greer RD, Dorow L, Williams G, et al. (1991) Peer-mediated procedures to induce swallowing and food acceptance in young children. Journal of Applied Behaviour Analysis 24(4): 348–58.

Gross RD, Mahlmann J, Grayhack JP (2003) Physiologic effects of open and closed tracheostomy tubes on the pharyngeal swallow. Annals of Otology, Rhinology and Laryngology 112(2): 143–52.

Gurnett CA, Bodnar JA, Neil J, et al. (2004) Congenital myasthenic syndrome: presentation, electrodiagnosis and muscle biopsy. Journal of Child Neurology 19(3): 175–82.

Hagberg B (1985) Rett's syndrome: Prevalence and impact on progressive severe mental retardation in girls. Acta Paediatrica Scandinavia 74: 405–8.

Haig D, Wharton R (2003) Prader-Willi syndrome and the evolution of human childhood. American Journal of Human Biology 15(3): 320–9.

Halper AS, Cherney LR, Cichowski K, et al. (1999) Dysphagia after head trauma: the effect of cognitive-communicative impairments on functional outcomes. Journal of Head Trauma Rehabilitation 14(5): 486–96.

Harris G, Booth IW (1992) The nature and management of eating problems in pre-school children. In Cooper PK, Stein A (eds) Feeding Problems and Eating Disorders in Children and Adolescents. Chur: Harwood Academic Publishers, pp. 61–85.

Harris G, MacDonald A (1992) Behavioural feeding problems in cystic fibrosis. Pediatric Pulmonology 8: 324.

Hart ZH, Jaslow RJ, Gomez MR (1965) The De Lange Syndrome. American Journal of Diseases in Children 109: 325.

Haslam RHA (1979) Facial diplegia, congenital. In Bergsma D (ed.) Birth Defects Compendium (2nd edn). National Foundation. March of Dimes, New York: Alar, R Liss.

Hawley PP, Jackson LG, Kurnit DM (1985) Sixty-four patients with Brachmann-de Lange Syndrome: A survey. American Journal of Medical Genetics 20(3): 453.

Helfrich-Miller KR, Rector KL, Straka JA (1986) Dysphagia: Its treatment in the profoundly retarded patient with cerebral palsy. Archives of Physical Medicine and Rehabilitation 67(8): 520–5.

Herbst JJ (1983) Development of suck and swallow. Journal of Pediatric Gastroenterology and Nutrition 2: S131–S135.

Hisa Y, Tatemoto K, Toyoda K, et al. (1989) A case of congenital laryngeal web with subglottic stenosis. Nippon Jibiinkoka Gakkai Kaiho 92(9): 1394–8.

Hislop AA (1997) Bronchopulmonary dysplasia: pre- and postnatal influences and outcome. Pediatric Pulmonology 23(2): 71–5.

Hofner G, Behrens R, Koch A, et al. (2000) Enteral nutritional support by percutaneous endoscopic gastrostomy in children with congenital heart disease. Pediatric Cardiology 21(4): 341–6.

Hollinger LD (1982) Treatment of severe subglottic stenosis without tracheostomy: a preliminary report. Annals of Otology, Rhinology and Laryngology 91: 407–12.

Howard RB, Herbold NH (1982) Nutrition in Clinical Care. 2nd edn. New York: McGraw-Hill.

Huckabee ML, Cannito MP (1999) Outcomes of swallowing rehabilitation in chronic brainstem dysphagia: A retrospective evaluation. Dysphagia 14(2): 93–109.

Hulsmann AR, Van den Anker JN (1997) Evolution and natural history of chronic lung disease of prematurity. Monaldi Archives of Chest Disease 52(3): 272–7.

Hyman PE (1994) Gastroesophageal reflux: One reason why baby won't eat. Journal of Pediatrics 125(6): 103–9.

Ida S (2004) Evaluation and treatment of gastroesophageal reflux in infants and children. Nippon Rinsho 62(8): 1553–8.

Illingworth RS, Lister LJ (1964) The critical or sensitive period, with special reference to certain feeding problems in infants and children. Journal of Pediatrics 65: 839–48.

Jackson M, Poskitt EM (1991) The effects of high-energy feeding on energy balance and growth in infants with congenital heart disease and failure to thrive. British Journal of Nutrition 65(2): 131–43.

Johnson DB, Cheney C, Monsen ER (1998) Nutrition and feeding in infants with bronchopulmonary dysplasia after initial hospital discharge: risk factors for growth failure. Journal of the American Dietetics Association 98(6): 649–56.

Jolley SG, McClelland KK, Mosesso-Rousseau M (1995) Pharyngeal and swallowing disorders in infants. Seminars in Pediatric Surgery 4(3): 157–65.

Kardon DE, Wenig BM, Heffner DK, et al. (2000) Tonsillar lymphangiomatous polyps: A clinicopathologic series of 26 cases. Modern Pathology 13(10): 1128–33.

Kaufman FL (1991) Managing the cleft lip and palate patient. Pediatric Clinics of North America 38(5): 1127–47.

Kawahara H, Dent J, Davidson G (1997) Mechanisms responsible for gastroesophageal reflux in children. Gastroenterology 113(2): 399–408.

Kelley RI, Hennekam RC (2000) The Smith-Lemli-Opitz syndrome. Journal of Medical Genetics 37(5): 321–35.

Kelly CP, Isaacman DJ (2002) Group B streptococcal retropharyngeal cellulitis in a young infant: A case report and review of the literature. Journal of Emergency Medicine 23(2): 179–82.

Kennedy CA, Heimbach M, Rimmell FL (2000) Diagnosis and determination of the clinical significance of type 1A laryngeal clefts by gelfoam injection. Annals of Otology, Rhinology, and Laryngology 109(11): 991–5.

Kenny DJ, Casas MJ, McPherson KA (1989) Correlations of ultrasound imaging of oral swallow with ventilatory alterations in cerebral palsied and normal children: Preliminary observations. Dysphagia 4(2): 112–17.

Keng WT, Cole T, Pilz D, et al. (2002) Food aversion and facial dysmorphism: a newly described syndrome? Clinical Dysmorphology 11(4): 249–53.

Khan MA, Hameed A, Choudhry AJ (2004) Management of foreign bodies in the esophagus. Journal of the College of Physicians Surg Pak 14(4): 218–20.

Kohda E, Hisazumi H, Hiramatsu K (1994) Swallowing dysfunction and aspiration in neonates and infants. Acta Otolaryngol 517: 11–16.

Koenigsberger MR, Pascual JM (2002) Neonatal myasthenic syndromes. Revista de Neurologica 34(1): 47–51.

Kosko JR, Moser D, Erhart N, et al. (1998) Differential diagnosis of dysphagia in children. Otolaryngologic Clinics of North America 31(8): 435–51.

Kovesi T, Rubin S (2004) Long-term complications of congenital esophageal atresia and/or tracheoesophageal fistula. Chest 126(3): 915–25.

Kramer S (1985) Special swallowing problems in children. Gastrointestinal Radiology 10(3): 241–50.

Kramer S, Monahan-Eicher P (1993) The evaluation of pediatric feeding abnormalities. Dysphagia 8(3): 215–24.

Krishna S, Puri V (2001) Infant botulism: case reports and review. Journal of the Kentucky Medical Association 99(4): 143–6.

Krishnamoorthy M, Mintz A, Liem T, et al. (1994) Diagnosis and treatment of respiratory symptoms of initially unsuspected gastroesophageal reflux in infants. Am Surg 60: 783–5.

Kumar D, Blank CE, Griffiths BL (1985) Cornelia de Lange Syndrome in several members of the same family. Journal of Medical Genetics 22(4): 296–300.

Kurzner SI, Garg M, Bautista DB, et al. (1988) Growth failure in infants with bronchopulmonary dysplasia: nutrition and elevated resting metabolic expenditure. Pediatrics 81(3): 379–84.

Lachman R, Funamura J, Szalay G (1981) Gastrointestinal abnormalities in the Cornelia de Lange syndrome. Mt. Sinai Journal of Medicine 48: 236–40.

Lambert JM, Watters NE (1998) Breastfeeding the infant/child with a cardiac defect: an informal survey. Journal of Human Lactation 14(2): 151–5.

Lancaster JL, Hanafi Z, Jackson SR (1999) Adult presentation of a tracheoesophageal fistula with co-existing laryngeal cleft. Journal of Laryngology and Otology 113(5): 469–72.

Lau C, Hurst N (1999) Oral feeding in infants. Current Problems in Pediatrics 29(4): 105–24.

Lee SW, Fang TJ, Hsu CW, et al. (2003) Microfibrillar collagen for hemostasis in laryngomicrosurgery of hypopharyngeal hemangioma. Chang Gung Medical Journal 26(1): 65–9.

Lee SS, Schwartz RH, Bahadori RS (2001) Retropharyngeal abscess: epiglottitis of the new millennium. Journal of Pediatrics 138(3): 435–7.

Li H-Y, Lo L-J, Chen K-S, Wong K-S, Chang K-P (2002) Robin sequence: review of treatment modalities for airway obstruction in 110 cases. International Journal of Pediatric Otorhinolaryngology 65(1): 45–51.

Lifschitz MH, Seilheimer DK, Wilson GS, et al. (1987) Neurodevelopmental status of low birth weight infants with bronchopulmonary dysplasia requiring prolonged oxygen supplementation. Journal of Perinatology 7(2): 127–32.

Limbrock GJ, Fischer-Brandies H, Avalle C (1991) Castillo-Morale's oro-facial therapy: treatment of 67 children with Down Syndrome. Developmental Medicine and Child Neurology 33(4): 296–303.

Lin AE, Ardinger HH, Ardinger RHJ, et al. (1997) Cardiovascular malformations in Smith-Lemli-Opitz syndrome. American Journal of Medical Genetics 68(3): 270–8.

Lindgren AC, Barkeling B, Hagg A, et al. (2000) Eating behaviour in Prader-Willi syndrome, normal weight, and obese control groups. Journal of Pediatrics 137(1): 50–5.

Linscheid TR (1992) Eating problems in children. In CE Walker, MC Roberts (eds) Handbook of clinical child psychology (pp. 451–73). New York: Wiley.

Lobo ML (1990) Parent-infant interaction during feeding when the infant has congenital heart disease. Journal of Pediatric Nursing 7(2): 97–105.

Lobo ML, Michel Y (1995) Behavioral and physiological response during feeding in infants with congenital heart disease: a naturalistic study. Progress in Cardiovascular Nursing 10(3): 26–34.

Loughlin GM (1989) Respiratory consequences of dysfunctional swallowing and aspiration. Dysphagia 3(3): 126–30.

Loughlin GM, Lefton-Greif MA (1994) Dysfunctional swallowing and respiratory disease in children. Advances in Pediatrics 41: 135–62.

Logemann JA, Pepe J, Mackay LE (1994) Disorders of nutrition and swallowing: Intervention strategies in the trauma center. Journal of Head Trauma Rehabilitation 9(1): 43–56.

Lucaya J, Garcia-Conesa A, Bosch-Banyeras JM, et al. (1981) The Coffin-Siris syndrome: a report of four cases and a review of the literature. Pediatric Radiology 11(1): 35–8.

Marcon M, Briani C, Ermani M, et al. (1998) Positive correlation of CTG expansion and pharyngoesophageal alterations in myotonic dystrophy. Italian Journal of Neurological Sciences 19(2): 75–80.

MacDonald A, Harris G, Rylance G, et al. (1997) Abnormal feeding behaviours in phenylketonuria. Journal of Human Nutrition and Dietetics 10: 163–70.

MacDonald A, Holden C, Harris G (1991) Nutritional strategies in cystic fibrosis: Current issues. Journal of the Royal Society of Medicine 18(84): 28–35.

Macie D, Arvedson J (1993). Tone and Positioning. In Arvedson JC, Brodsky L (eds) Pediatric Swallowing and Feeding. San Diego CA: Singular, pp. 209–48.

Mackay LE, Morgan AS, Bernstein BA (1999) Swallowing disorders in severe brain injury: risk factors affecting return to oral intake. Archives of Physical Medicine and Rehabilitation 80(4): 365–71.

Marie I, Hachulla E, Levesque H, et al. (1999) Intravenous immunoglobulins as treatment of life threatening esophageal involvement in polymyositis and dermatomyositis. Journal of Rheumatology 26(12): 2706–9.

Marques IL, DeSousa TV, Carniero AF, et al. (2001) Clinical experience with infants with Robin sequence: A prospective study. Cleft Palate-Craniofacial Journal 38(2): 171–8.

Martin RJ, Pridham KF (1992) Early experiences of parents feeding their infants with bronchopulmonary dysplasia. Neonatal Network 11(3): 23–9.

Mathisen B, Worrall L, Masel J, et al. (1999) Feeding problems in infants with gastro-oesophageal reflux disease: a controlled study. Journal of Paediatric Child Health 35(2): 163–9.

Mayer EA, Gebhart GF (1994) Basic and clinical aspects of visceral hyperalgesia. Gastroenterology 107(1): 271–93.

Mbakop A, Fouda-Onana A, Bengono G, et al. (1991) Laryngeal papillomatosis in Cameroon (Central Africa): Anatomical aspects. Annales d'oto Laryngologie et de Chirurgie Cervico Faciale 108(8): 484–6.

McColley SA, Carroll JL (1994) Pulmonary complications of impaired swallowing. In Tuchman DN, Walter RS (eds) Disorders of Feeding and Swallowing in Infants and Children: Pathophysiology, Diagnosis and Treatment. San Diego, California: Singular, pp. 209–29.

McCreery KM, Hussein MA, Lee AG, et al. (2002) Major review: the clinical spectrum of pediatric myasthenia gravis: Blepharoptosis, ophthalmoplegia and strabismus. Binocular Vision and Strabismus Quarterly 17(3): 181–6.

McElhinney DB, Jacobs I, McDonald-McGinn DM, et al. (2002) Chromosomal and cardiovascular anomalies associated with congenital laryngeal web. International Journal of Pediatric Otorhinolaryngology 66(1): 23–7.

McGhee EM, Klump CJ, Bitts SM, et al. (2000) Candidate region for Coffin-Siris syndrome. American Journal of Medical Genetics 93(3): 241–3.

McLean DE, Kaitz SE, Keenan CJ, et al. (1995) Medical and surgical complications of pediatric brain injury. Journal of Head Trauma Rehabilitation 10(5): 1–12.

McMaster P, Piper S, Schell D, et al. (2000) Journal of Paediatrics and Child Health 36(6): 596–7.

McPherson KA, Kenny DJ, Koheil R, et al. (1992) Ventilation and swallowing interaction of normal children and children with cerebral palsy. Developmental Medicine and Child Neurology 34(7): 577–88.

Mercado-Deane M-G, Burton EM, Harlow SA, et al. (2001) Swallowing dysfunction in infants less than 1 year of age. Pediatric Radiology 31(6): 423–8.

Metheny JA (1978) Dermatomyositis: a vocal and swallowing disease entity. Laryngoscope 88(1): 147–61.

Meyerson MD, Foushee DP (1978) Speech, language and hearing in Mobius syndrome: a study of 22 patients. Developmental Medicine and Child Neurology 20(3): 357–65.

Michaud LJ, Duhaime A-C, Batshaw ML (1993) Traumatic brain injury in children. Pediatric Clinics of North America 40(3): 553–65.

Milczuk HA, Smith JD, Everts EC (2000) Congenital laryngeal webs: surgical management and clinical embryology. International Journal of Pediatric Otorhinolaryngology 52(1): 1–9.

Miller RM, Groher ME (1997) General treatment of neurologic swallowing disorders. In Groher ME (ed.) Dysphagia: Diagnosis and Management. Boston: Butterworth-Heinemann, pp. 223–43.

Minde K, Minde R (1986) Infant Psychiatry: An Introductory Text. London: Sage.

Morgan AS (1992) Risk factors for infection in the trauma patient. Journal of National Medical Association 84(12): 1019–23.

Morgan AS (1994) The trauma center as a continuum of care for persons with severe brain injury. Journal of Head Trauma Rehabilitation 9(1): 1–10.

Morgan AT, Ward E, Murdoch B, et al. (2002) Acute characteristics of pediatric dysphagia subsequent to traumatic brain injury: videofluoroscopic assessment. Journal of Head Trauma Rehabilitation 17(3): 220–41.

Morgan AT, Ward E, Murdoch B, et al. (2003) Incidence, characteristics, and predictive factors for dysphagia after pediatric traumatic brain injury. Journal of Head Trauma Rehabilitation 18(3): 239–51.

Morgan AT, Ward E, Murdoch BE (2004a). Acute clinical characteristics of paediatric dysphagia following traumatic brain injury. Journal of Head Trauma Rehabilitation 19(3): 226–40.

Morgan AT, Ward E, Murdoch B (2004b) Clinical progression and outcome of dysphagia following paediatric traumatic brain injury: a prospective study. Brain Injury 18(4): 359–76.

Morgan AT, Ward E, Murdoch B (2004c) A case study of the resolution of paediatric dysphagia following brainstem injury: clinical and instrumental assessment. Journal of Clinical Neuroscience 11(2): 182–90.

Morgan D, Bailey M, Phelps P, et al. (1992) Ear-Nose-Throat Abnormalities in the CHARGE association. Archives of Otolaryngology Head and Neck Surgery 119(1): 49–54.

Morris SE (1982). The Normal Acquisition of Oral Feeding Skills: Implications for Assessment and Treatment. New York: Therapeutic Media Inc.

Morris SE (1989) Development of oral-motor skills in the neurologically impaired child receiving non-oral feedings. Dysphagia 3(3): 135–54.

Morris SE, Klein MD (1987). Pre-feeding Skills. Tucson AZ: Therapy Skill Builders.

Morton RE, Bonas R, Minford J, et al. (1997) Feeding ability in Rett syndrome. Developmental Medicine and Child Neurology 39(5): 331–5.

Morton RE, Bonas R, Minford J, et al. (1997) Respiration patterns during feeding in Rett syndrome. Developmental Medicine and Child Neurology 39(9): 596–606.

Morton RE, Wheatley R, Minford J (1999) Respiratory tract infections due to direct and reflux aspiration in children with severe neurodisability. Developmental Medicine and Child Neurology 41(5): 329–34.

Motil KJ, Schultz RJ, Browning K, et al. (1999) Oropharyngeal dysfunction and gastroesophaeal dysmotility are present in girls and women with Rett Syndrome. Journal of Pediatric Gastroenterology and Nutrition 29(1): 31–7.

Motion S, Northstone K, Emond A, et al. (2002) Early feeding problems in children with cerebral palsy: weight and neurodevelopmental outcomes. Developmental Medicine and Child Neurology 44(1): 40–3.

Munro FD (2003) Dysphagia in children: a paediatric surgical perspective. International Journal of Pediatric Otorhinolaryngology 67: S103–S105.

Nash M (1988) Swallowing problems in the tracheotomized patient. Otolaryngological Clinics of North America 21(4): 701–9.

Newman L (2000) Optimal care patterns in paediatric patients with dysphagia. Seminars in Speech and Language 21(4): 281–91.

Noerr B (2003) Current controversies in the understanding of necrotizing enterocolitis. Advances in Neonatal Care 3(3): 107–20.

Nowaczyk MJM, Waye JS (2001) The Smith-Lemli-Optiz syndrome: a novel metabolic way of understanding developmental biology, embryogenesis, and dysmorphology. Clinical Genetics 59(6): 375–86.

Nwokoro NA, Mulvihill JJ (1997) Cholesterol and bile acid replacement therapy in children and adults with Smith-Lemli-Opitz syndrome. American Journal of Medical Genetics 68(3): 315–21.

Odman C, Kiliaridis S (1996) Masticatory muscle activity in myotonic dystrophy patients. Journal of Oral Rehabilitation 23(1): 5–10.

Oley CA, Baraitser M, Grant DB (1988) A reappraisal of CHARGE association. Journal of Medical Genetics 25(3): 147–56.

Oliver RG, Jones G (1997) Neonatal feeding of infants born with cleft lip and/or palate: Parental perceptions of their experience in South Wales. Cleft Palate Craniofacial Journal 34(6): 526–32.

Orenstein SR, Magill HL, Brooks P (1987) Thickening of infant feedings for therapy of gastroesophageal reflux. The Journal of Pediatrics 110(2): 181–6.

Orenstein SR, Orenstein DM (1988) Gastroesophageal reflux and respiratory disease in children. Journal of Pediatrics 112(6): 847–58.

Orenstein SR, Putnam PE, Shalaby TM, et al. (1994) Symptoms of infantile reflux esophagitis using validated techniques for symptoms and histopathology [Abstract]. Gastroenterology 106: A153.

Orenstein SR, Shalaby TM, Cohn JF (1995) Reflux symptoms in 100 normal infants: Diagnostic validity of the infant gastroesophageal reflux questionnaire. Clinical Pediatrics 35(12): 607–14.

Orenstein S, Shalaby T, Putnam P (1992) Thickened feedings as a cause of increased coughing when used as therapy for gastroesophageal reflux in infants. Journal of Pediatrics 121(6): 913–15.

O'Reilly MFO, Lancioni GE (2001) Treating food refusal in a child with Williams syndrome using the parent as therapist in the home setting. Journal of Intellectual Disability Research 45(1): 41–6.

Osborne TE, Haller JA, Levin LS, et al. (1991) Submandibular cystic hygroma resembling a plunging ranula in a neonate: review and report of a case. Oral Surgery, Oral Medicine and Oral Pathology 71(1): 16–20.

Ouoba K, Diop EM, Diouf R, et al. (1994) Retropharyngeal abscess: 6 case reports. Medecine Tropicale Revue du Corps de Sante Colonial 54(2): 149–51.

Palmer S (1978) Down's syndrome. In Palmer S, Ekvall S (eds) Pediatric Nutrition in Developmental Disorders. Springfield IL: Charles C. Thomas, pp. 223–43.

Palmer S, Thompson RJ, Linscheid TR (1975) Applied behaviour analysis in the treatment of childhood feeding problems. Developmental Medicine and Child Neurology 17(3): 333–9.

Pandya AN, Boorman JG (2001) Failure to thrive in babies with cleft lip and palate. British Journal of Plastic Surgery 54(6): 471–5.

Papargyriou G, Kjellberg H, Kiliaridis S (2000) Changes in masticatory mandibular movements in growing individuals: a six-years follow-up. Acta Odontologica Scandinavica 58(3): 129–34.

Papazian O (1992) Transient neonatal myasthenia gravis. Journal of Child Neurology 7(2): 135–41.

Parkinson KN, Wright CM, Drewett RF (2004) Mealtime energy intake and feeding behaviour in children who fail to thrive: a population-based case-control study. Journal of Child Psychology and Psychiatry 45(5): 1030–5.

Penarrocha M, Bagan JV, Vilchez J, et al. (1990) Oral alterations in Steinert's myotonic dystrophy: a presentation of two cases. oral surgery, oral medicine, and oral pathology 69(6): 698–700.

Perlman AL (1999) Dysphagia: populations at risk and methods of diagnosis. Nutrition in Clinical Practice 14: 2–9.

Peruzzi WT, Logemann JA, Currie D, et al. (2001) Assessment of aspiration in patients with tracheostomies: Comparison of the bedside colored dye assessment with videofluoroscopic examination. Respiratory Care 463: 243–7.

Peterson-Falzone SJ, Pruzansky S, Parris PJ, et al. (1981) Nasopharyngeal dysmorphology in the syndromes of Apert and Crouzon. Cleft Palate Journal 18(4): 237–50.

Pinder GL, Faherty AS (1999) Issues in pediatric feeding and swallowing. In Caruso A, Strand E (eds) Clinical Management of Motor Speech Disorders in Children. New York: Thieme Medical Publishers, pp. 281–318.

Potsic WP, Wetmore RF (1990) Sleep disorders and airway obstruction in children. Otolaryngologic Clinics of North America 23(4): 651–63.

Potsic WP, Wetmore RF (1992) Practical aspects of managing the child with apnea. Journal of Otolaryngology 21(6): 429–33.

Prasad C, Marles S, Prasad AN, et al. (2002) Smith-Lemli-Opitz syndrome: New mutation with a mild phenotype. American Journal of Medical Genetics 108(1): 64–8.

Pridham KF, Martin R, Sondel S, et al. (1989) Parental issues in feeding young children with bronchopulmonary dysplasia. Journal of Pediatric Nursing 4(3): 177–85.

Putet G (1993) Energy. In Tsang RC, Lucas A, Uany R, et al. (eds) Nutritional needs of the preterm infant. Baltimore MD: Williams & Wilkins, pp. 15–28.

Putnam PE (1997) Gastroesophageal reflux disease and dysphagia in children. Seminars in Speech and Language 18(1): 25–37.

Qazi QH, Heckman LS, Markouizos D, et al. (1990) The Coffin-Siris syndrome. Journal of Medical Genetics 27(5): 333–6.

Qureshi MA, Vice FL, Taciak VL, et al. (2002) Changes in rhythmic suckle feeding patterns in term infants in the first month of life. Developmental Medicine and Child Neurology 44(1): 34–9.

Raidoo DM, Rocke DA, Brock-Utne JG, et al. (1990) Critical volume for pulmonary acid aspiration: reappraisal in a primate model. British Journal of Anesthesia 65(2): 248–50.

Ravid S, Maytal J, Eviatar L (2000) Biphasic course of infant botulism. Pediatric Neurology 23(4): 338–9.

Redford-Badwal DA, Mabry K, Frassinelli JD (2003) Impact of cleft lip and/or palate on nutritional health and oral-motor development. Dental Clinics of North America 47(2): 305–17.

Reed GK, Piazza CC, Patel MR, et al. (2004) On the relative contributions of non-contingent reinforcement and escape extinction in the treatment of food refusal. Journal of Applied Behaviour Analysis 37(1): 27–42.

Regev RH, Lusky A, Dolfin T, et al. (2003) Excess mortality and morbidity among small-for-gestational-age premature infants: a population-based study. Journal of Pediatrics 143(2): 186–91.

Reilly S, Carr L (2001) Foreign body ingestion in children with severe developmental disabilities: a case study. Dysphagia 16(1): 68–73.

Reilly S, Cass H (2001) Growth and nutrition in Rett syndrome. Disability and Rehabilitation 23(3–4): 118–28.

Reilly S, Skuse D (1992) Characteristics and management of feeding problems of young children with cerebral palsy. Developmental Medicine and Child Neurology 34(5): 379–88.

Reilly S, Skuse D, Poblete X (1996) Prevalence of feeding problems and oral motor dysfunction in children with cerebral palsy: a community survey. Journal of Pediatrics 129(6): 877–82.

Renault F, Flores-Guevara R, Soupre V, et al. (2000) Neurophysiological brainstem investigations in isolated Pierre Robin sequence. Early Human Development 58: 141–52.

Ricciardelli EJ, Richardson MA (1991) Cervicofacial cystic hygroma: patterns of recurrence and management of the difficult case. Archives of Otolaryngology Head and Neck Surgery 117(5): 546–53.

Rizos M, Negron RJ, Serman, N (1998) Mobius syndrome with dental involvement: a case report and literature review. Cleft Palate-Craniofacial Journal 35(3): 262–7.

Robin P (1923) La chute de la base de la langue consideree comme une nouvelle cause de gene dans la respiration naso-pharyngienne. Bull Acad Med Paris 89: 37–41.

Rode H, Millar AJ, Brown RA, et al. (1992) Reflux strictures of the esophagus in children. Journal of Pediatric Surgery 27(4): 462–5.

Rogers B (2004) Feeding method and health outcomes of children with Cerebral Palsy. The Journal of Pediatrics 145: S28–S30.

Rogers B, Arvedson J, Buck G, et al. (1994) Characteristics of dysphagia in children with cerebral palsy. Dysphagia 9(1): 69–73.

Rogers BT, Arvedson J, Msall M, et al. (1993) Hypoxemia during oral feeding of children with severe cerebral palsy. Developmental Medicine and Child Neurology 35(1): 3–10.

Romero R, Chaiworapongsa T, Espinoza J (2003) Micronutrients and intrauterine infection, preterm birth and the fetal inflammatory response syndrome. Journal of Nutrition 133(5): S1668–1673.

Rosenbek JC, Robbins JA, Roecker EB, et al. (1996) A penetration-aspiration scale. Dysphagia 11(2): 93–8.

Rosingh HJ, Peek SHG (1999) Swallowing and speech in infants following tracheotomy. Acta-oto-rhino-laryngologica belgica 53(1): 59–63.

Rowe LA (1999) Case studies in dysphagia after pediatric brain injury. Journal of Head Trauma Rehabilitation 14(5): 497–504.

Rozsasi A, Neagos A, Nolte F, et al. (2003) Critical analysis of complications and disorder in wound healing after tracheostomy in children. Laryngorhinootologic 82(12): 826–32.

Ryan AK, Bartlett K, Clayton P, et al. (1998) Smith-Lemli-Opitz syndrome: a variable clinical and biochemical phenotype. Journal of Medical Genetics 35(7): 558–65.

Saito Y, Honda H, Matsuoka Y (1995) Prognosis for myotonic dystrophy. Clinical Neurology 35(12): 1489–91.

Salvado A, Rodriguez K, Guarisco JL (2003) Hemifacial microsomia. Journal of the Louisiana State Medical Society 155(3): 136–41.

Sartoretti C, Sartoretti S, DeLorenzi D, et al. (1996) Intestinal non-rotation and pseudoobstruction in myotonic dystrophy: case report and review of the literature. International Journal of Colorectal Disease 11(1): 10–14.

Satter EM (1990) The feeding relationship: problems and interventions. Journal of Pediatrics 117(2): 181–9.

Schaefer RB, Stadler, JA, Gosain AK (2004) To distract or not to distract: an algorithm for airway management in isolated Pierre Robin sequence: An algorithm for airway management in isolated Pierre Robin sequence. Plastic Reconstructive Surgery 113(4): 1113–25.

Schinzel A (1979) The Coffin-Siris syndrome. Acta Paediatrica Scandinavia 68(3): 449–52.

Scheid SC, Spector AR, Luft JD (2002) Tracheal cartilaginous sleeve in Crouzon syndrome. International Journal of Pediatric Otorhinolaryngology 65(2): 147–52.

Schwaab LM, Niman CW, Gisel EG (1986) Tongue movements in normal 2-, 3-, and 4-year old children: a continuation study. American Journal of Occupational Therapy 40(3): 180–5.

Schwarz SM, Corredor J, Fisher-Medina J, et al. (2001) Diagnosis and treatment of feeding disorders in children with developmental disabilities. Pediatrics 108(3): 671–6.

Schurr MJ, Ebner KA, Maser AL, et al. (1999) Formal swallowing evaluation and therapy after traumatic brain injury improves dysphagia outcomes. Journal of Trauma 46(5): 817–21.

Shaker R, Milbraith M, Junlong R, et al. (1995) Deglutitive aspiration in patients with tracheostomy: Effect of tracheostomy on the duration of vocal cord closure. Gastroenterology 108(5): 1357–60.

Sheckman-Alper B, Manno CJ (1996) Dysphagia in infants and children with oral-motor deficits: Assessment and management. Seminars in Speech and Language 17(4): 283–309.

Shepherd R, Wren J, Evans S, et al. (1987) Gastroesophageal reflux in children: clinical profile, course and outcomes with active therapy in 126 cases. Clinical Pediatrics 26(2): 55–60.

Sher AE (1992) Mechanisms of airway obstruction in Robin sequence: Implications for treatment. Cleft Palate-Craniofacial Journal 29(3): 224–31.

Sherer DM, Anyaegbunam A, Onyeije C (1998) Antepartum fetal intracranial hemorrhage, predisposing factors and prenatal sonography: a review. American Journal of Perinatology 15(7): 431–41.

Shiao SY, Brooker J, DiFiore T (1996) Desaturation events during oral feedings with and without a nasogastric tube in very low birth weight infants. Heart Lung 25(3): 236–45.

Shprintzen RJ (1992) The implication of the diagnosis of Robin sequence. Cleft Palate Craniofacial Journal 29(3): 205–9.

Shreiner RL, McAlister WH, Marshall RW, et al. (1973) Stickler syndrome in a pedigree of Pierre Robin syndrome. American Journal of Diseases in Children 126: 86–90.

Singer L, Davillier M, Preuss L, et al. (1996) Feeding interactions in infants with very low birth weight and bronchopulmonary dysplasia. Journal of Development and Behavioural Pediatrics 17(2): 69–76.

Singer L, Martin RJ, Hawkins SW, et al. (1992) Oxygen desaturation complicates feeding in infants with bronchopulmonary dyplasia after discharge. Pediatrics 90(3): 380–4.

Sjogreen L, Andersson-Norinder J, Jacobson C (2001) Development of speech, feeding, eating, and facial expression on Mobius sequence. International Journal of Pediatric Otorhinolaryngology 60: 197–204.

Skuse D (1993) Identification and management of problem eaters. Archives of Disease in Childhood 69(5): 604–8.

Smith DW, Lemli L, Optiz A (1964) A newly recognized syndrome of multiple congenital anomalies. Journal of Pediatrics 64: 210–17.

Spender Q, Dennis J, Stein A, et al. (1995) Impaired oral-motor function in children with Down's syndrome: a study of three twin pairs. European Journal of Disorders of Communication 30(1): 77–87.

Spender Q, Stein A, Dennis J, et al. (1996) An exploration of feeding difficulties in children with Down Syndrome. Developmental Medicine and Child Neurology 38(8): 681–94.

St Guily JL, Perie S, Willig TN, et al. (1994) Swallowing disorders in muscular diseases: Functional assessment and indications of cricopharyngeal myotomy. Ear Nose and Throat 73(1): 34–40.

Stevenson RD, Allaire JH (1991) The development of normal feeding and swallowing. Pediatric Clinics of North America 38(6): 1439–453.

Stewart KB, Meyer L (2004) Parent-child interactions and everyday routines in young children with failure to thrive. American Journal of Occupational Therapy 58(3): 342–6.

Stoelhorst GM, Rijken M, Martens SE, et al. (2003) Developmental outcome at 18 and 24 months of age in very preterm children: a cohort study from 1996 to 1997. Early Human Development 72(2): 83–95.

Stolovitz P, Gisel EG (1991) Circumoral movements in response to three different food textures in children 6 months to two years of age. Dysphagia 6(1): 17–25.

Stromland J, Sjogreen L, Miller M, et al. (2002) Mobius sequence: a Swedish multidiscipline study. European Journal of Paediatric Neurology 6(1): 35–45.

Sugarman-Isaacs J, Murdock M, Lane J, et al. (2003) Eating difficulties in girls with Rett syndrome compared with other developmental disabilities. Journal of the American Dietetic Association 103(2): 224–30.

Sullivan PB (1997) Gastrointestinal problems in the neurologically impaired child. Bailliere's Clinical Gastroenterology 11(3): 529–46.

Takagi Y, Bosma JF (1960) Disability of oral function in an infant associated with displacement of the tongue: therapy by feeding in prone position. Acta Paediatric Scandinavia 49: S62–S69.

Takamatsu I (1996) Bilateral vocal cord paralysis in children. Nippon Jibiinkoka Gakkai Kaiho 99(1): 91–102.

Taniguchi MH, Moyer RS (1994) Assessment of risk factors for pneumonia in dysphagic children: significance of videofluoroscopic swallowing evaluation. Developmental Medicine and Child Neurology 36(6): 495–502.

Tellier AL, Cormier-Daire V, Abadie V, et al (1998). CHARGE Syndrome: Report of 47 cases and review. American Journal of Medical Genetics 76: 402–9.

Terry PB, Fuller SD (1989) Pulmonary consequences of aspiration. Dysphagia 3(4): 179–83.

Thilo EH, Rosenberg AA (1999) The newborn infant. In Hay WW, Hayward AR, Levin MJ, et al (eds.) Current Pediatric Diagnosis and Treatment. Stamford CO: Appletone & Lange, p. 58.

Thomas CE, Mayer SA, Gungor Y, et al. (1997) Myasthenic crisis: clinical features, mortality, complications, and risk factors for prolonged intubation. Neurology 48(5): 1253–60.

Thommessen M, Heiberg A, Kase BF (1992) Feeding problems in children with congenital heart disease: the impact on energy intake and growth outcome. European Journal of Clinical Nutrition 46(7): 457–64.

Tierney E, Nwokoro NA, Kelley RI (2000) Behavioural phenotype of RHS/Smith-Lemli-Opitz syndrome. Mental Retardation and Developmental Disability 6(2): 131–4.

Tierney E, Nwokoro NA, Porter FD, et al. (2001) Behaviour phenotype in the RSH/Smith-Lemli-Opitz syndrome. American Journal of Medical Genetics 98(2): 191–200.

Tilton AH, Miller MD, Khoshoo V (1998) Nutrition and swallowing in pediatric neuromuscular patients. Seminars in Pediatric Neurology 5(2): 106–15.

Tuchman DN (1988) Dysfunctional swallowing in the pediatric patient: clinical considerations. Dysphagia 2(4): 203–8.

Tuchman DN (1989). Cough, choke, sputter: the evaluation of the child with dysfunctional swallowing. Dysphagia 3(3): 111–16.

Tunnessen WW, McMillan JA, Levin MB (1978). The Coffin-Siris Syndrome. American Journal of Diseases in Children 132(4): 393–5.

Ungkanont K, Friedman EM, Sulek M (1998) A retrospective analysis of airway endoscopy in patients less than 1-month. Laryngoscope 108(11): 1724–8.

Ungkanont K, Yellon RF, Weissman JL, et al. (1995) Head and neck space infections in infants and children. Otolaryngology Head and Neck Surgery 112(3): 375–82.

Van den Elzen A, Semmekrot BA, Bongers EMHF, et al. (2002) Diagnosis and treatment of the Pierre Robin sequence: results of a retrospective clinical study and review of the literature. European Journal of Pediatrics 160(1): 47–53.

van Ravenswaaij-Arts CM, van den Ouweland AM, Hoogeboom AJ, et al. (2002) From gene to disease; Craniosynostosis, syndromes due to FGFR2-mutation. Nederlands Tijdschrift Voor Geneeskunde 146(2): 63–6.

Varan B, Tokel K, Yilmaz G (1999) Malnutrition and growth failure in cyanotic and acyanotic congenital heart disease with and without pulmonary hypertension. Archives of Disease in Childhood 81(1): 49–52.

Verspyck E, Mandelbrot L, Dommergues M, et al. (1993) Myasthenia gravis with polyhydramnios in the fetus of an asymptomatic mother. Prenatal Diagnosis 13(6): 539–42.

Vohr BR, Bell EF, Oh W (1982) Infants with bronchopulmonary dysplasia: growth pattern and neurologic and developmental outcome. American Journal of Diseases in Children 136(5): 443–7.

Volpe JJ (1997) Brain injury in the premature infant: from pathogenesis to prevention. Brain and Development 19(8): 519–34.

Wagener S, Rayatt SS, Tatman AJ, et al. (2003) Management of infants with Pierre Robin sequence. Cleft Palate-Craniofacial Journal 40(2): 180–5.

Wang Y, Zhang R, Ouyang Z, et al. (2002) Chinese Journal of Oncology 24(4): 394–6.

Ward RM, Beachy JC (2003) Neonatal complications following preterm birth. British Journal of Obstetrics and Gynaecology 110: S8–16.

Werle MA, Murphy TB, Budd KS (1993) Treating chronic food refusal in young children: Home-based parent training. Journal of Applied Behaviour Analysis 26(4): 421–33.

Werlin SL (2004). Antroduodenal motility in neurologically handicapped children with feeding intolerance. BMC Gastroenterology 4(1): 19.

Werlin SL, Dodds WJ, Hogan WJ, et al. (1980) Mechanisms of gastroesophageal reflux in children. Journal of Pediatrics 97(2): 244–9.

Willard HF, Hendrich BB (1999) Breaking the silence in Rett Syndrome. Nature and Genetics 23(2): 127–8.

PAEDIATRIC DYSPHAGIA465

Willging JP (2000) Benefit of feeding assessment before pediatric airway reconstruction. The Laryngoscope 110(5): 825–34.
Williamson D, Kelley ML, Cavell TA, et al. (1987) Eating and elimination disorders. In Frame CL, Matson JL (eds) Handbook of assessment in childhood psychopathology: applied issues in differential diagnosis and treatment evaluation. New York: Plenum, pp. 461–87.
Williams D, Thompson DG, Heggie L, et al. (1994) Esophageal clearance function following treatment of esophagitis. Gastroenterology 106(1): 108–16.
Wilson R, Morris JG, Snyder JD, et al. (1982) Clinical characteristics of infant botulism in the United States: a study of the non-California cases. Pediatric Infectious Disease 1(3): 148–50.
Wohlert AB, Smith A (2002) Developmental change in variability of lip muscle activity during speech. Journal of Speech Language and Hearing Research 45(6): 1077–87.
Wolf L, Glass RP (1992) Clinical feeding evaluation. In Feeding and Swallowing Disorders in Infancy. San Antonio, TX: Therapy Skill Builders, pp. 85–149.
Wolff PH (1968) The serial organization of sucking in the young infant. Pediatrics 42: 943–55.
Yellin SA, LaBruna A, Anand VK (1996) YAG laser treatment for laryngeal and hypopharyngeal hemangiomas: a new technique. Annals of Otology, Rhinology and Laryngology 105(7): 510–15.
Ylvisaker M, Logemann JA (1985) Therapy for feeding and swallowing disorders following head injury. In Ylvisaker M (ed.) Head injury rehabilitation: children and adolescents. Boston: College-Hill Press, pp. 195–215.
Zahid MA, Waqar SH, Shamsuddin S, et al. (2003) Leiomyoma of oesophagus. Journal of the College of Physicians and Surgeons 13(6): 347–9.

14 Assessment Techniques for Babies, Infants and Children

NATHALIE ROMMEL

INTRODUCTION

Chapter 13 has provided a detailed discussion of the clinical signs, aetiologies and characteristics of paediatric dysphagia. Before treatment and management can commence, however, there is a need for a thorough assessment of swallowing function. As detailed in Chapter 2, the infant swallow and the adult swallow are quite different and warrant individual discussions in their own right. Once cannot assume that assessment techniques that are suitable for adults will also be suitable for babies, infants and children. This chapter will discuss both (a) clinical assessments and (b) instrumental assessment techniques that are suitable for use with babies, infants and children.

CLINICAL ASSESSMENT

BACKGROUND

It is generally accepted that feeding difficulties in infants and children need to be assessed from multiple perspectives in order to determine the underlying causes (Rommel et al., 2003). The ultimate goal of the clinical oral assessment is to define the pathophysiology and the extent of the feeding difficulties. In this problem-solving process, the evaluation of the oral cavity and its functions by observation plays a major role, and should occur prior to instrumental assessment.

The feeding specialist must have a thorough understanding of normal function of the many interacting systems involved in feeding. In the clinical oral feeding evaluation, oral anatomy, motor skills, reflex activity, responsivity and swallowing are examined. With this information, referrals can be made for further diagnostic testing and multidisciplinary management where a specific treatment plan can be developed. The clinical oral examination should therefore always be the initial assessment scheduled in a team evaluation.

Dysphagia: Foundation, Theory and Practice.   Edited by J. Cichero and B. Murdoch
© 2006 John Wiley & Sons, Ltd.

CLINICAL ORAL FEEDING EVALUATION

Evaluation of oral structures

Oral anatomy in infants and children has been described extensively in anatomy text-books, developmental and rehabilitation literature and is summarized in Chapter 2 (Noback, 1923; Logan and Bosma, 1967; Bosma, 1985, 1992). Oral structures are examined for malformations and for abnormalities of muscle tone and muscle mass. The lips, cheeks, jaw, tongue, hard and soft palate are examined at rest and during spontaneous movement. Palatal and labial clefts, micrognathia, deviant dental occlusion, ankyloglossia and trismus are some of the most frequently seen anomalies.

Assessment of oral motor function

Oral motor skills have been described extensively in anatomy text books, developmental and rehabilitation literature (Morris, 1982). A brief discussion of the most clinically relevant oral reflexes in terms of infant sucking will be presented because the oral motor assessment in young infants occurs mainly by evaluation of the oral reflexes. These oral reflexes are defined as programmed responses to a specific sensory input, generally a tactile stimulus, and they become modified or integrated into functional activity with increased maturity. The expression of oral reflexes at any age can be quite varied, depending on a number of factors such as state of arousal or hunger. Eliciting specific oral reflexes during the clinical feeding evaluation provides information on the baby's neurological maturity or integrity as well as on the quality of its response to tactile input (Wolf and Glass, 1992). The interplay of the reflexes with the child's functional feeding skills is, however, more important than the presence or absence of specific reflexes (Ingram, 1962). Oral reflexes fall into two categories: temporary and permanent reflexes (see Table 14.1).

Permanent reflexes such as the transverse tongue reflex, gag, cough and swallow develop quite early *in utero* but remain present during an individual's lifetime. The cough and gag reflex are also called protective reflexes as they are designed to protect the airway during feeding and to expel aspirated foreign material. The cough, the most important protective reflex, is triggered by two mechanisms. The first is foreign material that actually enters the upper airway. This stimulates the laryngeal receptors and triggers a cough. The second mechanism to protect the airway is bronchial receptor stimulation by excessive secretions with the purpose of clearing the lower airways of foreign material or mucus. During the act of coughing, the mouth opens, the tongue protrudes and grooves. Consequently the velum elevates and the vocal folds adduct. It is important to observe the cough because the protective laryngeal cough is a prerequisite for safe feeding and excessive coughing suggests lack of suck-swallow-breath coordination. All infants and children periodically cough during feeding. One should note the subject's response, the recovery and coughing frequency. Although the presence of a cough is imperative for safe feeding, it does not guarantee that the subject is a safe feeder. Many children with swallow dysfunction cough sometimes, but do not when they aspirate during deglutition. This is called 'silent aspiration' (Wolf and

Table 14.1 Temporary and permanent oral reflexes

| | | | | Permanent | Temporary | | Outcome | |
				Present at	Present at	Extinction		
Oral reflex	Present	Absent	Not observed	Present at	Present at	Extinction	Normal	Pathological
Cough				birth	—	—		
Gag				18 wks GA	—	—		
Swallow				14 wks GA	—	—		
Transverse tongue				28 wks GA	—	—		
Phasic bite				—	28 w GA	9–12 months		
Tongue protrusion				—	birth	4–6 months		
Santmyer				—	34 w GA	1–2 years		
Palmomental				—	birth	3–4 months		
Rooting				—	32 w GA	3–6 months		
Suck				—	17 w GA	3–4 months		

GA = gestational age.

Glass, 1992). As coughing is the mechanism that protects the airway, the presence and effectiveness of the cough, and not the gag, needs to be considered in regards to safe oral infant feeding (Wolf and Glass, 1992).

The gag reflex is present at 18 weeks' gestational age (Inniruberto and Tajani, 1981; Tucker, 1985). The purpose of the gag reflex is to protect the baby from ingesting large items that can block the airway. It is elicited by touch pressure to receptors located on the tongue or pharyngeal wall causing a reverse peristaltic movement in the pharynx. The spot triggering the gag reflex moves with increasing age: in the newborn gagging is elicited in the mid-tongue area; when the baby matures, the gag gradually moves back to the pharyngeal wall or posterior portion of the tongue (Wolf and Glass, 1992). The status of the gag reflex does not predict the swallow ability as they are innervated independently but does provide information on the responsivity of the pharyngeal receptors (Dodds, 1989; Leder, 1996). The gag reflex is discussed in detail in Chapter 7.

The swallowing response has been observed in the foetus at 12 to 14 weeks (Inniruberto and Tajani, 1981) and is present throughout life. The transverse tongue reflex is triggered by unilateral stimulation of the anterior 1/3 lateral border of the tongue. Lateral tongue movement occurs towards the side of stimulation and should be elicited bilaterally. This reflex is easy to elicit and proves to be important in terms of chewing.

The *temporary oral reflexes*, which include rooting, sucking, palmomental reflex, Sandmyer reflex, and the phasic bite, assist in the acquisition of food, but disappear or are integrated by muscle function respectively at 3–6 months, 3–4 months, 1–2 years, 6–8 months and 9–12 months of age.

The rooting reflex is elicited by a stroke to the perioral area. This causes the baby to turn its head towards the stimulus and open the mouth. The purpose of the rooting reflex is to help the infant locate the food source. The presence of this response is quite variable and is based on factors such as state (e.g. hunger state) and satiation. An absent reflex may reflect poor tactile sensitivity or neural integration (Wolf and Glass, 1992).

Sucking is reflexive in the newborn with a gradual transition to full volitional control of sucking by 3 to 4 months of age. Its purpose is to ensure that the infant obtains nourishment. The elicitation of the reflex varies depending on the type of stimulus (nutritive or non-nutritive) and can be inhibited by factors such as state or satiation (Wolf and Glass, 1992). The sucking reflex is expanded upon in Chapter 2.

The palmomental (Babkin) reflex can be elicited by giving bilateral pressure to the palms resulting in mandible depression and sucking movements of the tongue.

A stimulus on the mandibular molar table leads to the elicitation of the phasic bite reflex resulting in rhythmic up and downward movements of the mandible (Sheppard, 1995). This reflex precedes chewing, together with the transverse tongue reflex.

The Santmyer reflex is a swallow as a response to administration of a puff of air to the perioral area in the face of an awake non-crying infant (Orenstein et al., 1988; Orenstein et al., 1992). This swallow triggers a normal primary peristaltic sequence but responses vary in children from 11 months to 2 years of age. This reflex should be absent in neurologically normal children after the age of 2 years (Arvedson, 1993).

ORAL SENSATION

An infant must have appropriate registration and perception of tactile input as well as appropriate responses to feed successfully. The baby must adapt to the tactile characteristics of tools (breast, bottle, spoon or cup) and food in order to perform correct motor responses (Wolf and Glass, 1992). Since oral motor and oral sensory based feeding disorders can be distinguished (Palmer and Heyman, 1993), a structured sensory examination in and around the oral cavity is essential to delineate difficulties with the tactile components of feeding. Both sensory and motor attributes are considered, however it is not possible to observe sensations, only the reactions to sensations (Arvedson, 1993). The child's ability to respond adequately to tactile input can be observed during a typical feeding situation or by a structured sensory examination. This is accomplished by graded sensory input. A sensory baseline on consistency, taste, temperature, tools, area of stimulation and amount needs to be established, which is defined as the level of tactile input that the child can tolerate without any discomfort (Palmer and Heyman, 1993). A wide range of tactile responses can be observed and these responses tend to form a continuum of function: absent responses, hyporesponsivity, normal tactile function, hypersensitivity and aversion (Wolf and Glass, 1992). When tactile responses are severely diminished or absent, a significant sensory impairment should be suspected and oral feeding may not be possible. In hyposensitivity, a strong stimulation is required, the responses are slow or partial. A hypersensitive response is exaggerated or out of proportion to the magnitude of the stimuli. While similar to hypersensitive responses, aversive responses are even stronger and more negative. Both hypersensitive and aversive responses can be part of a global tactile processing problem or be localized to the face and mouth

Table 14.2 Tactile responses – continuum of function

Absent tactile response	Hyposensitive tactile response	Normal tactile response	Hypersensitive tactile response	Aversive tactile response
• Suspect significant sensory impairment • Oral feeding may not be possible	• Suspect significant sensory impairment • Oral feeding may not be possible • Strong stimulation is required • Responses may be slow or partial		• Response exaggerated or out of proportion to magnitude of stimuli • Can be part of global tactile processing problem • Could be localized to face and mouth (often a certain part of the mouth, i.e. tongue)	• Response very exaggerated in regard to magnitude of stimuli and negative • Can be part of global tactile processing problem • Could be localised to face and mouth (often a certain part of the mouth, i.e. tongue)

or more specifically to a certain part of the mouth, most frequently the tongue. This continuum is summarized in Table 14.2.

ADVANTAGES AND DISADVANTAGES OF THE CLINICAL ASSESSMENT

The clinical assessment establishes the nature of the feeding problem, the readiness and need for further workup and possible management strategies. During the examination the assessor will be able to determine whether the parents reports and perceptions are matching the observations (Reilly et al., 2000). Although considered most valuable by many authors, the clinical assessment is not designed to substitute for the instrumental techniques. The clinical examination remains assessor dependent and cannot rule out with certainty the possibility that patient is at risk for aspiration. Ultimately, determination of the child's potential capacity for oral feeding needs to be based on data from both the clinical and instrumental assessment.

PUBLISHED CLINICAL ASSESSMENT SCALES

There are several published clinical assessment scales and checklists for paediatric dysphagia (Sheppard, 1987; Tuchman, 1989; Gisel, 1991; Wolf and Glass, 1992; Arvedson, 1993); however, few have a sound theoretical merit. Several multidisciplinary teams working with paediatric dysphagia have developed their own checklists, using the milestones of oral motor development as a reference to distinguish between normal and abnormal feeding skills. At present no universally accepted infant/paediatric feeding assessment tool exists (Arvedson, 1993). Therefore, knowledge of normal development and experience with oral motor and feeding function are often used as reference points for clinicians to evaluate children with abnormal functioning.

Infant assessment scales (0–2 years)

The Clinical Feeding Evaluation of Infants scale (CFEI) evaluates the baby's or infant's ability to suck on a bottle and/or breast (Wolf and Glass, 1992). It describes the child's feeding history, oral motor skills and tactile responses, suck-swallow-breath coordination, general motor control as well as the state and physiological control during feeding. The authors provide a most detailed and useful theory (evaluation and interpretation) behind the evaluated items as well as concordant therapy guidelines.

The Neonatal Oral Motor Assessment Scale (NOMAS) is an evaluation of nutritive and non-nutritive sucking in infants up to 3 months of age that discriminates normal from abnormal sucking and quantifies the degree of abnormality (Palmer et al., 1993). Tongue and jaw movements during sucking are classified into normal, disorganized (lack of overall rhythm of the total sucking activity) and dysfunctional (interruption of sucking by abnormal movements of tongue and jaw) (Braun and Palmer, 1985; Palmer et al., 1993). A revised NOMAS identifies different oral motor components, as efficient and inefficient feeders, in a sample of high-risk premature neonates (Case-Smith et al., 1989).

The Conway Shannon Infant Feeding Assessment Scale (CSIFAT) describes oral feeding behaviour, kinaesthetic behaviour, sensory behaviour and respiratory patterns during feeding. Each item is divided in subcategories and is described by exclusive characteristics forming a continuum from normal to abnormal (Conway, 1989).

Paediatric assessment scales (2–5 years)

The Pre-speech Assessment Scale is a rating scale that examines voice and swallowing in children from birth to 2 years of age. Lips, tongue and jaw movements and swallowing are rated separately for each type of food. The duration of meal, amount of intake, food consistencies, positioning, sucking from a nipple, sipping from a cup and coordination of suck-swallow-breath are rated. A summary provides an analysis of the quality of movement patterns and the developmental level of the observed behaviours (Morris, 1982).

The Oral-Motor/Feeding Rating Scale is a rating scale for adequacy of lip, cheek, tongue and jaw movement during a typical meal (Jelm, 1990). This scale is useful from children 1 year of age through to adult clients and the assessment takes less than an hour. It can be used for initial observations of skill levels or to re-evaluate previously observed skills.

The Multidisciplinary Feeding Profile was described as the first statistically based protocol for patients who are dependent feeders, particularly children with neurological deficits (Kenny, Koheil et al., 1989). Scaled numeric ratings are made for posture, tone, reflexes, general motor control, oro-facial structures, oro-facial sensory input, oro-facial motor control, ventilation and functional feeding assessment. The scales' numerical rating however does not rate the level of severity of the feeding problem.

The Assessment Scale of Oral Functions in Feeding rates the functionality of lip, jaw and tongue movement during liquid and solid foods. The scale assesses sipping from a cup, coughing, gagging, and hypersensitivity associated with swallowing (Ottenbacher et al., 1985). Abnormal oral structures, oral reflexes, positioning, diet, utensils and feeding time can be marked on the provided checklist.

The Preschool Motor Speech Evaluation (Earnest, 2000) is developed to assess oral motor and oral motor speech abilities in children from 18 months until 5 years of age. As well as focusing on speech and language development, this scale provides an oral motor examination at different levels of performance (spontaneous, imitation, cueing or elicitation) and oral sensory skills are screened at different age levels. The link is made between oral movements and respiration.

The Dysphagia Disorder Survey (DDS) (Sheppard, 2002) is a standardized screening tool originally developed to assess adults with developmental disability for dysphagia and related eating disorders. However, the DDS is applicable for different populations and is appropriate for use in assessing children from 2 years to 21 years of age. The survey consists of two major parts: related factors and swallowing competency. Related factors include body mass index or weight for height percentile, restrictions in food textures and viscosity, dependence in eating, need for special utensils or positioning strategies. Swallowing competence is assessed during liquid, chewable and non-chewable foods and addresses oral preparatory, oral, pharyngeal and oesophageal phases of swallowing.

It provides the user with a raw score that can be interpreted by using a percentile ranking. These percentiles refer to the level of competency and the higher percentile rank refers to the more severely deficient swallow. The statistical analysis and normative studies on the base of this screening tool are well documented and are unique amongst the current available paediatric assessment scales. The Dysphagia Management Staging Scale (DMSS) (Sheppard, 2002) is a five-level scale that designates the level of severity of the eating disorder depending on the special needs of nutritional and medical management of the disorder. The DMSS classification is identified during DDS screening. The percentile derived from the raw score on the DDS can be used to compare one individual with others at each level of severity. This allows the therapist to compare the patient to others with the same severity of disorder in regards to management needs.

It is generally accepted that the clinical examination has its main focus on the oral phase of swallowing. In addition to the assessment scales discussed above, checklists can be useful for systematizing observations (Herman, 1991; Arvedson, 1993). Examples of published checklists include: the Infant Feeding Evaluation (Swigert, 1998) and the Feeding Assessment Checklist in the Manual of Feeding Practice (McCurtin, 1997).

In general, published protocols and checklists evaluate many of the same variables but interpretation guidelines are lacking. Most of the scales imply that abnormal deglutition will be reflected in the functional movements of the oral preparatory phase. The scales do not localize the dysfunction or reveal their possible causes (Sheppard, 1995). Authors tend to provide practical and accessible assessment tools but most of the scales lack normative data, standardization and validation. The clinical examination often needs to be complemented with further instrumental assessment to reveal the underlying cause of the oral feeding problem.

INSTRUMENTAL TECHNIQUES TO ASSESS DEGLUTITION IN INFANTS AND YOUNG CHILDREN

As in any observational method, the quality of information from a clinical examination depends mainly on the examiner's perceptual skills. Instrumental assessment has the potential to document oropharyngeal function objectively if selected and applied properly. Many different functional tests are available to assess oropharyngeal function during swallowing. Most of these assessment techniques remain subjective in the interpretation of the results. However, recently a few new paediatric techniques which allow objective measurement of oropharyngeal function have been developed and will be discussed here in detail. The reality is that the use of one particular technique often depends on institutional experience, funds and its commercial availability rather than being based on clinical and theoretical considerations. Some of the techniques are at this stage used for research only. Their main premise is to provide precise understanding of the biomechanics of infant swallowing, which will ultimately lead to more specific therapeutic intervention. Medical tests used to assess oesophageal function, for example, will not be included in this chapter. The major instrumental assessments that will be discussed in this section include: ultrasound, fibreoptic endoscopic evaluation of swallowing (FEES), electomyography, cervical auscultation, videofluoroscopy or modified barium swallow, and manofluoroscopy.

ULTRASOUND

This technique, also called ultrasonography, relies on the propagation of sound energy through fluid or semifluid matter such as blood and tissues (Sonies, 1991). In infants and children, for the purposes of a swallowing assessment, the transducer is placed under the chin (submental) or on the cheeks (transbuccal) in case the teeth have not yet erupted (Benson and Tuchmann, 1994). The echoes or reflections of the returning signal are recorded: the send /receive time interval is coded as distance and the strength of the returning signal is seen as brightness (Shawker et al., 1984). Ultrasound describes oral preparatory, oral and parts of the pharyngeal phases of swallowing in a dynamic view and in multiple planes. This technique is well tolerated in children (Kenny, Casas et al., 1989; Benson and Tuchmann, 1994; Casas et al., 1995), can be applied repeatedly, used for a prolonged time period, and is useful for observing movements of soft tissue structures. It captures the salient features of tongue, hyoid and palate activity and bolus transport across the tongue into the hypopharyngeal area (Bosma et al., 1990; Lefton-Greif and Loughlin, 1996; Yang et al., 1997). The technique requires no contrast medium or radiation exposure. The test uses real liquid and food boluses. Because the trachea is an air-filled space, fluid penetration or aspiration cannot be visualized with ultrasound (Benson and Tuchman, 1994). Some authors have indicated the need to use both static and dynamic ultrasound during the (digital) analysis (Casas et al., 2002). According to some authors there is excellent soft tissue delineation (Yang et al., 1997), but definitive landmarks of the structures are currently lacking (Arvedson and Lefton-Greif, 1998a). Paediatric ultrasound data have shown that children with cerebral palsy have a longer oral transit time than normal children and that they manage solid boluses more easily than liquid bolus (Casas, Kennny and McPherson, 1994; Casas et al., 1995). They also tolerate small liquid bolus more easily than large liquid boluses (Casas et al., 1994).

FIBEROPTIC ENDOSCOPIC EVALUATION OF SWALLOWING (FEES)

This technique is used to view the pharyngeal phase of swallowing and laryngeal structures using a flexible laryngoscope (Aviv et al., 1998; Langmore, 2001). A flexible fibreoptic endoscope is passed via the nasal cavity to the oropharynx and or hypopharynx to allow a direct view of these areas during swallowing. The FEES technique is also discussed in Chapter 8. It allows dynamic viewing of the pharynx, larynx and glottis at rest, immediately before and after the pharyngeal swallow. This procedure documents pooling and detects velopharyngeal insufficiency, vocal fold abnormalities and aspiration. Direct stimulation of the mucosa innervated by the superior laryngeal nerve with a pressure-controlled and duration-controlled air pulse allows assessment of the laryngeal and pharyngeal sensation (Aviv et al., 1993; Link et al., 2000). It is a routine for the otolaryngologist and is often performed by a trained speech language pathologist for swallowing assessment (Association, 2002). No radiation exposure is required nor does anything need to be added to the real liquid and food boluses used in order to enhance contrast. In order to obtain an accurate representation of the swallow patient cooperation is needed, which may be a concern in paediatrics due to the invasive nature of the procedure. Successful application in children has been reported recently (Link et al., 2000). Fiberoptic endoscopic evaluation of swallowing does not show the interaction between oral, pharyngeal and cervical oesophageal structures during the actual swallow (Lefton-Greif and Loughlin, 1996), as can be determined from the videofluoroscopic swallow study (VFSS). However, when comparing FEES and VFSS, the two techniques are equally effective in discriminating between aspiration and penetration (Colodny, 2002) and the outcomes with respect to pneumonia incidence are similar (Aviv, 2000).

ELECTROMYOGRAPHY

Electromyography assesses the myoelectric activity of muscles (Palmer, 1989). To obtain accurate recording, good contact is required between probe (suction cups, needles or clips) and muscle. At present this technique is not indicated for routine evaluation of deglutition in infants and children (Benson and Tuchmann, 1994).

CERVICAL AUSCULTATION

Cervical auscultation is a non-invasive method that amplifies the sounds associated with breathing and swallowing (Bosma, 1986; Eichler et al., 1994). It involves placing the flat diaphragm of the stethoscope on the lateral side of the thyroid cartilage, adjusting placement until cervical breath and the pharyngeal phase of swallowing during feeding can be heard (Logan and Bosma, 1967; Arvedson and Lefton-Greif, 1998b). Cervical auscultation has been proposed as a clinical bedside technique to identify patients who aspirate and to improve the sensitivity of feeding evaluation (Newman and Petersen, 1999). The procedure is easy, safe and cost efficient. No preparation is required. Swallows can be sampled repeatedly and for prolonged time periods. The procedure requires no contrast and uses real food or liquid but does not offer a direct view of the swallowing mechanism or the aetiology of dysphagia (Lefton-Greif and Loughlin, 1996). Therefore, cervical auscultation is not envisioned as replacing direct imaging of the act of deglutition. Cervical auscultation is also discussed in detail in Chapter 7.

Aspects that may influence the usefulness of cervical auscultation are the acoustic characteristics of the stethoscope (Abella et al., 1992; Hamlet et al., 1994) and the placement of the diaphragm at the cervical site. The acoustic properties of different popular stethoscopes were compared for use in cervical auscultation of swallowing sounds (Abella et al., 1992; Hamlet et al., 1994). In infants and children, the use of an infant stethoscope is necessary because of its small diameter of the diaphragm (2.6 cm) (Rommel, 2002) which is placed on the lateral border of the trachea immediately inferior to the cricoid cartilage or on the midpoint between the centre of the cricoid cartilage and the site immediately superior to the jugular notch (Takashashi et al., 1994; Vice, Bamford et al., 1995). According to Takahashi et al. listening unilaterally is reliable and the acoustic characteristics of swallowing sounds should be evaluated from consecutive rather than from isolated swallows (Takashashi et al., 1994).

The inability to explain the cause of swallowing sounds and thus the lack of validation of the physiological source of the sounds heard was seen as a major limitation of the diagnostic potential of cervical auscultation for dysphagia assessment (Hamlet et al., 1990; Cichero and Murdoch, 1998). It was hypothesized that the characteristic sound of swallowing is generated by increased bolus velocity corresponding to the onset of pressurized flow into the oesophagus (Hamlet et al., 1990), by elevation of the larynx and bolus flow through the pharyngo-oesophageal segment (Sievers, 1997) or by the pharyngeal valves and pumps producing reverberations (Cichero and Murdoch, 1998). Correspondence between sounds and events remains difficult to study because many aspects of deglutition are silent (Logemann, 1983). Although trained clinicians will identify abnormal swallowing mainly by perception, normal and abnormal deglutition correlate with well defined acoustic parameters (Cichero and Murdoch, 2002; Rommel, 2002). Normative acoustic data for swallowing in adults are available and are variable according to age, gender and volume (Cichero and Murdoch, 2002).

The acoustic spectrum of swallowing in infants was first illustrated by Logan et al. (Logan and Bosma, 1967). The swallow sounds during bottle feeding were continuous and usually had two detectable components with the highest intensity in the frequency range below 1500 Hz. Their duration was brief: in the order of 20 ms to 30 ms. After a conspicuous pause, another swallow or respiration ensued (Logan and Bosma, 1967). Vice and colleagues (1990) found that swallow breath sounds were distinctively patterned, with discrete sounds preceding and following the bolus transit sounds. In their studies using cervical accelerometry with digital processing, bolus transit sounds varied in amplitude and pattern, in relation to postmenstrual age (Reynolds et al., 2002), medical pathology (Reynolds et al., 2003) and to the volume or consistency of the bolus (Vice et al., 1990).

VIDEOFLUOROSCOPIC SWALLOW STUDY

Videofluoroscopic swallow study (VFSS) is a qualitative, dynamic, radiological registration of deglutition, often considered the gold standard (Logemann, 1983; Arvedson and Lefton-Greif, 1998b). It primary purpose is to define the physiology of the pharyngeal phase of swallowing and to identify concomitant risk of aspiration

(Logemann, 1983). This technique has become widely available and requires patient cooperation, the ingestion of a contrast medium and exposes the patient to radiation (Lefton-Greif and Loughlin, 1996).

The paediatric literature reports on the methodology of VFSS (Arvedson and Lefton-Greif, 1998c; Zerilli, 1990; O'Donoghue and Bagnall, 1999) but only a limited number of studies address descriptive and qualitative assessment of swallowing in children (Morton et al., 1993; Mercado-Deane et al., 2001; Newman et al., 1991).

A number of videofluoroscopic studies of children with neurological disease emphasized the common occurrence of pharyngeal phase abnormalities including aspiration (Sloan, 1977; Helfrich-Miller et al., 1986; Griggs et al., 1989; Morton et al., 1993; Rogers et al., 1994; Wright et al., 1996; Schwarz et al., 2001; Sheikh et al., 2001; Morgan et al., 2002). Other studies on paediatric dysphagia have focused on cricopharyngeal dysfunctions and the impact of ear-nose-throat pathology such as tracheostomies and congenital pharyngeal paralysis (Utian and Thomas, 1969; Williams and Mitchell, 1980; Arvedson et al., 1994; Elmaleh et al., 1994; Mbonda et al., 1995; Eichler et al., 2000).

So far, and mainly because of ethics, the biomechanics of oropharyngeal patterns in normal children have not been determined (Rommel, 2002). However, improved understanding of normal oropharyngeal motility will enable clinicians to design more effective therapeutic strategies in cases of abnormality.

MANOFLUOROSCOPY

Manofluoroscopy allows the clinician to integrate both manometric and videofluoroscopic data to determine important parameters such as tongue driving force, pharyngeal contraction, pharyngeal shortening, upper oesophageal sphincter (UES) relaxation and the amplitude of the pharyngeal contraction. Manometry may be particularly helpful in instances where videofluoroscopic imaging demonstrates impaired or absent transit from the hypopharynx to the oesophagus (Benson and Tuchman, 1994). When this occurs, it may be difficult to distinguish between failure of the UES to relax or to open. Failure of UES relaxation can be documented by manometry. Upper oesophageal sphincter closure, despite relaxation results from poor pumping action of weakened pharyngeal musculature (Benson and Tuchman, 1994). The major aim of manofluoroscopy is to clarify the role of the pharyngeal wall in paediatric deglutition and to quantify the pharyngeal movements in relation to bolus passage and to the opening of the UES.

In order to perform manofluoroscopy in infants and young children, age adapted microcatheters (OD 2mm) are required, with sensors placed at the structures involved in swallowing. High resolution manometry (HRM) allows the measurement of pharyngo-oesophageal pressure and enables the direct assessment of the mechanics of flow during deglutition. It measures pressure across the length of pharyngo-oesphageal segment using a chain of closely spaced pressure sensors. This technique enables highly accurate spatiotemporal interpolation of dynamic pressure changes which can be visualized and interpreted in the form of a 'space time plot' (refer to

(a) Normal swallow T1   (b)
                                                              UES Achalasia T1

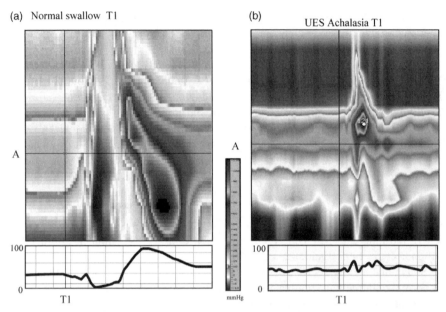

Temporal Pressure Profile at Axial Position A (UOS)

Figure 14.1a & b   Patterns of pressure during swallowing of a 1ml liquid bolus in a healthy subject (Figure 14.1a) and in a two-year old patient with UES achalasia (Figure 14.1b). Recordings were made with a high resolution manometry assembly and were performed simultaneously with videofluoroscopy. The vertical axis frame shows the position of pressure sensors, the horizontal axis shows time. The figures shown are high resolution spacio-temporal plots of pressure patterns during deglutition. The high resolution manometry allows (i) interpolation of pressure patterns over time at any given position. In this example, the pressure of the upper oesophageal sphincter is located at position 'a', and (ii) the interpolation of axial pressure profile at a given time, in this example the profile and time 't'

Figures 14.1a and b). It thus provides a detailed representation of the space-time pressure structure of the pharyngo-oesophageal segment, which can be used to define the biomechanics during normal or disordered transsphincteric bolus flow.

Manofluoroscopy requires a thin and flexible catheter and is more invasive than videofluoroscopy due to the placement of the nasopharyngeal catheter. Clinical experience, however, shows that the insertion and the positioning causes no problems and sedation is not required as only limited discomfort is experienced in order to obtain interpretable recordings.

Oropharyngeal transit time must be interpreted as a measure of the overall efficiency of bolus transit. Increased duration of the swallow is a marker for increased aspiration risk. Delayed oropharyngeal transit time is likely to occur when tongue action is limited. In adults, normal oropharyngeal transit time ranges from 2 s to 2.25 s (Arvedson and Lefton-Greif, 1998b). In infants, normal oropharyngeal transit time is reported to be 1.5 s (Newman et al., 1991) and in children 1.3 s to 2 s (Arvedson and Lefton-Greif, 1998b). The mean oropharyngeal transit time

Table 14.3 Oropharyngeal transit times: infants, children and adults

Normal infants	Normal children	Normal adults	Infants with feeding difficulties
1.5 s	1.3–2 s	2–2.25 s	0.5–4.3 s (mean 1.9 s)

in children with feeding difficulties ranged from 0.5 s to 4.3 s and averaged 1.9 s (Rommel, 2002). These times are summarized in Table 14.3. The videofluoroscopy analysis using quantitative parameters suggest that the epiglottis is moving in the infant pharynx, but not tilting during swallowing as the top of the epiglottis is not moving more than 48°. It has been suggested that the epiglottis has a specific function in nasal breathing during sucking but that its contribution in airway protection is limited (Rommel, 2002).

Two types of pharyngeal contractions facilitate bolus movement through the pharynx to the oesophagus (Miller et al., 1997). First, the pharynx shortens in the vertical dimension which decreases the distance a bolus must travel (Cook et al., 1989; Kahrilas et al., 1992). Vertical pharyngeal shortening is described in adult and geriatric patients and plays a major role in the formation of hypopharyngeal residue (Cook et al., 1989; Kahrilas et al., 1992; Dejaeger, 1995). In adults, pharyngeal shortening has been reported to be most pronounced between the valleculae and the arytenoids (Dejaeger, 1995). In children with feeding difficulties, pharyngeal shortening is not as pronounced in the lower pharynx as was observed in adults (Rommel, 2002). Secondly, the pharyngeal constrictors are activated in rostrocaudal sequence generating a propulsive contractile wave (Miller et al., 1997). Adult data show that when the bolus arrives in the pharynx, the widening occurs mainly on the anterior side of the pharyngeal wall. The posterior part stays practically immobile initially. After bolus transit, the pharynx closes, the anterior side resumes its initial position while the posterior side moves forward (Dejaeger, 1995). Manofluoroscopic data suggest that the contraction of the posterior pharyngeal wall occurs after bolus passage, which implies that the posterior pharyngeal wall has a clearing function. The data in infants with feeding difficulties indicate a similar mechanism of pharyngeal movement and demonstrate clearly that the movement of the anterior pharyngeal wall is followed by subsequent movement of the posterior pharyngeal wall at different levels in the pharynx (Rommel, 2002).

The first detailed reports on the UES motor function were those by Gybroski (1965), Moroz et al. (1976) and Sondheimer (1983). Recently, paediatric UES pressures have been studied with more accurate recording techniques. A micromanometric catheter with oval sleeve and perfused sideholes was used to account for the asymmetry of the UES (Davidson et al., 1991; Omari et al., 1999). Davidson et al. reported that UES resting pressure in children up to 42 months varied from 18 to 56 mmHg depending on the state of arousal (Davidson et al., 1991). Omari et al. (1999) found a UES resting pressure in healthy preterm infants ranging from 2 to 26 mmHg. Jadcherla and Shaker (2001) published that UES resting pressure in newborns averaged 46 mmHg as measured by a round micromanometric catheter.

Thus far, only limited paediatric studies are available on the UES motor function using orally administered liquid boluses. Rommel et al (2002) found that the UES resting pressures in between wet swallows are much higher than those reported in dry swallows of premature infants, normal children and children with gastro-esophageal reflux disease. In the literature, a distinction is made between UES resting pressure of a total manometric sequence and the UES resting pressure prior to relaxation (Omari et al., 1999). In the study on swallowing wet boluses (Rommel, 2002), the UES resting pressure of the whole sequence was calculated. Possible explanations for the higher resting pressures may be that in the other studies, no boluses were administered orally (Davidson et al., 1991; Omari et al., 1999; Jadcherla and Shaker, 2001), measures occurred during mid oesophageal infusion of air, water or apple juice (Jadcherla et al., 2000) or because manometry occurred post prandially in a less distracting situation than the manofluoroscopy setting (Davidson et al., 1991; Omari et al., 1999). Furthermore, UES pressures are known to be higher during straining in children (Willing et al., 1994). It can be hypothesized that UES resting pressures increase during deglutition.

An important pressure parameter of deglutition is the tongue driving force. It is the propagation force of the tongue and pharyngeal walls that transport the bolus from the oropharynx to the hypopharynx. Normal values average 1.8 mmHgs (SD = 1.0) in adults and 1.4 mmHgs in the elderly (Dejaeger, 1995). Tongue driving force is known to be influenced by stress, bolus size and place of measurement. In adults, tongue driving force values increase caudally. In a preliminary study in children with feeding difficulties, much higher tongue driving force values (mean: 10 mmHgs) were found (Rommel, 2002). As the paediatric pharynx is significantly more compressed in comparison to the adult pharynx, this anatomical configuration might influence the tongue driving force. Another probable explanation is that the upright position of the epiglottis limits the space in the pharyngeal cavity and thus causes higher pressure values. Because of the anatomical difference in the pharyngeal cavity where the parameter is measured, we renamed the 'adult' tongue driving force as 'infant tongue driving force' (Rommel, 2002).

Intra bolus pressure is a frequently reported deglutition parameter in adult swallow research. It is influenced by bolus volume, bolus consistency and position of the sensor (Kahrilas et al., 1993). In paediatric studies however bolus sizes are often not standardized as the infants are allowed to drink *ad libitum* according to their normal feeding pattern.

The amplitude of the pharyngeal contraction plays an important role in the formation of stasis in the adult and geriatric dysphagic population. The mean amplitude of pharyngeal contraction is 124 mmHg in adults and 145 mmHg in the elderly (Dejaeger et al., 1997). In normal infants, the amplitude of pharyngeal contraction was reported to be 74 cm/H2O (54 mmHg) and 66 cmH2O in infants with gastro-esophageal reflux disease (48 mmHg) (Sondheimer, 1983). These results are summarized in Table 14.4. In this report of Sondheimer (1983), the subjects were sedated during the study and the pharyngeal measurements were performed with water-perfused sideholes, which might have induced reflexive swallowing.

Table 14.4 Mean amplitudes of pharyngeal contraction in adults and children

Population	Mean amplitude of pharyngeal contraction (mmHg)
Normal infants	54
Infants with gastroesophageal reflux	48
Normal adults	124
Normal elderly	145

Recent data (Rommel, 2002) showed higher amplitudes of pharyngeal contraction (mean: 107 mmHg) than previous paediatric reports but lower values than in adults. Adult studies have proved a correlation between UES function and pharyngeal contractility. With lower UES compliance, stronger compensatory pharyngeal contractions have been demonstrated (Dejaeger et al., 1997). However, in young children, it was hypothesized that UES compliance in young children is higher as weaker pharyngeal contractions were documented to effectively clear the bolus (Rommel, 2002).

Qualitative analysis of deglutition on radiological dynamic recordings also revealed some different findings as compared to adults. The hyoid bone plays an important role in adult deglutition (Logemann, 1983). However, its role could not be specified in this paediatric population due to the poor visualization of the structure. It cannot be used consistently as a reference structure, although its traction may facilitate UES opening.

Although currently only used as a research tool, manofluoroscopy is feasible in infants and young children. The use of manofluoroscopy should be considered when paediatric patients aspirate or present with a lack of suck-swallow-breath coordination or nasal regurgitation. Its use is not indicated, however, in cases of isolated oral phase problems. At present, researchers are obtaining normative values for different paediatric age groups and evaluating the influence of bolus variables on infant deglutition.

SUMMARY

In summary, clinical assessment remains the starting point for investigation into the feeding and swallowing abilities of babies, infants and children. The outcomes of those preliminary assessments will determine whether further instrumental assessment techniques are required. Which instrumental assessment technique to use must be determined on a case-by-case basis. Combinations of assessments may also help to yield the best diagnostic picture to enable individualized treatment programmes. With a move away from treating infants as 'mini-adults', assessment techniques and protocols are now being designed with the requirements of babies, infants and children in mind. This area must continue to be developed in order to meet the specific needs of the paediatric population.

REFERENCES

Abella M, Formollo J, Penney D (1992) Comparison of the acoustic properties of six popular stethoscopes. Journal of the Acoustical Society of America 91: 2224–8.

Arvedson J (1993) Oral-motor and feeding assessment. In Arvedson J, Brodsky L (eds) Pediatric Swallowing and Feeding: Assessment and Management. San Diego: Singular, pp. 249–92.

Arvedson J, Lefton-Greif M (1998a) Instrumental assessment procedures used in pediatric dysphagia. Pediatric Videofluoroscopic Swallow Studies (pp. 2–13). San Antonio Texas: Communication Skill Builders.

Arvedson J, Lefton-Greif M (1998b) Instrumental assessment procedures used in pediatric dysphagia. In Arvedson J, Lefton-Greif M (eds) Pediatric Videofluoroscopic Swallow Studies. San Antonio Texas: Communication Skill Builders, pp. 2–12.

Arvedson J, Lefton-Greif M (1998c) Videofluoroscopic swallow procedures in pediatrics. In Arvedson J, Lefton-Greif M (eds) Pediatric Videofluoroscopic Swallow Studies. San Antonio Texas: Communication Skill Builders, pp. 72–116.

Arvedson J, Rogers B, Buck J, et al. (1994) Silent aspiration prominent in children with dysphaghia. Otorhinolaryngology 28: 173–81.

American Speech-Language-Hearing Association (2002) Knowledge and Skills for Speech-Pathologists Performing Endoscopic Assessment of Swallowing Procedures. ASHA, Suppl 22: 107–12.

Aviv J (2000) Prospective, randomized outcome study of endoscopy versus modified barium swallow in patients with dysphagia. Laryngoscope 110(4): 563–74.

Aviv J, Kim T, Thompson J, et al. (1998) Fiberoptic endoscopic evaluation of swallowing with sensory testing in healthy controls. Dysphagia 13(2): 87–92.

Aviv J, Martin J, Keen M, Debell M, Blitzer A (1993) Air pulse quantification of supraglottic and pharyngeal sensation: a new technique. Annals of Ototology, Rhinology and Laryngology 102(10): 777–80.

Benson J, Tuchmann D (1994) Other diagnostic tests used for evaluation of swallowing disorders. In Tuchmann D, Walter E (eds), Disorders of Feeding and Swallowing in Infants and Children: Pathophysiology, Diagnosis and Treatment (1st edn). San Diego: Singular, pp. 201–9.

Bosma J (1985) Postnatal ontogeny of performances of the pharynx, larynx and mouth. American Review of Respiratory Disorders 131: S10–S15.

Bosma J (1986) Development of feeding. Clinical Nutrition 5(5): 210–18.

Bosma J (1992) Pharyngeal swallow: basic mechanisms, development and impairments. Advances in Otolaryngology 6: 225–75.

Bosma J (1990) Ultrasound demonstration of tongue motions during suckle feeding. Developmental Medicine and Child Neurology 32: 223–9.

Braun M, Palmer M (1985) A pilot study of oral motor dysfunction in at-risk infants. Physical and Occupational Therapy in Pediatrics 5: 13–25.

Casas M, Kenny D, McPherson K (1994) Swallowing/ventilation interactions during oral swallow in normal children and children with cerebral palsy. Dysphagia 9(1): 40–6.

Casas M, Pherson M, Kenny D (1995) Duration aspects of oral swallow in neurologically normal children and children with palsy: an ultrasound investigation. Dysphagia 10(3): 155–9.

Casas M, Seo A, Kenny D (2002) Sonographic examination of the oral phase of swallowing: bolus image enhancement. Journal of Clinical Ultrasound 30(2): 83–7.

Case-Smith J, Cooper P, Scala V (1989) Feeding efficiency of premature neonates. American Journal of Occupational Therapy 43: 245–50.

Cichero J, Murdoch B (2002) Acoustic signature of the normal swallow: characterization by age, gender and bolus volume. Annals of Otology, Rhinology and Laryngology 111: 623–32.

Cichero J, Murdoch B (1998) The physiologic cause of swallowing sounds: answers from heart sounds and vocal tract acoustics. Dysphagia 13(1): 39–52.

Colodny N (2002) Interjudge and intrajudge reliabilities in fiberoptic endoscopic evaluation of swallowing (fees) using the penetration-aspiration scale: a replication study. Dysphagia 17(4): 308–15.

Conway A (1989) Young infants feeding patterns when sick and well. Maternal-Child Nursing Journal 18(4): 255–358.

Cook I, Dodds W, Dantas R (1989) Timing of videofluoroscopic, manometric event and bolus transit during the oral and pharyngeal phases of swallowing. Dysphagia 4: 8–15.

Davidson G, Dent J, Willing J (1991) Monitoring of upper oesophageal sphincter pressure in children. Gut 32: 607–11.

Dejaeger E (1995) Deglutition and deglutition disorders assessed with the use of new techniques: ultrasound and computer-assisted analysis of manofluorography. Unpublished PhD Medical Sciences, Catholic University Leuven, Leuven.

Dejaeger E, Pelemans W, Ponette E, et al. (1997) Mechanisms involved in postdeglutition retention in the elderly. Dysphagia 12: 63–7.

Dodds W (1989) The physiology of swallowing. Dysphagia 3: 171–8.

Earnest M (2000) Preschool Motor Speech Evaluation and Intervention. Bisbee, Arizona: Imaginart.

Eichler P, Donald-McGinn DM, Fox C, et al. (2000) Dysphagia in children with a 22q11.2 deletion: unusual pattern found on modified barium swallow. Journal of Pediatrics 137(2): 158–64.

Eichler P, Manno C, Fox C, et al. (1994) Impact of cervical auscultation on accuracy of clinical evaluation in predicting penetration/aspiration. Dysphagia 10(2): 133.

Elmaleh M, Garel C, François M (1994) Dysphagie de l' enfant: imagerie. Annals of Radiology 37(7–8): 488–93.

Gisel E (1991) Effect of food texture on the development of chewing of children between six months and two years of age. Developmental Medicine and Child Neurology 33: 69–79.

Griggs C, Jones P, Lee R (1989) Videofluoroscopic investigation of feeding disorders of children with multiple handicaps. Developmental Medicine and Child Neurology 31: 303–8.

Gryboski J (1965) The swallowing mechanism of the neonate: esophageal and gastric motility. Pediatrics, March: 445–52.

Hamlet A, Nelson R, Patterson R (1990) Interpreting the sounds of swallowing: fluid through the cricopharyngeus. Annals of Otology, Rhinology and Laryngology 99: 749–52.

Hamlet S, Penney D, Formolo J (1994) Stethoscope acoustics and cervical auscultation of swallowing. Dysphagia 9: 63–8.

Helfrich-Miller K, Rector K, Straka J (1986) Dysphagia: its treatment in the profoundly retarded patient with cerebral palsy. Archives of Physical Medicine and Rehabilitation 67: 520–5.

Herman M (1991) Comprehensive assessment of oral motor dysfunction in failure-to-thrive infants. Infant and Toddler Intervention 1(2): 109–23.

Ianniruberto A, Tajani E (1981) Ultrasonographic study of fetal movements. Seminars in Perinatology 5: 175–81.

Ingram T (1962) Clinical significance of the infantile feeding reflexes. Developmental Medicine and Child Neurology 4: 159–69.

Inniruberto A, Tajani E (1981) Ultrasonographic study of fetal movements. Seminars in Perinatology 5: 175–81.

Jadcherla S, Shaker R (2001) Esophageal and upper esophageal motor function in babies. American Journal of Medicine 111(8A): 64S–98S.

Jadcherla S, Zhang J, Shaker R (2000) Maturation of esophageal motor function. Neurogastroenterology and Motility 12(5): 483.

Jelm J (1990) Oral-Motor/Feeding Rating Scale. Tucson AZ: Therapy Skill Builders.

Kahrilas P, Lin S, Logemann J, et al. (1993) Deglutitive tongue action: volume accommodation and bolus propulsion. Gastroenterology 104: 152–63.

Kahrilas P, Logemann J, Lin S (1992) Pharyngeal clearance during swallowing: a combined manometric and videofluoroscopic study. Gastroenterology 103: 128–36.

Kenny D, Casas M, McPherson K (1989) Correlation of ultrasound imaging of oral swallow and ventilatory alternations in cerebral palsied and normal children: preliminary observations. Dysphagia 4: 112–17.

Kenny D, Koheil R, Greenberg J, et al. (1989) Development of a multidisciplinary feeding profile for children who are dependent feeders. Dysphagia 4: 16–28.

Langmore S (2001) Endoscopic Evaluation and Management of Swallowing Disorders. New York: Thieme.

Leder S (1996) Gag reflex and dysphagia. Head and Neck 18: 138–41.

Lefton-Greif M, Loughlin G (1996) Specialized studies in pediatric dysphagia. Seminars in Speech and Language 17(4): 311–30.

Link D, Willging J, Miller C, et al. (2000) Pediatric laryngopharyngeal sensory testing during flexible endoscopic evaluation of swallowing: feasible and correlative. Annals of Otology, Rhinology and Laryngology 109: 899–905.

Logan W, Bosma J (1967) Oral and pharyngeal dysphagia in infancy. Pediatric Clinics of North America 14(1): 47–61.

Logemann J (1983) Evaluation and Treatment of Swallowing Disorders. Austin TX: Pro Ed.

Mbonda E, Claus D, Bonnier C, et al. (1995) Prolonged dysphagia caused by congenital pharyngeal dysfunction. Journal of Pediatrics 126(6): 923–7.

McCurtin A (1997) The Manual of Paediatric Feeding Practise. Bicester: Winslow Press.

Mercado-Deane M, Burton E, Harlow S, et al. (2001) Swallowing dysfunction in infants less than 1 year of age. Pediatric Radiology 31(6): 423–8.

Miller A, Bieger D, Conklin J (1997) Functional controls of deglutition. In Perlman A, Schulze-Delrieu K (eds) Deglutition and its Disorders: Anatomy, Physiology, Clinical Diagnosis and Management. San Diego: Singular Publishing, pp. 43–98.

Morgan A, Ward E, Murdoch B, et al. (2002) Acute characteristics of pediatric dysphagia subsequent to traumatic brain injury: videofluoroscopic assessment. Journal of Head Trauma Rehabilitation 17(3): 220–41.

Moroz S, Espinoza J, Cumming W, et al. (1976) Lower esophageal sphincter function in children with and without gastroesophageal reflux. Gastroenterology 71: 236–41.

Morris S (1982) Pre-Speech Assessment Scale: A Rating Scale for the Development of the Pre-Speech Behaviors from Birth through Two Years. Clifton NJ: JA Preston.

Morton R, Bonas R, Fourie B, et al. (1993) Videofluoroscopy in the assessment of feeding disorders of children with neurologic problems. Developmental Medicine and Child Neurology 35: 388–95.

Newman L, Cleveland R, Blickman J, Hillman R, Jaramillo D (1991) Videofluoroscopic analysis of the infant swallow. Investigative Radiology 26: 870–3.

Newman L, Petersen M (1999) Clinical evaluation of swallowing disorders: the pediatric perspective. In R Carrau, T Murry (eds) Comprehensive Management of Swallowing Disorders. San Diego: Singular Publishing Group, pp. 43–6.

Noback G (1923) The developmental topography of the larynx, trachea and lungs in the fetus, newborn, infant and child. American Journal of Diseases of Childhood 26: 515–33.

O'Donoghue S, Bagnall A (1999) Videofluoroscopic evaluation in the assessment of swallowing disorders in paediatric and adult populations. Folia Phoniatrica et Logopedica 51(4–5): 158–71.

Omari T, Snel A, Barnett C, et al. (1999) Measurement of upper esophageal sphincter tone and relaxation during swallowing in premature infants. American Journal of Physiology, 277(Gastrointestinal Liver Physiology 40): G862–866.

Orenstein S, Bergman I, Proujansky R, Kocoshis S, Giarrusso V (1992) Novel primitive swallowing reflex: facial receptor distribution and stimulus characteristics. Dysphagia 7(3): 150–4.

Orenstein S, Giarusso V, Proujansky R, et al. (1988) The Santmyer swallow: a new and useful infant reflex. Lancet 13: 345–6.

Ottenbacher K, Dauck B, Gevelinger M, et al. (1985) Reliability of the behavioral assessment scale of oral functions in feeding. American Journal of Occupational Therapy 39: 436–40.

Palmer J (1989) Electromyography of the muscles of oropharyngeal swallowing: basic concepts. Dysphagia 3: 192–8.

Palmer M, Crawley K, Blanco I (1993) Neonatal Oral Motor Assessment Scale: a reliability study. Journal of Perinatology 8: 28–35.

Palmer M, Heyman M (1993) Assessment and treatment of sensory versus motor-based feeding problems in very young children. Infants and Young Children 6: 67–73.

Reilly S, Wisbeach A, Carr L (2000) Assessing feeding in children with neurological problems. In Southall A, Schwartz A (eds) Feeding Problems in Children. Oxford: Radcliffe Medical Press, pp. 153–71.

Reynolds E, Vice F, Bosma J, et al. (2002) Cervical accelerometry in preterm infants. Developmental Medicine and Child Neurology 44(9): 587–92.

Reynolds E, Vice F, Gewolb I (2003) Cervical accelometry in preterm infants with and without bronchopulmonary dysplasia. Developmental Medicine and Child Neurology 45(7): 442–6.

Rogers B, Arvedson J, Buck G, et al. (1994) Characteristics of dysphagia in children with cerebral palsy. Dysphagia 9: 69–73.

Rommel N (2002) Diagnosis of oropharyngeal disorders in young children: new insights and assessment with manofluoroscopy. Unpublished PhD, University of Leuven, Leuven, Belgium.

Rommel N, Meyer AD, Feenstra L, et al. (2003) The complexity of feeding problems in 700 infants and young children presenting to a tertiary care institution. Journal of Pediatric Gastroenterology and Nutrition 37(1): 75–84.

Schwarz S, Corredor J, Fisher-Medina J, et al. (2001) Diagnosis and treatment of feeding disorders in children with developmental disabilities. Pediatrics 108(3): 671–6.

Shawker T, Sonies B, Hall T, et al. (1984) Ultrasound analysis of the tongue, hyoid and larynx activity during swallowing. Investigative Radiology 19(2): 82–6.

Sheikh S, Allen E, Shell R, et al. (2001) Chronic aspiration without gastroesophageal reflux as a cause of chronic respiratory symptoms in neurologically normal infants. Chest 120: 1190–5.

Sheppard J (1987) Assessment of oral motor behaviours in cerebral palsy. Seminars in Speech and Language 8: 57–70.

Sheppard J (1995) Clinical evaluation and treatment. In Rosenthal S, Sheppard J, Lotze M (eds) Dysphagia and the Child with Developmental Disabilities: Medical Clinical and Family Interventions. San Diego: Singular, pp. 37–77.

Sheppard J (2002) Dysphagia Disorders Survey and Dysphagia Management Staging Scale (Revised). Lake Hopatcong NJ (USA edition): Nutritional Management Associates. Ryde (Australian edition): Center for Developmental Disability Services.

Sievers A (1997) Nursing evaluation and care of the dysphagic patient. In Leonard R, Kendall K (eds) Dysphagia Assessment and Treatment Planning: A Team Approach. San Diego: Singular, p. 47.

Sloan R (1977) The cinefluorographic study of cerebral palsy deglutition patterns. Journal of the Osaka Dental University 11: 58–73.

Sondheimer J (1983) Upper esophageal sphincter and pharyngoesophageal motor function in infants with and without gastroesophageal reflux. Gastroenterology 85: 301–5.

Sonies B (1991) Instrumental procedures of dysphagia diagnosis. Seminars in Speech and Language 12(3): 185–97.

Swigert NB (1998) The Source for Pediatric Dysphagia. East Moline IL: LinguiSystems.

Takashashi K, Groher M, Michi K-I (1994) Symmetry and reproducibility of swallowing sounds. Dysphagia 9: 168–73.

Tuchman D (1989) Choke, cough, splutter: the evaluation of the child with dysfunctional swallowing. Dysphagia 3: 111–16.

Tucker J (1985) Perspective of the development of the air and food passages. American Review of Respiratory Diseases 131: 7–9.

Utian H, Thomas R (1969) Cricopharyngeal incoordination in infancy. Pediatrics 43(3): 402–6.

Vice F, Bamford O, Heinz J, et al. (1995) Correlation of cervical auscultation with physiological recording during suckle-feeding in newborn infants. Developmental Medicine and Child Neurology 37: 167–79.

Vice F, Heinz J, Giurati G, et al. (1990) Cervical auscultation of suckle feeding in new born infants. Developmental Medicine and Child Neurology 32: 760–8.

Williams D, Mitchell D (1980) Pharyngo-esophageal dysphagia in infancy. International Journal of Pediatric Otorhinolaryngology 2: 231–42.

Willing J, Furukawa Y, Davidson G, et al. (1994) Strain induced augmentation of upper esophageal sphincter pressure in children. Gut 35: 159–164.

Wolf L, Glass R (1992) Clinical feeding evaluation. In Wolf L, Glass R (eds) Feeding and Swallowing in Infants and Children: Pathophysiology, Diagnosis and Treatment. San Diego: Therapy Skill Builders, pp. 85–147.

Wright R, Wright F, Carson C (1996) Videofluoroscopic assessment in children with severe cerebral palsy presenting with dysphagia. Pediatric Radiology 26(10): 720–2.

Yang W, Loveday E, Metreweli C, et al. (1997) Ultrasound assessment of swallowing in malnourished disabled children. British Journal of Radiology 70: 992–4.

Zerilli K, Stefans VA, DiPietro MA (1990) Protocol for the use of videofluoroscopy in pediatric swallowing dysfunction. American Journal of Occupational Therapy 44(5): 441–6.

15 Management of Paediatric Feeding Problems

SARAH STARR

INTRODUCTION

Managing infants and children with dysphagia can be both a challenging and satisfying experience incorporating a diverse range of health professionals, families, cultures and potential issues. Dysphagia management is both multifactorial and multidisciplinary. When a child has been referred with dysphagia it is essential to explore *all* the factors that influence the child's development, skills in feeding and how they play a role in the child's current feeding skills. It is only when we have a thorough understanding of these factors paired with an in depth clinical assessment and consultation with family and specialists and/or health professionals that can we positively assist in the management of dysphagia.

This chapter will outline the factors that need to be explored, the principles and rationales of management and discuss techniques appropriate in the management of feeding problems in infants and children. The aim is to guide the health professional to consider all the aspects of the child and family, to solve problems and select appropriate management options. However, all children are unique in terms of their problems, family dynamics, environmental factors and access to support and equipment and these issues are important in managing dysphagia effectively.

MULTIDISCIPLINARY MANAGEMENT

Dysphagia management requires a multidisciplinary approach (Wolf and Glass, 1992; Arvedson and Brodsky, 1993; Morris and Klein, 2000). It is essential that all relevant health professionals are either a part of the dysphagia team or can be sourced at appropriate times, as their involvement will assist in the total and appropriate management of the child with feeding problems (Arvedson and Brodsky, 1993). The specific health professionals to be involved will depend on the nature of the child's feeding difficulties, medical issues, nutritional issues, fine/gross motor skills and developmental and physical disabilities. This will also be influenced by the age of the child, parental needs, and the support required for a particular child and family. The following health professionals are commonly involved in the management of dysphagia:

Dysphagia: Foundation, Theory and Practice. Edited by J. Cichero and B. Murdoch
© 2006 John Wiley & Sons, Ltd.

- speech pathologist;
- nurse;
- lactation consultant;
- early childhood nurse;
- dietitian;
- paediatrician/general practitioner;
- occupational therapist;
- physiotherapist;
- gastroenterologist;
- social worker;
- other medical personnel.

The role of each professional is clearly different. However, at times roles may also overlap depending on the child's needs and the resources available in the workplace. The health professional's knowledge, experience and skills in dysphagia management will also play a part in role delineation, training and support that the health professional will need. Each team member's role and skills needs to be clearly identified, documented and discussed to ensure the child receives the best possible care (Speech Pathology Australia Dysphagia Position Paper, 2003).

MANAGEMENT OF CHILDREN VERSUS ADULTS

Although there are some shared principles when managing both paediatric and adult dysphagia there are some significant differences to consider and incorporate into management. Firstly, infant anatomy and physiology are significantly different from those of the adult (Morris and Klein, 2000; see also Chapter 2). The infant has primitive reflexes and different oromotor and feeding abilities to the adult that need to be considered (Christenson, 1989). The child's anatomy and physiology is evolving and the skills and abilities will change significantly over time in view of developmental changes that occur. These anatomical and physiological differences will play an important role in the choice of positioning, equipment and methods of feeding. For example, the choice of spoon for an infant may be smaller and flatter than that required for an adult.

Secondly, the child's neurological, physical, cognitive, oromotor, feeding, independence status and skills will be constantly changing. The child's development may also be affected by congenital or acquired disability (Christenson, 1989). In view of these changes, the therapeutic choices made, strategies employed, and support required for the child and family will need to be reviewed, modified and updated on a regular basis. The particular health professionals involved over time may also vary depending on the child's advancing age, development and needs.

Thirdly, as children are largely dependent on parents and caregivers it is crucial that the parent's and caregiver's skills in:

- positioning;
- setting the environment;
- selecting feeding choices and methods; and
- understanding of the feeding problem

be assessed, with appropriate support and training provided. The range of places and institutions where the child may be cared for such as home, hospital, daycare, pre-school, school, foster, respite facilities will need to be explored and often included in the management process. Management may need to incorporate liaison and visits to relevant environments where the child is, or will be, fed. Although inclusions of caregivers and family members is also relevant when managing adult clients with dysphagia, the actual knowledge, skills and needs of the family and caregivers will vary significantly from the child to the adult client.

In view of the differences in anatomy and physiology between the child and adult, and changes in the developmental status of the child, specialist knowl-edge and skills are required of the health professionals involved in paediatric dysphagia management. This is not to say that health professionals cannot work in both adult and paediatric areas; however, it is important that it is never assumed that the knowledge and skills are the same for adult and paediatric dysphagia management.

MANAGEMENT OPTIONS

When managing feeding problems in children the clinician has several treatment op-tions to consider often involving a combination of approaches depending on the age of the infant, the child's needs, family's needs and the child's problems. Dysphagia management often involves:

- nutritional considerations/decisions;
- the feeding environment and its impact on the feeding process and how it can be modified to facilitate feeding success;
- positioning of the child and parent/care giver;
- selection of appropriate feeding methods in accordance with the child's skills, age and needs;
- selection of appropriate timing, amount and type of food – these also depend on the child's age, skills and needs);
- scheduling and timing of meal;
- addressing and supporting parent's needs and skills;
- oral exercises and oral/facial support that will facilitate oral motor function and feeding skills.

These areas will be discussed in greater depth below.

NUTRITION

Whether the infant or child is breast, bottle, solid or tube fed, nutritional intake is crucial to facilitate the child's

- growth;
- cognition;

- motor skills; and
- organ, body and skeletal development (White et al., 1993; Young, 1993; Morris and Klein, 2000).

When children present with feeding difficulties they are often at risk of insufficient intake due to the increased time to feed, possible refusal patterns and physical, oro-motor or swallowing difficulties (Ganger and Craig, 1990; Kamal, 1990). They are also at risk for stunted skeletal growth, poor weight gain, anaemia, specific mineral and nutrient deficiencies and dental problems (White et al., 1993). Medications may also interfere with absorption of specific vitamins or minerals.

The speech pathologist is responsible for identifying the infant's or child's feed-ing skills. They must also practically relate these skills to the time taken to feed and how the child's nutritional requirements are met whilst also facilitating oromotor skills or swallowing function. This is done through specific food or liquid types, exercises and equipment. For example, a child who is breastfeeding and not putting on weight may need to be complemented with bottle feeds to facilitate weight gain. The child who is only just learning to bite and chew solids may need opportunities to practise chewing more challenging chopped food at the beginning of a meal or at snack times, whilst their nutrition may be *primarily* met through purees.

The therapist must consider that a full oral feed should be achieved within 40 minutes to 45 minutes for a newborn and by 30 minutes for a child above 6 months of age. This allows not only for adequate nutrition for growth and health but also allows the child to have normal sleep, wake times and developmental experiences. Mealtimes need to be scheduled to fit in and around family, environmental and social routines as much as possible. For some children fatigue factors also need to be considered, with these infants and children requiring shorter oral feeding times to ensure adequate nutrition and safe swallowing.

Many children with dysphagia may require supplementation of their oral intake (Ganger and Craig, 1990, White et al, 1993. This may be achieved through:

- small, frequent feeds;
- adding calories to feeds – e.g. commercial additives such as polyjoule or polycose;
- adding specific vitamins, minerals and nutritional supplements;
- natural food additives such as butter, thickened cream or cheese to feeds; or
- nasogastric or other tube feeding routes.

A dietitian and paediatrician should be consulted regarding the appropriate selection and method of nutritional supplementation. In doing so they will take into account the child's weight, age, growth, medical condition and nutritional needs. Through team discussions an appropriate balance of oral versus non-oral intake, amount of intake, timing and dietary supplementation can be achieved. This will then ensure optimum health and growth of the child, whilst facilitating oral intake and skills. Achieving this balance can be challenging and may need regular and ongoing modi-fication for the developing and changing needs of the child.

It is important for the speech pathologist to explain and document the child's individual oral feeding skills with the range of liquid and solid consistencies appropriate to the child's age. This will assist the dietitian's nutritional management including the range, type, amount and timing of foods/liquids offered.

THE FEEDING ENVIRONMENT

The feeding environment or actual physical place the child is fed can have an impact on both the parent and child during feeding. The aim is for the feeding environment to be a calm, rhythmical setting where the child is able to focus on feeding and swallowing. The therapist needs to explore aspects such as:

- Where the child is fed? Does this encourage the child's position and stability as these will have an impact on the child's self-feeding skills and oromotor or swallowing ability? Conversely, does the child's positioning or seating encourage negative positioning, e.g. head extension, general seating instability, inhibiting patterns such as asymmetrical tonic neck reflex (ATNR).
- Is the environment calming or distracting? Aspects such as lighting, sound, noise and visual objects and patterns need to be considered and possibly modified, removed or relocated in the environment. Pastel walls and softer lighting are often more helpful than environments that contain busy visual patterns or loud, inconsistent or distracting noises.

An environment may have a different impact on different children. The therapist needs to observe aspects of the environment such as lighting, visual elements, noise, and rhythm. The therapist should then determine whether these have a positive or negative impact on the child and make appropriate modifications as necessary.

Many children respond positively to the introduction of a rhythm. Our sucking and chewing mechanisms occur rhythmically and often the suck/swallow/breathe and chewing cycles are close to one cycle per second. Classical music with a moderate tempo that mirrors this rhythm of one beat per second can be helpful. Often in newborns, patting on the infant's back or gentle rocking during feeding can also assist feeding rhythm and coordination of sucking/swallowing and breathing. Music can also have a calming and focusing effect on the child and parent (Morris and Klein, 2000). Music may suit some children and their parents but not others. The positive and negative impacts of using music during feeding should, therefore, be evaluated.

POSITIONING AND SEATING

Many children who present with feeding difficulties may have abnormalities in their posture, tone and movement which may well result in abnormal gross or fine motor development. Children with neurological disorders (e.g. cerebral palsy) often have significant physical challenges that influence feeding (Morris and Klein, 2000).

Appropriate positioning and posture of the body, trunk, head, feet, neck and pelvis are vital in facilitating oromotor function, and developing safe feeding or swallowing skills.

Positioning and seating must take into consideration (a) the gross motor development of the child, and (b) the need to support stability. In addition, positioning should aim to inhibit abnormal tone and reflex movement so that normal movement patterns may be facilitated. Factors such as the child's respiratory status, age, needs, seizure activity, presence of gastroesophageal reflux and various medical conditions (e.g. cleft palate – see also Chapter 13) may also influence positioning of the child. Positioning and seating options will change depending on children's neuromuscular development, their age and size, their need for stability, feeding needs and level of independence. Sensory integration and responses to touch, pressure, posture and movement may also influence the therapist's choice in positioning and seating equipment and support.

The family also plays an integral role in positioning and seating. One must ensure that the carer will be in a comfortable and sustainable position to facilitate the child's oral motor function for feeding. The context of feeding needs to be considered:

- at home;
- when parents are out; and
- as children grow older, including seating arrangements at daycare, preschool and school.

Options and suitable arrangements may vary depending on the physical environment, caregiver skills and available support (Macie and Arvedson, 1993).

Access to equipment in a variety of settings will also need to be addressed as these may vary enormously. Children may be waiting for seating equipment or chairs and therefore interim and affordable measures may need to be investigated and provided. Simple, cheap and accessible resources may include, swaddling cloth, cushions, foam wedges, beanbags, rolled up towels, footstools, sports headbands, and car seats. These can then move to more sophisticated and expensive seating systems. (e.g. tilt in space chairs – see Figure 15.1). Cost, the temporary or long-term nature of the child's positioning and movement needs and accessibility of equipment will also influence choices.

The main aims when addressing positioning and seating are to facilitate:

- a relaxed and comfortable seating arrangement;
- a sustainable posture/position;
- balance, stability and mobility;
- efficient and safe swallowing;
- oromotor function and control;
- inhibition of abnormal movement patterns and reflexes;
- independent feeding.

These points will now be expanded upon. Children with abnormal tone and movement are particularly at risk for poorly coordinated and ineffective swallowing,

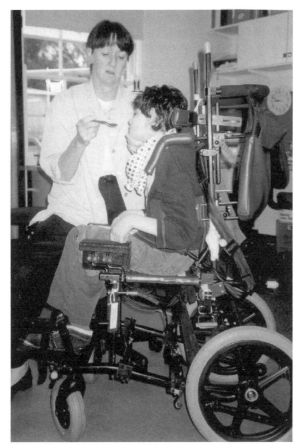

Figure 15.1   Mulholland seating system – tilt in space chair. Note the shoulder block to provide shoulder and trunk support (reproduced with kind permission of Allowah Presbyterian Children's Hospital)

resulting in aspiration of food and/or liquid into the airway, with possible consequent chest pathology. Supportive, correct positioning for feeding is essential to facilitate appropriate head and neck posture to achieve optimal oral and pharyngeal phases of swallowing and minimize the risk of aspiration (Wolf and Glass, 1992).

It is important then, that the posture or position chosen will reduce the likelihood of fatigue for both the child and caregiver. If a seating or positioning arrangement cannot be maintained easily it is either likely to be modified by the caregiver or will deteriorate with time. In both cases it is likely to be ineffective. Balance, stability and mobility are critical during child development. Movement and functional skills such as feeding, require that the child has a stable base (Morris, 1985). With increased stability there is a greater chance for mobility to develop (Alexander, 1987; Macie and Arvedson, 1993). Efficient use of the mouth for eating depends heavily on stability of the trunk, neck and head (Morris and Klein, 2000). Posture and stability must be viewed as a whole body continuum. Movement and instability in the feet, legs and pelvis influences what occurs in the trunk. The tone and movement in the trunk will affect function in the shoulder girdle. These then influence head and neck stability and then jaw, lip, cheek and tongue control (Morris and Klein, 2000). Development of movement control in one area of the body then significantly influences development of movement in other areas of the body (Wolf and Glass, 1992; Macie and Arvedson, 1993). If stability of the head and neck is facilitated and abnormal movements and reflexes are inhibited then normal feeding/swallowing movements and oro-motor functions are able to be facilitated in the developing child (Wolf and Glass, 1992). It is critical that oromotor function and control are optimized in the early years to facilitate long-term positive outcomes in terms of the child's feeding, oromotor and speech skills.

If abnormal patterns of movement are not inhibited the child's oromotor control functions and feeding may be negatively influenced. Positioning strategies and purposeful intervention that inhibit abnormal patterns allow the child more independent and volitional movement. It is crucial that inhibition of abnormal patterns occurs in the very early years to maximize long-term oral-motor and feeding outcomes. For example, if children are fed with the head in an extended posture, this will perpetuate and encourage jaw extension, which can often exacerbate tongue thrusting and poor feeding.

As the child's stability, motor control and movement develops and cognitive changes occur, the child is able to move to more independent feeding patterns. This may involve moving from the breast or bottle to spoon/ fingers/ cup and later knife and fork. Although we expect newborns and young children to be dependent or at least partially dependent on caregivers during feeding it is a normal phase of development and identification of one's self in society that we work towards independent function in our everyday lives (Morris and Klein, 2000). By facilitating assisted self feeding the child gains greater control over the feeding process, which may increase cooperation and alleviate possible behavioural problems associated with feeding. Positioning, seating and equipment selection should address the child's independence in eating and drinking over time. For example seating modification, correct tray placement, and elbow support that facilitates hand-to-mouth function and mouth opening will ultimately promote independent feeding.

Before proceeding further with positioning strategies it is important to emphasize that positioning needs to be a multidisciplinary process. The physiotherapist and occupational therapist are clearly vital team members to be consulted. It is also important for the speech pathologist to be an integral part of the process to facilitate oromotor function and efficient, safe swallowing. The individual child and their family also play a key role in individualizing treatment.

Seating supports, such as harnesses or strapping need to be safe for the child and abide by local and national safety standards, and occupational health and safety standards. Questions that should be asked include: 'Does the child need to be supervised at all times with the equipment or seating arrangements? Does it place the caregiver or child at risk of injury, compensatory posture or negative outcomes?'

POSITIONING PRINCIPLES

To achieve safe and efficient swallowing and to assist stability and appropriate movement patterns the therapist should aim to reduce hyperextension, minimize hyperflexion, and minimize further physical deformity (Macie and Arvedson, 1993). As mentioned earlier, positioning will vary for each child. The main focus areas that often need to be addressed and supported are as follows:

- *The pelvis and hips.* The newborn may need to be flexed into a curled position with hips bent and knees flexed. Similarly, to achieve a good sitting position the hips need to flexed and the pelvis titled slightly back.
- *The trunk* should be symmetrical and not rotated or side flexed. In a sitting position the trunk is often upright. In some cases it is marginally reclined to achieve a stable, erect and midline trunk position.
- *The shoulder girdle* should be slightly protracted (forward) to assist forward arm positioning and general flexion. This will also assist later propping of the elbows on the table or tray and independent use of the arms. Positioning of the shoulder girdle may be assisted by swaddling in the newborn or later by hand pressure or cuffing of the arms or wrists.
- *The legs* should be still during feeding and assist in the maintenance of hip flexion. This usually means the knees should be bent to inhibit extension in the hips and knees.
- *The head and neck* are often areas that need particular support during feeding. The head should be supported and maintained in a slightly forward posture with chin tucked. This will assist swallowing efficiency and airway protection as well as inhibiting abnormal extensor patterns, and will allow for more controlled and coordinated movements of the mouth for feeding. Care should be taken however, to ensure that the posture does not inhibit respiration and contribute to airway collapse.

Positioning of the newborn

Infants do not have stability and volitional control of their movement at birth. Their movements are largely whole body or whole mouth movements and heavily influenced by early reflex patterns (Morris and Klein, 2000). Newborn positioning techniques may include swaddling, specific positions and use of positioning aids. Swaddling the infant provides external stability, improved general body flexion and, assists in calming the infant which may allow for better oromotor function. Swaddling is demonstrated in Figure 15.2. In addition, specific positions may need to be incorporated. Positions such as side lying, prone or more upright positioning may be useful. For example, infants with micrognathia (a small mandible) or macroglossia (large tongue) often benefit from a side lying or prone position that facilitates a more forward tongue posture and improved respiratory status during feeding (see Figure 15.3). Children born with a cleft palate may be fed in a more upright position to minimize nasal regurgitation of milk into their nasal passage during feeding. Children with gastro-esophageal reflux are more often fed and slept in a more upright position to minimize their reflux and facilitate gastric emptying. Pillows, towels and footstools are common

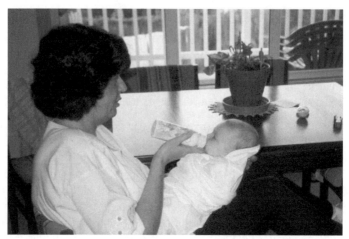

Figure 15.2 Infant swaddled on mother's lap with head and jaw support provided (reproduced with kind permission of Allowah Presbyterian Children's Hospital)

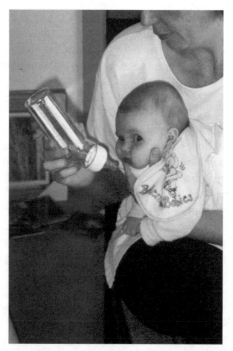

Figure 15.3 Child being fed in prone position (reproduced with kind permission of Allowah Presbyterian Children's Hospital)

pieces of equipment used in the early months to support arms, backs and feet of both the feeder and infant. Infants need maximum support to provide stability.

Positioning of the child in a seated position

Once the child is being fed solids or at the developmental stage to facilitate or achieve sitting, new positioning techniques to support this position may be incorporated.

A pelvic strap is often the first point of stability to assist with flexion at the hips. If the pelvis and hips are stabilized this acts as an axis point and stability for the rest of the body. The feet should be maintained in a flat position. The legs should bend at right angles. Feet often need to rest on a footplate and additional foot cuffs may be needed to secure and maintain feet positioning. The trunk may be supported in a symmetrical, upright position by lateral trunk supports or strapping in the form of harnesses individually tailored to the child's size, posture and disability.

The shoulder girdle may be assisted into forward rotation by cushioning placed behind the shoulder girdle. The head and neck may be supported by an arm or hand of the feeder around the neck, a hand under the chin or on the apex of the head (see Figure 15.4). Additional supports such as neck rolls or neck cushions may also be used. Care must always be taken with head and neck supports that they do not push the child's head back into hyperextension (see Figure 15.5a and 15.5b) or hyperflexion, which can have an immediate impact on oral and swallowing function.

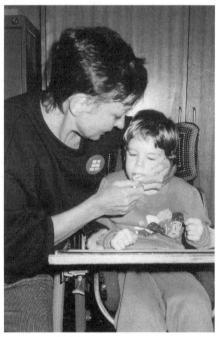

Figure 15.4 Child being provided with head support and full jaw and lip support during spoon feeding (reproduced by kind permission of Allowah Presbyterian Children's Hospital)

(a)

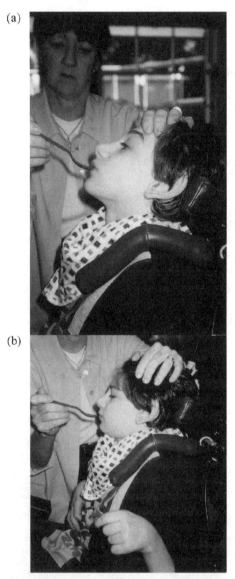

(b)

Figure 15.5   (a) Poor hand support by carer resulting in head extension (b) child receiving head support on the apex of the head to assist head position during feeding (reproduced with kind permission of Allowah Presbyterian Children's Hospital)

Positioning of the feeder

The position of the feeder will influence the success of positioning of the infant or child. In the early months the feeder provides optimum support and stability to the child through maximum body support and holding either in a 'madonna' hold, twin position on the breast or bottle or in front and facing the feeder on the lap. Certain conditions such as cleft palate may require more upright positioning by the feeder to minimize regurgitation into the nasal cavity. As children grow, lap feeding may become difficult for the feeder and not the optimum way of providing the best support to the child whilst feeding. The actual seating system selected for the child will often influence whether the feeder sits in front of or to the side of the child during feeding. For example, the size of the chair, the presence and depth of a tray will affect the location of the feeder relative to the child. The feeder needs to be aware of how their positioning will facilitate the child's posture, particularly head posture and eating or swallowing function as well as facilitating social mealtimes with others.

FEEDING EQUIPMENT

SELECTION OF FEEDING EQUIPMENT

When selecting the most appropriate equipment for an infant or child the therapist needs to consider many variables. Although the focus of this chapter is the management of dysphagia, it is well documented that oral-feeding, and communication skills and development are closely linked (Kent, 1984; Alexander, 1987; Selly et al, 1990). Careful selection of equipment ensures oral movements and early speech development are facilitated in conjunction with feeding skills (Starr S, 1995; Morris and Klein, 2000). For example, a flat spoon may be selected to facilitate inward upper lip cleaning of the spoon whilst also promoting the 'm, p, b' sounds that require this movement. A training cup with dribble lid (inverted into cup) may be selected to facilitate inward lip closure as well as labial sounds such as 'm, p, b'.

Other variables the clinician should consider include:

- the child's age and size;
- the anatomical relationships of the child's facial, oral and pharyngeal structures;
- the child's feeding skills/difficulties;
- the child's medical status or craniofacial abnormality if present, (see also Chapter 13);
- self-feeding and feeding independence;
- the motor and cognitive development of the child;
- disabilities and their influencing issues;
- the positioning and/or seating of the child;
- child and parental preferences;
- durability, cost and accessibility;
- oromotor and communication skills and development;
- nutritional guidelines; and
- the feeding goals.

These variables are detailed in Table 15.1.

Table 15.1 Factors affecting selection of feeding equipment

Factors affecting equipment selection	The clinician should consider
Child's age and size	• Size of handles for cups, spoons, forks. • Length, shape and depth of bowl and spoon. • Length and shape of spout. • Size of cup lips. • Teat lengths and widths. For example a long, fast-flow teat may be an inappropriate choice for a premature infant who is 6 weeks old (corrected age 36 weeks). More suitable choice may be a short, slow-flow teat design. Shorter teat may be more suitable as long teat may induce gagging because it extends beyond the posterior tongue area.
Child's feeding skills or difficulties	• Equipment should facilitate control and refinement and manintain swallowing safety. • Inhibit abnormal movement patterns. For example, the equipment should not facilitate, perpetuate or exacerbate gagging, a tonic bite reflex, tongue thrusting, coughing or aspiration. Rhythmical, controlled and safe feeding should be encouraged and facilitated.
Child's medical status (e. g. craniofacial abnormality)	• May require non-oral or alternative feeding (e.g. nasogastric, orogastric tube feeding). • If concurrent respiratory/cardiac abnormalities present, fatigue may need to be considered.
Self feeding and feeding independence	• Self-feeding readiness, abilities and goals should be considered. For example, some equipment may be used for primary nutrition (e.g. a bottle) and another piece of equipment may be trialled at particular times in the day (a) to transition the child gradually or (b) to teach new oromotor/ self feeding skills or (c) allow for a degree of independence.
Developmental level of the child	• Motor and cognitive development affects child's readiness and acceptability of equipment. • Some children may have restricted equipment experiences. For example, a 5-year-old child still drinking from a bottle and teat even when there may have been no physiological reason for not transitioning the child to mature cup drinking. The longer some children progress using immature or earlier feeding equipment (such as bottles) the more difficult it is to transition them to new equipment. Despite a lower cognitive level a child may still be ready to transfer to mature feeding options and equipment.
Disability	• Physical skills and limitations, visual skills/impairment, oral sensitivity, oromotor abilities, and abnormal reflex patterns may influence the feeding equipment as well as the need for assistance or support (e.g. handcuffing/strapping). For example, a child with visual impairment may benefit from equipment that is brightly coloured and when touch and verbal cueing is given.
Positioning/Seating of the child	• Reciprocal relationship exists between equipment and positioning. For example, consider a child who is seated in a wheelchair with minimal head support and without a tray. If this child is given a two-handled cup with open rim for mealtimes the therapist may notice poor arm and trunk stability and head.

Table 15.1 (*Continued*)

Factors affecting equipment selection	The clinician should consider
Positioning/Seating of the child (*Continued*)	extension during drinking. This child may need consideration for (a) head-and-neck support, (b) a tray to assist trunk stability, and (c) arm propping to facilitate independent cup drinking and better oral control and safer swallowing. A younger infant who is fed in a side lying position may need feeding facilitated by an angled bottle.
Child and parental preferences	• Does the child refuse particular equipment? If so, why is this occurring and does it influence equipment choices? • Does the parent feel the equipment is user friendly, practical, accessible, and understand the rationale behind equipment choices?
Durability, cost, accessibility	• Thorough investigation of the marketplace needs to occur. • Consider purchase price and availability, equipment durability, ease of washing and sterilization.
Nutritional needs	• Is the child's nutrition being met by the current feeding method and equipment? • Will the introduction of equipment support and ensure nutritional requirements? • There needs to be a practical balance of equipment choice, timing and frequency of feeds appropriate to the child's abilities, feeding duration, time taken and in order to meet nutritional needs. • Consider consultation with a dietitian, paediatrician and sometimes psychologist to assist decision making and management. For example, obviously in the newborn, breast milk and breastfeeding are the ideal nutrition and process. However, many infants may be bottle fed as a complimentary or alternative method for a variety of reasons such as poor weight gain, insufficient growth, allergies or intolerance (e.g. lactose intolerance), feeding and swallowing skills, medical conditions and parental preferences/choice. If a child has a 'new' cup, it may take several weeks and months before the child is able to ingest liquids effectively and completely with this method and so often the transition to the 'new' piece of equipment may be gradual and supported by more familiar or easier options. Very occasionally if some children are resistant to change, total removal of the 'old' equipment may by necessary for change to occur as long as liquid intake and nutritional needs can be met. An example of this could be a four-year-old who insists all liquids be taken via a teat-cup and resists efforts to sip/ try an open cup or more mature cup when it is known the child is capable with the 'new' cup. The child's liquid intake may be able to be sustained via pureed consistencies whilst the 'new' cup is offered only.
The feeding goals	• Equipment is chosen not only on age expectations and current skills, but also to facilitate new or more effective patterns of movement. For example, a child of 12–15 months who is unable to use the upper lip to move downwards to clean the spoon may need a flatter bowl of the spoon to assist with this upper lip movement. The therapist is focusing, then, on the next step in oral feeding development and selecting equipment and presentation that may facilitate these new movement patterns.

SPECIFIC FEEDING EQUIPMENT

Choices of equipment will vary from child to child in view of the numerous variables that impact on the therapist's selection. Selection needs to be based on the individual's needs and circumstances. There are however, some basic principles when selecting specific teats, bottles, pacifiers (i.e. dummies), cups, spoons and forks. These principles are listed below to guide the therapist in choosing from the vast array of commercially available equipment. It is important to emphasize that there is no 'one teat' or 'one cup' on the market that is the 'best'. Unfortunately market trends and availability of equipment change, which means that therapists need to keep up to date with these trends and with the resources that are available. It is also important that health professionals communicate regularly with equipment suppliers and distributors. Clinicians should indicate their needs so that suppliers can provide the required equipment, and assist in its availability to our clients.

BREAST, BOTTLES AND TEATS

Breastfeeding

As mentioned earlier, health professionals should be promoting breastfeeding and breast milk intake in the first 12 months of life (World Health Organization, 1989). There are many pieces of equipment available to support breastfeeding such as supply lines, nipple shields, breast pumps, etc. When using equipment with breastfeeding and bottle feeding the therapist needs to keep in mind that the infant's early oral reflexes are facilitated in the first four months of life (i.e. rooting, pouting and sucking reflexes), and rhythmical, coordinated and nutritive sucking is facilitated. For example, if an inappropriate teat or nipple shield is used, this may facilitate non-nutritive ('dummy') sucking, which will not be helpful.

If a child presents with a craniofacial, congenital, physical, oromotor abnormality or is born prematurely, breastfeeding should be considered in view of these issues. In some instances, breastfeeding may not be possible. Parents should then be provided with information regarding bottle feeding or even enteral feeding if indicated and assisted in making choices suitable to their child. Factors to consider when deciding whether to breastfeed are:

• Will it provide adequate nutrition alone or will supplementation be required?
• Is it is physically possible for the child to succeed successfully on the breast?
• What positioning needs arise from the child's condition/status?
• Is breastfeeding a *safe* method of nutritional intake in terms of the infants swallowing mechanism and cardiac/respiratory function?
• Is additional support required to assist in breastfeeding and/or expressing breast milk.
• Does the mother *want* to breastfeed.

It may be possible to breastfeed many infants either fully or partially at certain stages in their lives despite prematurity, craniofacial or other physical abnormalities. The introduction, timing and maintenance of breastfeeding will often depend on

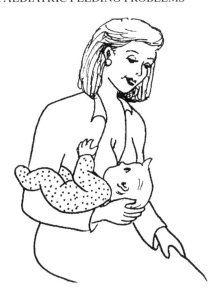

Figure 15.6 Diagram of infant feeding in 'football' hold or 'twin' hold position

- the nature of the infant's dysphagia and associated problems;
- the child's health status; and
- parental preferences.

Facilitating breastfeeding

There are many factors involved in successful breastfeeding including the child's condition/skills, the mother's breast status, the mother's diet, the emotional and physical state of the mother, support by family, and support through equipment, positioning and breastfeeding techniques. There are several texts available that address facilitation of normal and successful breastfeeding (Mackeith, 1981; Kitzinger, 1987; Laviners and Woessner, 1990). In view of the emphasis on dysphagia in this chapter, the focus will fall on facilitating breastfeeding in infants experiencing feeding difficulties. By careful positioning and by stimulating and normalizing the infant's early primitive oral reflexes involved in breastfeeding, the child's breastfeeding skills and success may be enhanced.

Positioning the child at the breast will be dependent on the infant's difficulties. The usual method of feeding is in the 'madonna' hold where the infant is held facing the breast and in a lying position across the mother's torso. For some infants with conditions such as macroglossia (large tongue) or tongue tie, the baby may be positioned in a more prone position in the 'madonna' hold to facilitate forward tongue posturing during breastfeeding. Children who have macroglossia or other conditions such as micrognathia (small jaw) will feed more efficiently in a more prone position where their tongue is brought forward so as not to occlude the pharyngeal airway during feeding. Other children may be best fed in a 'twin, football hold'. The twin feeding position is where the baby's body extends underneath the mother's arm. The position allows for two infants to be fed simultaneously, hence the name 'twin feeding position'. It has also been likened to a 'football hold', resulting in its other name (see Figure 15.6). Note that a more upright position may also better facilitate breast placement into the infant's mouth.

The mother assists the breastfeeding process by:

- supporting the infant's head, neck and trunk;
- shaping her breast to form a 'teat';
- eliciting the rooting reflex at the breast; and
- bringing the baby to the breast (rather than the breast to the baby).

The *rooting* reflex is stimulated by the breast or nipple touching the corner of the mouth. The baby turns the head to the side that was stimulated; the mouth simultaneously opens wide and the tongue moves forward, anchoring the tongue over the gum line. While this occurs, a central groove is created in the tongue and the gag reflex is inhibited in preparation to receive the breast. As the baby turns the head the lips make contact with the breast which elicits the *pouting* reflex where the lips pout into a flange. The infant receives the breast and stabilizes the jaw around the areola tissue approximately 1 cm to 2 cm outwards from the nipple. The aim is for the infant to take as much of the areola as possible into the mouth. The inner mucosa of the infant's lips seals onto the breast and the *sucking* reflex is initiated when breast tissue makes contact with the hard palate. The infant then sucks rapidly and continuously to facilitate the mother's 'letdown' of milk. The 'letdown' reflex occurs when the breasts are full of milk and sucking or the baby's hunger cries cause the release of the hormone oxytocin into the blood. The release makes the muscles around the milk glands contract, and the milk is forced into the milk ducts (Leach, 1988). The milk flows quite quickly initially. Once the let down occurs the baby will settle into a rhythmical nutritive suck-swallow-breathe pattern. That is, approximately one suck-swallow cycle occurs every second while there is a steady flow of milk (see also Chapter 2).

Many infants who are experiencing dysphagia and breastfeeding problems may have difficulty eliciting the primitive reflexes of rooting, pouting and sucking normally and may need these reflexes to be stimulated prior to feeding and at the feed time to facilitate good attachment and nutritive breastfeeding (Evans, 1977; Woolridge, 1986; Laviners and Woessner, 1990; Wolf and Glass, 1992; Shaker, 1990). Many infants have difficulty sucking efficiently, resulting in a delayed letdown of milk. Alternatively the infant may use several sucks prior to swallowing. Other infants may have difficulty initiating, and maintaining attachment and rhythmical sucking. Some may have difficulty achieving nutritive sucking and predominantly suck in a non-nutritive pattern (i.e. a rapid suck pattern with smaller jaw excursions and often not associated with swallowing of milk. It is often referred to as 'flutter' or 'dummy' sucking as it is similar to this.) Some infants may detach from the breast, cease feeding, or feed in intermittent bursts. Many infants may benefit from:

- additional positioning support or swaddling;
- external pacing to achieve a feeding rhythm (e.g. patting, rocking, music); or
- cheek, lip and/or jaw support to maintain adequate lip and jaw stability and closure during breastfeeding.

Specific head and facial supports will be discussed in the section on techniques and methods.

Bottles

Many children with significant dysphagia often need to be complimented with bottle feeds or are unable to successfully breast feed (see Figure 15.7). I will focus on bottle and teat selection in this section. The two main bottle shapes available widely are the standard width teat of 36 mm to 38 mm. or the wider neck bottles that fit wider teats of 50 mm to 52 mm diameter. There are also angled neck bottles that may facilitate head posture and swallowing in some babies (see Figure 15.3). Squeeze bottles or softer, pliable bottles (e.g. Douglas Bean, Cleft Pals, Mead Johnson varieties) are also available through specific distributors or support groups for very specific cases. There are generally two standard bottle sizes – 120 ml and 250 ml, often dependent on the child's intake and positioning needs. Recommendations for bottle selection include:

- it should be clear so movement of liquid can be seen easily;
- it should have clear markers denoting the amount (i.e. volume);
- it should be the appropriate size for the baby's requirements;
- it should be easy to clean and sterilize;
- it should facilitate good positioning and holding of the bottle;
- the size and neck width should be suitable for the teat selected.

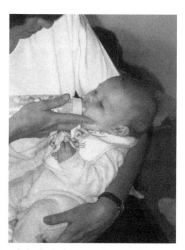

Figure 15.7 Child with hemiplegia being provided with cheek support (reproduced by kind permission of Allowah Presbyterian Children's Hospital)

Squeeze bottles may be selected but they must be used with care and thorough assessment of the child's feeding and swallowing skills. Squeeze bottles require demonstration to carers and ongoing monitoring. Squeeze bottles are generally used when the child has an ineffective suck or oral phase but an adequate and intact pharyngeal and laryngeal phase of swallowing (e.g. cleft palate). Occasionally they may also be used when a child has thickened fluids to assist flow into the mouth. A squeeze bottle is used to assist flow of the fluid into the infant's mouth.

Care must always be taken with squeeze bottles. Note, squeezing should be practised first prior to feeding the child. Squeezing should only occur *as* the infant sucks. Ideally squeezing should occur at the point of maximum jaw opening during the sucking cycle when milk flow is most abundant into the child's mouth. Squeezing may need to occur regularly or intermittently or at a particular time in the feed depending on the child's needs. Note, if the child is swallowing rapidly, gulping, coughing or gagging then the squeeze bottle flow may be too fast and inappropriate.

Squeeze bottles may be contraindicated in infants that have difficulty coordinating sucking – swallowing – breathing pattern and in certain client populations (see also Chapter 4 for a discussion of the interaction between swallowing and breathing). If squeeze bottles are used *inappropriately* or *ineffectively* then the following may occur:

- feeding refusal;
- gagging;
- aspiration of liquid into the trachea; or
- chest pathology and illness associated with aspiration.

Teats

There are a variety of teat sizes, shapes and flow rates. The three main shapes available include: a standard shape (width 36 mm to 38 mm diameter), a broader tip orthodontic variety (see Figure 15.8a,b) or a broad base variety (50 mm to 52 mm diameter). Teat selection is important in facilitating breastfeeding, early oral reflexes, effective nutritive sucking, good lip flanging, tongue posture and movement and jaw stability and movement.

The characteristics one should consider when selecting a teat are:

- it should fit the size and shape of the child's mouth:

  - a small mouth may need a small or shorter teat;
  - longer teats may elicit gagging and refusal if the mouth is small or the child has a hypersensitive gag reflex.

- The teat should facilitate lip flanging around the base of the teat, and lip closure.
- The teat should facilitate forward tongue posture just over the lower gum line and forward to backward tongue motion for sucking (i.e. suckling).
- The flow rate of the teat should suit the sucking ability and needs of the infant.

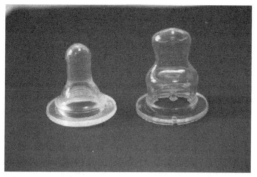

(a) Standard teats.

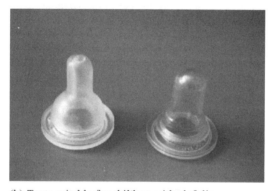

(b) Teats suitable for children with cleft lip.

Figure 15.8   (a) Teats from left: standard teat, orthodontic teat (b) specially designed cleft-palate teats: Chu Chu cleft teat (left), pigeon cleft teat (right)

- Although teats are often labelled and marked according to the child's age, the feeding abilities of an infant are more helpful in selecting a teat flow.
- For example, if the child has delayed initiation of or a poorly coordinated swallow then a slower flow may be more appropriate whereas a child that has an ineffective, weak suck but an adequate pharyngeal and laryngeal phase may benefit from a faster flowing teat (e.g. medium flow). Many different brands vary in flow rates.

- The teat should allow for pacing if needed.
- Teats may have open holes or be 'cross-cut' in design:

  - open-hole teats allow for a steady flow of liquid;
  - cross-cut teats require sucking to allow milk entry into the mouth;
  - the cross-cut teats can be effective when it is important for children to take rests to recover or breathe and without having ongoing milk flow into their mouth.

There are specialized teats designed for children with specific craniofacial abnormalities such as cleft palate. These cleft teats (see Figure 15.8b) are designed to assist the flow of milk onto the infant's mouth when their suck is ineffective, but the pharyngeal and laryngeal phases of swallowing are intact. Some infants who are unable to use or reject a teat may be tested on specific spouts or alternative bottle attachments to facilitate liquid intake. This may depend on the infant's skills and needs.

Spoons

Many spoons are available for use with pureed or mashed solids. (see Figure 15.9). The choice of spoon will often be influenced by the skills of the child, difficulties the child may be having and the oromotor or feeding movement that is to be facilitated. Factors to be considered for spoon selection are:

- A flat bowl may be useful in facilitating upper lip inward cleaning of the spoon.
- An unbreakable plastic spoon is often recommended as it won't adopt the temperature of the food, or 'bang' the child's gums as metal ones may. If the child has a bite reflex the plastic spoon will be more comfortable for the child.
- Consider the length, width, shape and weight of the handle.

  - Does the length facilitate appropriate spoon entry?
  - If the spoon handle or bowl is too long it may cause gagging in some children.

- Ensure that the size of the bowl is suited to the child's mouth, oral function and self feeding issues. For example, a child who is not yet lateralizing food pieces to the side of the mouth for chewing may be fed via a smaller size spoon into the side of the mouth (between the back molar area) (see Figure 15.11). If a child is

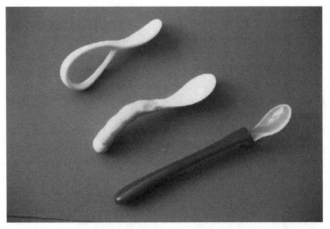

Figure 15.9 Variety of feeding spoons: Twinkle Tots self-feeding spoon (back), built up handled spoon (middle), Tommee Tippee soft scoop spoon (bottom)

self-feeding a larger, deeper bowl may be used so less is lost from the bowl to the mouth.
- Ensure that the spoon is easy to hold and facilitates self-feeding.

  - Does the handle facilitate a good hold and grip?
  - Does the spoon need to be modified with a built up handle or strapping to facilitate the grip?

- Ensure that the spoon is visually noticeable and appealing to the child.

Selecting a cup

Cups can be introduced as early as four months of age with assistance if (a) the child is ready, (b) supported with good positioning, head and facial support and (c) the appropriate liquid consistency is used. One of the biggest challenges in selecting cups is the trend in the market for sports bottles, 'popup' bottles and sipper cups. It is often difficult for therapists and families to find 'regular' cups that are not of the sucking or sipper/spout variety. Spout varieties have their place in management, however, a broader variety of non-spout cups would be useful for many children. The proliferation of spout cups makes these the norm, rather than more traditional cup types. The following are factors to be considered for appropriate cup selection:

- The cup should fit the size and shape of the child's mouth.
- A clear cup has the advantage of permitting the carer to observe its contents and allows control of the liquid.
- The cup should be capable of being tipped up to get liquid at the bottom without tipping the child's head back into extension.
- The cup should be of unbreakable plastic. An unbreakable cup allows for children who might bite down on the cup.
- The cup should facilitate lip closure and appropriate tongue posture and movement. Ideally the aim is to move towards good lip closure on the rim of the cup with the tongue held within the oral cavity. A deep cup lip with lip flange often assists this posture.
- Spouts and teats may be unhelpful for some children – they may exacerbate tongue thrusting, prolonged sucking behaviours or forward tongue posture.
- The cup should allow for a controlled flow of liquid. Lids are often useful as they assist in slowing liquid flow and make drinking tidier.
- The cup should facilitate independent self-drinking.
- Lids on cups are often appropriate. Handles should be an appropriate size and shape and the cup should be of an appropriate weight (see Figure 15.10).

Specially designed cups, e.g. Nosey cut-out cups or clear, flexible cups (see Figure 5.10) allow the carer to control and see fluid flow and encourage good head posture. Weighted or angled handles may also assist with self-feeding. It is recommended that the clinician consult with an occupational therapist when selecting appropriate feeding equipment to facilitate self-feeding.

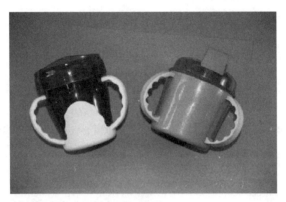

(a) The Heinz Baby basic cups.

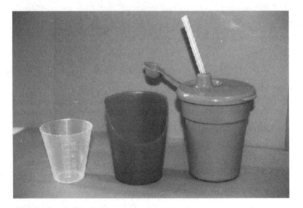

(b) Variety of cups.

Figure 15.10   (a) The Heinz Baby basic cup with dribble lid (left) and with spout lid (right)
(b) small flexible medicine cup (left), nosey cut-out cup (middle), straw cup (right)

Choice of cups can vary depending on the age, size and needs of the child. It is important that the choice of cup *should not* exacerbate (a) tongue thrusting, (b) a tonic bite reflex, (c) gagging/ coughing, (d) deterioration in the oral/ pharyngeal and laryngeal phases of swallowing or aspiration.

Choosing straws

Straw drinking may be used as a drinking method for children to

- facilitate liquid intake;
- develop oral movement, lip protrusion and jaw stability; and
- facilitate independent liquid intake.

Straw drinking requires a coordinated suck-swallow-breathe pattern (see also Chapter 3). Early on children often use a suckle pattern of forward-backward tongue movement and later are able to stabilize the jaw and isolate lip protrusion and closure from tongue movement.

Success in straw drinking will be affected by the child's age, sucking mainte-nance and strength. In addition, their coordination of suck-swallow-breathe pattern-ing will be critical. The overall swallowing skills, lip closure, protrusion and lip seal will also affect the success of straw drinking. The clinician should also bear in mind that the width of the straw will affect suck strength or pressure and lip closure. The child's interest and acceptance of the straw in their mouth will also be important.

In the early years, straws may be used, however the therapist needs to consider whether the straw is durable and made of strong plastic that is able to be cleaned thoroughly. They should also consider whether the straw facilitates oral function and development. If the use of the straw is likely to exacerbate tongue thrust, gagging or prolongation of the sucking reflex in the early years, then it may be avoided so more normal patterns can be facilitated through cup drinking.

SUMMARY ON FEEDING EQUIPMENT SELECTION

Equipment selection is an evolving process in paediatric dysphagia. The therapist will select, modify and change equipment as the child progresses in age, develop-ment, skills and needs. The role of the speech pathologist in the selection of feeding equipment may be summarized as follows. With any piece of feeding equipment chosen the therapist should clearly:

• assist in the access to equipment where possible;
• explain the rationale behind the equipment choice;
• demonstrate the appropriate use of the equipment;
• explain and demonstrate the method and timing of presentation of equipment;
• document the equipment use and provide written guidelines;
• explain the types of consistency to be offered with the particular equipment (e.g. thin versus thickened fluid, puree versus mashed solid);
• provide ongoing monitoring and review of equipment.

Too often parents have been referred to my clinic having been advised to use a piece of equipment without any demonstration or observation by the health professional as to the safety and usefulness of the equipment.

Equipment needs to be selected on the basis of promoting the child's nutrition, oromotor skills, feeding skills, safe swallowing, general safety, posture, physical, motor, cognitive development, communication skills. Equipment selection and use should be a team and family oriented approach that evolves over time.

Inappropriate equipment choices may have detrimental consequences. These may include:

• poor posture during mealtimes;
• refusal patterns by the child;
• gagging;

- poor intake, which consequently affects nutrition, weight gain and growth;
- reduced compliance and/or poor parental or carer acceptability and use of equipment;
- poor oral motor and feeding development;
- deterioration or inhibition of oromotor, feeding and swallowing skills; and
- possible aspiration into the trachea and lungs.

Equipment selection is, therefore, very important and another crucial element in successful management of dysphagia.

SELECTING APPROPRIATE FOOD AND LIQUID CONSISTENCIES

Children with dysphagia may require careful selection of liquid and food consistencies that ensure swallowing is safe and with a reduced risk of aspiration. In addition, it is imperative that nutritional requirements are met. Oral and feeding skills need to be facilitated in a timely manner and developmentally appropriate. Feeds or meals should be able to be completed in a reasonable time frame and fatigue factors should also be considered. The following sections discuss the liquid and solid consistencies the speech pathologist should be aware of in the treatment of dysphagia in infants and children.

LIQUIDS

Thin or regular liquids such as breast milk, formula milk, water, juices, cow's milk and other drinks require coordinated and effective oral, and pharyngeal phases and effective swallow-respiratory coordination for the child to control and execute swallowing in a timely and safe manner. Children may exhibit difficulties swallowing thin liquids. It may be appropriate to thicken or modify liquid consistencies under the following circumstances:

- pooling of liquid in the oral cavity;
- poor lip closure and associated liquid loss;
- poor tongue control, movement and coordination;
- delayed initiation of the oral and pharyngeal phases of the swallow;
- coughing/choking/gulping;

or the child presents with:

- clinical signs of aspiration (e.g. coughing, gurgling vocal quality, pooling of saliva and secretions, excessive drooling, significant feeding refusal);
- known evidence of aspiration (e.g. confirmed by modified barium swallow/video fluoroscopy x-ray) on thin fluids but not on thickened fluids;
- a history of chest infections or chest pathology associated with aspiration onto the lungs;
- gastroesophageal reflux and associated problems – e.g. aspiration.

Thickening techniques vary depending on the age, degree of thickening required and specific needs of the child and the child's preferences. Use of commercial thickening agents (e.g. Karicare, Resource Thickener) or other products such as cornflour, or rice cereal or the use of purees as thickeners, needs to be checked with the child's paediatrician and dietitian. This is to determine the suitability and tolerance of these thickening agents for the particular child's age, weight and condition.

In the newborn period, thickening of breast milk and commercial infant formulas is common when dysphagia or gastroesophageal reflux exists (White et al., 1993). There are prethickened infant formulas (e.g. S26AR). However, these have been developed at a particular thickness for treatment of gastroesophageal reflux. When thickening formula or breast milk to improve swallowing function and safety, it is usually recommended that the commercial thickener powder is added to the thin fluid with a predetermined amount of thickener powder per ml of liquid.

Transitional feeding has been discussed briefly in Chapter 2. From the age of 6 months, children may progress to boiled water or diluted juice and then, from 12 months, cow's milk may be introduced. When a child progresses beyond 6 months of age a follow-on formula, containing additional nutrients such as iron, is often recommended, particularly when solid intake is minimal. All of these liquids may be thickened with commercial thickeners but may vary in the amount of thickener required per liquid volume and trials of thickening is often required. If thickeners are being considered for use with infants and children, factors to be considered are:

- Suitable selection of bottles/teats/cups needs to occur. Modification of equipment may be necessary for sufficient and effective intake of the thickened liquid.
- Training, demonstrations and trials of thickening agents and new equipment should be provided.

  - Provision of clear thickening guidelines is important
  - Provision of amount of thickener in teaspoon or tablespoon measures per liquid volume is often advised, e.g. (2 teaspoons per 50 ml) and may need to be individualized.

- When the consistency is only described for example as 'nectar' or 'honey' consistency the margin for error is often increased and thickening will be variable across carers and environments.
- The amount of thickening powder required to achieve the same consistency may vary across different liquids. This needs to be investigated, documented and explained clearly to parents (see also Chapter 11). For example, breast milk often requires more thickening agent than formula milk.
- The stability of the consistency over time may vary across liquids (i.e. some thickeners continue to get thicker as the day goes on).
- Some thickeners and liquids are more stable than others.

Commercial prethickened milks and juices are available and often reduce the likelihood of inappropriate or inconsistent thickening. Unfortunately, the prethickened liquids available may be more expensive and may not be cost effective for families to meet all liquid intake requirements. Prethickened drinks are also usually full strength juices and cow's milk-based drinks and, therefore, their use needs to be checked to ensure it is appropriate for the age and condition of the child.

The thickening of liquids may improve the child's oral control of the liquid and the coordination of the oral and pharyngeal phases of swallowing and swallow-respiratory coordination. These may in turn improve the effectiveness and safety of the swallow, thereby reducing the risk of aspiration. The use of thickened liquids may also assist the development of lip, tongue and jaw movements and improve self-drinking abilities, thereby improving oral intake of liquid. Often thickened liquids are more easily controlled and safely swallowed which may have positive influence on the child's willingness to consume liquids.

Thickened liquids are denser than normal fluids and this characteristic may assist children with gastroesophageal reflux as they are more likely to remain in the stomach, reducing the likelihood of re-entry of stomach contents into the oesophagus. This may lead to increased willingness for oral intake, an increase in intake of liquid volume and reduced loss of fluid and nutrition through vomiting.

Thickening agents may be used as a temporary or long-term option for liquid intake. They may also be used at different times during the day or week. For example, a child who can be well seated, supported and facilitated may be able to swallow thin liquids safely and tidily when a carer provides full assistance. However, when the child is self-drinking with minimal carer assistance, the liquid may be thickened to facilitate the child's intake, oral control and safety in swallowing while encouraging independence.

The rationale for thickening liquids must be made clear, well explained and documented to parents and caregivers if compliance and appropriate use is likely to occur. As the child develops, the use and type of thickening agent needs to be reviewed.

SOLID CONSISTENCIES

The introduction of solid consistencies is often dependent on the child's age. According to the World Health Organization (1989) guidelines, infants are able to have their nutritional needs sufficiently met by breast or formula milk until the age of 6 months and do not require solid foods until this age. In practice, however, a solid *consistency* or puree may be given earlier than 6 months if liquid intake is poor and/or the therapist is facilitating development of oral/feeding skills. A 'solid' food may consist of thickened breast or formula milk to a solid consistency via commercial thickening agents if this is a way of providing safe and effective oral nutrition and practice from the age of three months.

In the normally developing population, solid foods are introduced based on the child's nutritional needs and oral/feeding skills and are generally recommended as follows (Carr, 1979; Stevenson and Allaire, 1991; Kleinman, 1994; Morris and Klein, 2000):

- 6 to 8 months – purees;
- 8 to 9 months – mashed lumpy/mixed textures (e.g. soft fork, mashed vegetables/fruit).

Finger food:

- 6 to 7 months onwards – rusks;
- 7 to 8 months onwards – toast/biscuits (e.g. arrowroot) or soft fruit;
- 10 to 11 months onwards – soft chopped food (e.g. cheese, bread, pasta, fish);
- 10 to 12 months onwards – firm finger foods (e.g. sandwiches);
- 15 months + – harder/chewy foods (i.e. foods that require sustained biting/chewing. Their introduction is usually dependent on the presence of teeth, especially middle incisors and molars for biting and chewing (e.g. chopped meat such as steak, fruit sticks, sultanas, raw carrot sticks).

Children may well be offered textures earlier than these guidelines, however, they run the risk of swallowing large pieces whole, which may cause gagging, refusal and disinterest of textures.

It is important to determine a dysphagic child's readiness for solid foods, not only based on age but also on present oromotor/feeding skills and the most appropriate method of presentation, timing and amount offered. Children may be ready to commence particular textures at the usual ages with specific techniques to assist the transition. Alternatively, they may need to commence particular textures at later stages depending on their experience and skills. Children who present with dysphagia may have particular difficulty with the transition to semi-solid (lumpy) and finger foods due to delayed oromotor skills and/or difficulty with isolating tongue movement, lateralizing the tongue to the side and chewing efficiently.

To ingest solids children usually require seating in a more upright or semi-reclined position. No solid foods should ever be offered in a lying position to infants or children, e.g. a baby bouncer. Solids should be given when the child is preferably well seated and not 'on the run' or during mobility when posture and swallowing skills may be compromised.

Purees

Commercial purees tend to be thinner and smoother than home purees. Both types of purees can provide adequate nutrition as long as the appropriate variety is offered. Choices of purees (i.e. commercial/home made) may depend firstly on the child's preferences for tastes/texture/temperature. They may also depend upon any displays of oral sensitivity. For example, if the child is *hypersensitive* to taste and texture, he or she may initially prefer commercial purees over home purees. The child who is *hyposensitive* may benefit from increased thickness, taste and temperature variations to improve sensation. The thickness of the puree also needs to be determined carefully for each child. For example, a child with poor tongue control of the bolus or tongue thrusting may benefit from a thicker puree that is easier to control. A child who gags easily may tolerate a thinner, smoother puree such as commercial 4 months puree, e.g. custard. Other factors to consider when choosing a puree include parental preferences, food allergies or intolerances if present and dietary preferences.

Semi-solids

Semi-solids consist of fork mashed or lumpy solids that contain a mixture of puree and lumps. For successful oral preparation of semi-solid food and chopped finger foods, the child needs to be able to hold lumps on the tip or blade of the tongue and transfer the tongue laterally to the sides of the mouth and the molar area. Initially gums are used for chewing and, later, teeth assist with firmer and chewier lumps. Efficient chewing needs to occur and then the tongue transfers the food back to the midline for swallowing. Many children with underlying oromotor disorders who have associated abnormal tone and/or movement difficulties may struggle with the transition to lumpy or chopped solids due to the more specific, coordinated and precise movement required. It is important to note, however, that children need exposure to semi-solid and solid food if they are to learn these new skills. The therapist must determine the child's readiness to commence these foods and explore ways of presenting them to facilitate the skills required.

Finger foods

Initially children may be offered soft chopped finger foods such as bread or strips of finger foods such as toast. They then progress onto firmer foods (e.g. biscuits) and then chewy foods (e.g. dried fruit). Introduction of finger foods is often based on the ability to:

- sustain a bite through the food offered;
- grade the jaw opening to achieve the appropriate bite pressure required;
- hold and transfer food to the side of the mouth with the tongue;
- chew efficiently for the particular texture eaten; and
- transfer food from the side to the middle of the mouth and then later across the midline of the mouth.

If the child does not have these skills then specific equipment and techniques may be employed to facilitate the required oromotor skills and intake of these foods (see the technique section). The presence of upper and lower middle incisor teeth assists with biting, and the presence of molar teeth assists with grinding and chewing chewier foods such as meat. Many children are able to ingest and chew semi-solid foods and softer chopped table foods successfully without the presence of teeth.

Critical period for the introduction of solid foods

The literature supports the notion that there is a critical period in the child's development when solid foods need to be introduced to ease transition as well as develop the appropriate oromotor and chewing/biting and eating skills (Thorpe and Zangwill, 1961; Illingworth and Lister, 1964; Illingworth, 1969; Stevenson and Allaire, 1991). The critical or sensitive period for introducing solid foods is reportedly between 6 months and 15 months and if introduction occurs beyond this period the transition is often more difficult and specific movements of biting, tongue lateralization and chewing will need to be learned (Thorpe and Zangwill, 1961; Illingworth and Lister, 1964; Illingworth, 1969; Stevenson and Allaire, 1991). This is important information for therapists and families in terms of intervention. If transition to solid textures can be facilitated within the critical learning period, then the transition may occur more naturally and successfully. If a child presents beyond the critical period for feeding therapy, such as the child of 18 months eating only pureed foods, who has had limited exposure to semi-solid and finger foods, then these oromotor movements are unlikely to occur with simple food exposure. The child may need more input in terms of the specific oral movements to be learned and even if the child is willing to ingest the new texture may have difficulty knowing how to orally prepare the texture prior to swallowing. Therapists therefore need to keep this critical period in mind when determining when and how to facilitate the introduction of more textured foods.

TECHNIQUES AND METHODS OF FEEDING

The importance of appropriate positioning and correct equipment was strongly emphasized in previous sections. This is complemented by the way in which the therapist uses and incorporates feeding equipment, positioning and facilitation techniques into the child's feeding routine. The method of presentation, timing and scheduling of presentation of liquids and solids also need to be planned, discussed, demonstrated and monitored with the family. Preparation for the feed or meal, how equipment is introduced and presented and when and how long equipment is used will affect the child's feeding success.

PREPARING THE CHILD FOR A FEED

Infants and children may need an opportunity to become calm and focused for a feed. The *hypersensitive* child who may easily refuse facial/oral touch and feeding equipment may need oral desensitization exercises to desensitize their body and mouth prior to a feed. This will settle their general posture and oral reactions and may facilitate acceptance of oral feeding, feeding equipment, and oral intake. The sleepy, *hypotonic* child may need stimulating input from the environment, to his/her face and oral area to prepare and ready the mouth to initiate and co-ordinate movement. The child who has *delayed*, *reduced* or *immature* feeding skills may be given oral exercises, mouthing or chewing activities prior to the meal to facilitate the skills desired for introduction of new food textures. Some exercises or activities to prepare the infant or child for a feed are:

- modifications to the feeding environment;
- ensuring appropriate positioning;
- oral desensitization exercises;
- oral stimulation exercises;

- mouthing of toys;
- touching and visual cueing before or at the meal;
- biting/chewing games;
- licking/tasting games;
- handling feeding equipment and/or food;
- role playing meals and feeding times such as feeding others or puppets, etc.;
- assisting in the preparation of the meal;
- role playing feeding, e.g. tea parties.

The choice of activity will depend on:

- the underlying problems that arise in assessment;
- the age of the child;
- the individual needs of the child and family; and
- the settings in which the child will be fed.

Two main areas in the treatment of oral preparation are *oral desensitization* and *oral stimulation* exercises. These will be discussed below.

ORAL DESENSITIZATION

Desensitization exercises are often introduced when a child demonstrates negative responses or overreaction to normal sensory stimuli, such as touch, taste, temperature, or texture (Rausch, 1981; Anderson, 1986). The child who displays these behaviours is often considered orally defensive or hypersensitive in the oral area. The child who is orally hypersensitive may limit oral exploration, which may lead to a lack of oral and feeding experiences that may have a further negative impact on their oral and feeding skills. Oral hypersensitivity is common among infants with:

- cerebral palsy;
- long-term oral feeding deprivation;
- a history of aversive input or trauma to the nose or mouth, e.g. enteral feeding such as nasogastric tube feeding, surgery;
- visual impairment;
- difficulty integrating sensory input/stimuli;
- a history of gastroesophageal reflux; and
- negative oral feeding experiences (Wolf and Glass, 1992; Morris and Klein, 2000).

The characteristics of children with oral hypersentivity are shown in Table 15.2.

   Desensitization exercises and activities should aim to provide a stimulus that is interesting, comfortable and acceptable to the child whilst gradually pushing back the child's abnormal threshold and building a more appropriate response and reaction (Morris and Klein, 2000). Desensitization exercises involve use of fingers, thumb, mouthing toys, toothbrush trainers, washers, dummies and other feeding equipment. It is important that the child is positioned comfortably, with the body

Table 15.2 Characteristics of orally *hyper*sensitive children and *hypo*sensitive children

Characteristics of oral *hyper*sensitivity	Characteristics of oral *hypo*sensitivity (Arvedson and Brodsky, 2002)
○ Avoidance of mealtimes (e.g. feigns sleep, withdraws, refuses, removes self from the environment). ○ Refuses the breast. ○ Refuses or gags on teats. ○ Refuses the dummy. ○ Displays a reticence/rejection of mouthing toys/objects. ○ Refuses a range of textures. ○ Avoids particular tastes/textures. ○ May also resist play and handling of food. ○ Affects the child's willingness or preference for self-feeding.	• Poor sucking and chewing. • Diminished response to sensory input. • Drooling. • Inclined to overfill mouth. • Enjoy foods of strong flavours and increased texture.

and head very stable. A calming environment and activity such as bathing, rocking or rhythmical music often helps to relax the child prior to the meal. The therapist then introduces firm but gentle rhythmical stroking movements. Most children are more accepting to input initially at their extremities (feet and hands). The therapist then moves the input to the head and shoulders, then to the face, outer mouth and then finally into the oral area. When reaching the face, the therapist provides stroking inwards towards the lips. Then touch is applied to the lateral and middle gum margins and very gradually to the hard palate and tongue (not further than middle of the tongue). Stroking or maintaining position or pressure may be suitable (Wolf and Glass, 1992; Morris and Klein, 2000).

Music, rocking or singing can provide an appropriate rhythm and often makes the touch or stimuli more acceptable. It is important at all times that the therapist observe the child's reactions to determine how rapidly the input moves to the head and face. Some infants may take several days, weeks or longer to tolerate touch into their mouth and onto the tongue. Tolerance is usually gained gradually and with regular daily practice by allowing the child to become mildly uncomfortable and then reducing the negative input. If the child becomes visibly upset, gags excessively, or cries, the input may have been too rapid or too intense. The therapist aims to push the child beyond their threshold of tolerance and then may return to a more acceptable area of the body whilst the child recoups. The aim over time is to achieve input into the mouth without discomfort, gagging or distress occurring. The therapist will need to demonstrate these methods carefully to the parent/care-giver and assist the parent in reading the child's cues and when to continue or cease the input. Usually these exercises may be for 1 or 2 minutes prior to a feed/meal or at other times in the day that fit the child and family routine.

During oral desensitization, for some children finger stroking is useful, for others the use of dummies, mouthing toys, toothbrush trainers may be more acceptable or appropriate depending on the child's age, tolerance and particular likes/dislikes. Desensitization games and activities can also include:

- gradual equipment and seating changes;
- gradual introduction to new tastes; and
- gradual introduction to a new food or liquid consistency.

The aim is gradually to assist the child's acceptance of new stimuli starting with the familiar and desired and gradually incorporating the new.

ORAL STIMULATION

The previous section has detailed ways of desensitizing the oral region. For some other children, oral stimulation may be required. The following section describes some of the exercises prior to feeds that can be useful in facilitating more normal reflexes in newborns and stimulating early sucking, chewing/biting skills.

It is always important for the therapist to have clear goals and rationales for introducing exercises. These need to be explained well to the parents/care-giver. It must also be stressed that children, particularly those with dysphagia and possibly other special needs are time consuming. Parents often do not have a great deal of spare time for 'separate exercises'. Stimulating input is often best incorporated either just prior to a feed or incorporated into other family routines such as nappy change, bathing and communication time. Stimulating exercises are usually selected on the basis of facilitating:

- muscle tone (i.e. resistance and strength of the muscle);
- movement of the lips, face, jaw, tongue and palate;
- more refined and mature feeding skills; and
- improved sucking, biting and chewing skills (Rausch,1981; Fetters, 1986; Wolf and Glass, 1992; Boshart, 1995; Morris and Klein, 2000).

Stimulation exercises appropriate for the newborn

When a child presents with poor rooting reflexes or a reduced sucking reflex in the first 4 months of life, stimulation of these reflexes prior to and during the feed will facilitate:

- improved head positioning;
- improved mouth opening to accept the breast or teat;
- forward tongue posturing and anchoring over the gum line;
- reduction and normalization of the gag reflex prior to breast/teat entry;
- sucking initiation; and
- lip flanging and closure.

To stimulate the rooting reflex prior to the feed, the clinician should ensure the child's body is well positioned and head supported. Then stroke the child's mouth from the corner of the mouth outwards towards the ear. This process should cause the head to turn to the stimulated side paired with jaw depression, forward tongue placement over the lower gum, and depression of the gag reflex. If the infant does not turn the head, or open the mouth, the head turn can be prompted by the therapist's or parent's hand supporting the head with gentle thumb pressure on the mentalis muscle/jaw to depress the jaw. Once the mouth is open, a gloved finger or clean finger can be inserted with pressure applied to the hard palate to stimulate sucking. This exercise should be repeated on both sides a few times to stimulate the reflex just prior to a breast/bottle feed when the child is hungry. At the feed, the reflex can be stimulated by forming a 'teat' with the breast or using the bottle teat and stroking the corner of the infant's mouth.

Stimulation exercises appropriate for the older infant and child

As the child develops, oral exercises may be used to inhibit abnormal patterns but particularly to stimulate oral movement patterns for facilitation of biting, chewing, tongue lateralization, cup drinking and spoon feeding skills. Mouthing toys and toothbrush trainers can be used as stimulating tools to facilitate oral musculature tone and movement (these are described below). For example, just prior to having lumpier/mashed food or chopped solids, a toothbrush trainer may be given to the child to hold (with assistance as necessary). This can be directed into the side of the child's mouth between the molar area to facilitate chewing and lateral tongue movement. The therapist can also assist elevation and depression of the mandible to facilitate vertical chewing movements. This can lead on to placement of lumpy texture into the side of the child's mouth or a piece of chopped finger-food placed between the back molars (see Figure 15.11).

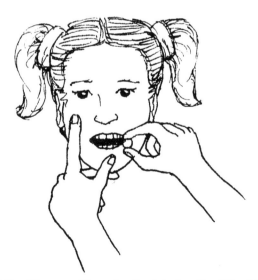

Figure 15.11 Diagram of finger feeding into the side of the child's mouth

Specific oral exercises can be given to stimulate contraction and strength of muscles in the infant and child (Wolf and Glass, 1992; Boshart, 1995). However, appropriate exercises rely on a thorough understanding of the facial and oral musculature and how the contraction of specific muscles will facilitate specific movements that relate to feeding movements. Stroking and stretching along the muscle to facilitate contraction is often best achieved by applying pressure from the origin to the insertion of the muscle. This can also be achieved by vibration, tapping and pressure (Wolf and Glass, 1992; Boshart, 1995). However, this process should be muscle specific rather than general. Muscle strength is often facilitated by resistance exercises where force is applied to the muscle and the child exerts force against pressure – e.g. finger, spatula, or mouthing object. Many diagrams and published oral exercises may not relate to oral facial musculature and, therefore, the benefit and validity of these exercises is in question. Exercises must always have an anatomical and physiological basis and be easily demonstrated and followed through by parents/caregivers (Boshart, 1995; Morris and Klein, 2000). If exercises are carried out incorrectly or infrequently the benefit may be negligible and possibly adverse.

The therapist needs to keep in mind the rationale for all exercises, explain this clearly to the parent/caregiver, demonstrate the exercise on several occasions and document in writing or by video to ensure correct carry over. It is important to determine that exercises are not only useful but how they can be incorporated into the family's routine and often demanding schedule. Children who have feeding difficulties often have a variety of other needs, often take longer to feed and place far greater demands on the family's time, resources and dynamics. It is crucial to incorporate practical, useful and relevant exercises that are going to have direct and beneficial outcomes for the child's oral musculature, feeding and speech production and that can be realistically carried out by the family.

FACILITATION

The word 'facilitation' has been used extensively in this chapter. Morris and Klein (2000) stated that facilitation is the incorporation of 'touch, pressure, taste, temperature, and support' to make movement 'easy'. Facilitation is often provided through:

- head, jaw, lip and facial support during feeding;
- texture changes;
- taste changes;
- food and equipment placement; and
- temperature modifications. (These are also discussed in Chapters 4 and 11.)

The aim of facilitation is to inhibit abnormal reflex patterns and movement and promote normal oral sensation, movement and feeding skills and oromotor/feeding development. The therapist provides input initially that stimulates normal oral posture and movement and with time and progression in skills the aim is to gradually reduce the input to allow for independent and self-controlled movement patterns.

Facilitation via head support

There are different ways of providing head support to the infant and child. The therapist can use his/her non-dominant arm to support around the back of the head, under the chin (Figure 15.4) or on the apex of the head to stabilize the head and maintain the appropriate head posture for feeding (Figure 15.5). Choices may be governed by the impact the support has on the child and parent/caregiver. One must determine whether the support does facilitate head position and is it comfortable and sustainable for the caregiver.

Facilitation via jaw and lip support

Jaw and lip support is often given when the child has difficulty with jaw stability, jaw grading, jaw opening and lip closure. (Figure 15.4). The use of the carer's fingers or hands to support the child's jaw or lips allows the child to learn:

- an appropriate jaw, tongue and lip resting posture;
- jaw stability;
- lip closure (reduce liquid loss);
- improved tongue posture and movement; and
- better initiation of the swallow.

Facilitation via cheek support

Support on the cheek area is often given to the newborn or infant during breast-feeding/bottle feeding (see Figure 15.6) or during later straw drinking if the child displays:

- poor lip flanging and protrusion;
- liquid loss from the mouth;
- poor control of the liquid bolus;
- poor tongue grooving; or
- asymmetrical facial, tongue or lip movement as in hemiplegia.

USING FOOD TO FACILITATE IMPROVED ORAL FUNCTION

Purees

Once the child has experienced pureed foods for 1 month to 2 months they often move from an early 'extension–retraction' tongue movement to a 'tongue-tip' swallow at approximately 6 months to 9 months (Morris and Klein, 2000). Children with dysphagia, however, may have difficulty with this transition and may retain early patterns of movement or display tongue thrusting, tongue retraction, reduced tongue movement or gagging. Some of the following strategies may be useful. The clinician could try thickening the puree to a firmer consistency. This may improve oral control of the puree and assist progression to a more mature tongue tip movement for swallowing. The carer should aim to ensure placement of the spoon onto the middle of the tongue with firm pressure using a firm plastic spoon (e.g. maroon spoon). If the child gags, a softer, smaller spoon may be more acceptable. Placement to the anterior entrance of the mouth or to the side of the mouth may be more acceptable to the child with increased gagging behaviour.

When spoonfeeding, children may need lip and/or jaw support as described above. Infants may display a bite reflex and bite down on the spoon making removal difficult and feeding uncomfortable for the child. When spoonfeeding it is often helpful to:

• start with a closed-mouth position assisted by jaw support if needed;
• tap the lower lip to cue the child of the spoon presence particularly if they do not automatically open in anticipation of the spoon;
• place the spoon well into the mouth – do not leave the spoon in for long when a bite reflex or gag is present as this often exacerbates the problem;
• press the blade of the spoon firmly down on the middle of the tongue, particularly when a child tends to tongue thrust;
• move the spoon up and out against the upper lip – avoid any contact with the teeth as this may encourage a bite reflex to be elicited; or
• provide jaw and lip support to assist jaw and lip closure and facilitate the swallow initiation.

Semi-solids (mashed/lumpy textures)

Transition to lumpier textures is facilitated by mouthing experiences, reduction in the gag reflex, and development of lateral tongue movements and chewing. Some children do not have the appropriate oral feeding experiences, and present with immature skills or oral/feeding difficulties, so they may not be able to extract the lump or piece of food in a mixed texture and take it to the side of the mouth to chew in the molar area. If children are unable to transfer food for chewing or do not chew efficiently for swallowing then they often demonstrate:

• gagging on lumpy textures;
• refusal of the texture;
• swallowing the texture with incomplete oral preparation, which can cause gagging or affect stomach and bowel function as food is less masticated before swallowing; or
• poor intake of the semi-solid texture.

As noted earlier, there is a critical period for the introduction of solid food. The therapist may therefore need to determine and introduce exercises and techniques that will facilitate intake of semi-solids when the child's skills may be immature or inadequate. It is also important that issues such as swallowing safety, timing and the nutritional aspects for the child are considered, which will guide the frequency, timing and the decision of whether to introduce more challenging solid food.

Children transitioning to mashed/lumpy textures may benefit from desensitization exercises when they have a history of oral hypersensitvity or refusal of semi-solid textures (see previous section). They may also benefit from oral exercises with toothbrush trainers to facilitate biting, chewing and tongue lateralization prior to semi-solid introduction (see previous section). Semi-solid food can be wrapped in fine cotton muslin or gauze and firmly secured. This can be placed into the side of the mouth to provide the taste and oral stimulation to facilitate chewing without the danger of swallowing large pieces in children that have poor oral preparatory skills. Food should be placed carefully into the side of the mouth using a small spoon when introducing lumpy textures. This often facilitates chewing and oral preparation of semi-solid food. If food is orally prepared better, the child is likely to swallow it, which will often reduce gagging and consequent refusal behaviours. If the child is prone to fatigue, then semi-solid textures may be best given at the beginning of the meal rather than at the end.

Finger foods

Finger-food transition in normal infants was described earlier. Many children with dysphagia may have physical, visual or developmental issues, which may mean that finger foods are difficult to see, hold or bring to the mouth, or may be difficult to bite, transfer to the side of their mouth with their tongue, and/or chew efficiently to swallow. The firmness and texture selected will often be influenced by the child's level of oral sensitivity and their biting and chewing strength and efficiency. Techniques to facilitate intake of finger foods include mouthing activities with a range of mouthing toys with respect to firmness, width, size and texture (these are described below). Toothbrush trainer exercises and chewing/biting stimulation may also be useful. As for semi-solids, food can be wrapped in fine cotton muslin or gauze and firmly secured. This can then be placed into the side of the mouth to provide the taste and oral stimulation to facilitate chewing without the danger of children who have poor oral preparatory skills swallowing large pieces. Soft finger food may be chopped into small pieces (i.e. approximately 1 cm square) and placed either with fingers or a spoon into the side of the mouth (see Figure 15.11). This will facilitate chewing and oral preparation prior to swallowing. Children who are able to chew but unable to transfer food laterally with their tongue may benefit initially from strips of food being placed to the side of the mouth where they can be bitten and easily chewed at the side. This can also be helpful for children who are unable to occlude their middle incisors to bite effectively but may be able to occlude effectively with their lateral incisor teeth.

Children may also need other techniques to assist their biting such as varying the width and firmness of food whilst maintaining a still head position and developing their sustained biting. Toothbrush trainer and other biting games may be useful in stimulating and facilitating biting strength. Some children will need to be cued or assisted in their handling of finger food and ways of bringing finger food to their mouth. The carer may assist this, or alternative equipment may be incorporated to facilitate it. Occupational therapists and specialized equipment suppliers for the disabled populations can often assist in these choices and assist in management.

ORAL EQUIPMENT USED TO FACILITATE ORAL MOVEMENT AND FEEDING SKILLS

Oral equipment other than feeding equipment may be incorporated into the child's routine or mealtimes to facilitate oral movement and feeding skills. These may include dummies/pacifiers, mouthing toys and toothbrush trainers.

Dummies/ pacifiers

Always discuss the use of dummies with parents as they will have their own preferences for their use. Dummies can be very useful in developing more rhythmical and efficient sucking or if an infant has a weak or dyscoordinate suck (Measal and Andrews, 1979; Bernbaum et al., 1983). They are particularly useful in the first 12 months of life for children who are born prematurely or who are receiving nasogastric/ gastrostomy tube feeds to encourage their sucking ability, association of sucking with a sense of fullness and facilitate gastric emptying (Bernbaum et al., 1983; Bazyk, 1990).

Dummies, like teats, come in a range of sizes, lengths and shapes. The size and shape should be selected on the basis of the child's oral cavity size, sensitivty, gag reflex, and sucking needs. For example, a premature infant may best suit a very small short dummy whereas a child with low tone who has poor lip closure and seal may benefit from a broader, wider dummy to assist lip closure and sucking.

Dummies are not usually recommended for children with a tongue thrust or prolonged sucking reflex (i.e. beyond 4 months) as they tend to exacerbate the problem (Wolf and Glass, 1992). Usually, when a child reaches 12 to 18 months, weaning from dummies is recommended. Extended or prolonged use of dummies is not recommended as it can be associated with forward tongue posture, dental problems (e.g. anterior open bite), articulation and speech problems. Examples are shown in Figure 15.12a.

Mouthing toys

Mouthing is a normal and extremely important period in the infant's early oral development, particularly between the age of 3 months and 12 months. Mouthing of toys, objects and fingers develops the infant's taste, depth perception, oral proprioception, oral spatial orientation, sensory processing and integration and assists the range, strength and coordination of oral movement. (Boshart, 1995; Morris and Klein, 2000). Many children with feeding difficulties, physical disability, sensory integration or oral hypersensitivity issues may not experience normal mouthing

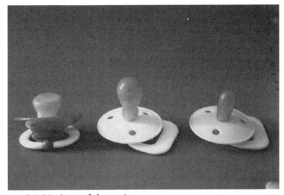

(a) Variety of dummies.

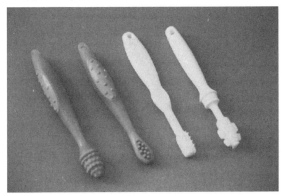

(b) Toothbrush trainers.

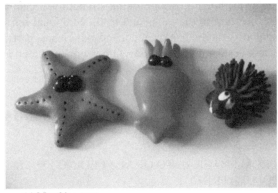

(c) Mouthing toys.

Figure 15.12 (a) Variety of dummies: Nuk orthodontic dummy (left), Happy Baby soother (standard shape) – small (middle), Happy Baby soother – premature (right) (b) variety of toothbrush trainers (c) variety of mouthing toys

experiences. This can have a negative impact on their oral awareness, oral sensitivity and sensory integration, oral movement, feeding and early communication skills (Boshart, 1995; Morris and Klein, 2000).

Selection of appropriate mouthing toys suitable to the child's age and needs can form an integral part of a child's feeding programme. Children who are particularly orally hypersensitive to touch, refuse oral feeding or who have reduced oral sensation and movement can benefit from mouthing experiences (Boshart, 1995). Mouthing toys come in a variety of shapes, textures, sizes and may be modified in temperature (Figure 15.12c).

Mouthing toy selection depends on the child's age, oral size, hand-to-mouth skills and specific needs. Lanco toys that are made of soft latex can be useful as they are visually appealing, varied in types and textures, and will squeak easily with minimal hand pressure. Some children may need a firm, smooth texture at first if they are hypersensitive to oral textures, whereas others who have reduced sensation may respond better to a more textured mouther or one that is colder or warmer. Mouthers that have pointed parts can be very useful for teaching early lateral tongue movements and chewing. Note, the pointed part should extend no further than the middle of the child's tongue otherwise it may induce gagging.

Toothbrush trainers

There are a variety of toothbrush trainer sets that are available commercially. These are very useful in facilitating mouthing, lateral tongue movements, biting and chewing skills. When a child has an ineffective bite, immature or weak chewing or poor lateral tongue movements during eating, toothbrush trainers may be effective prior to attempting semi-solid (lumpy/mashed) and solid food (chopped and finger food) or whilst the child is learning these skills. Sustained biting games between middle incisors or molar teeth can facilitate biting strength and chewing practice. By providing increased texture to the gums and teeth, additional sensory information can be provided that may facilitate movement and experience, particularly when the child is not ready to ingest, or to ingest safely, lumpier or solid food pieces. Examples are shown in Figure 15.12b.

PAEDIATRIC DYSPHAGIA MANAGEMENT – SPECIAL CONSIDERATIONS

TRANSITION FROM ENTERAL TO ORAL FEEDING IN THE PAEDIATRIC POPULATION

Enteral or tube feeding is required for infants when:

- their nutritional needs are not going to be met orally;
- they are at risk failure to thrive; or
- have already been placed in the category of 'failure to thrive' (see Chapter 13).

Many infants and children may be unable to successfully or safely orally feed due to numerous conditions that are detailed in Chapter 13.

The presence of orogastric or nasogastric tubes for enteral feeding, although necessary, may be associated with later oral feeding problems such as:

- The mouth and throat are not being stimulated normally in the developing infant.
- The presence of the tube may be uncomfortable, particularly if the child is attempting to feed orally whilst the tube is *in situ*.
- Negative associations with the mouth may develop due to the traumatic nature of enteral tube insertion and its constant presence with few pleasurable experiences occurring in the oral/pharyngeal region (Wolf and Glass, 1992; Morris and Klein, 2000).
- The routine and 'normality' of meals and feeding times are often changed, e.g. holding, bonding, sharing meals with family is often reduced (Bloch, 1987).
- Time for normal activities and stimulation of the child may be reduced due to the additional time associated with enteral feeding (Morris and Klein, 2000).
- The child may become orally hypersensitive, gag easily and associate general negativity with touch and equipment at or around the mouth (Bazyk, 1990; Wolf and Glass, 1992; Morris and Klein, 2000).
- The child may have reduced oral experiences and, therefore, be orally deprived of many normal oral feeding and swallowing experiences. This may result in poor oral skill and feeding development (Illingworth, 1969, Stevenson and Allaire, 1991), swallowing incordination, feeding refusal, and regression of or loss of early oral reflexes and feeding skills (Rausch, 1981; Sitzman and Mueller, 1988; Bazyk, 1990; Wolf and Glass, 1992).

Whilst the child is being non-orally or enterally fed the following techniques may be introduced to facilitate oral and swallowing skills. Pleasurable experiences should be encouraged – e.g. massage, kissing, touch to the face. Oral desensitization exercises, as described above can be used to reduce oral hypersensitivity or an increased gag reflex. These exercises will assist the child in allowing fingers, feeding equipment entering the mouth. In infants less than 4 months of age, oral stimulation exercises/activities to facilitate early primitive reflexes may be useful to stimulate tone and movement of the oral-facial region (Wolf and Glass, 1992; Morris and Klein, 2000). These may include specific exercises, dummies, or mouthing objects.

Parents of children who are being fed enterally need significant support and education on how they can support their children. Parents can often feel as though they have failed or are unable to care for their children when they are unable to feed them orally. It is important for the therapist to assist the parent in ways they can provide meaningful and therapeutic input to their child that will facilitate pleasure and movement in and around the mouth.

If the child is medically stable and can safely swallow a particular fluid or solid consistency (often supported by clinical review or objective assessment), the therapist must then carefully select appropriate positioning, equipment and techniques to facilitate not only safe but comfortable oral feeding. As noted above, children who have required enteral feeding over a long period may develop an aversion to oral touch and oral feeding so the transition to oral feeding can often be a slow and difficult process (Wolf and Glass, 1992).

Chest status and health should be monitored on a regular basis to ensure that optimum health is maintained during the transition process from enteral to oral feeding and also during feeding trials. The timing, frequency of oral feeds and consideration of fatigue during feeding will also need to be considered carefully (Cummings and Reilly, 1972). If a child who is being transitioned to oral feeding becomes ill, or his/her chest status deteriorates, then oral feeding may need to cease and enteral feeding may need to recommence. Reviews via chest x-ray and/or videofluoroscpopy modified barium swallow (see Chapter 14) may also need to occur regarding the ongoing safety of swallowing particular consistencies and the amount, type and frequency of oral feeding (Sorin et al., 1988; Griggs et al., 1989, Blitzer, 1990; Fisher, 1992; Arvedson, 1993).

As children develop, their swallowing status may change with maturation of their physical and neurological skills and regular reviews may need to occur to determine the type and amount of consistency a child may be able to ingest orally. Other children who may have been oral feeders or have been on a variety of consistencies but have had:

• repeated or deteriorating ill health;
• documented aspiration;
• severe gasteoesophageal reflux or gut abnormalities; or
• inadequate growth or weight gain over a period of time may be introduced to enteral feeding to assist their growth and health.

Alternative enteral feeding sites

Alternative enteral feeding sites may be discussed with the family when enteral feeding needs to be a longer term solution, when there are medical/anatomical reasons for different enteral feeding sites or the presence of oral/nasogastric tubes negates oral feeding transition. Gastrostomy tubes (often referred to as percutaneous gastrostomy or PEG) are a common alternative to oral or nasogastric tube feeding. A gastrostomy is a surgically created fistula through the abdominal wall and into the stomach. A tube is placed through the fistula and into the stomach (Wolf and Glass, 1992). As tubes are removed from the oral/nasal/pharyngeal area this often means that the oropharyngeal trauma and discomfort is lessened, which may facilitate oral feeding in some children. Gastoesophageal reflux may increase with gastrostomy tube feeds (Wolf and Glass, 1992) and this needs to be monitored closely as it may be associated with feeding aversion, reduced intake and associated respiratory consequences (e.g. aspiration). Children may be orally fed whilst also being fed via a gastrostomy tube; however, this needs to be decided carefully by the dysphagia team on the basis of swallowing safety and appropriate choice of fluids and solid consistencies appropriate for the child's status and age.

Enteral feeds need to be planned carefully to ensure that they facilitate normal family routines, e.g. meals, sleep. In addition, enteral feeds should be well timed, with appropriate amounts given to facilitate the child's nutrition but also to facilitate hunger and consequent oral intake and oral feeding where this is appropriate. Some children may be fed continuously or via bolus feeds depending on their condition and nutritional needs. This may affect their hunger and desire to orally feed. If bolus feeds are too large for a child they may cause gagging, vomiting, eye watering and discomfort in many children. Often enteral feeding needs to be reviewed regularly to ensure the correct and suitable type of feed and amount per feed can be determined. The timing of enteral feeds with oral feeds may be adjusted when needed, including whether the child has bolus or continuous feeds and whether feeds are given during the day or night. Children will differ with particular feed amounts depending on their age, disability, medical condition and whether oral feeding is being facilitated.

EPILEPSY

Some children with neurological disorders (e.g. cerebral palsy), congenital and chromosomal syndromes and developmental disability may also suffer from epilepsy. Fitting may occur during mealtimes. Consequently, epilepsy may be associated with dysphagia and possible aspiration due to alterations in awareness and movement during the oral or pharyngeal stages of swallowing, and lack of coordination of swallowing and respiration. Drowsiness following fitting episodes is common and can affect consequent awareness, swallowing ability and self-feeding. Epileptic medication, although necessary, may have adverse effects on the child (e.g. drowsiness) and influence muscle tone, which may have consequent negative influences on swallowing function.

The timing of meals and medications needs to be considered and planned carefully to avoid or minimize adverse effects. Children should also not be fed orally whilst fitting. Children with epilepsy may also be at nutritional risk and may need dietary guidance and supplementation (White et al, 1993).

MEDICATIONS

Children with dysphagia may be on medications for a variety of medical or nutritional reasons. Medications may have a negative impact on the child's feeding due to the associated adverse effects that medications may have including:

- sedation;
- drowsiness;
- dry mouth;
- fatigue;
- constipation;
- nausea;
- ataxia;
- hypersalivation;

- diarrhea;
- dizziness, or;
- anorexia (Poon, 1993).

Medications can also have an undesirable taste, which, if given close to a mealtime can cause negative associations with oral intake. Therapists managing children with dysphagia need to be aware of the current medications and their interactions. Provision of medication needs to be appropriately timed with mealtimes and parents and caregivers clearly informed on the manner they should be given, dependent on the child's swallowing skills. For example, if the child is on a thickened fluid regime then liquid medications should also be thickened. Many children are unable to swallow medications in tablet form and require medications given in liquid or crushable form. Discussion is recommended with a pharmacist or the child's doctor about the possible form of medication (e.g. tablet/liquid) and any adverse effects.

SUMMARY

This chapter has provided a comprehensive discussion of the management issues associated with paediatric dysphagia. The management of paediatric dysphagia requires a thorough knowledge of infant anatomy, physiology and the maturational changes that occur normally. An understanding and appreciation of normal oral/ feeding, motor, cognitive, and physical development and nutritional requirements provides a basis of therapeutic sequence for the therapist to aim towards and facilitate the child who presents with dysphagia and related physical, medical, cognitive issues (Alexander, 1987; Selly et al, 1990; Morris and Klein, 2000).

Important factors such as nutrition, positioning, environment, equipment, food/ liquid consistencies, exercises and methods have been discussed. These need to be individually considered and incorporated for each child and family. Incorporating all factors can be a challenging task and at all times the therapist needs to attempt to:

- Manage the child and family as a whole unit.
- Make the meal times practical, fit into a reasonable time frame, and incorporate the daily activities of the child and family.
- Make them pleasurable and comfortable for the child and parent.
- Offer children choices and options, particularly as they develop. This will allow them to have a degree of control and input into meal times and is more likely to foster acceptance. Therapists can have the best intentions, but often the child will guide the therapist and family (to some extent) regarding the acceptability of methods and equipment.
- Make meal times as natural and sociable as possible and an opportunity for normal communication.
- Share mealtimes with others at least for part of the day.
- Facilitate oral movement and mature feeding skills toward independent feeding behaviours.

To this end, two case reports are provided below to provide an example of the integrated management of children with dysphagia.

The therapist needs to consider factors that limit and influence oral feeding development such as the child's state, the effect of medications, negative influences on feeding (e.g. gastoesophageal reflux, enteral feeding), the child's health and emotional state, and the parent's emotional state and skills.

The primary role of the therapist is to assist the family to feed their child optimally and as successfully as possible (Arvedson, 1993). It is important that the therapist is sensitive to the family's and child's needs and aims to empower the family to confidently manage and assist in the monitoring of their child's feeding and swallowing skills.

Management of paediatric dysphagia is a process of ongoing assessment and monitoring. The child's maturation in age, cognitive, physical, nutritional needs, social skills, and independence will influence the ongoing revisions that therapists will need to make and the need for intervention and family support. The child's medical status, and ongoing health will also dictate needs and modifications. For example, if the child's condition or feeding deteriorates the therapist must constantly assess feeding intake and methods to determine whether further investigations and consultations with other teams members are necessary (e.g..repeat modified barium swallow, chest x-rays, blood tests, allergy testing).

Due to the reciprocal relationship between swallowing and breathing it is essential that children with dysphagia be closely monitored for any deterioration in health, particularly their chest status. When children are not managed appropriately their health and feeding progression may suffer and they are at risk of aspiration pneumonia (Loughlin, 1989; Terry and Fuller, 1989; Tuchman et al., 1989) and in the worst case scenario death (Terry and Fuller, 1989).

Feeding begins at birth and has an enormous impact on the child's development, health, growth and later social skills and independence. It is the earliest form of communication and provides the oromotor and functional basis for later speech production and communication. Early and appropriate feeding intervention facilitates the movements and coordination of the oral anatomy for speech production. Feeding plays a part in and influences other important areas of the child's communication, social, physical and cognitive development. Feeding is one of our basic needs and methods of survival. It also provides many opportunities for the child to develop independence and socialize in the community. As therapists we can play a very important role in supporting families and facilitating the most optimal outcome for the child with dysphagia.

CASE REPORT 1 – JAYDEN

Jayden was referred at the age of 4 weeks with the following concerns:

- poor weight gain;
- poor sucking on the breast and bottle;

- poor oral intake via the breast;
- irritability at and after feeds;
- waking and demanding feeds every 2 hours;
- vomiting after feeds.

When Jayden was assessed the following issues were noted:

- Jayden's facial and oral structures presented as symmetrical and intact including the soft palate. There was no evidence of tongue tie or any other oral structural abnormalities.
- A poor rooting reflex was elicited bilaterally with head turning occurring, but poor jaw opening and poor forward tongue placement. This meant that, at the breast, Jayden was not opening his mouth wide enough to accept the breast and was attaching around the nipple area. This was causing reported nipple soreness, with the mother finding breastfeeding too uncomfortable after 3 to 5 minutes. During sucking on the breast Jayden was noted to rapidly suck non-nutritively, with no swallowing noted during breastfeeding, indicating that a letdown had not occurred and there was not a sufficient flow of milk to initiate swallowing. After 4 minutes on the breast Jayden became restless and detached from the breast crying.
- On the standard bottle the family had been using with a standard slow flow teat, Jayden willingly received the teat and initiated sucking; however, he was noted to have a poor lip flange around the teat. He displayed rhythmical sucking but took only 20 ml of milk in 30 minutes suggesting an inefficient suck. A medium flow teat was trialed which Jayden tolerated well and displayed coordinated sucking and swallowing and took 50 ml in 15 minutes.
- At the end of the feed, Jayden began to cry and extend his body. He was difficult to settle. He then projectile-vomited after approximately 10 minutes of crying.

MANAGEMENT ISSUES

- Positioning of Jayden was explored initially. He was swaddled and flexed firmly in front of the caregiver. Prior to feeds, exercises to stimulate the rooting reflex were given. At the feed, Jayden was swaddled and held in a 'madonna' hold with support at the base of the neck. The body was held in a more upright position to reduce gastroesophageal reflux, if present. The rooting reflex was stimulated at the breast as well as jaw opening with the aim of achieving maximum jaw opening and forward tongue placement to attach Jayden. Once attached appropriately and sucking was initiated, Jayden's mother was shown how to manually express at the breast when Jayden was sucking to assist her letdown of milk. Once the letdown occurred she then ceased the manual expressing. Jayden was breast fed on each side of the breast whilst nutritive sucking occurred (i.e. sucking paired with swallowing). This was often for 5 minutes on each side initially. He was then detached and bottlefed. On the bottle, the rooting reflex was stimulated again to achieve better mouth opening and lip flanging. A medium flow teat was used initially with thickened expressed breast milk in view of the vomiting and suspected gastoesophageal reflux. After feeds, Jayden was kept in an upright, still position to minimize vomiting.

- The aim was that feeds would take no longer than 30 to 40 minutes in total (i.e. breast and bottle). Feeds were scheduled at 3 to 3.5 hourly intervals to assist weight gain and intake and to minimize vomiting.
- Weight and feeding methods were monitored once or twice weekly to ensure the appropriate feeding methods were being used. As Jayden improved in his breastfeeding and the amount of nutritive sucking at the breast, his bottle feeds were gradually reduced whilst monitoring his weight, urinary/bowel output and sleep patterns.
- Other approaches were incorporated such as calming Jayden's environment to keep him settled at and after feed times.
- Due to continued irritability after feeds and persistent vomiting he returned to his paediatrician for further advice and investigation of possible gastroesophageal reflux. This was confirmed via barium meal x-ray and he was placed on medication to alleviate his symptoms. This appeared to assist in settling Jayden after feeds and during sleep.
- Jayden will be monitored until his oral feeding improves and his nutrition is stable. He will then be monitored as to his progression to solid foods and speech development.

CASE REPORT 2 – AMELIA

Amelia was referred for a feeding assessment and advice:

- She is a 12-month-old girl who was diagnosed with Down syndrome soon after birth. She underwent cardiac surgery soon after birth for a congenital heart defect.
- She was tube fed nasogastrically for the first 4 weeks of life until she had undergone her surgery and was medically stable and oral feeding was established.
- At the time of assessment she was medically stable with respect to her cardiac and respiratory status.
- Despite her initial medical difficulties she was able to breastfeed fully by the age of 8 weeks and continued this until 6 months of age when she was weaned to a standard medium flow teat on a standard bottle.
- She was reportedly taking purees 'happily' and readily accepts and takes her bottles (i.e. 5×200 ml per day).
- Her parents' current concerns are that she is gagging and refusing more textured foods such as lumpy/mixed textures and finger foods. Although she is initially interested in these she will gag and consequently refuse to take any more. Amelia reportedly loves mouthing objects and will often put toys and other objects into her mouth during play.
- Her weight gain has been favourable and she is currently on the fiftieth percentile for weight for her age.

At Amelia's assessment the following was noted:

- Amelia was able to sit unsupported on the floor; however, in the highchair she often slumped her body to one side at mealtimes.
- During purees she happily opened her mouth for the spoon and displayed a mild tongue thrust during swallowing. She had not developed a tongue-tip swallow on pureed textures.
- On lumpy textures via the spoon, she was noted to display good anticipation of the spoon by opening her mouth and she displayed the same tongue thrust tongue movement during swallowing. Lumps were consequently swallowed whole with gagging occurring and distress. Neither lateral tongue movement nor chewing of lumps prior to swallowing was noted.
- Amelia held and mouthed both objects and strips of finger foods. She displayed some early munching and biting, which was successful on a soft biscuit. When pieces entered her mouth she mainly sucked these and swallowed large whole pieces without chewing.
- During drinking from the bottle Amelia displayed adequate seal and no liquid loss; however, her seal was achieved via her lips and with her tongue protruded. She sucked with a mild tongue thrust, however, appeared to control the liquid adequately for swallowing and no coughing or gagging was noted.
- Chopped finger food such as cheese was placed into the side of Amelia's mouth. This appeared to stimulate some chewing prior to swallowing.
- A training cup with dribble lid (not spout) was tested at the assessment. Amelia needed support to hold the two handles and bring the cup to her mouth. She displayed tongue protrusion under the rim of the cup and a suckling motion on the cup.
- Amelia was producing some early reduplicated babbling with labial sounds at her visit – e.g. 'mumum' and 'bubub'. She was not producing any chains of variegated babble or single words yet. She was not producing any tongue tip sounds such as 'd' or 'n'.

MANAGEMENT

The initial goals in therapy were to:

- *Improve positioning.* This was initially achieved by placing a seating insert into the highchair which gave better trunk support and a more midline body posture. A pelvic strap was also inserted into her current highchair to achieve a more stable seating arrangement.
- *Reduce tongue thrusting and improve lip closure and tongue tip movement for purees and drinking.* Initially Amelia's purees were thickened to a smooth 'mashed potato' consistency to achieve better tongue control and tip movement. Amelia was also provided with some jaw support to assist with her lip closure on the spoon and to minimize tongue thrusting. She was given a training cup with dribble lid for drinks at mealtimes. Full lip and jaw support was given to reduce tongue

protrusion and her tongue thrust and to encourage her tongue-tip movement. As her skills with the cup improved, weaning from the bottle was recommended as continued teat sucking would be likely to perpetuate her tongue thrust at this stage.

- *Improve lateral tongue movement and chewing skills.* This was achieved by introducing toothbrush trainers before mealtimes and prior to her meal. Chewing and biting strength exercises were demonstrated to facilitate her chewing and biting. Lateral placement of toothbrush trainers was used to encourage lateral tongue movement. Either soft chopped pieces of food or soft mashed food were given at the beginning of meals prior to her purees. These were placed into the side of her mouth either via fingers or small soft spoon. A small number of mouthfuls at this stage were given whilst Amelia developed her chewing skills. Pureed meals were given as the remainder of the meal and as the primary nutrition of solid foods. At snack times, Amelia was given rusks and 'dissolvable' finger foods such as a shortbread biscuits to try. Full supervision at all meals was suggested, especially with finger food. If pieces broke off into Amelia's mouth these were to be pushed across to the side of her mouth with the carer's finger to facilitate chewing and minimize swallowing of the whole piece.
- *Improve the range of speech sounds especially tongue tip sounds.* This would be encouraged by feeding activities that aim to reduce tongue thrusting and facilitate tongue tip movement and good lip closure. Activities requiring good lip closure and promoting tongue-tip movement include use of a cup and eating of purees. Additional exercises were also demonstrated, such as babbling games where the tongue was facilitated in to the mouth and firm tapping was given on the tongue tip. Oral imitation games would also assist Amelia gain control over her lips and, jaw and tongue for speech – e.g. blowing, raspberries, imitating babbling, car sounds, animal noises. Modelling of babbling with 'd' and 'n' was demonstrated. Additional signing and gesturing activities were also incorporated to facilitate object recognition and communication skills.

ACKNOWLEDGEMENTS

With thanks to Martin Taylor for drawing Figures 15.6 and 15.11.

REFERENCES

Alexander R (1987) Oral-motor treatment for infants and young children with cerebral palsy. Seminars in Speech and Language 8: 87–100.
Anderson J (1986) Sensory intervention with the preterm infant in the neonatal intensive care unit. American Journal of Occupational Therapy 40(1): 19–26.
Arvedson JC (1993) Management of swallowing problems. In Arvedson JC, Brodsky L (eds) Pedatric Swallowing and Feeding Assessment and Management. San Diego: Singular.

538

DYSPHAGIA: FOUNDATION, THEORY AND PRACTICE

Arvedson JC, Brodsky L (1993) Pedatric Swallowing and Feeding Assessment and Management. San Diego: Singular.

Arvedson JC, Brodsky L (2002) Pediatric Swallowing and Feeding: Assessment and Management (2nd edn). Canada: Thomson Learning.

Bazyk S (1990) Factors associated with the transition to oral feeding in infants fed by nasogastric tubes. American Journal of Occupational Therapy 44(12): 1070–8.

Bernbaum JC, Pereira GR, Watkins JK, et al. (1983) Non-nutritive sucking during gavage feeding enhances growth and maturation in premature infants. Pediatrics 71(1): 41–5.

Blitzer A (1990) Approaches to the patient with aspiration and swallowing disabilities. Dysphagia 5: 129–37.

Bloch AS (1987) Noctural tube feedings. Dysphagia 2: 3–7.

Boshart C (1998) Oromotor Analysis and Remediation Techniques (2nd edn). California: Speech Dynamics.

Carr J (1979) Oral function in infancy – its importance for future development. Australian Journal of Physiotherapy, Paediatric Monograph, December, pp. 103–14.

Christensen JR (1989) Developmental approach to pediatric neurogenic dysphagia. Dysphagia 3: 131–4.

Cummings WA, Reilly BJ (1972). Fatigue aspiration: a cause of recurrent pneumonia in infants. Radiology 105: 387–90.

Evans C (1977) Muscles involved in oral-motor function. In Wilson JM (ed.) Oral Motor Function and Dysfunction in Children. Chapel Hill, NC: University of North Carolina at Chapel Hill.

Fetters L (1986) Sensory-motor management of the high-risk neonate. In Wilson JM (ed.) The High-Risk Neonate: Developmental Treatment Perspectives. New York: Haworth Press, pp. 217–28.

Fisher M (1992) Aspiration and the Speech-Language Therapist. New Zealand STA Conference, Wellington.

Ganger D, Craig RM (1990) Swallowing disorders and nutritional support. Dysphagia 4: 213–19.

Griggs C, Jones P, Lee R (1989) Videofluoroscopic investigation of feeding disorders in patients with multiple handicap. Developmental Medicine and Child Neurology 31: 303–8.

Illingworth RS (1969) Sucking and swallowing difficulties in infancy: diagnostic problems of dysphagia. Archives of Disease in Childhood 44(238): 655–&.

Illingworth RS, Lister J (1964) The critical or sensitive period, with special reference to certain feeding problems in infants and children. Journal of Pediatrics 65(6): 839–46.

Kamal PL (1990) Nutritional assessment and requirements. Dysphagia 4: 189–95.

Kent RD (1984) Psychology of speech development: Coemergence of language and a movement system. American Journal of Physiology 246: 888–94.

Kitzinger S (1987) The Experience of Breast Feeding (3rd edn). Victoria, Australia: Penguin Books.

Kleinman RE (1994) Learning about dietary variety: the first steps. Pediatric Basics 68: 2–11.

Laviners J, Woessner C (1990) Counselling the Nursing Mother. A Reference Handbook for Health Care Professionals and Lay Counsellors. Avery Publishing, part 6, pp. 197–231.

Leach P (1988) Baby and Child: From Birth to Age Five. London: Penguin.

Loughlin GM (1989) Respiratory consequences of dysfunctional swallowing and aspiration. Dysphagia 3: 126–30.

Macie D, Arvedson J (1993) Tone and positioning. In Arvedson JC, Brodsky L (eds) Paediatric Swallowing and Feeding: Assessment and Management. San Diego: Singular.

Mackeith J (1981) Mackeith's Infant Feeding and Feeding Difficulties. London: Churchill-Livingstone, pp. 78–123.

Measal EP, Anderson GC (1979) Non-nutritive sucking during tube feeding: effects on clinical course in premature infants. Journal of Obstetric, Gynaecological and Neonatal Nursing 8(5): 265–72.

Morris SE (1985) Developmental implications for the management of feeding problems in neurologically impaired infants. Seminars in Speech and Language 6(4): 304–9.

Morris SE, Klein MD (2000) Prefeeding skills: a comprehensive resource for mealtime development (2nd edn). Therapy Skill Builders/Harcourt.

Poon CY (1993) Pharmacology. In Arvedson JC, Brodsky L (eds) Paediatric Swallowing and Feeding Assessment and Management. San Diego: Singular.

Rausch PG (1981) Effects of tactile and kinaesthetic stimulation on premature infants. Journal of Obstetrics, Gynaecological and Neonatal Nursing 90: 34–7.

Selly NG, Ellis RE, Flack FC, et al. (1990) Coordination of sucking, swallowing and breathing in the newborn: its relationship to infant feeding and normal development. British Journal of Disorders of Communication 25: 311–27.

Shaker CS (1990) Nipple feeding premature infants: a different perspective. Neonatal Network 8(5): 9–17.

Sitzmann J, Mueller R (1988). Enteral and parental feeding in the dysphagic patient. Dysphagia 3: 38–45.

Sorin R, Somers S, Austin W, et al. (1988) The influence of videofluoroscopy on the management of the dysphagic patient. Dysphagia 2: 127–35.

Speech Pathology Association of Australia (2003) Dysphagia Position Paper. Melbourne: SPA.

Starr S (1995) Feeding and Oral Development: Birth to 2 Years (video). Sydney, Australia: Western Sydney Area Health Service.

Stevenson R, Allaire J (1991) The development of normal feeding and swallowing. Pediatric Clinics of North America 38(6): 1439–53.

Terry PG, Fuller SD (1989) Pulmonary consequences of aspiration. Dysphagia 3: 179–83.

Thorpe WH, Zangwill OL (1961) Current Problems in Animal Behaviour. Cambridge: Cambridge University Press.

Tuchman DM (1989) Cough, choke, sputter: the evaluation of the child with dysfunctional swallowing. Dysphagia 3: 111–16.

White KR, Mhango-Mkandawire RD, Rosenthal SR (1993) Developmental disability. In Arvedson JC, Brodsky L (eds) Paediatric Swallowing and Feeding: Assessment and Management. San Diego: Singular.

Wolf LS, Glass RP (1992) Feeding and Swallowing Disorders in Infancy: Assessment and Management. Arizona: Therapy Skill Builders.

Woolridge MW (1986) The anatomy of infant sucking. Midwifery 2: 164 –71.

World Health Organization (1989) Protecting, Promoting and Supporting Breastfeeding. The Special Role of Maternity Services. Geneva: WHO Press.

Young C (1993) Nutrition. In Arvedson JC, Brodsky L (eds) Paediatric Swallowing and Feeding Assessment and Management. San Diego: Singular.

Recommended web site for current information on paediatric feeding:
http://www.new-vis.com

Part V Measuring Outcomes of Swallowing Disorders

16 Oropharyngeal Dysphagia Outcome Measurement

JOHN ROSENBEK and NEILA DONOVAN

INTRODUCTION

Oropharyngeal dysphagia (hereafter to be called dysphagia) is defined as difficulty swallowing resulting from abnormalities of structure or movement of the oral cavity, (including lips, jaw and tongue), the oropharynx, velopharynx, hypopharynx, larynx, and upper oesophageal sphincter (McHorney and Rosenbek, 1998; Chen et al., 2001). Dysphagia can occur at any time during the lifespan, but adult dysphagia is the focus of this chapter. Dysphagia treatment procedures have generally been organized according to physiological principles and selected to treat specific physiologic problems (Huckabee and Pelletier, 1999). Conclusions about what works, for whom, and under what conditions have generally been supported by changes in the biomechanics of swallowing. The traditional biomechanical assessment of dysphagia for diagnostic, treatment planning, and outcomes measurement purposes has traditionally been the videofluoroscopic swallowing examination (VFSE), a radiological procedure allowing visualization of the relationship of radiopaque boluses to oral, velopharyngeal, laryngeal, and pharyngeal structures and movements. The resulting images are evaluated perceptually, sometimes from remote locations aided by the Internet (Perlman and Witthawaskul, 2002) using simple or computer-assisted visual analysis (Dengel et al., 1991; Robbins, 1992). Predictably, pre- and post-treatment VSFEs have become the standard treatment outcome measure in many centres.

Dissatisfaction with the hegemony of this approach is increasingly common for a number of reasons. The first is that the goals of dysphagia management include but are not limited to improved biomechanics. The main goals of dysphagia management are safe, adequate, independent, and satisfying nutrition and hydration. It is at best naïve to assume that understanding mechanics allows prediction of safety, adequacy, independence, and satisfaction. Indeed changes in biomechanics of swallowing may be only weakly related to these conditions. Therefore, the myriad goals of dysphagia management have accelerated the search for additional outcome measures. Second, the number of activities that can appropriately be called treatment is expanding. Indeed management rather than therapy or even rehabilitation is the increasingly popular name for the multidisciplinary practices presently being employed with

Dysphagia: Foundation, Theory and Practice.   Edited by J. Cichero and B. Murdoch
© 2006 John Wiley & Sons, Ltd.

dysphagic persons (Huckabee and Pelletier, 1999). Third, patients, caregivers, and third-party payers are increasingly vocal about the need for outcome measurements that are functional and important to the patient, and even for measures from the patient's point of view. The fourth and most important is the emerging popularity of two types of models because they provide direction for thinking about what has been accomplished in dysphagia and what needs to be done. The first type includes models of what can be called 'enablement' and the second includes models created to identify all relevant domains of healthcare outcome measurement. The World Health Organization International Classification of Functioning, Disability, and Health (ICF) (WHO, 2001), and the National Center for Medical Rehabilitation Research (NCMRR) model of enablement (NIH, 1993) are examples of the first. The Health Care Value Compass (Batalden et al., 1994) is an example of the second.

Some members of the world community of dysphagia scientists recognized early on that a broader repertoire of outcomes was required if the full impact of dysphagia treatments was to be understood. The result is that a modest repertoire of outcomes in addition to the biomechanical ones is available. It is among this chapter's purposes to review this repertoire, to suggest bases for deciding which approach is best in individual clinical and research circumstances, and to advocate for additional measurement approaches. This chapter's first purpose, however, is to review the three aforementioned models for it is these that provide a structure for thinking about what has and needs to be done.

MODELS OF ENABLEMENT AND HEALTHCARE OUTCOMES

Conceptual models are designed to order and categorize conceptual elements and attempt to define the relationships among those elements. Models can impose order on extremely complex issues such as developing and selecting the appropriate measure of a treatment's effect. If done well, a model allows the researcher, clinician, or policymaker to understand and sometimes to discover previously unknown relationships among conceptual elements.

In 2001, the WHO presented the ICF to replace the International Classification of Impairment, Disability and Health (ICIDH) first proposed in1980. One of the most compelling reasons to employ the new ICF model rather than its predecessor or other models lies in its improved 'biopsychosocial' design. The ICF integrates aspects from both the traditional medical model and the newer social model of functioning and health to produce a dynamic, interactive picture of 'the person in his or her world' (National Committee on Vital and Health Statistics, 2001: 9). Moreover, the ICF model is designed so that health states are dynamic and interactive, rather than linear (National Committee on Vital and Health Statistics, 2001). There is another reason to adopt it as well. One of the complaints lodged against the earlier ICIDH model was that the terms *handicapped* and *disabled* resulted in stigma toward people who were trying to regain independence after disease or injury or while coping with chronic health problems. In recognition of the negative connotations the terminology carried, the ICF replaced the terms *impairment, handicap*, and *disability* with *impairment, activity limitation*, and *participation restriction* (WHO, 2001). *Impairment* is defined as the impact of disease or illness on the organ or organ system of the body structure and function. *Activity limitation* is defined as the difficulty a person has in executing an activity as a result of the impairment. *Participation restriction* is defined as the problem an individual has in performing an activity in life situations. In addition to changes in terminology, the ICF model recognizes the contextual factors that may positively or negatively influence a person's health state by adding *environmental* and *personal factors.*

One limitation of the ICF model in the eyes of some researchers is that it contains only two components: (a) body functions and structure and (b) activities, thereby potentially obscuring differences in the performance and experience of illness that can affect the outcomes of healthcare. The ICF model is an internationally recognized model and is frequently the model of choice in rehabilitation research but other models identify an expanded set of domains. A model with expanded domains may be more useful for conceptualizing the potential array of dysphagia outcome measures and for capturing significant differences among patients in response to treatment.

One of these is the NCMRR Model of Disability (NIH, 1993). The NCMRR was established in 1993 under the National Institute of Child Health and Human Development (NICHD) at the National Institutes of Health (NIH). Its mission is to enhance the quality of life for people with disabilities. To accomplish that mission, NCMRR developed a conceptual model of disability, somewhat similar to the WHO model of that time, the ICIDH. The NCMRR model recognizes rehabilitation as a dynamic process, with varying lengths and types of treatment resulting in different outcomes. The NCMRR model has five domains, defined as:

- *pathophysiology* – an interruption of or interference with normal physiological and developmental processes or structures;
- *impairment* – a loss or abnormality at the organ or organ level of the body;
- *functional limitations* – restriction or lack of ability to perform an action or activity in the manner or range consistent with the organ or organ system's purposes;
- *disability* – a limitation in performing tasks, activities and roles to levels expected within physical and social contexts;
- *societal limitations* – restrictions to social policy or barriers (structural or attitudinal), which limit fulfillment of roles or deny access to services and opportunities associated with full participation in society (NIH, 1993: 5).

The relationships among these domains can be quite complex. Performance in one does not necessarily predict performance in another; however, disruption of one can magnify disruptions in one or more of the others in sometimes quite idiosyncratic ways.

In addition, the NCMRR model was the first of the models to emphasize individuals and their successful reintegration into communities as the central purpose of the medical rehabilitation process. Its developers were apparently also the first to conceptualize the rehabilitation process in a non-linear way and to recognize the various extrinsic and intrinsic factors that can affect the person or the rehabilitation process. They identified the following factors that may affect the rehabilitation process:

- personal background – including organic, psychosocial, and environmental factors that may influence a person's response to a situation;
- quality of life after rehabilitation – emphasizing restoration of the individual to a productive and fulfilling life, including issues of survival, productivity, and social and work relationships;
- lifespan factors – such as recognizing that both habilitation and rehabilitation needs will vary with age.

By emphasizing the domains and their sometimes complex relationships and the presence of a set of equally complex extrinsic and intrinsic contributory factors to human performance in and outside treatment, the NCMRR model added an additional and much needed layer of complexity to the study of the rehabilitation process. Hence, terms such as 'the person served', 'stakeholders', and 'functional outcomes' emerged, and the rehabilitation industry was left with the onus of developing and implementing ways to operationally define and measure extremely complex concepts such as function and disability. How well dysphagia scientists have done in each of the model's domains will be described in a subsequent section.

There is yet another useful model to guide an analysis of what has been accomplished in outcomes measurement in dysphagia and of what remains to be accomplished. This is the Health Services value compass (Batalden et al., 1994). The value compass (Figure 16.1) has four broad classes of outcomes: clinical status, patient satisfaction, costs and utilization, and quality of life. It is designed to recognize that each class of outcome may stand alone, but that having information simultaneously

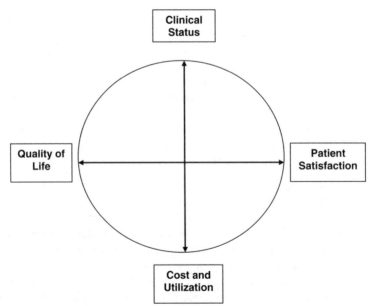

Figure 16.1   Health Service Value Compass
Source: Batalden et al., 1994

from all four will lead to a more complete picture of dysphagia treatment outcomes. The compass is added as an organizing model for this chapter because three of its four points – clinical status, patient satisfaction, and costs and utilization – are not unequivocally included in the other models. In addition, the final point – quality of life – is a better known label than functional limitation and disability for aspects of living with and without disease.

THE STATUS OF OUTCOMES MEASUREMENT IN DYSPHAGIA

Two kinds of search produced the material for this discussion. Dysphagia treatment articles published in English since the 1960s were reviewed to determine what outcome measures were being employed. The second source of information, again only in English, was published measurement tools. All the results will not be identified for two reasons:

- there is considerable redundancy especially in impairment domain measurement using videofluoroscopy, and
- many measures fail to meet even minimum standards of psychometric quality.

What has been retained is organized according to the NCMRR's five domains and the four points of the value compass. Some liberty has been taken with the operational definitions of certain domains so as to fit the widest possible array of outcome measurements into the outline.

PATHOPHYSIOLOGY

Three research efforts help to define this domain and to demonstrate the power of measurement within it. Robbins (1992) used magnetic resonance imaging (MRI) to measure lingual muscle fiber before and after a muscle-strengthening programme. Muscle changes paralleled changes in function. Mann is using similar technology to evaluate the influence of an oropharyngeal exercise programme for patients undergoing radiation treatments for head-neck cancer. Data are limited but promising (personal communication, 2003). This kind of work is critical if we are to understand the appropriate intensity and duration of the myriad exercise programmes advocated for dysphagic adults.

Probably the effects of these and other treatments depend upon different mechanisms during treatment's course (Huckabee and Cannito, 1999). Early, virtually immediate effects can often be attributed to what is commonly called the placebo effect but which might more accurately be called the information effect (Moerman and Jonas, 2002). Moerman and Jonas argue that it is impossible to treat or do research with humans without conveying information – to which humans will inevitably attach meaning, and that the meaning ultimately affects the outcome, rather than the placebo itself, which is by definition, inert. Examples from the medical literature include reports of differences in outcomes based on colour and number of pills people receive (Blackwell et al., 1972); physician dress (Blumhagen, 1979); physician-conveyed level of enthusiasm (Uhlenhuth et al., 1966) and some argue diagnosis and prognosis (Chistakis, 1999). After decades of trying to control this effect it is time to begin understanding it and measurement within this domain promises to contribute to that understanding. Other early effects may represent some variation of increased effort or background of physiological support, and these effects may well be in addition to the information effect. Electromyography (EMG) may be a significant outcome measurement tool for resolving such questions.

Some changes, both early and late, may result from central nervous system reorganization. The Manchester group's use of transcranial magnetic stimulation to establish the locus and extent of cortical controls of oropharyngeal swallowing is especially noteworthy (Fraser et al., 2002). They have demonstrated that different intensities and durations of electrical stimulation to the oropharynx can have different effects on cortical control of swallowing. With the correct intensity and duration, the cortical region associated with swallowing can be expanded, an expansion that is accompanied by improved swallowing. The wrong intensity and duration suppress the swallowing response. Thus, in addition to providing evidence in support of cortical reorganization as at least one part of the basis for a treatment effect, such research helps refine treatment approaches: the timing, duration, and intensity of treatment matter.

IMPAIRMENT

Psychometrically sound impairment domain measures abound. Most have been developed for measuring images from videofluoroscopy or endoscopy. Logemann and her colleagues (1993) led the way in the measurement of VFSE images. In general such measures are designed to capture four kinds of data:

- the timing of bolus and oropharyngeal and laryngeal structures during swallowing, yielding a variety of measures such as delay in swallow initiation or reduced duration of opening of the upper oesophageal sphincter;
- completeness of bolus passage with location and even amount of residual being scored;
- direction of bolus, with the major signs of an abnormality of direction being penetration in which material enters the larynx but does not pass below the vocal folds and aspiration in which material passes below the vocal folds, and
- abnormalities of structural function, as when the epiglottis fails to invert, or appearance, as when a swallow is disrupted by osteophytes or bony growths on the cervical vertebrae.

The Penetration–Aspiration Scale is a psychometrically sound tool for quantifying penetration and aspiration events (Rosenbek et al., 1996). The scale comprises eight points to summarize three variables:

- whether or not material enters the airway;
- the level to which material descends if it enters the airway – in other words whether it is penetrated or aspirated; and
- whether and how successfully the swallower responds to penetration or aspiration.

Its documented ordinality and intervality allow it to be used as a measure of severity of penetration aspiration events (McCullough et al., 1998).

Impairment domain measures can also be derived from other instrumented approaches. Simultaneous videomanometry and fluoroscopy is promising, as Bulow et al. (2002) demonstrated in their study of three swallow techniques: supraglottic swallow, effortful swallow and chin tuck. Equally promising is simultaneous videofluoroscopy and breathing function measurement as evidence of the importance of respiratory dysfunction to abnormal swallowing increases (Palmer and Hiiemae, 2003) and treatments such as exhalatory muscle strength training, move out of the laboratory and into the clinic (Sapienza et al., 2002). Endoscopy is an increasingly popular alternative to videofluoroscopy (Langmore, 2000). Cervical auscultation also has its advocates (Cichero and Murdoch, 2002) as does pulse oximetry (Sellars et al., 1998). While unavailable to most clinicians, ultrasound imaging of the oropharynx can also be used to measure treatment effects as Frattali et al. (1999) did in studying the effects of medication on the swallow of patients with progressive supranuclear palsy. For appropriately outfitted clinics and laboratories, simultaneous electromyographic and electroglottic measurement are equally promising, as demonstrated by Ding's group (2002) who used the procedures to measure the effects of the Mendelsohn manoeuvre.

Problems of reliability in judging events portrayed on VFSE and potential solutions for increasing reliability have been reasonably well studied for videofluoroscopy. Clinicians have difficulty making judgements, especially about the presence of such obviously important signs as aspiration (Wilcox et al., 1996). The solution is training (Scott et al., 1998). Without training, measures of treatment effect derived from VFSE may well be unreliable, as would any subsequent conclusion about treatment effect. Users of other instrumented approaches probably face the same challenge but data have been slower to arrive.

The clinical swallowing examination occupies an odd place in the array of impairment measures. Mostly it has been criticized for its presumed insensitivity to aspiration and it has been treated as if it were merely a screening examination to determine if a patient needed an instrumental examination. As an outcome measure the criticism has been that it is – at least as used by most practitioners – a qualitative rather than quantitative measure. Quantification is straightforward. For example McCullough and his colleagues (2001) have established the approach's sensitivity and specificity when used to predict aspiration on a subsequent VFSE. MASA: The Mann Assessment of Swallowing Ability is another answer to the problem of quantification (Mann, 2002). Twenty-four signs such as dyspraxia, dysarthria, reduced voluntary and reflexive cough, and delayed swallow initiation are scored with 5- and 10-point scales. The maximum score is 200 and varying levels of performance are associated with the presence and severity of dysphagia, the likelihood of aspiration on a subsequent VFSE, and even with diet recommendations. It can reasonably be argued that moving, as a result of treatment, from a lower to a higher score on the MASA, which has been standardized on a large sample of stroke patients, is a sign of treatment effect.

We must avoid the danger of assuming that one can use an impairment score to predict performance in other domains. One rationale for expanding the repertoire of outcome measures is that tests from the different domains are likely to be only modestly related. If that were not the case then a major reason for domains would disappear. Indeed if two measures presumably from different domains are highly correlated it is likely they are not from different domains at all.

FUNCTIONAL LIMITATIONS

The outcry for more functional measures echoes in all professions and for the study of dysphagia it is no different. Unfortunately the definition of *functional* as used in outcomes is sometimes confused with *functioning* leading to the conclusion that any measure of function is a functional measure. In this chapter, functional limitation is defined as limitation in the ability to eat and drink safely, adequately, independently, or with pleasure. Other researchers share the emphasis on eating and drinking and other outcome measures have been created. Often the approach is a questionnaire like that employed by Moerman et al. (2003), which allows patients to report on type of diet, eating tempo, length of time to chew, and other functional dimensions. Others have taken a more quantified approach. Logemann et al. (1992) measured:

- duration of tube feeding;
- date of first oral intake;
- date premorbid diet was resumed; and
- date of normal swallow.

To quantify mode of supplying nutrition, Aguilar et al. (1979) used a simple three-point scale: 1) oral, 2) oral plus tube and 3) tube alone. This scaling could have been made more elaborate by quantifying the percent of oral nutrition taken in the combined oral/tube condition. Huckabee and Cannito (1999) did use such a refined scale as seen in Table 16.1.

Table 16.1 Functional scale of feeding status developed by Huckabee and Cannito (1999)

Level	Description
1	Feeding tube only, no oral intake
2	Feeding tube for primary nutrition, oral intake secondary
3	Oral intake for primary nutrition, feeding tube secondary
4	Oral intake only, feeding tube removed, restricted diet texture
5	Oral intake only, feeding tube removed, minimal texture restriction

Table 16.2 Dysphagia Outcome and Severity Scale developed by O'Neil et al. (1999)

Level	Description
1	Severe dysphagia: NPO.
2	Moderately severe dysphagia: maximum assistance, partial PO only.
3	Moderate dysphagia: total assist, strategies, 2 or more consistency restrictions.
4	Mild/moderate dysphagia: intermittent supervision/cueing required, one or two diet consistencies restricted.
5	Mild dysphagia: distant supervision, one diet consistency restricted.
6	Within functional limits/modified independence, extra time required, no penetration or aspiration.
7	Normal diet in all situations. No strategies or extra time required.

A different approach is to assign numerical values to the types of food preparation a patient can eat. For example, the List et al. (1990) scale assigns 100 points for the ability to eat any diet, 90 points for the ability to eat peanuts, and lesser values for the ability to swallow other items. A score of 10 is assigned if one can only drink cold water, and 0 is assigned for tube feeding. Other common scales (Hillel et al., 1989) also assign fewer points for NPO (nil by mouth) and pureed diet, more points for soft and mechanical diets and the most for a normal diet.

The Dysphagia Outcome and Severity Scale (DOSS) (O'Neil et al., 1999) is described modestly as a "possible measure of functional outcomes in dysphagia" (O'Neil et al., 1999: 144). It comprises seven points as seen in Table 16.2. It was developed by having clinicians view videotaped swallows and make judgements about the impact of this performance on need for supervision, whether nutrition should be oral or non-oral, and on the appropriate diet.

The DOSS is useful but it exposes two weaknesses inherent in most functional measures. The first is that clinicians make the judgements and the second is that the judgements are usually based on performance on VFSE. The problem is one of validity. Evidence is slim that adequacy and safety of nutrition require the approaches to diet selection that clinicians recommend. Admittedly, such data are difficult to collect. Doing so requires patient input and, more critically, measurement of the patient's safety, adequacy, independence, and pleasure with a variety of diets. In other words it would involve letting them eat and drink what they think they can manage. Groher (1995) has already demonstrated that many nursing home patients do not need to be on the restrictive diets prescribed. More data of this sort are necessary. In the interim, Huckabee and Cannito (1999: 97) have published a reasonable compromise. Their judgements were based on VFSE and on 'functional ability to safely consume oral intake'.

Another step forward would be reliance upon formal assessments of eating and drinking in a more naturalistic environment. Progress is being made. Lambert et al. (2003) developed the McGill Ingestive Skills Assessment (MISA), a 44-item battery divided across five domains for assessing eating/swallowing in the elderly. Table 16.3 summarizes the domains and selected items from each. Testing requires

Table 16.3 Domains and selected items from the MISA (Lambert et al., 2003)

Domains	Selected items
Positioning	Maintains symmetry of posture
	Has adequate head control for feeding
Texture management	Accepts textures based on judgment and discretion
Feeding skills	Sets up tray independently
	Able to grasp utensil functionally
Liquid ingestion	Seals lips on cup
	Demonstrates same voice quality after drinking
Solid ingestion	Opens mouth in anticipation
	Retains food in mouth

a professional to observe the patient during a meal without intervening with such activities as tray setup or positioning. Observations are made in five domains: positioning, texture management, by which is meant identification of textures a patient will accept, feeding skills, liquid ingestion, and solid ingestion.

This measure may point the way toward improved decision making about diet. It is increasingly hard to defend use of an instrumented exam no matter how exquisite, not because instrumented examinations are flawed but because they were not developed to provide the basis for such decisions. This issue of validity must be addressed experimentally if the profession is to begin controlling the number of pureed diets with thickened liquids, amount of supervision, and imposition of postures and procedures now being recommended world wide in the name of safety. Almost inevitably these recommendations are at the expense of pleasure and independence and sometimes even at the expense of adequacy.

DISABILITY

Disability is defined as performance in context. Measures of performance in context are limited. The Eating in Public subscale of the List et al. (1990) scale assigns points for the environment in which one eats. To get one hundred points a person must report no restrictions where or with whom he eats. Despite the origins of dysphagia in healthcare where clinical and laboratory tests are the *sine qua non,* it is surprising that so few psychometrically sound disability measures have appeared. One instrument designed to measure swallowing disability with published validity and reliability is the Royal Brisbane Hospital Outcome Measure for Swallowing (RBHOMS) (Ward and Conroy, 1999). The RBHOMS is a four-stage, 10-point scale tested on a sample of 285 hospitalized individuals with various medical diagnoses and dysphagia.

Although Ward and Conroy (1999: 10) suggest that the RBHOMS is a measure of disability designed to 'identify and monitor difficulties with everyday performance of swallowing function, based on clinical indicators of swallowing, not specific diet/fluid consistencies', some would argue that it is, rather, a measure of functional

Table 16.4 RBHOMS stages, and described levels (Ward and Conroy, 1999)

Stage	Level	Description
A	1	Patient aspirates secretions
	2	Difficulty managing secretions but protecting airway
	3	Coping with secretions
B	4	Tolerates small amounts of thickened/thin fluids only
C	5	Commencing/continuing modified diet-supplementation is being provided
	6	Commencing/continuing modified diet – no supplementation provided
	7	Upgrading of modified diet
D	8	Swallowing function at patients optimal level
	9	Swallowing function at premorbid/preadmission level
	10	Swallowing function at better than premorbid/preadmission level

limitation because it assesses dysphagia in the hospital context, and does not address the participation restrictions of dysphagia or the related impact on quality of life.

Cardol et al. (2000: 27) remind us: 'Rehabilitation treatment in chronic illness ultimately aims to restore a person's participation in society, despite persistent sequelae of illness, such as impairments and disabilities.' Selected subscales of the SWAL-QOL to be reviewed in the section on quality of life address this issue (McHorney and Rosenbek, 1998; McHorney et al., 2000a, b et al., 2000, 2002).

SOCIETAL LIMITATIONS

Bickenbach et al. (1999) underline the importance of the societal limitations domain. They say, 'while there is a medical facet to disablement, far more important is the salient role played by features of the world built and designed by people in the creation of the disadvantages that people with disabilities experience' (Bickenbach et al., 1999: 1173). Their example of a person in a wheelchair prevented from entering a building because there is no ramp provides a trenchant example of the shift in thinking required by this social perspective. They say the problem is in the building not in the person's legs. A similar scenario is that facing a dysphagic patient on a pureed diet who loves to eat out but can find only one restaurant willing to puree his food. Those who believe that the social model of disability is at least as important as the medical model would argue the problem lies with restaurants, not with his swallowing.

'Features of the world' include policies, guidelines, laws, and regulations. Much of what happens in treatment of persons with dysphagia is determined in part or in whole by these variables. Consider that in the US individuals with certain disabilities and those over age 65 are entitled to medical benefits, which were designed to include the evaluation and treatment for dysphagia. The Social Security Act 42 U.S.C. 1395d, 1965 states:

> The insurance programme for which entitlement is established provides basic protection against the costs of hospital, related post-hospital, home health services and hospice care in accordance with this part for (1) Individuals who

are age 65 or over and are eligible for retirement benefits under title II of this Act (Social Security Act) or under the railroad retirement system, (2) individuals under age 65 who have been entitled for no less than 24 months to benefits under title II of this Act.

Medicare Intermediary Manual, Pub. 13 states:

Speech pathology services are covered under Medicare for treatment of dysphagia, regardless of the presence of a communication disability. Patients who are motivated, moderately alert and have some degree of deglutition and swallowing functions are appropriate candidates for dysphagia therapy. Design all programmes to ensure swallowing safety of the patient during oral feeding and maintain adequate nutrition.

In 1997 the US Congress instituted significant changes in the Medicare reimbursement system due to a decade of increasing rehabilitation claims. One of these changes placed limits on outpatient therapy services for evaluation and treatment of dysphagia. Physical therapy and speech therapy outpatient services were capped at $1,500 combined, and occupational therapy service was capped at $1,500. This action meant that, regardless of diagnosis, severity, length of inpatient stay, or discharge disposition, a person could expect Medicare to pay 80% of $3,000 worth of outpatient therapy. If a person were to receive therapy from all three disciplines three times a week, at a rate of $150 per hour, he would reach the limit in less than three weeks of treatment. A moratorium was placed on these therapy limits in 2000, in part because of negative public reaction to the arbitrary reduction in benefits.

During the same timeframe, a study on outpatient therapy utilization for physical therapy, occupational therapy, and speech-language pathology was being conducted. The results were presented to the Center for Medicare Services (CMS) in 2002 (Olshin et al., 2002). Findings of this report should have important implications for therapists, payers and policy makers alike. Here are a few examples:

- For speech-language pathology the most frequently reported claim diagnoses were 787 (dysphagia) and 436 (acute stroke) (Table 46).
- Neurological diagnoses remained disproportionately represented among those conditions more likely to be found in patients in the category 'top 5% most expensive patients'. The top three diagnoses included hemiplegia/hemiparesis, acute stroke, and late effects of stroke. Parkinson's disease was ranked seventh (Table 50).
- The 'top 5% most expensive patients' were disproportionately older (80+), female, rural, and included twice the number of racial minorities compared to the overall Medicare population. 'Examination of the most costly therapy outpatients suggested that payment policy should consider patient demographic information such as age, gender, race, geographic location and medical condition, as well as the interaction between these variables. Policy decisions that do not address such variables may have unintended consequences' (Olshin et al., 2002: 108).

Bickenbach et al. (1999) admitted the difficulty of designing research in this area while simultaneously demanding that ways of answering important questions about such matters be discovered or developed. Our examples are drawn from the US, but our prediction is that limitations on what is 'necessary' exist in all countries.

SUMMING UP

The NCMRR model's domains are only one way of classifying the types of outcome measurements. The value compass divides outcomes differently. One of its points – quality of life – is superordinate comprising the NCMMR domains of functional limitation and disability and, to a degree, even societal limitations. The compass's value is that it also provides an additional structure for describing and expanding the repertoire of outcome measures in dysphagia. Please refer to Figure 16.1.

CLINICAL STATUS

Clinical status measures continue to be compelling outcomes. Aspiration pneumonia, dehydration, malnutrition and death will be reviewed. Also included in this section are surrogate health status variables; length of hospital stay, number of re-hospitalizations, and the necessity of special medical procedures such as feeding tube placement.

Aspiration pneumonia: dysphagia programmes decrease the incidence of aspiration pneumonia in acute stroke patients (Doggett et al., 2001). This finding is cause for celebration, however, the complications of using aspiration pneumonia as an outcome should be recognized. Diagnosing aspiration pneumonia, especially in the elderly, is difficult (Feinberg et al. 1990, 1996). Help in the accurate diagnosis is provided by the clinical, radiological, and laboratory criteria summarized by Martin and colleagues (1994) and summarized in Table 16.5.

Another complication is aspiration of refluxed gastric contents (Feinberg et al., 1990) and infected saliva (Finegold, 1991). These are among the reasons why those on tube feedings are in some instances more likely than those eating by mouth to develop aspiration pneumonia (Johnson et al., 1990). A third complication is that dysphagia is an inadequate explanation for the presence of aspiration pneumonia in many populations (Langmore et al., 1998). Other critical factors include dependence, oral health, number of medical diagnoses and medications, and smoking. Therefore, a treatment can have a significant effect on swallowing physiology and fail to prevent aspiration pneumonia. One additional challenge to the use of aspiration pneumonia as an outcome measure is the low rate of this illness in many populations, making it difficult to obtain large groups for clinical trials that would demonstrate the influence of dysphagia treatment.

Mortality

Smithard and colleagues (1996) are but one group to include death among their outcomes. They completed a clinical bedside swallowing examination within 24 hours of onset of dysphagia in 121 stroke patients. When possible a VFSE was completed

Table 16.5 Criteria for having aspiration pneumonia (Martin et al., 1994)

Criteria	Descriptors
Gravitational segment infiltrate on chest x-ray film	Recumbent patients: posterior segment of upper lobes with or without superior segments of lower lobes
	Upright patients: basilar segments
Observed aspiration	
Predisposing conditions for aspiration	Mental status change, poor dentition, neurologic disease, vomiting
Gastric contents suctioned from the endotracheal tube	
Microbiology	Anaerobes isolated from empyema fluid
	Sputum gram stain: 4 + polys, no epithelial cells, mixed bacteria
	Anaerobes from blood culture in appropriate setting
Radiographic lung abscess	Greater than 2 cm cavity

within 72 hours. Dysphagia on bedside testing but not on VFSE was associated with increased risk of death, perhaps because the sickest patients were not given the instrumented examination. DePippo et al. (1994) included death as an outcome in their study of what they called three levels of clinician-directed treatment for inpatient stroke patients. No differences in death rate were discovered but a careful reading of the study makes this lack of a difference predictable. Severe patients were excluded from the study; all patients were eating by mouth and presumably carefully supervised, and treatment intensity and duration were limited. Evidence that treatment influences mortality would be powerful support for treatment programmes and approaches. The challenges to using it as an outcome mirror those for aspiration pneumonia.

Nutrition and hydration

Dysphagia clinicians include adequate nutrition and hydration among their most cherished outcomes. Serum albumin, as a measure of nutritional status, and serum sodium and blood urea nitrogen BUN as measures of hydration, were included in the repertoire of outcomes employed by DePippo and her colleagues (1994). Smithard et al. (1996) used hematocrit, plasma sodium, urea, and osmolality to evaluate hydration, weight and body mass indices, and total protein, albumin, and globulins for nutritional status. Reasons for abnormalities in these laboratory values have nothing to do with dysphagia or its management abound, thus their interpretation as outcome measures is challenging. Smithard et al. (1996) cope with this challenge by comparing values not with normative data but within patients at different times. Zachary and Mills (2000) provide a variety of solutions.

Hospital stay, disposition, and rehospitalization

Duration and frequency of hospital stays and whether discharge is to home or to another care facility are potentially useful, if imperfect, surrogate measures of health status. Odderson et al. (1995) studied 124 consecutive stroke patients admitted to an urban hospital and given a clinical swallowing examination as part of clinical pathways approach to stroke management, which specified the types and timing of tests and the treatments that follow. Outcomes included aspiration pneumonia, length of stay, and disposition after hospitalization. Length of stay was significantly shorter for non-dysphagic patients, and the likelihood of discharge home was greater.

Croghan et al. (1994) included the following outcomes for hospitalized patients who had undergone VFSE: feeding tube placement, rehospitalization within one year, and prolonged nursing home care. Dysphagia with aspiration documented on VFSE was associated with a higher probability of rehospitalization within one year and with placement of a feeding tube. Teasell et al. (2002) confirmed the significantly longer length of hospital stay after brain stem infarction for dysphagic than for non-dysphagic patients. None of these studies had a treatment focus.

But data do exist. Low et al. (2001) completed a retrospective cohort study of 140 hospitalized patients who received 'advice on dysphagia management' (Low et al., 2001: 123). Non-compliers who tended to be younger and discharged home rather than to an institution had higher rates of rehospitalization and were more likely to die, with aspiration pneumonia being a frequent cause of death.

QUALITY OF LIFE

Miller and Langmore (1994: 1261) say dysphagia is a 'quality of life impediment'. Clinicians tacitly agree, without in many cases knowing more than intuitively what is meant by 'quality of life' (QOL). Morton (1995: 1029) describes it as 'the perceived discrepancy between the reality of what one has, and what one wants, or expects, or has had' (p. 1029). It is usual to think of quality of life as comprising a number of constructs (Katz, 1987) associated with the gap between what one has and what one wants. The number of, and names for, these constructs differ from researcher to researcher. The usual ones include functional status, ability to perform a variety of roles, psychological status, including sense of wellbeing, and even symptom status. Ekberg et al. (2002) provide evidence of dysphagia's assault on QOL. Their study of 360 dysphagic patients from five European countries is informative. Only 45% found eating pleasurable, 41% were anxious while eating, and 36% avoided eating with others. Among their conclusions is that formal measures of these QOL-related conditions are mandatory and that treatment should be directed toward their amelioration.

With the publication of SWAL-QOL, a psychometrically sound measure comprising 44 items sampling 10 (or 11 when symptom status is included) domains is available for clinical and research use (McHorney and Rosenbek, 1998; McHorney et al., 2000a, b; McHorney, et. al., 2002). See Table 16.6 for the domains and items.

Scoring is with five-point Likert scales. For example, the first item in the social domain is 'I do not go out to eat because of my swallowing problem.' The five-point

Table 16.6 The SWAL-QOL's domains and items

Domains	Items
Burden	Dealing with my swallowing problem is very difficult
	My swallowing problem is a major distraction in my life
Eating duration	It takes me longer to eat than other people
	It takes me forever to eat a meal
Eating desire	Most days, I don't care if I eat or not
	I don't enjoy eating anymore
	I'm rarely hungry anymore
Symptom frequency	Coughing
	Choking when you eat food
	Choking when you take liquids
	Having thick saliva or phlegm
	Gagging
	Having excess saliva or phlegm
	Having to clear your throat
	Drooling
	Problems chewing
	Food sticking in your throat
	Food sticking in your mouth
	Food/liquid dribbling out your mouth
	Food/liquid coming out your nose
	Coughing food/liquid out your mouth
Food selection	Figuring out what I can eat is a problem for me
	It is difficult to find foods I both like and can eat
Communication	People have a hard time understanding me
	It's been difficult for me to speak clearly
Fear	I fear I may start choking when I eat food
	I worry about getting pneumonia
	I am afraid of choking when I drink liquids
	I never know when I am going to choke
Mental health	My swallowing problem depresses me
	I get impatient dealing with my swallowing problem
	Being so careful when I eat or drink annoys me
	My swallowing problem frustrates me
	I've been discouraged by my swallowing problem
Social	I do not go out to eat because of my swallowing problem
	My swallowing problem makes it hard to have a social life
	My usual activities have changed because of my swallowing problem
	Social gatherings are not enjoyable because of my swallowing problem
	My role with family/friends has changed because of my swallowing problem
Fatigue	Feel weak
	Have trouble falling asleep
	Feel tired
	Have trouble staying asleep
	Feel exhausted

scoring system is: 1 = strongly agree, 2 = agree, 3 = uncertain, 4 = disagree and 5 = strongly disagree. As but one more example, the first item in the fatigue domain is 'How often in the last month have you felt weak?' Scoring is 1 = all of the time, 2 = most of the time, 3 = some of the time, 4 = a little of the time and 5 = none of the time. SWAL-QOL is to be completed by the patient if possible and it can be completed in less than 30 minutes. The tool differentiates dysphagic from normal swallowing persons, oral from tube feeders, and among those taking a variety of diet textures from normal to puree. Research is under way to measure its sensitivity to change with treatment.

PATIENT SATISFACTION

Patient satisfaction measures are viewed with scepticism in many medical centres for the predictable reason that patient judgement is thought to be easily manipulated, ephemeral, and unquantifiable. Psychometrically sound measurement is possible and the scores are important (McHorney and Rosenbek, 1998). Patient satisfaction is related to compliance and what is called doctor shopping or hopping. SWAL-CARE was developed simultaneously with SWAL-QOL as a measure of patient satisfaction and quality of care as perceived by the patient (McHorney et al, 2002). SWAL-CARE comprises 15 items in three domains: clinical information, general advice, and patient satisfaction. The 15 items appear in Table 16.7.

The advice items are scored with identical six-point Likert scales in which 1 = poor, 2 = fair, 3 = good, 4 = very good, 5 = excellent, and 6 = outstanding. Instructions to the patient are: 'Think about the advice your swallowing clinician may have given you. How would you rate the advice you've received in the following

Table 16.7 Items in SWAL-CARE (McHorney et al., 2002)

CLINICAL INFORMATION AND GENERAL ADVICE
  Foods I should eat
  Foods I should avoid
  Liquids I should drink
  Liquids I should avoid
  Techniques to help get food down
  Techniques to help me avoid choking
  When I should contact a swallowing clinician
  My treatment options
  What to do if I start to choke
  Signs that I am not getting enough to eat or drink
  Goals of the treatment for my swallowing problem

PATIENT SATISFACTION
  Had confidence in your swallowing clinician
  Swallowing clinicians explained treatment to you
  Swallowing clinicians spent enough time with you
  Swallowing clinicians put your needs first

---

areas?' Statistical relationships between SWAL-QOL and SWAL-CARE are predictably modest. Both kinds of data are critical components of responsible care. One of the authors of this chapter (JR) was part of the team that developed these tools. Discovering his patients' perceptions of how little advice he had provided changed his approach to education and treatment orientation nearly immediately. Patient satisfaction has little to do with popularity and much to do with practising humanely and competently. SWAL-CARE is a psychometrically sound measure of how individual clinicians are doing from the patient's point of view.

COSTS AND UTILIZATION

McHorney and Rosenbek (1998: 240) observe: 'The value compass approach to outcomes assessment underscores that cost savings should not take place at the expense of clinical or patient-based outcomes.' Neither, of course, should costs and utilization be ignored. It is probably safe to say that the process of health care, which includes issues of cost, utilization, access, timeliness, and a host of other variables, is less interesting to clinical researchers than are other outcomes. Nonetheless data are emerging. Teasell and colleagues (2002) confirmed a shorter length of hospital stay for brain stem stroke patients without dysphagia. Odderson et al. (1995) evaluated the economic impact of a stroke pathway in acute care. A clinical swallowing examination was shown to be cost-effective because of the demonstrated effect of reducing pneumonias and thereby reducing length of stay for hospitalized dysphagic patients. Assumptions of such cost savings are also supported by Doggett et al.'s (2001: 279) conclusion that 'implementation of dysphagia programmes is accompanied by substantial reductions in pneumonia rates'.

CHOOSING THE RIGHT MEASURE

In clinical practice the first influence on what tool(s) one uses is one's philosophy of evaluation and treatment. Clinicians dedicated to biomechanics are likely to use instrumented evaluation and progress testing. They are also likely to assume that improved biomechanics translate into improvements in other domains, therefore measurement in other domains risks being incomplete or perfunctory. Clinicians dedicated to what might be called a rehabilitation science perspective are as likely to measure biomechanics as their colleagues with a narrower focus, but are more likely to measure carefully in other domains and much more likely to have a broader treatment approach. As one example: they are likely to know intuitively, even if they have not read the literature, that participation in society is rehabilitation's goal for those with chronic disease and that depression rather than impairment is the largest influence on participation in a variety of populations (Cardol et al., 2002). Therefore, their treatment plans and outcome repertoires, when appropriate, will include attention to depression and other psychological variables related to quality of life. Interestingly, performance on SWAL-QOL is strongly predictive of depression (McHorney et al., 2002).

A second major influence on selection of the right measure is one's specific clinical goal, which is usually some amalgam of what the patient wants and what the clinician thinks is reasonable and appropriate (assuming of course the two points of view are different). Improved biomechanics can only be demonstrated with biomechanical measures. Similarly, improved quality of life cannot be measured with surrogates and thus a quality of life measure is mandatory.

Regardless of philosophy or clinical goals, reliability and validity are major influences on choosing an outcome measure. Sonies (2000) is among those to observe that the majority of available measures are of uncertain psychometric integrity. Unreliable or invalid tools may miss treatment effects when they are present. This is potentially disastrous for practitioners and programmes because it may suggest treatment effects when none are present. That, in turn, may lead to adverse effects for patients who are treated by the next generation of clinicians applying treatments mistakenly thought to work.

Even psychometric soundness does not guarantee a measure's usefulness, of course. In dysphagia, condition specific measures can be important. Consider the difference between dysphagia secondary to stroke and head-neck cancer. Stroke patients may find solids easier than liquids and the opposite may be true for those made dysphagic by cancer. The tool List et al. (1990) developed is appropriate for the latter but not the former. This is not to say that generic outcome measures are to be avoided. Data from measures such as the SF-36 may allow clinicians to compare their patients on general quality of life dimensions to samples from other populations (Ware et al., 1995).

FUTURE NEEDS

It is axiomatic that every field in healthcare requires more data as the basis of decision-making. Equally important, however, is discussion about coping with uncertainty and opacity. These are the conditions faced daily by clinicians in dysphagia. Humility about what one knows is part of coping. Keeping abreast of the literature, despite its limits is another. Developing a clinical practice paradigm governed by reliance on informed clinical practice that treats patients as experiments, use of the best available models and measures, along with pristine measurement of response to treatment is yet another. Finally there is a need for patience, data are arriving at blistering speed.

The need is for an expanded repertoire of outcome measures across the model domains. Increasingly sophisticated measures of nervous system functioning are available in pathophysiology. The challenge facing functional magnetic resonance imaging (fMRI) may serve as a guide. The resulting pretty pictures yielded by this technology catch everyone's eye. The result sometimes is data collection that is not conceptually driven. The 'where' questions – where does the brain light up? – predominate over the more important 'why' questions. Models of swallowing motor control and hypotheses about the mechanisms of response to treatment can guide more intelligent data gathering.

The field has an embarrassment of riches in the impairment domain. Reducing their number to those of greatest significance is a legitimate goal to answer particular questions. For example, what measures represent the greatest value to the patient or are mostly strongly correlated with the variety of QOL concepts? Improving the psychometrics of functional measures and discovering ways to validate clinician decisions about diet are important needs in the domain of functional limitations. Psychometrically sound measures of disability may be the field's greatest need for it is participation that is the goal of rehabilitation for those having chronic illness. Expanding the population of dysphagia researchers to include more sociologists and healthcare economists would advance knowledge in the domain of societal limitations as it would in the area of costs and utilization. Substituting single-case designs in which each patient serves as his/her own control or utilizing group studies with sufficient subjects and power to discover differences in treated and untreated patients would also strengthen the science. This is particularly important when clinical status measures such as pneumonia are among the primary outcomes. Finally more condition-specific quality of life (QOL) and quality of care (QOC) measures would be welcome.

IN CONCLUSION

Practice in dysphagia has leapt forward in the last two decades to the benefit of patients and practitioners. The repertoire of treatments and of measures to establish what works, for whom, and under what conditions continues to expand. This chapter's purpose was to provide a structure for understanding that portion of the expansion related to measurement and then to review the extant measures, how they can be selected, and how they can be improved. With continued development of the repertoire of outcome measures dysphagia clinicians will come to know more about persons with swallowing problems. The more we know the better and more efficiently we will do it.

REFERENCES

Aguilar NV, Olson ML, Shedd DP (1979) Rehabilitation of deglutition problems in patients with head and neck cancer. American Journal of Surgery 138: 501–7.

Batalden PB, Nelson EC, Roberts JF (1994) Linking outcomes measurement to continual improvement: The serial 'v' way of thinking about improving clinical care. Journal of Quality Improvement 20: 167–80.

Bickenbach JE, Chatterji S, Badley EM, Ustun TB (1999) Models of disablement, universalism and the international classification of impairments, disabilities and handicaps. Social Science and Medicine 48: 1173–87.

Blackwell B, Bloomfield SS, Buncher CR (1972) Demonstration to medical students of placebo responses and non-drug factors. Lancet 1: 1279–82.

Blumhagen DW (1979) The doctor's white coat: the image of the physician in modern America. Annals of Internal Medicine 91: 111–16.

Bulow M, Olsson R, Ekberg O (2002) Supraglottic swallow, effortful swallow, and chin tuck did not alter hypopharyngeal intrabolus pressure in patients with pharyngeal dysfunction. Dysphagia 17: 197–201.

Cardol M, deJong BA, Van den Bos G, et al. (2002) Beyond disability: perceived participation in people with a chronic disabling condition. Clinical Rehabilitation 16: 27–35.

Center for Medicare Services (2003) New Medicare Limits on Therapy Services. Publication NO. CMS-10988, June 2003. Washington DC: US Department of Health and Human Services.

Chen AY, Frankowski R, Bishop-Leone J, et al. (2001) The development and validation of a dysphagia questionnaire for patients with head and neck cancer: the MD Anderson dysphagia inventory. Archives of Otolaryngology Head Neck Surgery 127: 870–6.

Christakis NA (1999) Death Foretold: Prophecy and Prognosis in Medical Care. Chicago: University of Chicago Press.

Cichero JAY, Murdoch BE (2002) Detection of swallowing sounds: methodology revisited. Dysphagia 17: 40–9.

Croghan JE, Burke JM, Caplan S, et al. (1994) Pilot study of 12-month outcomes of nursing home patients with aspiration on videofluoroscopy. Dysphagia 9: 141–6.

Dengel G, Robbins J, Rosenbek JC (1991) Image processing in swallowing and speech research. Dysphagia 6: 30–9.

DePippo KL, Holas MA, Reding MJ, et al. (1994). Dysphagia therapy following stroke: a controlled study. Neurology 44: 1655–60.

Ding R, Larson CR, Logemann JA, et al. (2002) Surface electromyographic and electroglottographic studies in normal subjects under two swallow conditions: normal and during the Mendelsohn maneuver. Dysphagia 17, 1–12.

Doggett DL, Tappe KD, Mitchell MD, et al. (2001) Prevention of pneumonia in elderly stroke patients by systematic diagnosis and treatment of dysphagia: an evidence-based comprehensive analysis of the literature. Dysphagia 16, 279–95.

Ekberg O, Hamdy S, Woisard V, et al. (2002) Social and psychological burden of dysphagia: Its impact on diagnosis and treatment. Dysphagia 17: 139–46.

Feinberg JJ, Knebl J, Tully J (1990) Prandial aspiration and pneumonia in an elderly population followed over 3 years. Dysphagia 11: 104–9.

Feinberg JJ, Knebl J, Tully J, et al. (1990) Aspiration and the elderly. Dysphagia 4: 61–71.

Finegold SM (1991) Aspiration pneumonia. Review of Infectious Diseases 13(Suppl. 9): S737–S742.

Fraser C, Power M, Hamdy S, et al. (2002) Driving plasticity in human adult motor cortex is associated with improved motor function after brain injury. Neuron 34(5): 831–40.

Frattali CM, Sonies BC, Chi-Fishman G, et al. (1999) Effects of physostigmine on swallowing and oral motor functions in patients with progressive supranuclear palsy: A pilot study. Dysphagia 14: 165–8.

Groher ME, McKaig TN (1995) Dysphagia and dietary levels in skilled nursing facilities. Journal of the American Gerontological Society 43: 528–32.

Hillel AD, Miller RM, Yorkston K, et al. (1989) Amyotrophic lateral sclerosis serverity scale. Neuroepidemiology 8: 142–50.

Huckabee ML, Cannito MP (1999) Outcomes of swallowing rehabilitation in chronic brainstem dysphagia: A retrospective evaluation. Dysphagia 14: 93–109.

Huckabee ML, Pelletier CA (1999) Management of adult neurogenic dysphagia. San Diego: Singular Publishing.

Johnson ER, McKenzie SW, Sievers A (1993) Aspiration pneumonia in stroke. Archives of Physical Medicine and Rehabilitation 74: 973–6.

Katz S (1987) The science of quality of life. Journal of Chronic Disability 40: 459–63.

Lambert HC, Gisel EG, Groher ME, et al. (2003) McGill ingestive skills assessment (MISA): development and first field test of an evaluation of functional ingestive skills of elderly persons. Dysphagia 18: 101–13.

Langmore SE, Terpenning MS, Schork A, et al. (1998) Predictors of aspiration pneumonia: how important is dysphagia? Dysphagia 13: 69–81.

Langmore SE (2000) Fiberoptic endoscopic evaluation of swallowing. In Vogel D, Cannito MP (series eds.), Mills RH (Vol. Ed.) Evaluation of Dysphagia in Adults: Expanding the Diagnostic Options. Vol 11. For Clinicians by Clinicians. Austin: Pro-ed, pp. 145–78.

Langmore SE, Skarupski KA, Park PS, et al. (2002) Predictors of aspiration pneumonia in nursing home residents. Dysphagia 17: 298–307.

List MA, Ritter-Sterr C, Lansky SB (1990) A performance status scale for head and neck cancer patients. Cancer 66: 564–9.

Logemann JA, Pauloski JC, Rademaker A, et al. (1992) Impact of the diagnostic procedure on outcome measures of swallowing rehabilitation in head and neck cancer patients. Dysphagia 7: 179–86.

Logemann JA, Pauloski JC, Rademaker AW, et al. (1993) Speech and swallow function after tonsil/base of tongue resection with primary closure. Journal of Speech and Hearing Research 36: 918–26.

Low J, Wyles C, Wilkinson T, et al. (2001) The effect of compliance on clinical outcomes for patients with dysphagia on videofluoroscopy. Dysphagia 16: 123–7.

Mann G (2002) MASA: The Mann Assessment of Swallowing Ability. Clifton Park, NY: Thomas Delmar Learning.

Martin BJW, Corlew MM, Wood H, et al. (1994) The association of swallowing dysfunction and aspiration pneumonia. Dysphagia 9: 1–6.

McCullough GH, Rosenbek JC, Robbins JA, et al. (1998) Ordinality and intervality of a penetration-aspiration scale. Journal of Medical Speech-Language Pathology 6: 65–72.

McCullough GH, Wertz RT, Rosenbek JC (2001) Sensitivity and specificity of clinical/bedside examination signs for detecting aspiration in adults subsequent to stroke. Journal of Communication Disorders 33: 1–18.

McHorney CA, Bricker DE, Kramer AE, et al. (2000a) The SWAL-QOL outcomes tool for oropharyngeal dysphagia in adults: I. Conceptual foundation and item development. Dysphagia 15: 115–21.

McHorney CA, Bricker DE, Robbins J, et al. (2000b) The SWAL-QOL outcomes tool for oropharyngeal dysphagia in adults: II. Item reduction and preliminary scaling. Dysphagia 15: 122–33.

McHorney CA, Robbins J, Lomax K, et al. (2002) The SWAL-QOL and SWAL-CARE outcomes tool for oropharyngeal dysphagia in adults: III. Documentation of reliability and validity. Dysphagia 17: 97–114.

McHorney CA, Rosenbek JC (1998) Functional outcome assessment of adults with oropharyngeal dysphagia. Seminars in Speech and Language19(3): 235–47.

Medicare Intermediary Manual (1997) Speech pathology services furnished by a hospital or by others under arrangements with a hospital or under its supervision. Publication 13:section 3101.10A(1). Washington DC: US Department of Health and Human Services.

Miller RM, Langmore SE (1994) Treatment efficacy for adults with oropharyngeal dysphagia. Archives of Physical Medicine and Rehabilitation 75: 1256–62.

Moerman DE, Jonas WB (2002) Deconstructing the placebo effect and finding the meaning response. Annals of Internal Medicine 136(6): 471–6.

Moerman M, Fakimi H, Celeen W, et al. (2003) Functional outcome following colon inter position in total pharyngoesophagectomy with and without laryngectomy. Dysphagia 18: 78–84.

Morton RP (1995) Evolution of quality of life assessment in head and neck cancer. Journal of Laryngology and Otolaryngology 109: 1029–35.

National Committee on Vital and Health Statistics Subcommittee on Populations (2001) Classifying and Reporting Functional Sstatus. Washington DC: US Department of Health and Human Services, pp. 1–17.

National Institutes of Health Publication No. 93-3509 (1993) Research Plan for the National Center for Medical Rehabilitation Research. Washington DC: US Department of Health and Human Services.

Odderson IR, Keaton JC, McKenna BS (1995) Swallow management in patients on an acute stroke pathway. Archives of Physical Medicine and Rehabilitation 76: 1130–3.

Olshin JM, Ciolek DE, Hwang W (2002) Study and report on outpatient therapy utilization: physical therapy occupational therapy, and speech-language pathology services billed to Medicare part b in all setting in 1998, 1999, and 2000. Deliverable #7-Final report on utilization, Contract 500-00-0009. Washington DC: US Department of Health and Human Services.

O'Neil KH, Purdy M, Falk J, et al. (1999) The dysphagia outcome and severity scale. Dysphagia 14: 139–45.

Palmer JB, Hiiemae KM (2003) Eating and breathing: interactions between respiration and feeding on solid food. Dysphagia 18(3): 169–78.

Perlman AL, Witthawaskul W (2002) Real-time remote tellefluorographic assessment of patients with dysphagia. Dysphagia 17: 162–7.

Robbins J (1992) The impact of oral motor dysfunction on swallowing: from beginning to end. Seminars in Speech and Language 13: 55–69.

Rosenbek JC, Robbins J, Roecker EB, et al. (1996) A penetration-aspiration scale. Dysphagia 11: 93–8.

Sapienza CM, Davenport PW, Martin AD (2002) Expiratory muscle training increases pressure support in high school band students. Journal of Voice 16(4): 495–501.

Scott A, Perry A, Bench J (1998). A study of interrater reliability when using videofluoroscopy as an assessment of swallowing. Dysphagia 13(4): 223–7.

Sellars C, Dunnet C, Carter R (1998) A preliminary comparison of videofluoroscopy of swallowing and pulse oximetry in the identification of aspiration in dysphagic patients. Dysphagia 13(2): 82–6.

Sitzmann JV (1990) Nutritional support of the dysphagic patient: methods, risks, and the complications of therapy. Journal of Parenteral Enteral Nutrition 14: 60–3.

Smithard DG, O'Neill PA, Park PC, et al. (1996) Complications and outcome after acute stroke. Stroke 27: 1200–4.

Sonies BC (2000) Assessment and treatment of functional swallowing in dysphagia. In Worrall LE, Frattali CM (eds) Neurogenic Communication Disorders: A Functional Approach. New York: Thieme, pp. 262–75.

Teasell R, Foley N, Fisher J, et al. (2002) The incidence, management, and complications of dysphagia in patients with medullary strokes admitted to a rehabilitation unit. Dysphagia 17: 115–20.

Uhlenhuth EH, Rickels K, Fisher S, et al. (1966) Drug, doctor's verbal attitude and clinical setting in the symptomatic response to pharmacotherapy. Psychopharmacologia 9: 392–418.

Ward EC, Conroy AL (1999) Validity, reliability and responsivity of the Royal Brisbane Hospital outcome measure for swallowing. Asia Pacific Journal of Speech, Language and Hearing 4: 109–29.

Ware JE, Kosinski M, Bayliss MS, et al. (1995) Comparison of methods for the scoring and statistical analysis of SF-36 health profile and summary measures: summary of results from the medical outcomes study. Medical Care 33(4 Suppl.): AS264–79.

Wilcox F, Liss JM, Siegel GM (1996) Interjudge agreement in videofluoroscopic studies of swallowing. Journal of Speech and Hearing Research 39(1): 144–52.

World Health Organization (2001) International classification of functioning, disability and health: ICF. Geneva: World Health Organization.

World Health Organization (1980) International classification of impairment, disability, and handicap (ICIDH). Geneva: World Health Organization

Zachary V, Mills RH (2000) Nutritional evaluation and laboratory values in dysphagia management. In Vogel D, Cannito MP (series eds) and Mills RH (vol. ed.) Evaluation of Dysphagia in Adults: Expanding the Diagnostic Options. Vol. 11. For Clinicians by Clinicians. Austin, TX: Pro-ed, pp. 179–205.

Index

Dysphagia: Foundation, Theory and Practice. Edited by J. Cichero and B. Murdoch
© 2006 John Wiley & Sons, Ltd.